1,000,000 Books

are available to read at

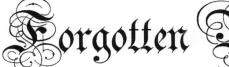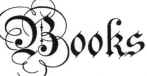

www.ForgottenBooks.com

Read online
Download PDF
Purchase in print

ISBN 978-0-332-08534-0
PIBN 11213112

English
Français
Deutsche
Italiano
Español
Português

www.forgottenbooks.com

Mythology Photography **Fiction**
Fishing Christianity **Art** Cooking
Essays Buddhism Freemasonry
Medicine **Biology** Music **Ancient**
Egypt Evolution Carpentry Physics
Dance Geology **Mathematics** Fitness
Shakespeare **Folklore** Yoga Marketing
Confidence Immortality Biographies
Poetry **Psychology** Witchcraft
Electronics Chemistry History **Law**
Accounting **Philosophy** Anthropology
Alchemy Drama Quantum Mechanics
Atheism Sexual Health **Ancient History**
Entrepreneurship Languages Sport
Paleontology Needlework Islam
Metaphysics Investment Archaeology
Parenting Statistics Criminology
Motivational

of

Laboratory and Clinical Medicine

VICTOR C. VAUGHAN, M.D., Editor-In-Chief
UniVersity of Michigan, Ann Arbor

ASSOCIATE EDITORS

Pharmacology
DENNIS E. JACKSON, M.D.
University of Cincinnati, Cincinnati

Bacteriology
HANS ZINSSER, M.D.
Columbia University, New York

Immunology and Serology
FREDERICK P. GAY, M.D.
UniVersity of California, Berkeley

Physiological Pathology
PAUL G. WOOLLEY, M.D.
Detroit

Physiological Chemistry and Clinical Physiology

J. J. R. MACLEOD, M.B.
UniVersity of Toronto, Toronto

ROY G. PEARCE, M.D.
Akron, Ohio

Clinical Pathology
W. C. MacCARTY, M.D.
Mayo Clinic, Rochester, Minn.

Internal Medicine
WARREN T. VAUGHAN, M.D.
Harvard Medical School, Boston

Tuberculosis
GERALD B. WEBB, M.D.
Cragmor Sanatorium, Colorado Springs

VOLUME V
OCTOBER, 1919—SEPTEMBER, 1920

ST. LOUIS
THE C. V. MOSBY CO.
1920

The Journal of Laboratory and Clinical Medicine

| VOL. V. | ST. LOUIS, OCTOBER, 1919 | No. 1 |

ORIGINAL ARTICLES

AN EXPERIMENTAL INVESTIGATION OF THE PHARMACOLOGIC PROPERTIES OF THE ACTIVE PRINCIPLE OF COMMERCIAL PITUITARY EXTRACTS, AND OF THE COMPARATIVE ACTION OF HISTAMINE*

BY D. E. JACKSON, M.D., AND C. A. MILLS, B.A., CINCINNATI, OHIO

SOME years ago while performing some experiments on the lungs, one of us observed what appeared to be a notable difference between the action of pituitrin and that of histamine ("ergamine," β-iminazolylethylamine) on the bronchioles of the dog. The later adoption of histamine in the U. S. Pharmacopœia as a standard to be used in the testing of commercial preparations of the infundibular portion of the pituitary gland served to again call attention to the previous (unpublished) observation. And during the progress of the work here reported, the publication of an especially interesting and valuable article by Abel and Kubota[1] has again served to add interest to the work.

The literature on this subject is very extensive, but we need to refer here in detail to only a few articles. A very comprehensive review (also bibliography) of the current knowledge of the action of extracts of the hypophysis has recently been published by Houssay[2] in his excellent monograph on that subject. McCord,[3] Roth,[4] Hamilton and Rowe,[5] Dale and Laidlaw,[6] Barger and Dale[7] and Abel and Kubota[1] (bibliography) have also made very valuable contributions to that phase of the subject with which we are especially interested in this article.

Figure 1 illustrates graphically the nature of the observation originally made with reference to the relative action of commercial "pituitrin" (Parke, Davis & Co.) and that of histamine ("ergamine" of Burroughs Wellcome &

*From the Department of Pharmacology of the University of Cincinnati Medical School, Cincinnati, Ohio.

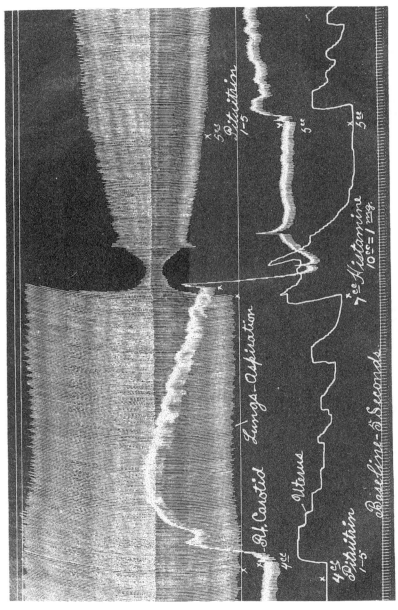

Fig. 1.—For discussion see text.

Co.). In this tracing a pithed dog of 7.2 kilos weight was arranged for the recording of uterine contractions (uterus in situ), blood pressure (mercury manometer, right carotid artery), and bronchiole contractions. The method[9] used in recording the latter has been fully described previously and need not be discussed here further than to briefly indicate that a special instrument (lung plethysmograph) was inserted air-tight into the sectioned anterior wall of the chest. This instrument held the chest wall rigidly expanded and a special artificial respiration machine was used to aspirate air from the chest intermittently. This partial exhaustion of the chest cavity caused air to rush into the lungs through the trachea and expand the lungs. The drum tracing was made by means of a tambour connected to the side tube of the tracheal cannula. The record thus obtained shows by its amplitude the amount of air passing into and out of the lungs at each inspiration and expiration. Contraction of the bronchioles reduces this amount of (tidal) air and simultaneously reduces the amplitude of the lung tracing.

In Fig. 1 it is seen that the intravenous injection of 4 cubic centimeters (from a burette into the femoral vein) of a 1 to 5 dilution of Parke, Davis & Company's *commercial* pituitrin caused a contraction of the uterus, a very considerable and prolonged rise in blood pressure, but scarcely any appreciable effect on the bronchioles. Whatever effect the tracing may show in this case on these we believe to be due entirely to some obscure changes in the volume of blood in the lungs (thus probably slightly changing their degree of elasticity), or to changes in the relative dilatation of the heart. In this case we believe that no true contraction of the bronchial musculature due to a direct action of the pituitrin occurred.

After the effects of the pituitrin had mainly worn off another injection of 7/10 of one milligram of histamine (ergamine) was made. This produced a more marked contraction of the uterus, a sharp fall in blood pressure and a considerable contraction of the bronchioles. This contraction of the bronchial musculature tended to pass off but slowly, so that a later injection of 5 cubic centimeters of pituitrin (1 to 5) was made in order to determine whether or not the pituitrin would counteract the action of the histamine. This produced contraction of the uterus and a rise in blood pressure, but no perceptible increase in the previous slow rate of dilatation of the bronchioles. Obviously this indicates that *commercial* pituitrin does not possess much power toward counteracting the constricting influence of histamine on the bronchioles.

It would appear that certain conclusions might be drawn from this experiment, but we have refrained from proceeding too hastily in the matter in the hope that a variety of experiments might throw a different light on the problems here involved. We may, therefore, refer to Fig. 2 in which two (separate) tracings, both taken from the same animal, are shown. Here a contraction of the uterus in situ was produced in the first case by 1/15 of a milligram of histamine (ergamine). This is practically 1/15 of the ordinary therapeutic dose of this material as placed on the market in hypodermic tablets by the Burroughs Wellcome Co. The second part of the tracing shows a contraction of the uterus produced by 1/2 cubic centimeter of pituitrin (Parke, Davis & Co.) diluted 1 to 5 with distilled water. Both injections were made into the femoral vein. In both instances the uterus was relaxed (after a brief primary contraction) by the injection of 1/4 cubic centimeter of adrenaline (1 to 10,000). These two tracings show that 1/15 of a therapeutic "dose" of histamine produced a little greater contraction of the uterus in this particular animal than 1/10 of a therapeutic "dose" of pituitrin. While these "doses" are not sufficiently accurate to serve as a basis for exact scientific conclusions, they are still useful here as a means of giving some approximate estimation of the relative activity of different amounts of the two substances on the uterus in situ in a dog in which the organ (in this instance) was especially sensitive to both drugs. By comparison with Fig. 1 it will be seen that in that tracing 8/10 of a therapeutic "dose" of pituitrin caused a somewhat less contraction of the uterus than did 7/10 of a "dose" of histamine. But the action on the bronchioles is quite different in these two instances. That the injection of pituitrin in this case (4 c.c. of 1 to 5 dilution)

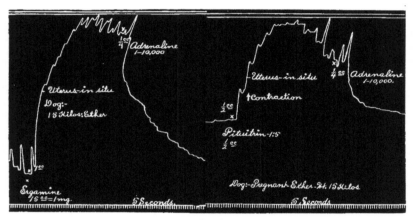

Fig. 2.—For discussion see text.

was sufficient to elicit the ordinary pharmacologic reaction of the drug is shown by the very marked rise in blood pressure.

A variety of methods and of animals have been used by previous workers in studying the action of pituitary extracts on the bronchioles. The conclusions of these observers may be briefly summarized as follows: P. Titone,[10] working with isolated bronchial muscle, found no action produced by hypophysin and pituitrin. In guinea pigs, Froehlich and Pick[11] found pituitary extracts to produce fatal broncho-spasm which they believed was of peripheral origin and could be prevented by atropin, while in perfused guinea pigs' lungs Baehr and Pick[12] found that after perfusion with pilocarpine and adrenaline the later perfusion of "pituglandol" (Hoffmann-LaRoche—4 c.c. per 100 c.c. Tyrode's solution) through the lungs for 20 minutes failed to contract the bronchioles, while immediately following this, perfusion with histamine (1 mg. to 100 c.c. Tyrode) caused broncho-spasm in one minute, and this was relieved by perfusion with adrenaline (1 to 100,000) for two minutes. But in a freshly prepared animal

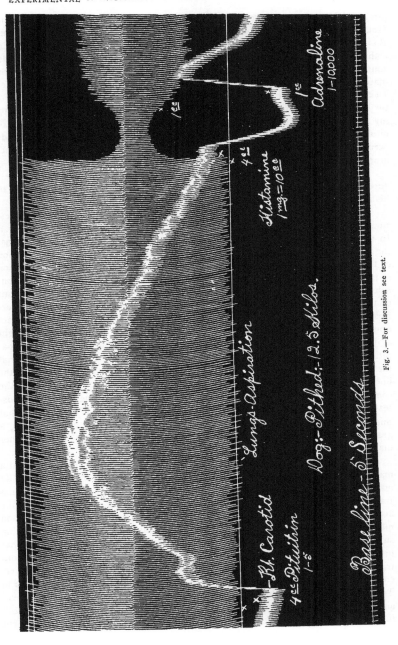

Fig. 3.—For discussion see text.

pituglandol produced bronchoconstriction (Lungenstarre) after a short time. Houssay[13] observed bronchoconstriction in guinea pigs, while Borchardt[14] and Bourgeois[15] have attempted to use pituitary extract in the treatment of bronchial asthma, and Zueblin,[16] and Bensaude and Hallion[17] have studied the action of the combination of pituitrin and adrenaline in asthma. Lanari[18] has induced asthmatic attacks by the administration of pituitary extract. Jackson[19] has published (without discussing) a tracing showing a contraction produced in the lungs of a turtle by the injection of pituitrin into the circulation (heart), and another tracing showing a slight bronchoconstriction in a dog when a dose of 5 c.c. of pituitrin (1 to 5) was injected intravenously. Both of these results have already been quoted in the literature[20] as evidence that pituitary extracts will produce bronchoconstriction.

It will thus be seen that the literature is somewhat inconsistent with reference to the action of pituitary extracts on the bronchi. Regarding the action of histamine on the bronchi, however, there is no difference of opinion.

In Fig. 3 are shown the comparative actions on the bronchi and blood pressure of 4 c.c. of pituitrin (1 to 5) and 4 c.c. of histamine solution (4/10 mg.). In the recent paper by Abel and Kubota the interesting suggestion is made that the plain muscle stimulating and depressor constituent of the posterior portion of the pituitary gland is really histamine. We have kept this valuable suggestion in mind while we have been carrying out a portion of this work. The very considerable financial gain to laboratory and clinical workers which observations of this kind foreshadow is a matter of much interest to all. And we have performed some experiments with the special object of studying the comparative action of pituitrin and histamine on the bronchi in order to gain as much light as possible regarding the presence of histamine in ordinary *commercial* preparations of the pituitary gland. While the foregoing experiments indicate that the pituitary extracts possess practically no action on the bronchi either in the line of contraction or dilatation, we must state, however, that with some of the commercial products the presence in minute quantities of some substances possessing a histamine-like action is very evidently indicated. We have felt that this could best be demonstrated by introducing a number of tracings showing a gradual gradation from practically no effect at all on the bronchi to a rather marked bronchoconstriction.

Figure 4 shows an injection of 3 c.c. of pituitrin (1 to 5) which produced a marked uterine contraction, a considerable rise in blood pressure, but practically no effect on the bronchi. The slight shortening of the amplitude of the lung tracing here is almost certainly due to blood volume changes in the lungs, or to the action of the drug on the heart (McCord.) In this case, as in Fig. 1, the conclusion might easily be drawn that the uterine contracting and the blood pressure raising substance was one and the same. But on the other hand it might be supposed that histamine present in the commercial pituitrin was responsible for the uterine contraction and that the blood pressure raising principle was powerful enough to overcome the action of the histamine on the blood pressure. But it has been shown in Tracings 1 and 3 that the bronchioles are exceedingly sensitive to very small amounts of histamine (much more sensitive than is the uterus in dogs). In order to explain the failure of the pituitrin to contract the bronchi in Fig. 4 then, it might be presumed that the pressor substance stimulated the endings of the broncho-dilator nerves (sympathetic) and thus counteracted the direct muscular con-stricting action of the histamine. We might suggest here that atropine does not change any of these reactions, so that the vagus nerve is probably not concerned in them. The later failure of adrenaline to cause any perceptible dilatation of the bronchi in Fig. 4 shows that no special contraction had been produced by the previous pituitrin injection. (This very slight progressive shortening for a

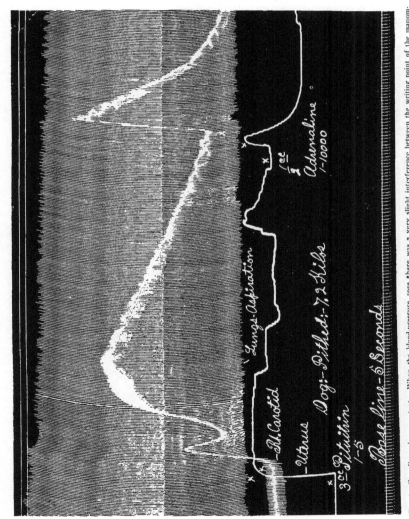

Fig. 4.—For discussion see text. When the blood-pressure rose there was a very slight interference between the writing point of the manom-eter and that of the lung tambour. The tambour was accordingly moved slightly to the right.

time in the amplitude of the lung tracing is often seen with this method in normal animals, when no drugs at all are given.)

Figure 5 shows a slightly different type of action. In this case 2½ c.c. of
infundin (Burroughs Wellcome & Co—1 to 5 dilution) were injected and caused
a marked effect on the blood pressure. This evidently consisted of a mixture
of pressor and depressor effects. The heart was evidently also involved in
this (the medullary centers were, of course, not concerned, as the brain and most
of the cord were destroyed). But in this case there is more evidence
of a bronchoconstrictor action. It is perhaps observable here that the most
marked period of bronchoconstriction coincides with the position of the greatest

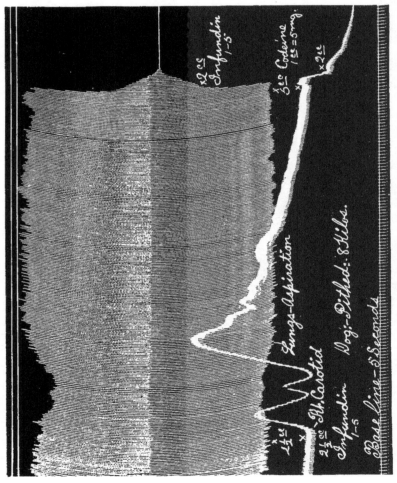

Fig. 5.—For discussion see text.

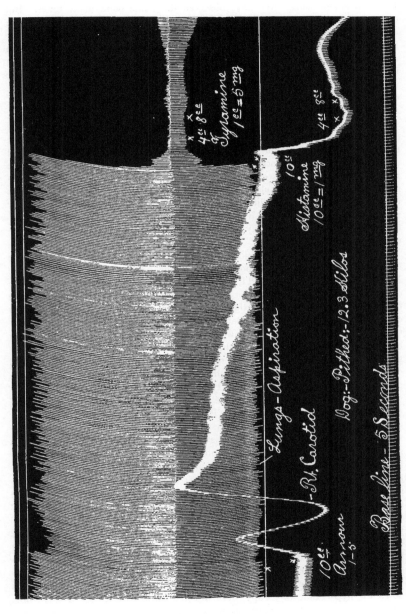

Fig. 6.—For discussion see text.

fall in blood pressure. We have observed this same point many times. But coinciding with the point of greatest rise in blood pressure in the tracing there appears to be a fairly evident dilatation of the bronchi. This may be due to the better circulation washing out any constrictor substance which might have been acting on the lungs. Or it might be due to the pressor substance stimulating the bronchodilator nerves. This possible action of pituitary extracts to dilate the bronchioles we have kept carefully in mind, as it might entirely explain the difference in action on the bronchi between pure histamine and pituitary extracts. We have therefore devised several experiments to test this point. Consequently in the last part of Fig. 5 we injected 25 milligrams of codeine sulphate to produce a bronchoconstriction (direct muscular effect), and then attempted to inject 2 c.c. of infundiu (1 to 5) to determine whether or not the extract could cause an active bronchodilatation. But the dose of codeine was too large for this animal which was evidently exceedingly sensitive to substances producing a direct muscular stimulation of the bronchi. Consequently no conclusions could be drawn here regarding a possible dilator action of the infundin. By reference to Fig. 1, however, it will be seen that 5 c.c. (1 to 5) after the injection of histamine failed entirely to produce any active increase in the slow rate of relaxation of the bronchi.

In Fig. 6, ten c.c. of Armour's "pituitary liquid" (1 to 5 dilution) were injected. Two phases to the blood pressure changes are markedly produced (see McCord: Arch. Int. Med., 1911, viii, 609). A notch is also formed in the top of the lung tracing. This does not, however, have quite the appearance of a true bronchoconstrictor effect, but rather seems due to other causes which are almost certainly connected with the circulation. Later in the tracing 1 milligram of histamine is injected and this is followed by two injections of tyramine, the object being to determine whether or not this body (which Abel and Kubota have suggested may be quite similar to the pressor principle in pituitary extracts) could cause a dilatation of the bronchi sufficiently powerful to prevent a histamine contraction if both histamine and tyramine (para-hydroxyphenylethylamine) should be acting in combination at the same time on the lungs. In this experiment the dilator action of tyramine (Burroughs Wellcome & Co.) was entirely too feeble to overcome the bronchoconstriction produced by the histamine. Possibly it might be questioned here whether or not the proper doses had been selected to give a fair test to the combination as it (histamine plus some unknown pressor body) might exist in pituitary extracts. The proportion of histamine to tyramine here was 1 to 60, but we have tried a variety of other proportions of this combination both when the drugs were injected separately and when mixed before injection. It might be mentioned here that Baehr and Pick[21] have described a bronchoconstriction as being produced in perfused guinea pigs' lungs by tyramine dissolved in Tyrode's solution. Amyl nitrite removed this constriction. One of us has previously observed that tyramine caused a slight bronchodilatation in dogs (Jour. Pharm. and Exper. Therap., 1913, iv, p. 307) and we have confirmed this observation again in this work.

In Fig. 7, two c.c. of pituitrin, *full strength* (i.e., two maximum human doses for hypodermic injection) were injected intravenously into a small dog. The usual blood pressure reactions occur, but in addition there is a moderate

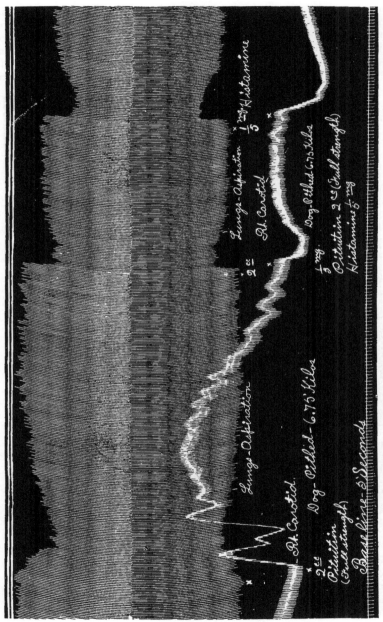

Fig. 7.—For discussion see text.

bronchoconstriction. Again this constriction coincides with the point of fall in blood pressure after the first primary rise. The character and general appearance of this bronchoconstriction should be directly compared with that produced by the second injection into the animal of 2 c.c. of pituitrin (same as the initial dose) but to which 1/5 of a milligram of histamine had been added before the pituitrin was injected (by means of a hypodermic syringe into the intact femoral

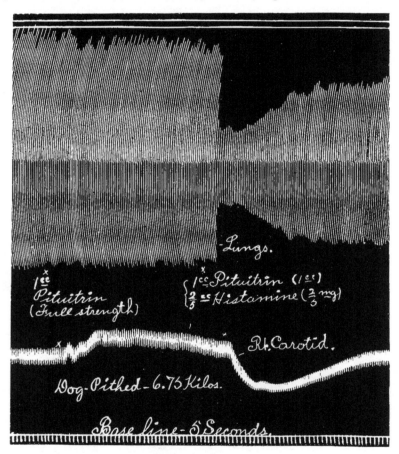

Fig. 8.—For discussion see text.

vein). Here a moderate, abrupt, and rather persistent bronchoconstriction is produced. In this case it might be suggested as possible that the pituitary pressor principle tended to counteract the bronchoconstrictor action of the histamine and thus reduced the normal action of the histamine on the bronchi. To further test this point we next injected 1/5 milligram of histamine (same as previous dose) again. But the bronchoconstriction produced in this case is almost identical both in form and extent with that produced by the combined dose of histamine and pituitrin. We have considered the possibility that histamine might be loosely combined in some unknown fashion with the pressor principle of the pituitary extract. In this case it would be necessary to presume that some tissues (uterus, e.g.) could suddenly break down this combination and react to the liberated histamine while perhaps not responding to the pressor principle. On the other hand we should then be compelled to assume that the bronchioles of the dog possessed practically no power either to break down the combination or to react to the combination as a whole. This explanation does not seem very plausible to us, but it might be considered by others. And we are inclined to believe that Fig. 7, in which a mixture of pituitrin and histamine exercised practically exactly the same action on the bronchioles as a separate dose of the same amount of histamine alone, shows exactly the nature of the reactions here involved. It is to be noted that in this experiment very large doses of pituitrin are used. This was done in order to determine whether or not the doses ordinarily used were simply too small to produce bronchoconstriction. This suggestion probably involves an element of truth as later tracings will show.

Figure 8 is taken from the same animal as Fig. 7 and follows it directly. (The bronchi were in the meantime dilated back to normal by mechanically increasing for a moment or two the force of aspiration from the chest. The previous force of aspiration was then resumed.) In this tracing (8) one c.c. of pituitrin (*full strength*) is injected. The bronchial effect is exceedingly slight. This is followed by a second injection of 1 c.c. of pituitrin to which 2/5 of a milligram of histamine had previously been added. The bronchoconstrictor effect is almost exactly twice that which was produced by the two previous injections (Fig. 7) each amounting to one-half as much histamine as that given in Fig. 8. A further point should be noted here. The first injection of pituitary extract into an animal often gives a suspicious-looking bronchial tracing which might at once be taken to indicate a very mild degree of contraction. Later injections may, however, especially if they be of only ordinary quantities, show no trace whatever of a bronchoconstriction. By comparison of Figs. 7 and 8 it will also be seen that whereas the pressor effect of pituitrin tends to become less and less with repeated injections, the bronchoconstrictor effect of the same sized doses (or larger ones) of histamine tends to remain almost exactly the same. If ordinary commercial preparations of the pituitary gland are mixtures of histamine and some unknown pressor substance, then when repeated doses of commercial pituitary extracts are injected into dogs, and the pressor effects are gradually lost, then the response of the bronchioles to the histamine should probable become more and more relatively accentuated. This gives the pressor principle the benefit of the doubt as to whether or not it (if it could act alone) would possess a dilator action (as would be expected from the nature of its reactions on the blood vessels) on the bronchi, and assuming that the point of action of the substance here lost its susceptibility to the drug simultaneously as the pressor effect was lost. We do not think this is very probable, and experimentally the slight initial bronchoconstriction sometimes produced by ordinary doses of "pituitrin" rather tend to become less with repeated injections (and are very generally entirely ab-

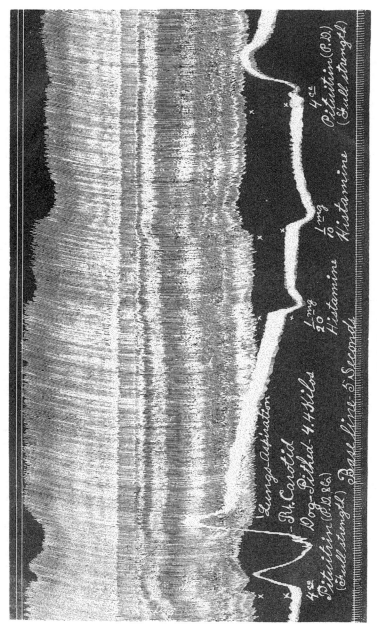

Fig. 9.—For discussion see text.

sent after the first dose). This leads us to suggest that we believe that the circulatory reactions to the drug are entirely responsible for such slight bronchoconstrictor effects as moderate doses of ordinary extracts may produce.

In Fig. 9 an enormous dose (4 c.c., full strength) of pituitrin was injected into a very small dog. The direct object here was to test the effect of large doses on the bronchi. The point which we had in mind was the possibility that a very small amount of histamine might be contained in these extracts. If this were the case a very large dose might contain enough to cause a bronchoconstriction. In this case the 4 c.c. did cause some bronchial contraction, and we are not sure as to the nature of this. We believe that the vascular changes probably account for most of the constriction. But there is a small, sharp notch just at the beginning of the contraction which looks very much as though it *might*

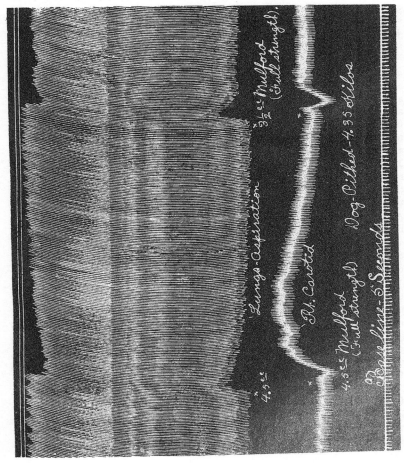

Fig. 10.—For discussion see text.

have been caused by a very small dose of histamine. To gain further light on this point we later gave two separate injections of 1/20 milligram and 1/10 milligram of histamine. The effects of these on the bronchi are quite obvious, and by comparison of all three injections we should estimate that the *apparent bronchoconstriction* produced by the 4 c.c. of full strength pituitrin corresponded approximately to about what we should have expected from a dose of 1/15 milligram of histamine at that stage of the experiment, i.e., there is indicated a bare possibility that each cubic centimeter of the pituitrin may have contained about 1/60 milligram of histamine. This gives the view that this sample of *commercial pituitrin* might contain histamine the benefit of all doubt in the matter, and we have proceeded from this point to reason as to whether or not this very small proportion of histamine could account for all the (histamine-like) therapeutic actions which the pituitrin is believed to possess. It is with a certain sense of regret that we have been compelled to conclude that the evidence is too small to substantiate the point. And it is interesting to observe that a second injection of 4 c.c. of full strength pituitrin following shortly after the last injection of histamine produced rather dilatation than contraction of the bronchi.

Figures 10 and 11 were both made in direct succession from the same animal. The primary injection into the animal was 4½ c.c. of Mulford's pituitary extract, full strength. The animal weighed only 4.35 kilos and both the brain and the entire cord were fully destroyed (eliminating all central influence). The animal had been etherized, but much of this had escaped before the first injection was made so that the presence of ether did not influence the tissues. The first injection raises the blood pressure (note the slight initial fall) and causes a direct and unmistakable contraction of the bronchi. A second injection of only 3½ c.c. of the same preparation caused a greater initial fall of pressure followed by only a slight rise. This shows quite well the usual loss of susceptibility of the vascular system to repeated doses of pituitary extracts. This second injection, however, produces a very evident and persistent contraction of the bronchi. And this contraction with a smaller dose than the first is more marked on the bronchi than is the constriction produced by the first injection. Evidently the substance which produces the bronchoconstriction does not simultaneously produce a loss of susceptibility as occurs with the pressor effect, but rather the reverse.

Passing now at once to Fig. 11 we see the result of the third injection into the animal of 3¾ c.c. (full strength) of the pituitary preparation sold by Heister. This produces a considerable rise in blood pressure, but without any special initial fall. We might suggest here that a great preponderance of pressor effect probably overcame the slight tendency for a primary fall which was almost certainly present. A slight but unmistakable bronchoconstriction is produced, but this is slightly less than that produced by a somewhat smaller dose of Mulford's extract in the last part of Fig. 10.

We now come to an injection of 4 c.c. (full strength) of pituitary (infundibular) extract of Burroughs Wellcome & Company. The immediate drop in blood pressure and the perfectly *typical bronchoconstriction* which this injection produces leaves practically no room for doubt, in the light of the recent splendid experimental work of Abel and Kubota, but that this preparation con-

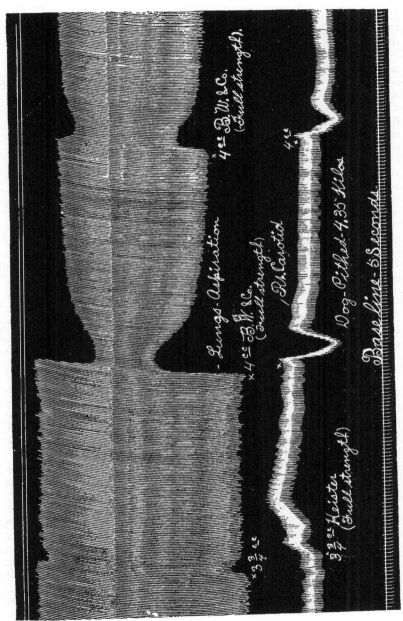

Fig. 11. For discussion see text.

tained a considerable proportion of histamine ("ergamine"). We should here compare with great care the results of this first injection of 4 c.c. of the B. W. & Co. preparation with that of the 3¾ c.c. of the Heister preparation shown in the first part of the tracing. It seems obvious here that the blood pressure lowering principle must certainly be the same as that which causes the bronchoconstriction and the blood pressure raising principle probably has no action at all on the bronchi. The reader should now compare these results with those shown in Figs. 1, 3, and 4 in which it is shown that a dose of pituitrin which will cause a marked uterine contraction may produce no effect whatever on the bronchioles. But when histamine is injected into the same animal both the uterus and the bronchioles contract. This is a matter of special interest, and we have repeatedly returned to the laboratory to do over again various experiments concerning the results of which we felt that some uncertainty might have arisen. We have worked here with ordinary *commercial preparations,* but these have been the freshest products we could buy, and always stamped by the manufacturer as being active to a much later date than that at which we used them. It may be possible, of course, that a few samples had undergone some deterioration. We do not believe, however, that this had occurred to any material extent. We have considered that point especially in the case shown in Fig. 11. But when we consider that the presence of the substance which caused the great bronchoconstriction would with practical certainty cause a marked uterine contraction, and that the material is sold with its obstetrical use directly in mind, the chances for this substance to have resulted from decomposition in the sealed ampules does seem especially great. It should be particularly emphasized here, however, that 4 c.c. of the full strength extract is an enormous dose for a 4.35 kilo dog. Only a very small amount of histamine need be present in each therapeutic (human) dose in order to make the combined quantities in the four maximum human doses sufficient to produce a very evident effect on the bronchioles which are very sensitive to histamine.

Some commercial preparations contain preservatives, especially chloretone. It was shown by Roth that the presence of this substance did not affect the action of the drug in the tests performed by him. And we feel that in all probability this is true in our experiments also. The very small quantities of chloretone in 3 or 4 c.c. of pituitrin, when injected into a dog of 4 to 12 kilos weight would not be likely to have any detectable results whatever.

Before leaving the discussion of Fig. 11 we should add that later injection of histamine showed that in this animal the bronchioles gave a very obvious contraction when 1/40 of a milligram was injected, but no perceptible contraction was produced by 1/80 of a milligram, so that the limit of the sensitivity of the bronchioles in this case was probably about 1/60 of a milligram. And in this same animal 1/20 of a milligram of histamine mixed with 1 c.c. of pituitary extract sold by Heister gave almost exactly half as big a contraction of the bronchi as did 1/10 of a milligram of histamine alone. That is, the pituitary extract had practically no power whatever toward influencing in any way the normal action of histamine on the bronchi.

We wish now to present briefly some further evidence regarding a possible bronchodilator action of pituitary extracts which might counteract the constrict-

ing action of histamine and thus neutralize its action on the bronchi, while leaving it free to cause uterine contractions.   Fig. 12 shows a bronchoconstriction
produced by 10 c.c. of histamine solution (½ milligram). Following this there
was quickly injected a dose of 2½ c.c. of pituitrin (diluted 1 to 5), i.e., approximately one-half of a therapeutic dose. Time was given for this to reach the
lungs, but it failed entirely to dilate them. Consequently a small injection of
adrenaline was given to dilate the bronchi a little and thus save the animal from

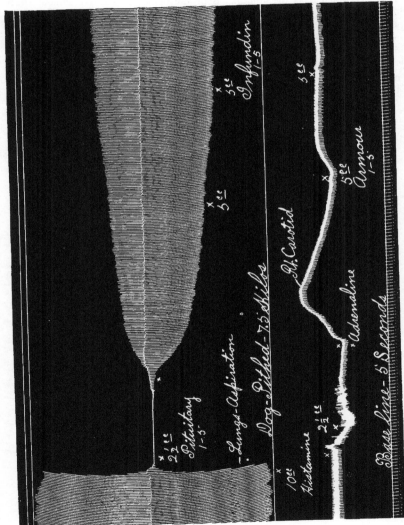

Fig. 12.—For discussion see text.

dying of asphyxia. Following this 5 c.c. of Armour's extract (1 to 5) and 5 c.c. of infundin (1 to 5) were given, but these were wholly without any dilating influence on the bronchi. Practically this same thing is shown again with another animal in Fig. 13.

The matter is approached from a little different angle in Fig. 14. Here 20 milligrams of codeine sulphate were used to produce a bronchoconstriction and two injections of infundin were given in order to determine whether or not the substance would relax the bronchi. Both injections were entirely without effect on the lungs. It should be noted here that these doses of the extract were considerably smaller than the ones used in Figs. 9, 10, and 11, although the doses used in Fig. 14 were fully ample to produce the usually recognized effects of the drug.

We turn now to another phase of the subject, namely, the possibility of making mixtures of histamine and tyramine which would possess approximately the same action as pituitary extracts. This possibility has been suggested by Abel and Kubota, and they quote the patent of A. Hoerlein (U. S. Patent,

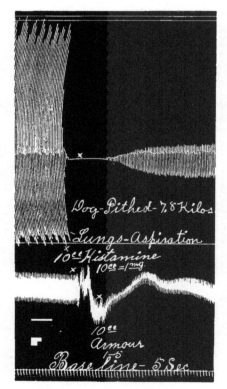

Fig. 13.—For discussion see text.

1,178,720, April 11, 1916). which introduces a combination of parahydroxy-phenylethylamine and histamine in the proportions of 1-4 to 30 in aqueous solution as a substitute for ergot.

Figure 15 shows the result of injecting a mixed dose consisting of 7/10 milligram of histamine and 28 milligrams of tyramine, i.e., a mixture of 1 to 40. Obviously no such result as this can be obtained by the injection of ordinary commercial pituitary extracts. We consequently tried a new set of proportions with the results shown in Fig. 16. Here 1 milligram of histamine was mixed with 80 milligrams of tyramine, i.e., a proportion of 1 to 80. Fig. 17 shows the result of injecting ½ milligram of histamine and 50 milligrams of tyramine (i.e., 1 to 100) into another dog. Obviously these results in nowise resemble those produced by pituitary extracts, and we are inclined to suspect that no combination of histamine and tyramine would be likely to produce such action, for if the histamine was in small enough proportion not to affect the bronchi, it would probably be too small in amount to act sufficiently on the uterus. There is an-

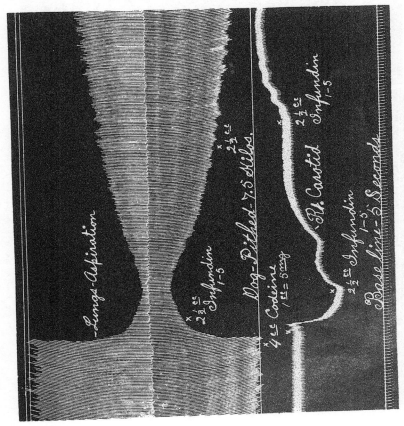

Fig. 14.—For discussion see text.

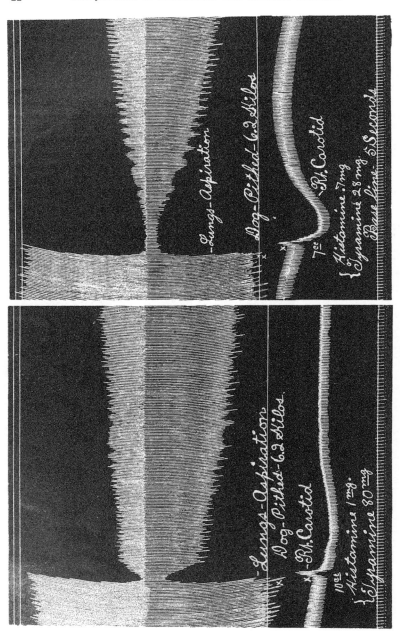

Fig. 15.—For discussion see text.

Fig. 16.—For discussion see text.

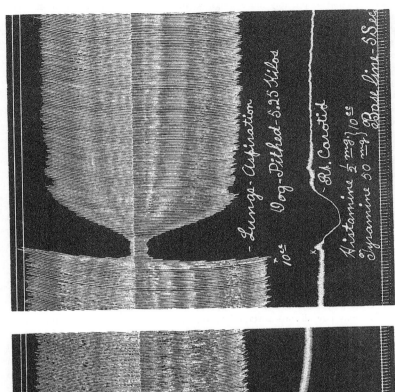

Fig. 17. For discussion see text.

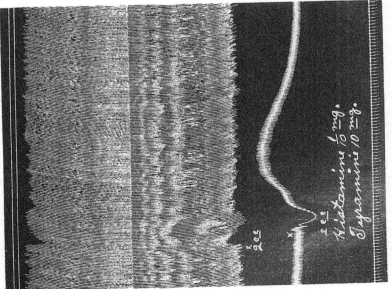

Fig. 18. For discussion see text.

other objection of possibly more weight than this also to the combination. We have found that when an animal has been injected repeatedly with a mixture of tyramine and histamine so that it has lost its susceptibility to the combination (somewhat after the manner of pituitary extracts) then the injection of pituitary extracts may produce practically the normal type of blood pressure rise. (The reverse of this experiment also holds good.) This test was described long ago by Barger and Dale for various sympatho-mimetic amines. Before leaving this subject, however, we wish to emphasize the fact that we have some evidence indicating that combinations of histamine and tyramine may readily be made which certainly resemble the action of pituitary extracts in many particulars. Fig. 18 is typical in this respect. Here 1/10 of a milligram of histamine and 10 milligrams of tyramine (proportion 1 to 100) produced a rise in blood pressure and a very slight, sharp, transient bronchoconstriction which certainly greatly resembles some pituitary tracings. Without further study one might at once conclude that this combination (1 to 100) was the proper proportion to use in making artificial pituitary extracts. There is, however, one serious objection as will be seen by comparing this tracing with Fig. 17 which was made also from the same animal by a mixture of 1 to 100 histamine and tyramine, but with a dose five times as large. It is seen at once that the increased bronchoconstriction is in almost direct mathematical proportion to the increase in the quantity of histamine injected. Consequently if pituitary extracts consisted of such combinations, then increase in dosage should immediately produce marked increases in the extent of bronchoconstriction. We have shown that that does not occur with some preparations, but does apparently to some slight extent with others.

We may now discuss certain features of the results described in this paper. As it appears to us there are two features which demand special scrutiny. These are the matter of dosage, and the method which we have used to record bronchial contractions. Regarding the first point we may say that we have tried even a much larger range of separate doses and of combinations than we believed to be really necessary. We are sorry that the limit of space prevents us from publishing many other tracings which we have at hand, and which would undoubtedly explain more fully many points which we have barely mentioned herein. There is one point which has especially concerned us. That is the question, is it possible for a combination of histamine and a pressor substance to be made (as a simple mixture) in such proportions that the amount of histamine will be too small to contract the bronchi (which in the dog are exceedingly sensitive to the drug) but will at the same time be sufficient in amount to contract the uterus? The effect of such a combination on the blood pressure and the other smooth musculature we omit from the discussion at present. The only way to obtain evidence on this question is by pharmacologic experiment, and we believe that the results presented above prove that at least some *commercial* pituitary extracts can not be such mixtures. Figs. 1 and 4 probably show completely that the particular extract used in these experiments was not such a mixture of histamine (in appreciable amount) and some pressor substance. While it is possible that some objection might be brought against these experiments, perhaps in regard to the matter of relative dosage, still we have been unable to conceive of any evidence which would demonstrate the matter any more clearly than it is shown in these two experiments. With reference to certain other commercial pituitary extracts we may say at once that we feel assured that some of these undoubtedly contain histamine, and in all probability in a few preparations the amount is sufficient to be of some therapeutic importance. This histamine we regard rather as an accidental impurity for which ordinary commercial methods are responsible, or else as an added product which is intended to increase the oxytoeic action of the product, rather than as a necessary component of all extracts which are efficient in producing contractions of the uterus. In Fig. 1 it is shown that 7/10 of a milligram of histamine produced only a little greater uterine contraction than did the 4 c.c. of (1 to 5) pituitrin. And the histamine here has the advantage of the increase in irritability which the preceding injection of pituitrin produced. Consequently these two doses are fairly comparable so far as their uterine action is concerned. But the action on the bronchi is so wholly at variance that it is practically impossible to reconcile the two results. There can be no doubt but that we are here dealing with two entirely different substances. Histamine is a profound constrictor of the bronchial musculature, but the true active principle of the posterior portion of the pituitary gland is almost, if indeed not entirely, without any action whatever on the bronchial muscles. This holds for the dog. We are unable to say what action pituitary extracts may have on the bronchioles of other animals. But that is immaterial so far as the present point is concerned.

Regarding our method of recording bronchial contractions we may simply say that it is effective in demonstrating the action of exceedingly small doses of histamine, and we have been unable to think of any special reason why it should fail to show a contraction with pituitary extract, if such contraction really occurred.

If the results and conclusions which we have presented above are correct, then it follows as a matter of the greatest probability that the true active principle of the posterior portion of the pituitary gland exerts its action in the body by stimulation of certain nervous elements. This is contrary to the ordinary view which assumes that the drug acts directly on the muscle fibers. It will be recalled by older workers in this field that almost exactly this same history was repeated in the early work on adrenaline. There are now a variety of instances known in which the action of pituitary extracts can be much more plausibly explained on the basis of an action on nerves than of one directly on muscle fibers. Perhaps the most striking of these is the observation by Paton[22] and Watson that pituitrin lowers the blood pressure in birds (duck), and that after repeated injections the fall becomes less and less and may even be finally replaced by a slight rise, i. e., exactly the reverse of the action in mammals. Atropine does not change these results. We may advantageously quote here from Paton and Watson's article (page 419): "The antagonism of pituitrin and barium salts would seem to confirm Dale's contention that the action of the former is upon muscle fibers (it raises blood pressure after ergotoxine) beyond the neuromuscular junction, but on the other hand the way in which adrenaline antagonizes pituitrin (on the blood pressure in the duck), would rather point to the action being upon these terminations." Another example has been noted by Shamoff[23] and also by Hoskins.[24] Shamoff worked with excised loops of rabbit intestine and found that a variety of pituitary preparations caused relaxation and inhibition. Hoskins did the same thing with intact dogs and got "a clean cut depression of tonus and peristalsis" in five cases out of six. He used commercial "pituitrin," but in three other instances he used saline extracts of old preparations of desiccated gland and got similar results. While we merely mention these few observations, all workers in these fields will readily collect other examples of obscure actions (or lack of actions) on the part of pituitary extracts (such, for example, as its probable failure to produce abortion in the human until very late in pregnancy, and the peculiar and varying reactions of the pupil in different species). And adrenaline itself shows so many striking similarities to the action of pituitrin that a similar pharmacologic basis seems exceedingly probable.

Regarding the nature of nervous structures on which pituitrin might act we can only suggest that possibly some portion of the sympathetic mechanism may be involved, but we suspect that some nervous elements whose course and nature are as yet unknown may be concerned. Pharmacologists are already familiar with such cases, as for instance the action of atropine in checking the marked peristalsis produced by pilocarpine, but failing to prevent vagus stimulation from producing normal peristalsis. (For discussion and references see Cushny, Pharmacology and Therapeutics, 1918, p. 326). And while none of these observations prove that pituitary extracts act on nervous structures to produce smooth muscle contractions, still we believe this view is much more plausible and more in keeping with modern methods of thought than is the older notion of being compelled to assume some peculiar difference in the chemistry of each portion of widely distributed systems of smooth muscle. Even the observation—if it be correct—that histamine itself fails to cause contraction of the rat's uterus is of interest here. And those who are familiar with the widely varying and capricious character of the action of the many sympatho-mimetic amines (Barger and Dale: Journal of Physiology, 1910, 41, p. 19) will be able to appreciate our views on this matter at once.

We feel that the above results probably justify us in suggesting the following conclusions:

1. The true active principle of the posterior portion of the pituitary gland is a simple body of the sympatho-mimetic amine type, which in the dog produces contraction of the uterus but fails to contract the bronchi. With the other smooth musculature we are not especially concerned in this paper.

2. This is in all probability due to an action of the substance on certain nervous elements and not to a direct muscular action.

3. Certain commercial preparations of the pituitary gland apparently contain very small and very variable proportions of histamine, and the amount of this substance is probably great enough in some samples to exert some therapeutic action. But it is in nowise a necessary constituent of first-class preparations of the posterior portion of the pituitary gland.

It is exceedingly probable that the action of histamine on the bronchioles of spinal dogs can be used as a commercial test for the presence of small amounts of this substance in ordinary commercial extracts of the pituitary gland. We presume that excised bronchial rings might be used as a very poor substitute for the method which we have here employed.

5. If the findings reported in this paper are substantiated, then there are very obvious clinical advantages in favor of the pituitary extracts rather than of the very intense broncho-constricting and blood-pressure lowering histamine for obstetrical uses. But in all probability very small amounts of histamine would not be of any serious disadvantage in these preparations.

BIBLIOGRAPHY

[1]Abel, J. J., and Kubota, S.: Jour. Pharmacol. and Exper. Therap., 1919, xiii, 243.
[2]Houssay, B. A.: La Acción Fisiológica de los Extractos Hipofisiarios, 1918, Buenos Aires.
[3]McCord, C. P.: Arch. Int. Med., 1911, viii, 609.
[4]Roth, G. B.: U. S. Pub. Health Service, Hygienic Laboratory Bull., 1914, No. 100, and 1917, No. 109.
[5]Hamilton, H. C., and Rowe, L. W.: Jour. Lab. and Clin. Med., 1916, ii, 120.
[6]Dale, H. H., and Laidlaw, P. P..: Jour. Physiol., 1919, lii, 355.
[7]Barger, G., and Dale, H. H.: Jour. Physiol., 1910, lii, 355.
[8]Jackson, D. E.: Jour. Lab. and Clin. Med., 1917, iii, 63.
[9]Jackson, D. E.: Jour. Pharmacol. and Exper. Therap., 1914, v, 479. Also (in detail) Jackson: Experimental Pharmacology, 1917, St. Louis, Mo., C. V. Mosby Co., p. 287.
[10]Titone, P.: Pflüger's Arch., 1913, clv, 77.
[11]Froehlich, A., and Pick, E. P.: Arch. f. exper. Path. und Pharmakol., 1913, lxxiv, 92.
[12]Baehr, G., and Pick, E. P.: Ibid., 1913, lxxiv, 41.
[13]Houssay, B. A.: Loc. cit., p. 139.
[14]Borchardt, L.: Therapie der Gegenwart, 1914.
[15]Bourgeois: Prog. Méd., 1917, 3 février.
[16]Zueblin: Med. Rec., 1917, xci, No. 9.
[17]Bensaude, R., and Hallion, L.: Presse Méd., 1918, No. 20, p. 185.
[18]Lanari, A.: Argentina Medica, 1913, 6 set., No. 36, p. 710.
[19]Jackson, D. E.: Experimental Pharmacology, pp. 388 and 391.
[20]Houssay, B. A.: Loc. cit., p. 140. MacLeod, J. J. R.: Physiology and Biochemistry in Modern Medicine, 1918, St. Louis, Mo., C. V. Mosby Co., p. 769.
[21]Baehr, G., and Pick, E. P.: Arch. f. exper. Path. und Pharmacol., 1913, lxxiv, 41.
[22]Paton, D. Noel, and Watson, A.: Jour. Physiol., 1912, xliv, 414.
[23]Shamoff, V. N.: Am. Jour. Physiol., 1916, xxix, 268.
[24]Hoskins, R. G.: Jour. Am. Med. Assn., 1916, lxvi, 733.

REPORT ON EPIDEMIC AND INFECTIOUS DISEASES IN CAMP DEVENS, MASS*

By Paul G. Woolley, M.D., Cincinnati, Ohio

Formerly Major, M.C., U. S. A., Camp Sanitary Inspector and Epidemiologist, Camp Devens, Mass.

THE following preliminary section will serve to indicate the general conditions in Camp Devens and in its environment. The various points are but briefly considered but they will make clear that the diseases which have been observed in the camp personnel were not closely, at least, related to faults of drainage, water supply, sewage disposal, food supply, or insects, and were not apparently related to the geographical location of the camp except as that is related to climate.

Moreover these paragraphs relate especially to cantonment conditions and not to those, inherent or developed, in the extra-cantonment area in which there was much to be desired in the matter of general sanitation.

SECTION I

Camp Devens is situated in Middlesex County, Mass., about 14 miles from Fitchburg, Mass., and about 2 miles from Ayer, Mass., 42 deg. 32 min. North latitude, and 17 deg. 37 min. East of Greenwich. The country is rolling and largely wooded with second growth hard-wood trees. In the camp proper there are occasional clumps of trees and in the open places which are used as drill grounds, the turf has been worn away exposing the underlying sand and gravel. About the camp and especially along the Nashua River, and in the region between the camp and Ayer, there are many marshy places in and about which the undergrowth is vigorous and abundant. In these areas there are many mosquitos which breed in the damp grass and the pools of standing water. Within the camp there is considerable flying dust in dry windy weather, but because of the porous nature of the soil there is but little mud to be carried upon the feet even in very wet weather. The roads are all of tar-bound macadam and so are quite free from dust. In situations where, because of the nature of the roads, the dust would be detrimental, as for instance about the bakeries, the roads and their margins are kept thoroughly oiled.

The camp was designed as a receiving and training camp for New England soldiers. It was planned for the accommodation of a complete division and a depot brigade. In the latter recruits were received, housed, and partially trained, and from it they were later transferred into more permanent organizations, chiefly into units of the 76th Division which from the earliest days of the camp occupied the divisional area. Later, when the 76th Division had gone overseas, men were transferred to the 12th Division which succeeded the 76th at Camp Devens. The 76th Division was, from the start, a replacement division in which partially seasoned and trained men completed training before being transferred to combat divisions. The camp as a whole, then, was devoted to receiving, examining, sort-

*Authority for publication granted by the Surgeon-General's Office, Washington, D. C.

ing, and training, enlisted and drafted troops. After the armistice the camp became a demobilization center and was thereafter devoted to inspection, examination and discharge, of New England troops, and to inspection, examination and transfer of troops belonging in other sections of the country than New England. In its early days the camp was what it planned to be—a New England camp. Later, because of transfers in and out, it became more cosmopolitan.

From the start the camp was overcrowded, sometimes, more, sometimes less, but always some. In certain periods this was general; at other times it was local. It was planned that the area should accommodate approximately 35,000 troops, but this figure was often exceeded. Especially was this true during August and September, 1918. At other times the crowding was due to lack of proper distribution of troops, and was almost constant in the case of the black troops. An early reason for this was that portions of barracks were set aside for recreation rooms—an arrangement which was totally unauthorized, and which was corrected. Also in the early days the Remount Depot and the Public Utilities were badly overcrowded, conditions which were very slowly met by construction of additional buildings. In the Engineer Section overcrowding was noticeable, but was later corrected. The guard houses were generally overcrowded. Even in the early part of January, 1918, there was a deplorable lack of hot water which resulted in lack of use of the bathing facilities.

Despite the overcrowding the health of the whole command did not seem to be very noticeably affected except in the case of measles. The early outbreak of this disease which began in 1917 rapidly exhausted itself and in February had reached a,—what might be called,—fairly normal average. In this period pneumonia was rising, but it was not until the negro troops from Florida entered the camp that it reached anything like epidemic proportions.

The climate is characteristic of New England; i.e., generally and moderately cold in winter with spells of severe cold, and moderately warm in summer with some acutely hot days which are often almost unendurable because of the humidity. The season of 1918-19 was exceptionally mild.

The surface drainage of the camp is naturally good and takes place, as a rule, into the Nashua River or its tributaries. The character of the soil permits of rapid seepage. Originally there were many ponds and pools within the camp area but these have been filled or drained. Those which have not been drained or filled were kept thoroughly oiled, and drip cans for oil were placed at the heads of all streams passing through the camp. The result of all this has been that despite the presence of many mosquitos without the camp area there are very few within it. No anopheles were found within the camp, but in the wooded places along the Nashua River close to the camp specimens have been seen.

On January 1, 1918, the sewage system of the camp was incomplete as regarded the disposal. The collection system was complete, but, lacking a disposal plant, the sewage of the camp was drained directly into the Nashua River, a condition of affairs which added to the size of that already large open sewer. Early in the year the whole system was completed.

Since the completion of the plant the sewage has been disposed of by applying it to sand beds. A main plant of 20 acres receives the sewage of the camp proper, and two smaller plants receive the flow from the Base Hospital. There were pit latrines located at various places within the camp not convenient to existing sewers and others at the various ranges and at other places used by troops, for instance at Hell Pond,—the authorized swimming place. The sewage flows by gravity to a receiving well the capacity of which is 237,000 gallons. From there it is sent by a centrifugal pump to the twenty sand beds situated on a knoll of sand and gravel above the Nashua River about two miles north of the camp and a few hundred yards north of the corrals of the Remount Depot. The liquid is spread on the beds by wooden flumes. Because the knoll is formed of sand and gravel, no under-drains were provided, the effluent sinking into the soil at the rate of 85,000 gallons per acre. During July, 1918, the flow did not exceed 1,400,000 gallons per day and at that rate of dosage the liquid disappeared so rapidly that the beds were but rarely fully covered. The mat formed on the surfaces of the beds was raked off at intervals of 10 days or two weeks and the beds were then harrowed with a horse drawn harrow. The mat was hauled away and burned. There was but little odor connected with the beds and there were few flies on them. The material taken from the screens at the receiving well is hauled away and buried. It consists largely of rags and paper. The larger of the two Base Hospital plants, about an acre and a half in size, is similar to the main plant but owing to its position the sewage flows into the well from which it is discharged directly by a siphon at the rate of about 72,000 gallons per day. The beds of this plant are underdrained and the effluent flows almost directly into the Nashua River, entering below the surface. Mat forms quickly at this plant and the solid waste is not so thoroughly broken up as at the large plant. The rakings were used for filling low places near the beds and were thoroughly oiled to prevent fly breeding. The second Base Hospital plant, about an acre in extent, receives sewage at the rate of about 24,000 gallons per day, and is underdrained into a creek which flows into the Nashua River.

The garbage of the camp was separated and collected in covered galvanized iron cans, and was sent, daily, to the transfer station where it was delivered to the contractor who removed it. It was presumed that these cans were thoroughly cleansed at the transfer station, but the presumption was erroneous. They were merely cleaned as thoroughly as the water-heating facilities would permit. The result was that flies were more numerous at the transfer station than at any other place in the camp. Manure from the stables and picket lines was hauled away daily and delivered at the railway where it was taken over by the contractor. The stables were kept clean and were not inhabited by any number of flies. There were, however, numerous rats and mice in these buildings.

The water supply of the cantonment is secured from shallow wells on the bank of a small pond just on the east side of the camp. One dug well twenty-eight feet deep and fifty feet in diameter, cased in wooden sheet piling and covered with tar paper covering wood, furnishes the bulk of the supply. During the winter of 1917 the quantity of water from this well was not sufficient for the needs of the camp and so in July, 1918, an auxiliary system of forty driven points, two and one-half inches in diameter and forty feet deep, was completed. These points are spaced thirty feet apart along the bank of the pond near the dug well. The water from the driven points is siphoned into the driven well by exhausting the air in the suction line. The capacity of the system is estimated at from 2,500,-

000 to 3,000,000 gallons per day. The water from the well is pumped against a head of 200-240 pounds into four 100,000 gallon wooden tanks, from which it is distributed to all parts of the camp by gravity. The water was originally pure and the drainage area was practically free from pollution, but occasionally the bacterial counts indicated a leak, probably from the adjacent pond into the well. Therefore the water was consistently dosed with varying small, but sufficient amounts of chloride of lime, or later treated with liquid chlorine. Other sources of water supply were used by troops outside the camp and at the several ranges. The spring and wells from which these waters come were inspected and examined at frequent intervals and posted to indicate whether they might or might not be used for drinking purposes. When the water was of doubtful potability and yet must be used it was treated with hypochlorite in a Lister bag. Bathing facilities were excellent. Showers, hot and cold, were provided in lavatories adjacent to each barrack. In warm weather outdoor bathing was authorized in Hell Pond, a deep lake filled with clear, clean water, situated near the camp.

The milk supply of the camp was, in general, a good one, and if, in certain instances it was not what it should be, the defects were remedied rapidly. The bulk of the milk came from large modern dairies and was packed and delivered under excellent conditions. Twice each week samples of milk were taken from the delivery wagons as they entered the camp and were sent to the laboratory of the Base Hospital for complete examination. The dairies themselves were subject to systematic inspections by the assistant camp veterinarian and were scored. Scores were filed with the dairies, and with the Camp Sanitary Inspector. All milk entering the camp was pasteurized. All meats and vegetables were inspected before they were permitted to enter the camp.

The heating of the buildings was accomplished by means of steam. The system was successful and there was no difficulty in preserving a comfortable warmth even in the coldest weather. Unfortunately this system was not completed until after the onset of the cold weather, in 1917.

The buildings forming the camp were of pine, lined with wall-board. This makes a comfortable house but it becomes most inconvenient in case of infection with cimex.

Kitchens were furnished with hot and cold water and with sinks which drain into grease-traps outside the building. The grease and sediment were collected from the traps frequently enough to keep them in good condition. It was supposed that the original traps were sufficient to care for the grease carried toward the sewers in the waste water from the kitchens. Late in the summer it became evident that unless some change were made, the grease which was being carried past the grease traps would clog the filter-beds, and put them out of commission. Accordingly a new type of trap was authorized and ordered installed. The installation was completed some weeks after the signing of the armistice.

At the main well and at the grenade field on the water shed incinerator latrines were in use, and were completely satisfactory.

The buildings and roadways were well lighted with electricity.

The laundry facilities of the camp were bad in certain particulars until late in the spring of 1919. There was no camp laundry and therefore all articles that required washing, such as those from the Base Hospital, and those from other sources, were sent to private concerns. It was the rule that these articles were packed in large canvas bags and hauled away by trucks which later returned the washed articles in the unwashed sacks. There was therefore a constant chance of infection and cross infection. In the summer of 1918 however, the bags were discarded at the request of the Camp Sanitary Inspector and were replaced by large baskets which were lined with fresh paper before the clean clothes were placed in them. Still later the camp laundry was put in operation and has been an improvement.

The camp was policed by members of the various organizations and by the Camp Sanitary Squad. The general sanitary condition was kept at a high level, as a rule.

Early in 1918 there was a shortage of warm clothing and as a consequence many men suffered, often severely, from cold. There were many cases of frost bite, epecially of the fingers and ears. Provision was gradually made to remedy this very essential defect. In the meantime there was a very large amount of bronchitis and coryza.

At the time when troops began to return to Camp Devens from overseas the facilities for delousing were absent, though plans were under way, late in the summer, for the construction of a complete delousing plant. Pending the completion of this plant temporary methods were used which served fairly efficiently so far as lice were concerned, but which were exceedingly inefficient so far as clothing was concerned. Much of the clothing handled by the extemporized methods was ruined and could not be reissued.

SECTION II

The following paragraphs relate to problems connected with infectious diseases in the cantonment and are based upon reports made by the Epidemiologist, and by members of the medical staff of the Base Hospital, and upon various miscellaneous reports in the Office of the Camp Surgeon.

Methods of Control.—(a) Measles cases were removed from their organization and sent to the Base Hospital where they were cared for in measles wards. The whole organization was sometimes placed in quarantine for 15 days during which time physical inspections are made at frequent intervals in order that new cases may be caught at an early date. Sometimes only the other members of the same squad were placed in quarantine, and sometimes a whole squad was isolated. The latter method was used to the exclusion of the others during the winter. Recently the squad method has been used with just as good results. Transfers, from one organization to another have been permitted provided that men transferred from an infected unit were sent to an infected unit in their new organization.

(b) Meningitis cases were immediately removed from their organizations and sent to the Base Hospital where they were isolated. Immediately the organization in which the cases belonged were placed in quarantine until the members were cultured. All positive culture cases (carriers) were sent to the Base Hospital. The other members of the organization were kept segregated for a week during which they were treated with chlorazene or dichloramin-T, or a mild disinfectant.

(c) Scarlet fever cases were sent immediately to the Base Hospital. The organization to which the case belonged was quarantined for eight days during which time each member was subjected to careful inspection twice daily.

(d) Diphtheria cases were sent to the Base Hospital. The organization to which the case belonged, or the squad room in which he lived was quarantined and each individual in the organization or squad room was cultured and "schicked." Carriers were sent to the Base Hospital for treatment. Suggestive "schicks" were given an immunizing dose of antitoxin, and quarantine was raised.

(e) German measles cases were treated in the Base Hospital. No quarantine was kept.

(f) Pneumonia cases were sent to the Base Hospital. Nothing was done in the squads or organizations to which the cases belonged. This seems to be something of an anomaly when such particular pains were taken to prevent the spread of the disease in the wards of the hospitals. Much could be done it seems in the way of prevention of serious complications if the men of an organization or of a command were treated prophylactically in such a manner as to limit the flora of the upper respiratory passages to but one type of organism at most. If the streptococci in the noses and throats of the men could be limited a great gain would be made. The figures which Major Spooner obtained at the Base Hospital are exceedingly suggestive in this connection. He found that practically 100 per cent of the persons examined by him harbored streptococci and that from 5 per cent to 71 per cent of these persons harbored streptococci of the hemolytic type. Lt. Grav and the writer suggested that special care be given to the earliest possible diagnosis of pneumonia. it would be much more to the point to pay especial attention to prophylaxis. With this in view it may be urged that men reporting at sick call with a cough or cold be treated with the object of at least reducing his respiratory flora and if possible of doing away with it. Too often such men are treated by giving them a placebo or a laxative, which is all very well in its place but which does not directly attack the trouble. A man's first sick call is the time to get busy with a possible pneumonia. Men who do not report at sick call and who at the same time have troublesome coughs,—and they are many,—should be sent to the infirmary for treatment. In the absence of such an individual method the only alternative is to treat whole organizations by means of sprays. This can be done and it was done in organizations of more than a thousand men, and done daily at Camp Green with apparently good results. The individual method is preferable.

(g) Incoming recruits were kept segregated for two weeks during which time they were inspected frequently for infectious diseases. Outgoing troops were carefully inspected for signs of infectious diseases and suspicious cases were held. A statement of the condition of the command is sent to the Commanding Officer at their destination.

2. The first infectious diseases (exclusive of venereal diseases) to appear in this camp were pneumonia, measles, mumps, diphtheria. and German measles. There was a single case of typhoid fever and two cases of malaria recognized during October but no other cases of typhoid appeared until the following July, 1918, when the draft brought in two others. Two additional cases of malaria were seen in November and these were the last to be found until the next Spring. From the beginning of the camp there was a gradual, though slow, increase in the incidence of the various infectious diseases through October and November. During this period the men were out of doors during a fair proportion of the time. Later they were more constantly confined to the barracks, or, at least, they chose to occupy their quarters for a larger part of their free time. In the case of measles and German measles the epidemic rise was sharp. In the case of the mumps it was lower. The top of the curve for measles and German measles was reached in January; for mumps, in February. Secondary peaks following the arrival of southern negroes and other recruits appeared in May. The secondary rises were sharper than the primary ones because at this time there was a tremendous amount of overcrowding which acted disastrously upon the sick rate in the blacks especially. Pneumonia on the other hand increased with much greater slowness and reached its maximum in admissions after the measles rise. The pneumonia curve seemed to follow after the curve of upper respiratory infections. Meningitis, diphtheria, scarlet fever, typhoid and paratyphoid fevers, and malaria were at no time epidemic.

Pneumonia seems to have been related not so much to mere opportunity for infection, such as exists in the camp environment, as to previous respiratory affections. Perhaps both factors are essential. Measles, German measles. and mumps appeared. on the other hand, to depend entirely upon multiplied opportunities for infection.

3. Recruiting was most active in October, April, May and June. At various other times in the course of the year small numbers of recruits arrived in camp in numbers of

from 200 to 2000. Following each accession there was an increase in the sick rate from all causes, and in the infectious disease rate, that was roughly proportional to the number of new men. In October the men sent to camp were all becoming accustomed to a completely new life with which few of them had ever had the slightest experience. Cold weather was coming on. The heating plant was not finished. Still conditions were such that they did not have to spend too much time huddled together for warmth. Therefore disease spread slowly. Later as they were more and more confined to their barracks infection spread more rapidly, and this was not confined to the specific diseases but included also the nonspecific infections of the air passages. So we find in December a total of 1013 cases of acute bronchitis, pharyngitis, laryngitis, and tonsillitis treated at the Base Hospital, a number of which indicates an enormous number of other cases treated and untreated in the regimental infirmaries. During December, January, February and March there were more than 3300 such cases treated at the Base Hospital, a figure that is worthy the greatest consideration in studying the pneumonia and empyema situation.

The data relating to the common acute upper respiratory tract infections, are shown in Table I.

TABLE I

	December	January	February	March	Totals
Bronchitis, acute	459	256	182	287	1184
Pharyngitis, ac.	248	196	198	380	1022
Laryngitis, ac.	148	33	11	18	210
Tonsillitis, ac.	158	251	206	290	905
Totals	1013	736	597	975	3321

The figures in the table apply only to cases admitted to hospital. The total for the Camp at large would be far larger. The tonsillitis figures suggest a connection between this infection and the empyema and streptococcus pneumonias.

4. Beside the factor which we call exposure and in which we include general housing conditions, lack of sufficient clothing, as well as direct exposure to weather, stands the factor of fatigue, a rather indefinite one, and one difficult of estimation. In one instance we believe we were able to see that fatigue was definitely associated with an increase in the sick rate. This was in the case of the 303rd Infantry. This regiment was one in which the sick rate had been rarely, if ever, high, and one in which the rate ran at a fairly constant level, without great variation. On May 15th this organization took a practice march to Concord, Mass., an exercise which occupied it until the 18th of May. Previous to May 15th the sick rate had not been above 26.0. The day after the regiment got back from its hike the rate rose and reached 28 on May 20th. On May 21st the rate was 26.6 showing that the increase of sickness was transient though there was still more than a normal amount. The weather was excellent during the whole period. After the 21st of May the sick rate was profoundly modified by additions of new men into the organization so that the further effect of the march can not be seen. It seems that the rise in the sick rate of this regiment on May 20th and 21st was due to fatigue and to exposure which expressed itself in upper respiratory troubles such as coughs and colds and bronchitis. An additional factor to be considered is the dust of the roads, which in this instance was an unimportant one it seems, since, for the most part, the roads over which the men passed were well oiled.

5. The sick rate and rate due to infectious disease was consistently lower among commissioned officers than among enlisted men except in the cases of meningitis and diphtheria. No deaths occurred from infectious diseases among officers except in meningitis which caused one death.

SECTION III

The following paragraphs relate to facts, chiefly statistical ones, associated with the different infectious diseases studied in Camp Devens.

The infectious diseases observed in the Camp were influenza, measles, mumps, pneumonia, meningitis, scarlet fever, diphtheria, German measles, typhoid, malaria, smallpox, chicken-pox and the venereal diseases. Of these influenza, pneumonia, measles, mumps, and German measles were epidemic. Meningitis and scarlet fever showed immature symptoms of becoming epidemic at one time but progressed no further. They and the other diseases were consistently sporadic. Tables II and III are illustrative. In the first, mumps, German measles and venereal diseases are not tabulated.

TABLE II

1918	Jan.	Feb.	Mar.	Apr.	May	June	July	Aug.	Sept.	Oct.	Nov.	Dec.
Influenza	0	0	0	0	0	0	0	0	14000	664	59	61
Pneumonia	44	52	110	160	89	39	24	112	2595	243	65	71
Measles	252	55	50	18	83	69	56	59	43	126	90	32
Scarlet fever	5	12	13	19	6	2	2	2	1	1	2	4
Diphtheria	0	1	4	5	5	1	4	3	0	0	1	1
Meningitis	1	2	2	3	2	5	1	1	8	18	1	2

TABLE III

1917-1918	Oct.	Nov.	Dec.	Jan.	Feb.	Mar.	Apr.	May	June	July	Total	Rate 1000
Pneumonia	11	8	16	44	52	110	160	89	39	24	533	22.4
Measles	5	29	168	252	55	50	18	83	69	56	785	31.4
G. Measles	1	8	57	140	30	13	0	0	7	1	257	10.3
Mumps	1	4	8	32	65	62	156	233	160	57	778	31.0
Scarlet fever	0	0	2	5	12	13	19	6	2	2	61	2.4
Diphtheria	1	4	1	0	1	4	5	5	1	4	26	1.04
Meningitis	0	0	0	1	2	2	3	2	5	1	16	0.60
Typhoid	1	0	0	0	0	0	0	0	0	0	1	0.04
Malaria	2	2	0	0	0	0	0	1	1	3	9	0.36
Total	22	55	252	474	217	254	361	419	284	148	2486	99.4

Generally speaking, the health of the Camp was excellent. Taken as a whole the incidence of disease, except during the epidemic of influenza and pneumonia was what may be called normal as compared with other camps and the mortality was low. During the influenza epidemic the death rate compared very favorably with that of other large camps. In certain exceptional instances both incidence and mortality were high, as for example in the cases of pneumonia in southern negro troops. The rule was that all infectious diseases were most frequent in new recruits, especially in those from rural districts, and in overcrowded troops.

Measles was from the start a disease of unseasoned rural troops. The only epidemic of any proportion was that which began in the latter part of 1917, after the weather condition forced men to remain indoors. This epidemic persisted through January and exhausted itself in February, in which month it reached a normal level. With each accession of new troops the number of cases increased. The disease showed relatively fewer complications in this camp than it did in many others.

Measles:
Period, 43 weeks from October 1, 1917, to July 31, 1918
Average strength of command   30,124
Total cases   785
Annual rate per 1000   31.4
Average non-effective rate per 1000   30.03
(There were no deaths due to measles.)

Causes of the epidemic:
Infection from civil community.
Susceptibility.
Housing (crowding).
Importation from other camps.
Weather.

With the exception of mumps, measles furnished the largest number of cases of infectious disease during the period under discussion,—in all 785. Taking it by and large the disease was not severe, and, of itself, in uncomplicated cases, it gave rise to no mortality. On the other hand, the complications which followed it were severe, at least in the case of pneumonia, which was frequently followed by empyema. The fact that the largest proportion of complications occurred during January and February appears to mean that the measles was not the immediate cause of the complications but rather the contributing cause, with which was associated the then prevalent respiratory infections, the effects of which were accentuated and rendered more severe by the secondary infection of measles. The records of the camp indicate that the first cases of measles appeared in recent recruits and that later cases were often imported from outside the camp. More recent records (August) showed that the cases of measles which were reported from day to day were, without exception, in recruits, and the daily reports from the U. S. Public Health Service showed cases of measles in most of the surrounding towns. In not a single case observed in this late period was there record that the man had been on leave or pass since coming into the service. All recruits were held in quarantine for two weeks after their arrival. It is therefore evident that all the cases observed in August were men who had been in camp less than two weeks and that the measles was brought into the camp with them. These new men formed foci from which the disease spread to other susceptible persons. Under conditions such as existed during the winter the spread was rapid. In August there was practically no spread. It might be suspected that had the general weather conditions during June and July been similar to those of the preceding winter we should have had a real epidemic. Under these later conditions the complications were fewer and less severe. Therefore it seemed not unreasonable to lighten quarantine in order that as many susceptible men as possible might contract the disease under the best possible conditions. It was believed that such a method of dealing with the disease during the summer months would react favorably upon the amount of sickness and upon the pneumonia incidence and mortality "over there," and also "over here" during the winter. In the absence of permission from the Surgeon General this suggestion was not carried out. Except for pneumonia, the complications of measles were relatively unimportant and resulted in no mortality. Likewise the sequelae were mild. In the last 24 cases there were three pneumonias, all lobular and all mild. It is probable that German measles should be included with measles in discussing the disease because it is one with which the average practitioner is not sufficiently well acquainted to make a certain diagnosis. Even the expert is prone to err, and so it happens that mild cases of measles are called German measles and very frank cases of German measles are called measles. All that seems necessary to be said at this time is that in the cases called German measles at this camp the rate per 1000 was 10.3 for the ten months, that there were no complications of note, and that the days of hospitalization were few.

Pneumonia played a very large part in the morbidity and mortality rates of the camp. In a report from the Base Hospital it was estimated that pneumonia could be held accountable for 45 per cent of all sick days. It has also been estimated that, exclusive of influenza-pneumonia, the mortality rate at this camp was about half that to be expected in a civilian population. The disease attacked both officers and men but was four times as frequent in the men. No empyema complicated the disease in officers. Medical officers suffered more frequently, but no medical officer, nurse, or orderly attending pneumonia cases contracted the disease. Lobar pneumonia was more frequent in negroes, lobular (broncho) pneumonia in white men. The empyemas were predominantly pneumococcic, but the mortality was highest in those due to or complicated by streptococci.

TABLE IV
PNEUMONIA (STATISTICAL TABLE)

Period of 43 weeks from October, 1917, to July 31, 1918.	
Average strength of command	30,124
Total number of cases	533
Annual rate per 1000	21.3
Total deaths	72
Annual rate per 1000	2.8
Case mortality	13 %
Average noneffective rate per 1000	30.03

Pneumonia furnished 21 per cent of the cases of infectious diseases during the above period, and Lt. Gray, in his report on pneumonia and empyema, has estimated that this disease accounted for 45 per cent of all sick days. Also, Lt. Gray suggested that the mortality rate from pneumonia in Camp Devens was about one-half of that to be expected in civilian population under the usual circumstances. This low rate was due to several factors: (a) The excellent general physical condition of the men of the command; (b) The absence of very young and very old persons; (c) the early diagnosis and treatment of sick. The disease attacked both officers and men, but the rate among the men was nearly four times as great as that among the officers. Also there were no cases of empyema and no deaths among officers, a state of affairs determined by (a) the better physical condition of the officers and their previous experiences in other camps, (b) less exposure and less crowding; (c) better attention to ventilation. Medical officers suffered twenty times as often as line officers, but no medical officer, nurse or orderly attending pneumonia cases was attacked by the disease. Organizational incidence of pneumonia can not be interpreted. The Field Artillery had the highest rate, and was followed by Infantry, Depot Brigade, Engineers, and Machine Gun Battalions. There were no cases in the Sanitary Train or the Base Hospital Detachment. Empyema was the one great cause of pneumonia deaths, accounting for 89 per cent of the black mortality and 68 per cent of the white. It appeared in lobar pneumonia, in black men, in but one-third as many cases as in white men, and in one-half as many cases of lobular pneumonia in blacks as in whites. Lt. Gray thinks this was due to the fact that the negroes resisted the pulmonary infection less well than the whites and they therefore did not live long enough to develop complications. It may also be that blacks were not so frequently carriers of streptococci as whites. Among the blacks 94 per cent were of the lobar type; among the whites 74 per cent were lobar. It is an interesting fact that pneumonia has not been, as a rule, a disease of very recent recruits. In Gray's series 14 per cent of the cases appeared in men who had been in the service for four months and 10 per cent were in men who had been in the service for two months, figures which indicate that the ground was being prepared for the attack of pulmonary invaders. This has been interpreted to mean that the upper respiratory tract infections (including measles) were essential factors in the whole situation and that exposure to weather, and defects of ventilation were the fundamental controlling, or better, predisposing factors—the ones which account for the tremendous incidence of the so-called coughs and colds,—which, beginning as acute processes, become chronic, and frequently purulent with the passing of time. This conception is borne out, in a way, by the fact that twenty-four of the first hundred cases of pneumonia followed measles, while in the second hundred cases of pneumonia only nine followed measles. The first hundred cases of pneumonia occurred during the period between September 27, 1917, and February 13, 1918, a period during which the weather conditions were at their worst. If measles had been the controlling factor there should have been as many postmeasles pneumonias in the second hundred cases as in the first. Of the 485 cases studied by Gray only forty-one followed measles, and of these thirty-three occurred during the severest part of the winter. Of these forty-one cases thirty-two per cent died. Of 588 cases of measles only about 7 per cent contracted pneumonia. In 44 per cent of the cases of pneumonia, taking Gray's series as a basis for discussion, the organism causing the disease was not determined. In 44 per cent the pneumococcus was found, the streptococcus alone in 9 per cent, and both pneumococcus and streptococcus in 3 per cent. But 49 per cent of the streptococcus cases died, 36 per cent of the mixed cases died, and only 12 per cent of the pneumococcus cases died.

There were seventy-seven cases of empyema, 53 per cent of which were due to streptococcus. Seventeen per cent of the cases showed a mixed infection. The mortality in the pneumococcus group and in the two groups of streptococcus and mixed infection were about equally divided, the pneumococcus having a little the advantage. In judging these cases, however, one must take into consideration the marked lack of resistance of the colored men to the pneumococcus. But even so the great importance of the streptococci must be realized. A special report on pneumonia in white and black men was made in 1918, at which time it was believed that change of climate, exposure and overcrowding were the essential causes of the pneumonia incidence in blacks. At the present time when it is being discovered that a very large number of the southern blacks are subjects of malaria, or hookworm, or both, the feeling grows that these multiple infections may have played an important part in bringing about lack of resistance which has been commented upon. How important syphilis is in this connection can only be surmised. It is interesting to note that the pneumonia mortality was highest during the first three months of the camp. Commencing with October, the percentage figures are as follows: 27, 25, 16, 11, 12, 11, 9, 13, 12—an interesting series which suggests either that treatment improved or that a certain immunity to the prevalent infections was developed.

In April, May, August, and October, the bulk of pneumonia cases occurred among the negroes. In April some 2000 southern negroes were received at the camp and from that time on the pneumonia rate of the camp remained above what it would otherwise have been.

The following statistical tables explain themselves. The data relate only to the months of April and May, 1918, because it is only in these months that the comparison between black men and white can be drawn. The black men arrived in camp on March 31 and the following few days of April and there have been practically no additions to their number until a much later time.

Total Cases (Black and White).

Period of nine weeks from March 31 to May 31, 1918:

Average strength of command for the period	35029
Total number of cases in the period	259
Annual morbidity rate per 1000	42.7
Total number of deaths	29
Annual mortality rate per 1000	4.7
Case mortality	11.2%
Average noneffective rate per 1000	42.1

The comparative data for the complete period covered in this table are as follows:

	White	Black
Average strength for the period	33131	1898
Total cases during the period	94	165
Annual morbidity rate per 1000	13.3	501.3
Total deaths from the period	6	23
Annual mortality rate per 1000	1.1	69.8
Case mortality	6.2%	13.9%

The comparative data for April are as follows:

	White	Black
Average strength for April	29402	1927
Total cases	71	99
Annual morbidity rate per 1000	29.1	623.3
Total deaths	4	16
Annual mortality rate per 1000	1.66	99.8
Case mortality	5.6%	16.1%

The comparative data for May are as follows:

	White	Black
Average strength for May	36861	1870
Total cases	23	66
Annual morbidity rate per 1000	6.9	414.3
Total deaths	2	7
Annual mortality rate per 1000	0.6	44.4
Case mortality	8.7%	10.6%

The meaning of the facts given above in tabular form will be more striking, perhaps, if they are stated in this form: If the morbidity rate for the negroes had existed among the white men of the camp there would have been 2849 cases of pneumonia in this group. If, on the other hand, the white rate had existed among the negroes this group should have had but five cases of pneumonia. These figures are based upon the estimate that 8.6 per cent of the 1898 negroes had pneumonia, as against 0.28 per cent of the 33,131 white men.

. When it is found that while the negroes formed 5.4 per cent of the average population of the camp, they furnished 63.7 per cent of the pneumonias, it at once becomes apparent that an explanation of the conditions is needed. A careful going-over of the situation indicated that there were two main factors to be considered. One of these is that which takes into account change of climate, by which we mean to a certain extent exposure, and the other is bad housing conditions; i.e., overcrowding in barracks. Undoubtedly the change of climate and exposure was the primary factor in leading up to the conditions, but it is just as certain that the element of overcrowding accentuated and tended to make permanent the high morbidity rate among the negroes from Florida. The fact that in some barracks white men were crowded together emphasizes the factor of change of climate and exposure in the blacks. At the same time it is reasonable to suppose that had there been no overcrowding the pneumonia rate would have been lower, not only among the blacks, but also among the whites. In the barracks of the Engineer Battalions the cots were so close together that there was barely room to pass between them, and occupying these cots were men, 75 per cent to 80 per cent of whom (according to the medical officer) had chronic coughs most troublesome at night. Observation indicated that the estimate of the medical officer was reasonably close to the facts.

Influenza and pneumonia in epidemic form caused the most serious condition. It invaded the camp at a period when there was most crowding and came completely unheralded. The result was that in the course of a week or ten days the Base Hospital and the infirmaries were almost overwhelmed. There were too few doctors, nurses and enlisted men of the medical department to meet the emergency and it was only after considerable delay that the personnel deficiency was met. Throughout the hospital and throughout the camp all cots were screened and throughout the days and nights very frequent medical inspections were made. By the time the disease had exhausted itself more than 14,000 cases had occurred, complicated in 2817 instances by pneumonia, and with 787 deaths. The case mortality was approximately 28 per cent. During the influenza epidemic the morbidity and mortality rates were lowest in the 36th Infantry, in the Remount Depot and in the Quartermaster Corps. The reasons for this seemed to lie in the larger proportion of seasoned men in the 36th Infantry, in lack of crowding (Remount and Q. M. C.) to outdoor work (Remount and Q. M. C.), to early screening of the cots (36th Infantry), and to methods of washing mess kits (pooling method—Remount). The Quartermaster Corps and 36th Infantry messes used graniteware dishes which were washed in bulk and not individually.

It is worthy of note that immediately after the order, prohibiting individual washing of mess kits and dishes, went into effect, the incidence of infectious disease as a whole dropped. The effect upon the measles rate seemed especially brilliant.

A complete study of the epidemic has been published in this Journal, 1919, Vol. 14, No. 6.

Meningitis has been relatively uncommon. The only time when it seemed to be taking on epidemic characters was immediately after the influenza epidemic. These cases appeared within a relatively short period in patients in the Base Hospital and in certain organizations in the Depot Brigade. After the personnel of the Base Hospital and of the affected organizations in the camp had been cultured, and the carriers isolated, the total personnel of all organizations was treated with applications of argyrol in nose, throat, and eye. After this no further cases appeared. Several carriers were discovered in the Base Hospital personnel, including two ward surgeons, one nurse, two ward orderlies, and one member of the Medical Detachment.

Following is a statistical table which indicates the extent of meningitis in the camp:

Period of 43 weeks from October 1, 1917, to July 31, 1918
Average strength of command   30,124
Total number of cases   16
Annual rate per 1000   0.5
Total deaths   6
Annual rate per 1000   0.19
Case mortality   37.5%

The essential factors in the cases, all of which were sporadic, seemed to be those indefinite things included in the term individuality, and overcrowding, which in respect to the last six cases seemed almost dominant.

Mumps:
Period of 43 weeks from October 1, 1917, to July 31, 1918
Average strength of command   30,124
Total number of cases   788
Rate per 1000   31.5

Mumps was not a serious feature of the disease problem except as it influenced the noneffective rate. The number of cases was fairly large and luckily so when one considers the effect these same cases would have had on the noneffective rate overseas. It seems a wise thing to allow mumps to run its course in a command so long as the facilities for treatment are good. Just what the number of complications has been can not be said until the records are completed, but it has certainly been small. No disability following the disease has been reported.

Scarlet fever:
Period of 43 weeks from October 1, 1917, to July 31, 1918
Average strength of command   30,124
Total number of cases   61
Annual rate per 1000   2.4

Scarlet fever was not epidemic in this camp and was as a rule a disease only of recent recruits. Of fifty-one tabulated cases 33 per cent were in men of less than two months' service. Very commonly it happened after a period during which there had been no cases in the camp that a new case would be found in a man arrived from another camp, or in one entering the camp from civilian life. The same phenomena were observed at Camp Green during the early months of 1918. The disease was exceedingly mild. It is perhaps this lack of virulence which accounts for the fact that it did not become epidemic. Most of the men may have been at least relatively immune to the disease and so either escaped it entirely or acquired it in such a mild form that they went unnoticed. If this be true then many of the men have acquired an active immunity.

Diphtheria was mild and readily controlled. Its incidence has been consistently low, giving a rate of 1.04 per 1000. One case died. This was a man who came from a western camp to Camp Devens with a detachment with no medical officer. The man was attacked by the disease shortly after entraining, and after two days en route was taken to the Base Hospital, where, in spite of treatment, he died.

Typhoid and paratyphoid did not originate in a single instance within the camp. The three cases which have been reported were all of external and civilian origin, and were admitted to the Base Hospital almost directly from civilian life. Therefore, like malaria, these diseases were imported. With but one exception all of the few cases of malaria were in men from the southern states. The one exception was of eastern Massachusetts origin.

TABLE V
SUMMARY

RATES (ANNUAL ADMISSION) FOR SIX MONTH PERIODS IN 1918		
	Ending June 28	Ending Dec. 27
Pneumonia	25.5	171.9
Influenza	0.0	760.3
Dysentery	0.0	0.05
Malaria	0.1	0.85
Venereal	91.1	75.6
Measles	39.6	24.7
Meningitis	1.0	1.8
Scarlet fever	2.8	0.6
Annual admission rate per 1000 (disease only)	970.7	1715.6
Noneffective rate	39.28	57.5

THE "DELAYED NEGATIVE" WASSERMANN REACTION*

By Guthrie McConnell, M.D., (Cleveland, Ohio) Major, M.C., U.S. Army

IN CARRYING out the Wassermann reaction the usual custom is to employ at least two antigens, one of which is a plain alcoholic extract of tissue, generally beef or human heart. The purposes of such a procedure are several. It must be remembered that the Wassermann method for the detection of syphilis is not a true immunity reaction in that the so-called antigen is not a true antigen. Its activity being in no way dependent upon its being obtained from syphilitic tissues. Consequently methods for the original diagnosis should not be used if they are so delicate that there is a danger of obtaining positive results when the products of the activities of the organism of syphilis are not present. Yet there are instances in which a more delicate reaction is of great value.

For ordinary diagnostic purposes the plain alcoholic antigen is probably the best, it being taken for granted that the condition has never been diagnosed and has never had any antiluetic treatment. Under such conditions a definitely positive reaction can be relied upon. The difficulty, however, lies in the proper interpretation of a negative result with the above-mentioned antigen. Unfortunately the statements of patients, particularly in the army where so much depends upon a disability being "in line of duty," can not always be relied upon. Consequently it becomes a matter of importance to obtain as accurate information as is possible.

In the Laboratory, Base Hospital, Camp Devens, Mass., since the middle of February two antigens have been employed: one a plain alcoholic, the other cholesterinized extract. As is well known the latter is a much more sensitive antigen, in fact so much so that it is rather unwise to make a positive diagnosis based on it alone. It has been recognized that this antigen if it gives any reaction at all, commonly gives a well-marked one. Its chief value, therefore, lies in the information that it gives concerning the effect of treatment upon the disease. By its means we can follow quite closely the results that are being obtained, determine when the treatment may be discontinued temporarily, and also when the case may be considered cured. It may, also, be of value when carefully correlated with the case history and clinical findings in picking up individuals who have been concealing important data. In relation to this matter come those reactions which for convenience sake may be referred to as "delayed negatives."

In performing the Wassermann reaction the textbooks, with but very few exceptions, state that after adding the hemolytic system, the tubes should be thoroughly shaken and then placed in the water-bath or incubator for from one to two hours; the general impression obtained being that the tubes are not to be disturbed until it is time for them to be examined finally. In the Medical War Manual No. 6, the directions state that the tubes should be shaken every fifteen minutes, but no reasons are given for so doing other than hastening hemolysis.

*From the Laboratory of the Base Hospital, Camp Devens, Mass.
Authority to publish granted by the Surgeon-General's Office, Washington, D. C.

Several years ago in the course of routine Wassermann examinations it was noted that every now and then there would be a specimen of blood that up to a half hour after having had the hemolytic system added and being placed in the incubator would remain as a strongly positive reaction. Very shortly after that time the blood would very quickly hemolyze and well before an hour had passed would show no traces of unhemolyzed cells. In the few cases observed at that time it was found that although no clear evidence of syphilitic infection could be obtained, yet there was a history of syphilis or a positive Wassermann in some other member of the family. These cases were picked up on account of the habit of shaking the tubes every fifteen minutes. About this same time G. M. Olson published a brief article (*Journal of Laboratory and Clinical Medicine*, 1916, i, *p*. 704) entitled "The 'Delayed Negative' Wassermann Reaction" in which he called attention to the same phenomenon. He commented on its importance from the diagnostic point of view in cases of suspected primary sores, and also in the tertiary stage when so many patients give negative reactions. No reference, however, is made in regard to the frequency of the "delayed negative" reaction.

Since February 5, 1919, a close watch has been maintained on all Wassermanns to determine, if possible, the significance of these delayed negatives, as well as the frequency of their occurrence. During the months of February, March, and April, 1793 Wassermann tests were made and of that number there were 18 that were considered delayed negatives. In every case cholesterinized and plain alcoholic antigens were used. A sheep cell hemolytic system was employed and the tubes placed in a water-bath at a temperature of 37° C. after having been well shaken. After this they were examined every fifteen minutes. In this report by delayed negative is understood one in which the tube containing the cholesterinized antigen showed no hemolysis at the end of thirty minutes but had completely cleared by the time of the following examination fifteen minutes later. In none of these cases was there any such delay in the tube containing the plain alcoholic antigen. In them, hemolysis was complete before the half hour period terminated. If no other antigen than the alcoholic had been used, or if the tubes had not been examined until they had been in the water-bath for an hour the report would have gone in as a negative Wassermann.

The difficult part in these instances is the proper interpretation of the findings. Are they to be reported as negative or positive, or shall they be reported as negative with the alcoholic, and positive with the cholesterinized antigen, and the attending physician allowed to draw his own conclusions? As a rule the majority of consultants will wish a definite expression of opinion from the laboratory as to the significance of such results.

In the hope of coming to some definite conclusion the above mentioned 18 delayed negatives have been studied as carefully as possible. It has been found that they can be placed in one of three classes. First, those that give a frank history of syphilis, either of long standing and little or no treatment, or of more recent infection with treatment. Second, those that might be considered as questionable on account of their generally loose sexual relations. Third, those in whom there can be obtained no history of venereal infection, and who give no clinical symptoms. In the actual number of cases the classes come in the order mentioned.

Of the eight in class one giving a positive history of luetic infection, seven of them have had antisyphilitic treatment, varying from one injection of some arsenic compound to a prolonged course of neosalvarsan and mercury. The eighth case had syphilis eight years ago, but no information relative to treatment was obtainable.

In Class II, the six questionable cases, all denied having had syphilis, but each man had or had had gonorrhea. Of these, three were colored men and their statements are distinctly unreliable. If any of them have had a sore on the penis it is nearly always referred to as a "hair cut," and the diagnosis is rendered more difficult by the fact that the skin lesions are frequently so inconspicuous as to be easily overlooked by the patient. Two other cases were admitted and under treatment for gonorrhea. The sixth man had had gonorrhea ten months previously, but at the time of entering the hospital he had no symptoms of any venereal infection. He was admitted as a case of acute bronchitis.

In Class III are four cases in which delayed negative reactions were obtained, but in which no history of luetic infection was obtainable. One of these was a man who was a chronic alcoholic and who had been admitted to the hospital for bronchitis and alcoholism. Knowing the inhibiting action of alcohol it might be that a strongly positive reaction would have appeared after the effects of the alcohol had passed off. A second case, who denied infection, had been in the ward for a week suffering from acute cholangitis. Of the other two, one had been admitted for lobar pneumonia and one for influenza.

As a matter of checking up the results of treatment it would appear that the delayed negative is a matter of some importance. By examining the tubes every fifteen minutes such reactions will be noted and a better record kept of the condition of the patient. In this way a case that is still in need of treatment will not be overlooked. Seven of the positive cases first mentioned give in each instance a distinct history of infection with subsequent treatment, which although evidently beneficial was not sufficient to eradicate the disease.

In the second group of six cases one feels almost justified in considering the three colored men as positive cases, their statements to the contrary notwithstanding. Their ages were twenty-four, twenty-five, and twenty-six and there is no question as to their having been exposed frequently, particularly as each had had gonorrhea, one of them claiming that he had had it for ten years. The remaining three had had gonorrhea and there is no question as to frequent exposures.

Of the four in group three it is difficult to come to any definite conclusions. They are all considerably older than the average of the other groups, each man being 29 or over, old enough and experienced enough to realize the disadvantages of telling too much about themselves. One of them had been admitted to the hospital for acute alcoholism, but in the others there was nothing found in the history that would tend to incriminate them. Consequently they must be given the benefit of the doubt and be considered as negative cases.

In regard to the frequency of delayed negatives, 1 per cent of all Wassermanns is what is indicated by these figures. Of the total number, approximately 0.44 per cent give a definite history of syphilitic infection, 0.33 per cent were probably syphilitic, leaving 0.23 per cent as probably negative.

To briefly summarize it would seem advisable that readings should be taken every fifteen minutes after the hemolytic system has been added and the tubes placed in the incubator or water-bath. By so doing there will be a certain number, about 1 per cent, that will give a so-called "delayed negative" reading. Of these nearly three-fourths will give either a positive or a very suspicious history in regard to venereal infection. Although such reactions are few and far between, very little additional labor is required, and information about the occasional case is frequently important.

CLASS I—POSITIVE CASES

H. F., 26, Colored, Florida.	Syphilis 8 years ago, gonorrhea 4 months ago. Feces negative, malaria negative. Admitted for follicular tonsillitis.
J. R., 26, Colored Florida.	Chancre 1910. Gonorrhea August, 1918. Undergoing treatment with arsenobenzol.
B. R., 28, White, Italy.	Infected January 1918. Received 8 injections of neosalvarsan from July to November, 1918, also 9 injections of mercury.
A. G., 27, Colored, Georgia.	Syphilis and gonorrhea 4 years ago. States that he had had one injection by way of treament.
S. S., 21, Colored, Iowa.	Denies syphilitic infection but admits that he has had three injections of "606."
A. L., 29, White, Italy.	Chancre 10 years ago. Chronic gonorrhea at present, also pulmonary tuberculosis. Has been given "606" and mercury.
C. B., ?, White, ?	General paresis. Positive Wassermann with spinal fluid. Amount of treatment unknown. ·
L. C., 26, White, Penna.	Had sore on lower lip during Aug. and Sept., 1918. Urethral discharge Sept.-Nov., 1915. Had eight salvarsan treatments in France in June, 1917, and Dec., 1918.

CLASS II—SUSPICIOUS CASES

J. McP., 22, Colored, Florida.	Denies syphilitic infection. Has had gonorrhea twice. Feces negative. Malaria negative. Admitted for influenza and bronchopneumonia.
E. C., 25, Colored, Indiana.	Gonorrhea 8 years ago. No luetic history.
N. J. G., 24, Colored, Florida.	Gonorrhea 1909. Says that it lasted ten years. No luetic history. Admitted for bronchopneumonia.
C. B., 25, White.	Gonorrhea 18 months ago, and acute attack at present.
J. P., 24, White, Macedonia.	Gonorrhea ten months ago. No history of lues. Admitted for acute bronchitis.
F. P., 25, White, Kentucky.	Gonorrhea for past month. No luetic history.

CLASS III—NEGATIVE CASES

M. M., 31, White, Ohio.	Denies all venereal infection. Admitted for bronchitis and alcoholism.
R. F., 31, White, Michigan.	Denies all venereal infection. Admitted for influenza.
F. T. D., 29, White, Arkansas.	No venereal history. Admitted for lobar pneumonia.
L. E. D., 31, White, Canada.	No venereal history. Admitted for acute cholangitis. Also has a Trichuris trichiura infection.

FURTHER OBSERVATIONS ON THE RELATION OF AORTIC INSUFFICIENCY TO THE WASSERMANN TEST*

By Julien E. Benjamin, Capt. M. C., (Cincinnati, Ohio), and Sydney J. Havre, 1st Lieut. M. C., (Akron, Ohio), Camp Funston, Kansas

I T IS noteworthy that the cause of insufficiency of the aortic valves in young adults, uncomplicated by any other valvular lesion, is attributed to a syphilitic infection in the large majority of cases. According to the following authors the incidence is expressed as follows:

Longcope,[1] in summing up the situation, says that 75 to 80 per cent of all aortic insufficiencies give positive evidence of syphilis, and also that signs of aortic insufficiency unassociated with any other valvular lesion in an individual under fifty are practically pathognomonic of syphilis.

Collins and Sachs[2] found 84 per cent of all cases of this disease due to syphilis.

Citron,[3] in fortifying his work by the Wassermann test, found a positive reaction in 60 per cent of his cases.

Cabot[4] has recently stated that he believes it possible for a primary rheumatic aortic insufficiency to occur with the preservation of the integrity of the mitral valve, but that such an event is a rare one.

From these figures, it is very evident that the most careful observers find a very close relationship between these two phenomena; syphilis and uncomplicated aortic regurgitation. The results which are reported in this paper fail to bear out the observations noted above, for a positive Wassermann reaction was obtained only in 11 per cent of the thirty-three cases referred for the test. Major Broman, who supervised the reactions at the Base Hospital at Fort Riley, Kansas, states that the element of error is no more than is to be usually expected. Further, the positive and doubtful reactions occurred in those subjects who gave an undoubted history of syphilis in its various manifestations. In the remaining number there was absolutely no knowledge of an existing cardiac condition, and it was only by close questioning that a history of predisposing infection could be obtained. From the appended tabulations, it will be seen in how many cases a definite history was related. It was because the histories coincided so closely to the laboratory findings that a report of this kind was considered justifiable.

The observations were conducted in each instance on recruits during their entrance examinations. The venipunctures were made by one of the cardiac examiners at the time of the examinations so that no unnecessary time was lost in rejecting the individual. The usual cardiovascular history was taken in each case.

Thus in Table I there are recorded 19 cases which give undisputed histories of rheumatism; 2 with doubtful histories, as against 3 cases in which reliable histories of lues were obtained, and one doubtful. In all 4 cases with positive histories of syphilis, the Wassermann reaction coincided. These cases of pure aor-

*Authority to publish granted by the Surgeon-General's Office, Washington, D. C.

tic insufficiency were found in the course of examination of 44,018 recruits over a period of three months.

TABLE I

TABULATIONS OF CASE HISTORIES AND WASSERMANN REACTIONS

CASE	NAME	AGE	PREDISPOSING HISTORY	OCCUPATION	REACTION (WASSER-MANN)
1.	C.B.	21	Rheumatism for six months at 13 Frequent attacks of tonsillitis	Farmer.	Neg.
2.	J.W.K.	21	Frequent attacks of tonsillitis.	Farmer.	Neg.
3.	F.F.M.	21	Rheumatism six weeks at 20. Frequent attacks of tonsillitis.	Farmer.	Neg.
4.	J.R.S.	25	Rheumatism at 13. All of diseases of childhood.	Farmer.	Neg.
5.	P.R.	26	History absolutely negative	Farmer.	Neg.
6.	C.N.B.	21	Rheumatism at 15. Frequent tonsillitis, pneumonia at 13.	Rancher.	Neg.
7.	G.R.	26	Typhoid and pneumonia at 18. Indefinite rheumatic history 10 years.	Farmer.	Neg.
8.	E.N.B.	27	History absolutely negative.	Farmer.	Neg.
9.	O.J.	25	Pneumonia at 17 and 18. Rheumatism 3 months at 23.	Cook.	Neg.
10.	A.E.F.	27	Rheumatism at 19. Frequent tonsillitis diseases of childhood.	Laborer.	Neg.
11.	C.T.C.	30	Rheumatism for past six years.	Laborer.	Neg.
12.	O.T.H.	22	Typhoid fever at 8. Diphtheria at 18.	Clerk..	Neg.
13.	W.W.	21	Rheumatism (?) Syphilis at 18.	Farmer.	Pos.
14.	H.G.F.	22	Rheumatism for 8 years.	Farmer.	Neg.
15.	G.S.	25	Rheumatism 4 years. Frequent tonsillitis. Pneumonia at 23.	Laborer.	Neg.
16.	J.R.	24	Tonsillitis frequent. Syphilis at 17.	Farmer.	Pos.
17.	V.D.S.	31	Diphtheria as child. Malaria at 24. Chancroid (?) 1910.	Laborer.	Neg.
18.	A.H.H.	29	Rheumatism at 27 and 29. Measles at 27 years.	Farmer.	Neg.
19.	A.A.T.	24	Rheumatism at 22 for five weeks.	Steam-fitter	Neg.
20.	H.J.E.	24	Rheumatism at 14 for 4 months. Measles at 20.	Farmer.	Neg.
21.	V.L.E.	22	Rheumatism at 16 for 8 weeks	Farmer.	Neg. (pos.)
22.	E.H.B.	23	Rheumatism at 10, 11, 12, and 13 yrs. Measles at 13.	Farmer.	Neg.
23.	R.N.B.	24	History absolutely negative.	Cook.	Neg.
24.	R.P.	22	Rheumatism at 17. Frequent tonsillitis.	Driver.	Neg.
25.	R.E.R.	28	Frequent tonsillitis.	Laborer.	Neg.
26.	A.C.S.	29	Rheumatism at 23 and 27.	Carpenter.	Neg.
27.	N.P.	24	Rheumatism at 21 and 24. Measles at 22.	Farmer.	Neg.
28.	S.C.S.	25	Syphilis at 23	Teamster.	Pos. Pos.
29.	A.A.W.	30	Indefinite history of rheumatism.	Farmer.	Neg.
30.	V.T.	31	Rheumatism at 27.	Porter.	Neg.
31.	C.E.G.	25	Syphilis ?	Farmer.	Neg. Pos.
32.	W.B.	22	Rheumatism at 14.	Farmer.	Neg.
33.	F.T.	24	Tonsillitis and measles at 23.	Farmer.	Neg.

TABLE II

THE RELATION OF AORTIC INSUFFICIENCY TO OTHER VALVULAR LESIONS IN 44,018 CASES

1. Total number cases examined	44,018	
2. Total number cases of valvular disease	147	.33% of 1
3. Total number cases of Aortic Insufficiency (Pure)	33	22. % of 2
4. Total number of Aortic Insufficiencies with other lesions	51	34. % of 2

TABLE III

GENERAL TABULATIONS OF RESULTS

In 33 cases of aortic insufficiency.

Wassermann reaction, positive	4	11%
Positive history of rheumatism	19	57%

Occupations.

Farmers	19.	58%
Laborers	5.	15%
Cooks	2.	6%
Miscellaneous		21%

Age.

Average	24 years
Youngest	21 years
Oldest	31 years

Race Of 44,018 recruits examined,

Colored	14,009
White	30,009

Of these, aortic insufficiency occurred as sole lesion in,

White	28	84%
Colored	5	16%

CONCLUSIONS

A report is hereby made of 33 cases of aortic insufficiency unassociated with any other organic cardiac disease from a clinical standpoint.

Wassermann reactions, taken in each case, were positive in only 11 per cent as against the reported higher rates of other writers.

Undisputed histories of rheumatism were obtained in 57 per cent of cases. Questionable histories of rheumatism and histories of frequent attacks of tonsillitis were noted in 15 per cent.

A tabulation of results as regards occupation, age, race, and incidence is reported.

BIBLIOGRAPHY

[1]Longcope, Warfield T.: Bulletin Ayer Clinic Laboratory, 1910, p. 60.
[2]Collins and Sachs: Am. Jour. Med. Sc., 1909, cxxx, viii, 344.
[3]Citron: Berl. klin. Wchnschr., 1908, xii, 2142.
[4]Cabot, Richard C.: Physical Diagnosis, New York, Wm. Wood & Co.
     Additional references:
Denke: Deutsch. med. Wchnschr., 1909, xxxv, p. 2148.
Oigaard: Arch. De Mal. De. Couer., 1910, iii, p. 478.
Clough: Bull. Johns Hopkins Hosp., 1910, xxi, p. 7.
Warthin: Am. Jour. Med. Sc., 1916, ciii, p. 508.

A REVIEW OF THE RECENT LITERATURE BEARING ON THE FUNCTION OF THE THYMUS GLAND

By W. E. Blatz, M.A., Toronto, Canada

THE study of the glands of internal secretion has occupied much attention in the past decade and many theories have been offered concerning their functions.

Of all of these glands, probably the thymus is the least understood, and this brief review of the most important work is offered in the hope that it may prove useful to those who are unfamiliar with the original papers in which it appears.

This work has been concerned with the anatomy of the gland, with the physiologic effects produced by extirpation, and by feeding with the gland substance, and with clinical observations, including the effects of x-ray.

Some uncertainty prevails as to whether the thymus is an epithelial or a lymphoid gland in so far as its activities are concerned. Wallin claims that the branchial epithelium of the lamprey has the *general* property of forming lymphocytes, which would explain the presence of the small thymic cells. Fulci maintains that "the small round cells of the thymus (the lymphocyte-like cells) are elements of epithelial nature, which following successive modifications evolve from the epithelial cells. * * * they are not capable of differentiating into eosinophiles or plasma or mast cells." On the other hand Bell maintains that the Hassal's corpuscles are connective tissue cells. Hammar explains the presence of the small thymic cells by an infiltration of leucocytes which have ultimately gone through a physiologic involution to their present form. Maximaw demonstrated the lymphatic nature of the thymic cells in amphibians and selachiens. Pappenheimer in a series of sera experiments developed small thymic cells from lymphocytes. Douchakeff showed that "granulocytoblasts" were developed only from lymphoid elements and that thymic cells were formed therefrom.

It is known that the thymus gland undergoes a normal involution, but it is remarkable how little the various authors agree as to the extent or time of this process. Baum in dogs gives the ratio between thymus and body-weight as follows: newborn 1 :125; two weeks 1 :170; two months 1 :1600; two to three years present. According to these figures involution begins immediately after birth. Basch gives the above ratio as 1 :300 in 3 to 4 weeks and Tongu gives 1 :189 in the first to second week. Klose and Vogt say that involution begins in the fourth week. On the other hand Tongu says that gross and microscopic involution does not begin until the fourth month and Hammar claims that it does not begin until the second year. Matti considers involution to begin when the period of most active growth occurs. Hoskins from a compilation of human statistics states that "Although the thymus reaches its greatest absolute size at about the time of puberty, nevertheless relatively * * * it is seven times as large at birth as at puberty" also that "in the growth of the thymus after birth the connective tissues make up an increasing amount of the entire organ." Quoting again from

Hoskins, 'Anatomists make an allowance of from 100 to 700 per cent in the normal weight of the thymus at different ages." Can there be any greater confusion than in the consideration of the above figures? One should moreover not overlook the significance of the frequent persistent thymus.

Before considering the literature bearing on the results of extirpation of the gland, there are certain points which should be kept forcibly in mind. The operation is necessarily severe and it is difficult to dissociate the immediate results of shock, etc., from the physiologic effects of loss of thymus influence. The mere fact that the organ does normally involute makes the time of operation of utmost importance. The presence of accessory thymus bodies predicates a serious complication when interpreting results. Only experiments which include a sufficient number of "successful" operations with proper controls should be considered. As before, we shall discuss first one view and then the opposite.

Basch with dogs two days old and controls from the same litter demonstrated a change in the skeletal state at the end of the third week after operation. The bones were softer and more pliable. There was a delayed growth and indications of diminished intelligence. Klose and Vogt found the greatest effect when the extirpation was performed on the tenth day after birth. He divides his results into three periods: a latent period of two to four weeks; an adipose stage of two to three months; a cachectic period of three to fourteen months. Matti corroborates this. Schimizu by injecting a serum, specifically cytolytic for thymus, has succeeded in causing early involution of the thymus accompanied by "all the symptoms commonly attributed to thymectomy." Weymersch records an increased leucocyte count and growth increase after atrophy of the thymus. Gilliberti attributes general symptoms such as collapse to thymectomy.

All observers do not, however, agree that thymectomy has such different effects. In contradistinction to the above the following results are significant. Fischl did not observe any effects of thymectomy with dogs, goats or rabbits. Hart and Nordmann, who operated on the fourth week also obtained negative results. Renton and Robertson performed extirpation experiments on puppies at different ages and found that rickets developed as quickly in controls as in the operated animals. (The controls were puppies of the same litter operated similarly to the *bona fide* operated animals, but without extirpation of the thymus). Renton observed no apparent symptoms in guinea pigs after thymectomy. Park discusses the presence of accessory thymus bodies at great length and made as complete an extirpation as possible and found no change from controls (as above) in procreative abilities, growth or condition of endocrine glands, no rachitic changes. Allen showed complete sexual differentiation in thymectomized tadpoles.

Probably the most complete work on thymectomy has been done by Tongu with a large number of dogs of various breeds and ages, with admirable controls and careful tests extending over a number of years. The following table is worth considering (no doubtful cases were included). Clinical and laboratory tests after operation showed:

I. Body weight—no influence after thymectomy.
II. Growth—no effect—Klose and Vogt 3 stages not shown.
III. Nervous, psychic—no effect.

IV. Blood corpuscles—no effect—number or differential.
V. Change in opsonic index—no change inexplicable by operation results.
VI. Blood pressure—results conflicting.
VII. Histologic—no change—sometimes found thymus accesssory bodies, but they did not seem to affect the result.
VIII. Skeletal system—no change in length, structure, calcium content, callus formation after fracture, etc.
IX. Changes in other organs—none.

Thus we see that there is slight preponderance of evidence indicating that thymectomy is not followed by any definite physiologic effects.

Many experiments have been performed on the influence of feeding thymus gland extract either to normal animals or to patients. We are concerned here rather with the physiologic than the clinical aspect, which will be dealt with later.

Gudernatsch fed thymus extract to tadpoles and produced an increase in size (growth), but a delay in development (metamorphosis). Uhlenhuth on feeding thymus extract to young salamanders observed tetanic convulsions (vide infra). In contradistinction to these authors E. R. Hoskins failed to show any constant effect of feeding thymus, and Swingle, taking two groups of individuals, frog larvæ, fed one, thymus extract and the other, liver, and could observe no difference in the growth or metamorphosis of either group. Uhlenhuth, in later papers, also divided his subjects (tadpoles) into two groups feeding one group thymus and the other worms. There was a differentiation,—seemingly an inhibition of metamorphosis with those fed on thymus, but when he added to the thymus other energy-producing bodies, i. e., ordinary food substances, the inhibitory effects of thymus disappeared. Thus he showed clearly that thymus does not contain sufficient substances to maintain growth, and its effects when fed alone are due to malnutrition.

The inclusion, in the past, of the thymus among the internal secretory glands naturally intimates some close relationship between the latter and the former. Let us briefly discuss this phase of the question.

Henderson reports that castration in cattle is accompanied by hypertrophy of the thymus and Paton observed an unusually severe disruption of the whole organism when thymectomy and ganodectomy were both performed. Hewer's work intimates a compensatory effect between thymus and testis based on feeding experiments. Thymus-fed animals, he says, show a delay in development of testis (vide supra).

Wulzen obtained a retardation in growth of thymus in birds during pituitary feeding. Maxwell reports evidence against any relation between these two organs.

Uhlenhuth theorizes that the thymus produces a substance that tonically raises the sensitivity of the central nervous system and that the parathyroid secretion inhibits this action normally. His proof for this is as follows. · In tadpoles there is no tetany in feeding thymus because the parathyroids have already developed, but in young salamanders, in which animal the parathyroids are developed late, thymus feeding does produce tetany.

Kahn wished to show a correlation between thymus and thyroid, using feeding experiments as evidence, but Uhlenhuth contradicts his results by stating that "the inhibitory effect of thymus is not due to a specific inhibiting substance in the thymus, but to the absence from the thymus of a substance required to develop the thyroid to the secretory stage."

From the above we can conclude that the only relation which seems worthy of consideration is that between thymus and testis, but both these glands are normally so susceptible to any changes in the organism that more evidence is necessary to make their interrelation conclusive.

In considering the clinical evidence of thymus function it should be borne in mind that it is much more difficult to judge the value of clinical data because of the relatively few observations and because important information is often omitted. Hammar in an excellent and exhaustive article is convinced that the so-called "thymus death" is not of thymic origin. Herrick calculates that the thymus can not compress the trachea sufficiently to cause death by suffocation.

Hoxie details a method for percussing the enlarged thymus and claims to have relieved cases by thyroid and adrenal feeding. Haneborg reports cases of chorea in which he has obtained relief from convulsions after thymus feeding. He expresses doubt at the end of his paper as to his results, however.

Clinical symptoms may always be verified by x-ray, the technic of which is given in great detail by Cook and Simpson. Hewer caused atrophy of thymus by prolonged treatment. Friedland reports that x-ray treatment, as a routine measure, clears up "thymus diseases" dissipating the dyspnea, suffocation, cyanosis, stridor, etc., (?).

It is clear from a review of the literature bearing on the thymus that it is impossible to attribute any function to the gland. The work of Hammar who has recently made an exhaustive study of the thymus function both chemically and experimentally concludes with the remark that in his estimation the thymus is not an organ of internal secretion. And E. R. Hoskins considers that "the thymus functions as a lymphoid organ in infancy and childhood when a large number of lymphoid cells and leucocytes are needed to combat infections," a view which is upheld by a comparison of the graphs showing the curve of involution of the thymus. These closely approximate the curve of the decrease in the number of lymphocytes in the blood with increasing age.

Elsewhere the author states that "whatever the real function of the thymus, certain it is that its production of an internal secretion has not been proved." If we might be permitted to express an opinion, we would suggest that the thymus is a lymphoid organ like an enlarged tonsil which involutes when its presence is no longer necessary.

BIBLIOGRAPHY

Baar: Endocrinology, 1917, i, 170.
Basch: Ztschr. f. exper. Path. u. Therap., 1906, ii.
Bell: Am. Jour. Anat., 1905, xiv, 86.
Cook: Boston Med. and Surg. Jour., 1916, clxxv, 483.
Donchakeff: Jour. Exper. Med., 1916, xxiv, 87.
Fischl: Ztschr. f. exper. Path. u. Therap., 1905, i.
Friedlander: Am. Jour. Dis. Child., 1917, xiv, 41.
Fulci: Deutch. med. Wchnschr., 1913, xxxvii.
Gilliberti: Ibid.
Gudernatsch: Am. Jour. Anat., 1913-14, xv, 431; Anat. Rec., 1917, xi, 357.
Hammar: Endocrinology, Abst., 1917, i, 88.

Haneborg: Ibid., 1917, i, 13.
Herrick: Surg., Gynec. and Obst., 1916, xxii, 333.
Henderson: Jour. Physiol., 1904, xxxi, 222.
Hewer: Jour. Physiol., 1914, xlvii, 1916, l.
Hoskins, E. R.: Jour. Exper. Zoology, 1916, xxi, 295; Endocrinology, 1918, ii, 241.
Hoxie: New York Med. Jour., 1916. liii, 676.
Kahn: Pflüger's Arch., 1916, clxiii, 384-404.
Klose and Vogt: Beitr. z. klin. Chir., 1910, lxix.
Matti: Ergeb. d. inner. Med. u. Kinderheil., 1913, x, 1.
Maximow: Compt. rendu. Soc. de Biol., 1917, lxxx, 235-237.
Maxwell: Univ. of Calif. Pub. Physiol., 1916, v, 5.
Müller: Physiological Abstracts, 1917, ii, 615.
Park: Jour. Exper. Med., 1917, xxv, 129.
Pappenheimer: Jour. Exper. Med., 1914, xix, 319.
Renton: Glasgow Med. Jour., 1916, lxxxvi, 14.
Renton and Robertson: Jour. Path. and Bacteriol., 1916, xxi, 1-13.
Ritchie: Jour. Path. and Bacteriol., 1908, xii.
Schimizu: Mitt. a. d. Med. Fakultät., 1913-14, ii, 261.
Simpson: South Med. Jour., 1916, ix, 857.
Swingle: Biol. Bull., 1917, xxxiii. 70.
Tongu: Mitt. a. d. Med. Fakultät z. Tokio, 1916-17, xvi, 539-605.
Uhlenhuth: Jour. Exper. Zoology (Balt.), 1918, xxv, 135; Jour. Gen. Physiol., 1919, i, 305;
    ibid., 1919, i, 23.
Wallin: Am. Jour. Anat., 1917, xxii, 127-159.
Wulzen: Jour. Biol. Chem., 1916, xxv, 625.

TYPHOID AND PARATYPHOID FEVER AT MESVES HOSPITAL CENTER*

By Frank Mock, M.D., (Chicago, Ill.)
1st Lieut., M. C., U. S. A.

SUMMARIZING the work on enteric diseases done at the Center Laboratory of Mesves Hospital Center, France, the figures total as follows: stool examinations, 506; urine examinations, 402; blood cultures, 201. Of this number there were 37 positive stools, 6 positive urines, and 12 positive blood cultures, a total of 55 positive results on 45 patients. Two more were diagnosed at autopsy and from one of these the B. typhosus was isolated from the spleen and bile sac. The 45 positive cases were distributed as follows: stools 29, or about 64½ per cent; blood, 10 or 22⅕ per cent; urine, 6 or 13⅓ per cent. Twenty-one cases were clinically positive, but could not be proved by laboratory findings.

Twelve cases came to the Center which had been diagnosed at evacuation hospitals at the front.

Only six specimens of feces were found positive the second time and two the third time examined. Two blood cultures were found positive on the second examination. There were no duplications of positive urines. In one case the blood, feces and urine were positive, in five cases the blood and feces, and in one case the feces and urine.

The organisms isolated were B. typhosus in 38 cases, B. paratyphosus A in two cases and B. paratyphosus B in four cases. In one of our earliest cases we found the Shiga bacillus. In one case, sent in from Camp Hospital of the 85th Division at Sancerre, we got an atypical paratyphoid bacillus from a patient with

*Authority to publish granted by the Surgeon-General's Office, Washington, D. C.

clinical typhoid. This organism did not agglutinate in the patient's serum, or in our diagnostic sera. Probably the same organism was obtained from two carriers and a sample of milk at the hospital. Another atypical paratyphoid bacillus was obtained from a carrier in Evacuation Hospital No. 24. The B. paratyphosus B was obtained from a carrier at B. H. No. 54 who was relieved of his duties as mess sergeant. No cases could be traced to him. There were four organisms that were culturally typhoid but did not agglutinate. Nine organisms failed to agglutinate after having been previously positive, one failed to agglutinate when first isolated, but afterwards became positive, and one agglutinated twice, then failed to agglutinate, and again agglutinated when the fourth culture was isolated. The titer in the positive cases ranged from 1:400 to 1:25,800.

Agglutinations were done with typhoid and paratyphoid A and B organisms against the serum of sixteen men, four of whom were not patients but were used as controls. From the patients we obtained three typhoid, one para A and two para B reactions, and from the controls only one typhoid reaction. The titer of these sera which agglutinated ranged from 1.20 to 1:2560. The higher titered reactions corresponded with those of the organisms isolated from the patients' stools. Six patients and three controls were negative throughout. The reactions in general seemed to indicate that the patients' vaccination had run out, and the reading corresponded to those of Widal reactions in unvaccinated patients. The average time since the patient had received his vaccination was about one year.

Ten of the proven cases originated on the Verdun front, ten in various hospitals of this Center, four in the Argonne, one each at Marcony, Toul, and St. Mihiel. The origin of the others is not known to us. Of those which originated in this Center, probably half were infected before they arrived. Of the clinically positive cases, eight originated at Verdun, five at this Center, and one each in the Argonne, at Varennes and Dunn-sur-Meuse.

The atypical paratyphoid bacilli in some cultures resembled the B. typhosus, that is, they did not form gas, and fermented all sugars except lactose and saccharose, but in most cultures they resemble the paratyphoid bacilli, forming gas and failing to ferment dextrin as well as lactose and saccharose. They did not agglutinate in antiparatyphoid A or B sera, neither did they agglutinate in the patients' own sera. One man who harbored an atypical organism had clinical typhoid, one had no typhoid symptoms except diarrhea, which he had before he entered the hospital, and two others were true carriers and not patients.

CONCLUSION

These atypical paratyphoid organisms probably are involution forms of the true typhoid or paratyphoid bacilli. This presumption seems to be verified by the fact that some changed their cultural characteristics while others changed their agglutinating characteristics. These organisms, both typhoid and paratyphoid, after agglutinating with a high titer (in some cases as high as 1:6400), failed to agglutinate at all. The fact that one culture should show the characteristics of the B. paratyphosus and a transplant of the same culture the characteristics of the B. typhosus, and a third transplant revert back to that of the B. paratyphosus, demonstrates the very close relationship between these organisms.

THE ACTION OF ALCOHOL ON THE HEART AND RESPIRATION*

BY EMRY G. HYATT, CHICAGO, ILL.

MOST of the experimental work on alcohol has been done on animals under an anesthetic. As is well known anesthetics act in a manner very similar to alcohol. For this reason the initial action of alcohol which is the only point when the action is disputed is obscured. In the investigation of alcohol, therefore, it is highly desirable to work without an anesthetic. To do this in an acceptable manner, a method must be devised which is painless and which will not excite the animal, since these conditions may be as obscuring as an anesthetic. Brooks[1] devised such a method for the study of alcohol without using an anesthetic. By introducing a pressure cannula into the neck of an animal under an anesthetic he was able to get tracings several days after the return to normal without apparent pain to the animal. While he states that there was no excitement and no pain connected with the recording of the tracings, one is doubtful about the degree of such absence, and must consider that while there was relatively little, it is still a question of relativity. This is especially true when the alcohol is administered with a hypodermic, or into a recently prepared gastric fistula. The same criticism may be applied to the work presented here although in the present case the circumstances are those in which alcohol has been given therapeutically, as a stimulant for heart or respiration.

The work corroborates the findings of Brooks and is recorded briefly.

METHOD

In order to eliminate the use of an anesthetic and at the same time to avoid pain when obtaining blood pressure tracings or when giving alcohol injections, the following method was employed: A large healthy dog was selected and anesthetized with ether and the spinal cord severed about the level of the 11th thoracic vertebra. This was done by making a short deep incision just to one side of the spine into which a probe was inserted between the 11th and 12th vertebræ thus completely severing the cord. The dog was then placed in a comfortable cage and allowed until the *next day* to recover. The operation was performed under aseptic conditions and no infection resulted which would have produced fever and other complications in a day or two afterwards.

The blood pressure was then recorded from the femoral artery by means of a mercury manometer and the alcohol was injected into the femoral vein.

One of the very important factors in obtaining a blood pressure tracing is that of keeping the animal absolutely quiet, and comfortable. In our case this was accomplished by feeding the dog before placing him upon the operating table, by carefully padding the table, and by covering his eyes when connecting him to the blood pressure apparatus or when giving him injections of alcohol.

The dog was entirely devoid of sensation in the hind legs and lay perfectly still during the operation and following the injection of alcohol. We feel con-

*From the Laboratory of Pharmacology, University of Illinois, College of Medicine, Chicago, Ill.
[1]Brooks: Jour. Am. Med. Assn., 1910, lv, 372.

fident, therefore, that the results obtained and reported below, were due specifically to the action of alcohol and not to outside factors such as ether, chloroform, movement, or excitement of the animal.

RESULTS

I. By Mouth.—Five c.c. of 25 per cent alcohol when given produced a slight rise in pressure followed by an immediate return to normal. That this rise was due to stimulation of the gustatory nerves and swallowing movements and not to any specific action of the alcohol was shown by the fact that a similar action was obtained by the same amount of normal one-tenth HCl.

II. By Injection.—Further proof that the rise in pressure was caused by local action and not to the action of the alcohol is shown by the fact that alcohol injected slowly into the femoral vein in doses of 5 c.c. and in concentrations from 5 per cent to 40 per cent produced no change in blood pressure. An amount equal to 60-75 c.c. of 40 per cent alcohol (the approximate strength of whiskey) was given during a period of one hour. To rule out the possibility of habituation playing a part in the results, initial doses in varying concentrations were given to different dogs with the same results.

III. By Infiltration.—Forty to 80 per cent alcohol was allowed to flow from a burette into the femoral vein of a dog at the rate of 2 c.c. per minute until the dog died. In different dogs this took place after the injection of from 50 to 150 c.c. of 40 per cent alcohol. The blood pressure in most instances remained constant almost until the time of death, at which point there was an abrupt drop.

When the alcohol was forced rapidly into the vein there was observed a fall in pressure followed by a rapid return to the normal. This was due perhaps to direct action on the central nervous system because when the vagi were cut a similar fall was not observed.

The effect of alcohol on the heart and respiration was also studied on the normal animal by counting. The animal was placed in a comfortable position and 40 per cent alcohol injected into the femoral vein. With careful work there is but the slight pain of the hypodermic needle. In this case the animal showed no detectable reaction to it. An anesthetic dose of alcohol may be given in this way without any apparent stimulation of the heart or respiration. The following experiment illustrates this:

Dog 25 lbs.	Time	Normal Heart	Normal Respiration
16 c.c. 40% alcohol injected.	11:00	94	17
	to		
	11:03	92	18
	11:15	78	15
	11:19	76	14
	11:26	74	15
	11:30	74	16
injected 10 c.c.	11:43		20
	11:47	88	
	11:55	74	15
	12:00		16
	12:10	74	16

Respiration increased in volume but not in number.

Heart is slowed.

In this experiment 26 c.c. of 40 per cent alcohol was injected into vein of leg without apparent effect on heart or respiration.

IV. By Stomach.—Forty per cent alcohol in doses varying from 5 to 16 c.c. when introduced slowly by means of a stomach tube produced no change in blood pressure.

Respiration.—No effect on rate was observed when the alcohol was injected gradually by the intravenous method or given by the stomach tube, although the respirations seemed deeper in quality. At the time of death a change was necessarily obtained.

We are confident that the volume of fluid introduced into the circulation was not sufficient to overcome any slight fall in pressure that might otherwise have been noted. To show this a control was made in which an equal amount of normal saline was injected in place of the alcohol without obtaining any change in pressure. To eliminate the possibility that the vaso-motor system might be unresponsive as the result of the severing of the spinal cord, adrenalin and nitrites were injected and characteristic curves obtained.

SUMMARY

From the results of the experiments performed above, we believe that alcohol has the following effects on heart and respiration when administered to an unanesthetized animal:

1. By mouth there is a rapid rise and an immediate return to normal. This is due to local action.

2. Intravenously.

(a) Given gradually in quantities sufficient to kill in one to two hours, there is no effect until just before death, when a rapid fall of pressure takes place.

(b) Given rapidly there is a sudden fall followed by an immediate return to the normal. There is no effect if the vagi are cut.

3. By stomach; when introduced by means of a stomach tube there is no effect.

4. When alcohol is introduced without excitement intravenously in the normal dog, there is no stimulation of the heart or respiration.

LABORATORY METHODS

THE EFFECT OF ADRENALIN ON THE BLOOD CATALASE*

By W. E. Burge, Urbana, Ill.

A S a result of the work of Blum,[1] Vosburgh and Richards,[2] Dreyer,[3] Oliver and Schaefer,[4] Cannon and de la Paz,[5] it is now considered that during combat the adrenals are stimulated to an increased output of adrenalin and that this produces a constriction of the small blood vessels of the abdominal viscera, thus increasing the blood supply to the heart, skeletal muscles, and nervous system; that it hastens the coagulation of the blood, and increases the output of sugar from the liver. It is evident that the purpose of diverting the blood from the abdominal viscera into the heart, skeletal muscles, and nervous system during combat is to render conditions more favorable for the increased action of those organs; that the hastening of the coagulation is to stop more quickly the bleeding from any superficial wound that may be inflicted, and that the flushing of the blood with sugar is to insure a plentiful supply of oxidizable material to the muscles. While the preceding explains certain phases of adaptation of the organism for combat, it does not explain how increased oxidation is brought about which gives rise to the energy for the fight.

We[6] had found that whatever increased oxidation in the body produced a corresponding increase in catalase, an enzyme possessing the property of liberating oxygen from hydrogen peroxide by stimulating the alimentary glands, particularly the liver, to an increased output of this enzyme, and that whatever decreased oxidation produced a corresponding decrease in catalase by diminishing the output from the liver and by direct destruction of the enzyme. It was found, for example, that the ingestion of food produced increase in the catalase of the blood parallel with the increase in oxidation, and that protein (meat), in keeping with its greater stimulating effect on oxidation, produced a larger increase in catalase than did fat or carbohydrate. On the other hand, narcotics decreased catalase parallel with the decrease produced in oxidation, chloroform being more effective in this respect than a less powerful anesthetic, such as ether. The object of the present investigation was to determine whether the introduction of adrenalin into the blood stream would stimulate the liver to an increased output of catalase. If this is found to be true, then it may be assumed that the increase in adrenalin during combat stimulates the liver to an increased output of catalase and that this, in turn, increases oxidation, thus giving rise to the energy for the fight.

The animals used were dogs. The adrenalin was introduced into the portal vein. The amounts will be given in the description of the individual experiments. The catalase was determined by adding 0.5 c.c. of blood to diluted hy-

*From the Physiological Laboratory, University of Illinois.

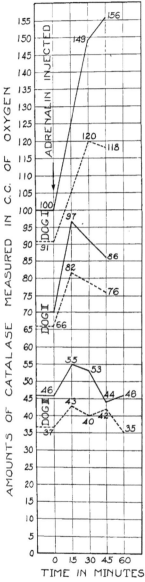

TIME IN MINUTES

drogen peroxide at approximately 22° C. in a bottle and the amount of gas liberated in ten minutes was taken as a measure of the amount of catalase in the 0.5 c.c. of blood.

After exposing the jugular vein and opening the abdominal wall, with the use of ether anesthesia, 3 c.c. of a 1:1000 solution of adrenalin chloride were introduced into the portal vein in Dog III, Fig. 1; 5 c.c. in Dog II. In these two dogs, the solutions were injected as quickly as could conveniently be done. In Dog I, 10 c.c. of a 1:1000 adrenalin solution diluted to 50 c.c. were injected at a rate of approximately 2 c.c. per minute, requiring about 30 minutes for the injection. The catalase in 0.5 c.c. of blood taken directly from the liver and the jugular vein was determined before, as well as at fixed intervals after the injection of the adrenalin. The blood of the liver was collected from a superficial incision made in this organ. The results of the determinations are given in Fig. 1. The figures (0-155) along the ordinate represent amounts of catalase measured in cubic centimeters of oxygen, and the figures (0-60) along the abscissa, time in minutes. The solid line curves were constructed from data obtained from blood of the liver and the broken-line curves from the blood of the jugular vein.

It may be seen in Dog I, that previous to the introduction of the adrenalin into the portal vein, 0.5 c.c. of blood from the liver liberated 100 c.c. of oxygen from hydrogen peroxide in ten minutes, while 0.5 c.c. of blood from the jugular liberated 91 c.c. At the end of the injection of the adrenalin, which required 30 minutes, the catalase of the blood of the liver and jugular vein was greatly increased as is indicated by the increase in the amount of oxygen liberated from hydrogen peroxide. The catalase of the blood of the liver was increased to a greater extent than that of the jugular vein. This is taken to mean that adrenalin was stimulating the liver to an increased output of catalase. It may also be seen in Dogs II and III that a single injection of smaller amounts of adrenalin produced an increase in the catalase of the blood.

The introduction of adrenalin into the portal vein stimulates the liver to a greatly increased output of catalase. This fact suggests that the increase in adrenalin during combat may stimulate the production of catalase and in this way aid in bringing about the increase in oxidation characteristic of great muscular exertion.

BIBLIOGRAPHY

[1] Blum, F.: Arch. f. d. gas. Physiol., 1902, xc. 617.
[2] Vosburgh and Richards: Am. Jour. Physiol., 1903, lx, 29.
[3] Dreyer: Am. Jour. Physiol., 1899, ii, 283.
[4] Oliver and Schaefer: Jour. Physiol., 1895, xviii, 230.
[5] Cannon and de la Paz: Am. Jour. Physiol., 1911, xxviii, 64.
[6] Burge and Neill: Am. Jour. Physiol., 1918, xlv, No. 4, 388; ibid., 1919, xlviii, No. 2, 133.

A SIMPLE METHOD FOR DETERMINING THE REACTION OF FECES

By W. J. Bruce, New York City

WHILE doing routine examinations of feces, I was impressed by the lack of a proper indicator for the reaction. No doubt, most technicians have at some time or other been confronted with a specimen the reaction of which it was impossible to determine correctly. The present method of using either litmus paper or litmus solution has, therefore, room for improvement.

When testing the reaction of feces that is very dark in color, using red litmus paper as the indicator, it is almost impossible to say whether the bluish color often obtained is a chemical reaction, or a stain from the specimen. Practically the same results are obtained with neutral litmus solution. The use of phenolphthalein as an indicator is also limited when testing feces.

Most textbooks recommend litmus paper. Faught states regarding the reaction of feces, "This is quite difficult to get with the ordinary paper. It can be easily obtained by dropping a little softened fecal matter into 5 or 10 c.c. of weak watery solution of neutral litmus solution, shaking it and noticing its color reaction." This method involves a most disagreeable piece of technic, that of getting the feces into a test tube and besides cleansing the glassware used for such an examination is objectionable to the person who takes care of such apparatus.

By the use of the method which I am about to describe, the reaction can be determined on the ordinary glass slide, or better still on a piece of white porcelain about 6 inches long and 1 inch wide. As soon as the reaction is decided, the slide is easily dropped in the disinfecting jar, thereby removing the menace of infection.

Prepare a 1 per cent aqueous solution of alizarin. Place two small drops of the indicator on a glass slide about one and a half inches apart. Dip a glass stirring rod into the liquid part of the specimen (or if the feces is formed, merely puncture the mass). By this means a sufficient amount of feces will be obtained for the test. Mix thoroughly in one of the drops, using the other drop as a control. An alkaline reaction is indicated by a reddish violet to violet color, neutral no change, and acid to a light yellow color. The density of these colors, of course, will depend on the amount of acid or alkali present. By placing the slide upon a piece of white paper, the depth of color can be more easily determined. After a few observations, it is easy to detect any abnormality in the reaction. The use of the white porcelain is much more satisfactory, and is strongly recommended. A suitable opaque glass or white porcelain may be easily obtained at any local plate glass store, or at a sign writing shop.

During the last year or so, we were unable to procure a proper quality of red litmus paper to use in the examination of urine, but this indicator was substituted and gave satisfactory results. It can also be used in determining the reaction of human milk.

Although some biochemists and physiologists state that the reaction of feces has very little value, I believe a great deal of this feeling is due to the present unsatisfactory methods of obtaining it.

THE PRESERVATIVE FOR WASSERMANN REAGENTS
CHLOROFORM THE BEST PRESERVATIVE

By Clarence Emerson, M.D., Lincoln, Nebraska

ONE of the chief causes of difficulty in the performance of complement-fixation tests is the great tendency for decomposition of the reagents by the action of bacteria. The various sera employed furnish a splendid culture media for many saprophytic bacteria and their presence engenders putrefactive decomposition which inactivates certain sera and makes others not inactivated disagreeable to work with because of the odors. Some of the reagents in the various complement-fixation tests must be freshly prepared, some keep indefinitely under ordinary conditions and without special treatment, while others will undergo putrefaction and lose strength unless some measures are enforced for preservation. Since the alterations are usually dependent chiefly upon bacteria and putrefaction, most of the efforts to preserve the reagents have had as their object the retardation of bacterial growth. Two methods have been mainly followed:

1. Cold storage.
2. Chemical antibacterial agents.

It is my intention in this article to report the deductions from my experience with various methods of preserving certain of these reagents and especially to lay stress upon the great value of chloroform as a preservative for these sera.

I have not seen in the literature any previous reference to the use of chloroform for this purpose, and its value so far exceeds any other agent that I am familiar with that I believe a general recognition of its efficiency would be a valuable addition to the technic of the complement-fixation tests. I shall consider separately the various reagents used in the tests.

1. ANTIGEN

Little need be said as to the preservation of antigen except in regard to the aqueous extract of luetic livers. Wassermann's original antigen was an aqueous extract and it was necessary to keep it in the ice chest and to avoid exposure to light. I have never used this form of antigen and since the alcoholic extracts are almost universally used and are preserved for an indefinite period because of the presence of alcohol, it seems that the preservation of antigen has reached a satisfactory stage of perfection.

2. RED CELLS

Red blood cells of the animal against whose blood an amboceptor has been developed are best preserved by keeping in cold storage after thoroughly washing with a salt solution that is one and one-half times as strong as normal salt solution. The cells, after washing until the supernatant liquid is clear, are finally centrifuged until sedimented and most of the supernatant fluid is poured off. To dry the cells completely and then reemulsify in salt solution increases fragility, while an excess of fluid favors autolysis. This is the usual recommendation with the exception of the strength of the salt solution. Often red cells from the sheep will hemolyze in normal salt solution, but will not break up in the stronger solution and the test is not in any way interfered with by the additional salt. I am also convinced that complement-fixation tests performed with red cells that are older than one week are unreliable. As soon as the red cell emulsion loses its bright red color and changes to a dark purple hue it is no longer serviceable for the test. If kept in the ice chest this usually will not take place before one week; however, if at room temperature it may occur in 24 hours. A few drops of chloroform retards this action, but reliance should be placed on freshness of the specimen rather than on any method of preservation known at the present time.

3. AMBOCEPTOR

An immune serum retains its amboceptor activity for a long time if kept in a suitable cold-storage. The common ice chests of small size are usually not cold enough to prevent bacterial growth and putrefactive changes. This activity, however, can go on in an immune serum even to the extent of producing cloudiness and putrefactive odor without complete loss of its combining qualities. There is a gradual loss of strength and finally such weakness that the serum is discarded. It is in the preservation of amboceptor that I have been especially pleased with the use of chloroform because it prevents putrefaction, the serum remains potent for months with almost uniform strength and the disagreeable odors are never present. The chloroform evaporates soon after the amboceptor is diluted for test purposes and does not in any way interfere with the complement-fixation tests. I have treated separate parts of the same amboceptor with chloroform, thymol, phenol and other antiseptics and compared them with an untreated specimen kept under the same conditions for several months and found that the chloroform preserved amboceptor much more potent and pleasant to work with than any other. In fact amboceptor with chloroform added may be kept at room temperatures for weeks without appreciable change. I usually add about 5 or 6 drops of chloroform to 10 c.c. of amboceptor, although I have made stronger proportions without any deleterious effect on the amboceptor or the test. The chloroform precipitates a whitish fine precipitate soon after addition, which does not carry with it any of the amboceptor qualities of the serum. It is not harmful to leave this precipitate and draw off the clear serum above as needed. From time to time if the chloroform seems to have evaporated as evidenced by the odor, I add more.

4. SUSPECTED AND CONTROL SERA

A most important consideration in complement-fixation tests is that of the handling of the suspected serum and control sera previous to the test. Of special importance are certain factors involved in the collection and mailing of blood to a distant laboratory. To collect blood in a bottle and send to a laboratory without special care as to the method will often make the test valueless. If the serum is not separated from the clot it may acquire antihemolytic qualities in 24 hours, and a complement-fixation test becomes impossible. Another important point is to be sure that the needle and syringe which may have been sterilized in boiling water just previous to use are thoroughly dry before blood is withdrawn because the water though small in amount may cause hemolysis and interfere with the test. Bacterial growth of course is detrimental and the addition of chloroform to the separated serum is a valuable procedure.

I would suggest the following instructions for physicians who desire to send blood to a laboratory for examination when the interval of time between securing the specimen and reaching the laboratory is apt to be 24 hours or more.

A. Collect 10 to 15 c.c. of blood in a clean dry homeopathic vial by inserting a sterile dry large-calibre hypo needle into a vein. The needles that come with record syringes are of such caliber that the blood will come through without suction by a syringe.

B. Immediately place the vial on its side with the mouth slightly elevated so the blood will clot with a proportionately greater surface. Separation of the serum is thus favored.

C. After a few hours when the clear serum has separated, draw it off with a clean, dry pipette and transfer to another vial. Add to this a few drops of chloroform.

In this form the serum may be shipped in an ordinary mailing case, without packing in ice and it will be serviceable for test purposes even after several days.

The control, normal, and syphilitic sera can be kept for a much longer period if chloroform is added.

5. COMPLEMENT (GUINEA PIG SERUM)

Guinea pig serum is probably universally used for complement and the necessity of having a source of supply is one of the trials of the Wassermann test. Various means have been suggested from time to time to prolong the period of activity of complementary serum, but my own observation has led me to reject all of them. Diluting with highly concentrated salt solution, preservation in potassium acetate, drying on filter paper, etc., may prolong the activity to some extent, but I have not found any of them to sufficiently preserve complement to warrant their use. I am of the opinion that for dependable complement-fixation work a clear serum kept in cold storage and less than four days old, is an essential.

The fact should not be lost sight of that the distilled water that is used in the making of salt solution for the test serves as a medium for the growth of bacteria and molds and that some of these may have anticomplementary or antigenic properties and interfere with tests. The water should be freshly distilled.

To epitomize—the alcoholic extract of antigen keeps indefinitely. Red blood cells may be serviceable up to one week after collecting if sedimented in salt solution and kept in the ice box. Complementary serum must be not over four days old and kept in the ice box. The amboceptor, suspected sera, and control sera are much better preserved and are active for a greater period of time if a few drops of chloroform are added as a preservative. No test is of undoubted value if performed on sera kept in contact with the clot longer than 24 hours.

As confirmatory of the value of chloroform in preserving these sera and its innocuousness in the performance of the test I will say that Dr. Miles Brewer, of Lincoln, who was laboratory technician in charge of Wassermann work at Base Hospital No. 49 in France reported to me that he had used my method of chloroform preservation of amboceptor and sera throughout an extensive experience there with very satisfactory results.

The Journal of Laboratory and Clinical Medicine

Vol. V.   OCTOBER, 1919   No. 1

Editor-in-Chief: VICTOR C. VAUGHAN, M.D.
Ann Arbor, Mich.

ASSOCIATE EDITORS

DENNIS E. JACKSON, M.D.	CINCINNATI
HANS ZINSSER, M.D.	NEW YORK
PAUL G. WOOLLEY, M.D.	CINCINNATI
FREDERICK P. GAY, M.D.	BERKELEY, CAL.
J. J. R. MACLEOD, M.B.	TORONTO
ROY G. PEARCE, M.D.	CLEVELAND
W. C. MACCARTY, M.D.	ROCHESTER, MINN.
GERALD B. WEBB, M.D.	COLORADO SPRINGS
E. E. SOUTHARD, M.D.	BOSTON

EDITORIALS

Some Recent Work on the Control of the Respiratory Center

FROM the moment the animal is born until death, breathing proceeds with a rhythm which is occasionally broken for brief periods of time by voluntary holding of the breath or by participation of the respiratory musculature in the various expulsive acts of the body, or in phonation and singing. The respiratory movements involve the harmonious activities of greatly diverse muscular groups, some of them contracting, while others relax, but always in so perfect a synchronism that the movement produced alters the capacity of the thorax in the manner which will most effectively ventilate the pulmonary alveoli. During inspiration, for example, the muscles which elevate the thoracic cage and those which depress the diaphragm contract at the same time that the muscles of the abdominal walls relax to make more room for the depressed viscera.

The excitatory or inhibitory nerve impulses which control these movements come finally, of course, from the cells of the lower neurones and these are scattered along the cerebrospinal axis from the level of the nerve centers for the muscles of the alæ nasi in the pons to those of the abdominal muscles in the lumbar region of the spinal cord. But it is plain that these centers can not in themselves be more than local executives for a higher command which must have its headquarters in some more or less localized group of nerve cells. This chief respiratory center, as it is called, is usually considered to be situated in the me-dulla oblongata but there is good reason for believing that its upper limits extend for some distance into and perhaps beyond the pons.

It is clear that the fundamental problems of respiratory control must be directed to ascertain the conditions which excite or alter the activity of this center, and it is around this question that much important work has been contributed during recent years, particularly by the Oxford School of Physiologists led by J. S. Haldane[1] and the Copenhagen School led by August Krogh.

There are in general two ways in which the activities of a center might be caused to alter. These are by changes in the chemical composition of the blood supplying it and by nerve impulses derived from other parts of the nervous system.

Confining our attention for the present to the former class of influences, it may be said that tendency is to consider the hydrogen-ion concentration (C_H) of the blood that bathes the center as chiefly responsible. According to this view alterations in C_H furnish the respiratory hormone.

While there can be no doubt that the respiratory center is extremely sensitive to the slightest changes in C_H of the blood, indeed, it is probably safe to say that there is no more sensitive indicator of changes in C_H than the respiratory center, yet many serious objections can be raised against the view that the ordinary physiologic alterations in respiratory activity are brought about in this way. Because of the fact that the center is sensitive to changes in C_H which can not be measured by any known laboratory method it is impossible to furnish direct proof for or against the hypothesis. All the evidence is of an indirect nature and in many cases it is dependent upon assumptions and analogies which may possibly be erroneous.

It has long been known that respiratory activity can be excited by experimentally raising C_H of the blood, through the injection of mineral acids intravenously, but this does not necessarily mean that ordinary (physiologic) alterations in that function are due to the same cause. A great part of the indirect evidence is based on the observation that the tension of carbon dioxide (CO_2) in the blood bears a relationship to C_H of this fluid and to the degree of pulmonary ventilation. This is the case because CO_2 in solution is a weak acid and therefore cooperates with the other acids of blood to maintain C_H. It possesses one advantage over the other acids in that it is volatile and consequently can readily be got rid of through the alveoli. Whenever, therefore, there tends to be an increase in C_H of the blood some of the CO_2 which is in simple solution in the plasma is got rid of so that the tension declines and the percentage of CO_2 in the alveolar air becomes lower. The tension of CO_2, in other words, declines so as to make room in the blood for other acids. When the adjustment is perfect, the condition is often called *compensated acidosis,* but when there is too much fixed acid, so that C_H is slightly raised, it is called *uncompensated acidosis.* In the former case there is no respiratory disturbance when the person is at rest, but such is readily induced by the slightest exertion because there is a deficiency of basic substance available in the blood and tissues to combine with the increased CO_2, and other acids, produced by the active muscles; the *buffer action* of the blood is said to be depressed. In the latter case, on the other hand, there is hyperpnea even at rest.

The H-ion concentration may obviously be raised by a process which is fundamentally the reverse of that just considered; namely, by an increase in the CO_2 tension while the other (fixed) acids of the blood remain constant. In this case acidosis will occur and there will be hyperpnea along with a higher percentage of CO_2 in the alveolar air; this condition is styled carbonic acid[2] and it occurs in uncompensated cardiac cases and to a certain extent in asphyxial conditions and during strenuous muscular exertion.

In all of the foregoing instances the interpretation of the respiratory excitement which has almost universally been adopted is that C_H of the blood has become raised, but if we pause to consider all the facts, it will be seen that the conclusion is by no means inevitable. It may as well be that it is the free CO_2 as such, or more precisely the anion HCO'_3 (for $H_2CO'_3$ will dissociate into $H \cdot \rightarrow HCO'_3$) that is the really important hormone instead of the cation $H \cdot$. In the cases of carbonic acid acidosis this is easy to understand; in cases of uncompensated acidosis it may be explained if we remember that there is now no sufficient amount of base to take up and fix as carbonates the CO_2 as it is produced, so that the free CO_2 in the cells of the respiratory center, as in other cells, is not adequately removed. There is a certain amount of experimental support for this view of which the following may be cited: Hooker, Wilson and Connett[3] succeeded in retarding death in the basal regions of the brain sufficiently so that respiratory movements were still present and they found that these movements became more markedly excited at a certain C_H of the perfusion fluid when the acid present was mainly H_2CO_3 than when it was any other acid. R. W. Scott[4] found that the respiratory movements in decerebrate cats were increased in proportion as the percentage of CO_2 in the respired air was raised. Examination of the arterial blood by the colorimetric method showed that C_H also became increased under these conditions, an observation which in itself, might support the view that it is really elevation of C_H that furnishes the stimulus to the respiratory center. That this is not the sole, if even the main, stimulus was shown in further experiments in which amounts of alkali were first of all injected intravenously so that decided depression in C_H of the blood was established. On now causing these "alkalosis" animals to respire in CO_2-rich atmospheres it was found that the respirations were excited practically to as great a degree as in the animals with normal C_H; although this became raised, it had not nearly attained the level at which it stands in normal blood even when very marked hyperpnea was present. Increase in CO_2 tension, quite independently of increase in C_H above the physiologic level, had quite clearly afforded the stimulus to the center. It will be necessary to repeat the observations by the use of the electrometric method for measuring C_H of the blood.

If further investigation should confirm the hypothesis that CO_2 tension is a more effective stimulus for the respiratory center than C_H it will mean that, unlike the rhythmic action of the heart which is highly susceptible to cations the rhythmic action of the respiratory center is so to anions. The excitability of the respiration center towards certain concentrations of the CN-ion is of great interest and significance in this connection although the action is differently explained by its discoverer, Loevenhart. The rhythmic contractions of the isolated small intestine are also highly susceptible to the influence of anions.

Apart from their theoretical interest the foregoing facts are of undoubted practical importance since they show that a certain tension of CO_2 must exist in the blood which bathes the respiratory, and very likely other centers, in order that the physiologic activity may be maintained. The observations recall the old hypothesis of Mosso that certain perversions of physiologic function may occur when the tension of CO_2 is subnormal (acapnia).

One of the most important questions in connection with the hormone control of the respiratory center concerns the influence of a deficiency of oxygen in the inspired air. It has long been known that dyspnea usually supervenes in atmospheres which are decidedly deficient in this gas. There are two well-known types of observation which illustrate this fact. The first of these is the laboratory experiment in which a person is caused to breathe in and out of a large spirometer or rubber bag provided with soda lime to absorb carbon dioxide, dyspnea develops, becoming very marked when the oxygen has fallen below 14 per cent. The other is afforded by watching the respiration at high altitudes, it is hyperpneic so that the alveoli are more thoroughly ventilated and the supply of oxygen in them becomes more frequently replenished in order to compensate for the decreased percentage in the atmosphere. There is therefore no doubt that deficiency of oxygen excites the respiration; the question is whether the stimulus is the oxygen deficiency *per se* or whether it is dependent upon some condition which is set up by this deficiency. In considering this question it is important to distinguish between extreme and moderate degrees of oxygen deficiency. When it is extreme the respiratory center, like all other centers, becomes depressed apparently without any preliminary stimulation, and breathing ceases. Such a condition occurs when the blood supply to the medulla is seriously interfered with and in cases of respiration in poisonous gases, like carbon monoxide or methane. A similar depression of the respiratory center due to oxygen deficiency may possibly be the cause of death in such diseases as acute pneumonia and edema of the lungs. It is of decided practical value to know that it is possible to restore a center rendered inactive through deficiency of oxygen by increasing the percentage of this gas in simple solution in the blood supplying the medulla. We have observed this restorative power of oxygen inhalations very strikingly in the case of decerebrate cats (Fraser, Lang and Macleod). These animals breathe with perfect regularity as long as there is an adequate supply of oxygen to the medulla, but if this be curtailed, as by temporarily clamping the vertebral arterioles, the respirations gradually cease but return immediately the circulation is restored. Sometimes, especially when the arterio corpora quadrigemina are destroyed, the breathing in the decerebrate animals becomes irregular and gradually ceases entirely, though the heart is still beating and there is a fair arterial blood pressure. In such cases normal respiration is promptly restored by raising the partial pressure of oxygen in the alveolar air which is most conveniently done by introducing pure oxygen low down in the trachea through a catheter and interrupting the stream rhythmically at about the same rate as the animal breathes. The restored breathing continues for some time after discontinuing the oxygen inhalations.

In view of the results it is possible to explain the beneficial effects which often follow the administration of oxygen in cases of pneumonia, in coal gas poisoning, etc. The inhaled oxygen raises the tension of this gas in the alveolar air so that a sufficient amount of it becomes dissolved in the plasma to keep the center alive, independently—in the case of CO-poisoning at least—of the formation of more oxyhemoglobin. That nerve centers and other tissues can be kept alive by physiologic saline in which excess of oxygen is dissolved is a well-established fact and it should be our aim, when treating cases of asphyxia, to raise the partial pressure of this gas in the alveolar air as high as possible. The dissolved oxygen supplied to the centers in this way must be maintained until the mechanism of which the supply is normally ensured, namely, by dissociation of the oxygen bound to hemoglobin, has been restored to normal. The resuscitation afforded by increasing the percentage of oxygen in the alveolar air, although it can only be temporary, may serve to tide over a crisis and so permit the normal mechanisms by which oxygen is transported to the tissues to become restored.

With regard to the second method of respiratory control, namely, that through afferent nerve impulses only a few of the most outstanding facts can be referred to here. The older work seemed to show the most important of these impulses to be transmitted to the center along the vagus nerves and the hypothesis was formulated that the rate of the respiratory movements depends fundamentally on the fact that towards the end of each inspiration an impulse set up by the distention of the alveoli, is transmitted to the center where it inhibits the rhythmic discharge and so brings on an expiration. Without these inspiration inhibitory impulses respiration is much slower and deeper than normal. There is a growing mass of evidence which goes to show that these afferent impulses, as well as others derived from the afferent nerves of the thoracic parietes (including muscular sense impressions) are important in harmonizing the action of the respiratory musculature much in the same way that afferent impulses from the extremities are important in the synthesis of the complicated muscular activities necessary for the maintenance of the erect posture and for locomotion (Pike,[5] Boothby and Berry[6]).

That the respiratory center is influenced by afferent impulses which are set up by the degree of distention of the lungs has been shown in experiments by Lois Fraser, Lang and Macleod.[7] The experiments were performed on decerebrate cats. When these animals were caused to breathe into wide-bore tubing provided with bottles containing soda lime to absorb the carbon dioxide it was found that the respiratory volume became markedly increased while there was still practically no reduction in the percentage of oxygen in the inspired air. This evidence, furnished by registration of the volume of respired air (by a Gad-Krogh spirometer) was confirmed by observing the behavior of the respiratory quotient of the alveolar air. Immediately the breathing into the tubing was started the quotient rose considerably. sometimes to 2.0, indicating that CO_2

was being washed out of the blood by the more thorough ventilation of the alveoli. When the animal was allowed to breathe in outside air again the breathing respiratory volume quickly returned to the normal and the respiratory quotient fell to a very low level showing that the blood was now taking up the CO_2 it had lost.

This experiment recalls the experience of every one who has tried to breathe through tubing into a spirometer or gas absorbing apparatus; a certain degree of hyperpnea is always set up which is usually attributed to a conscious sense of effort. But the foregoing observations show clearly that the reaction is independent of the higher centers and that it must be purely reflex through the respiratory center, the afferent stimulus being the state of distention of the lungs or thorax. The stimulus which excites the hyperpnea may persist indefinitely or it may subside after a time. In cases in which it does not subside it will lead to an overventilation of the alveoli and consequently to a depletion of the free CO_2 of the blood (acapnia). It is possible that it is because of this condition that prolonged respiration through a gas mask or into a respiratory apparatus frequently becomes unbearable on account of the sense of bodily discomfort which develops (mask staleness).

BIBLIOGRAPHY

[1]Haldane, J. S.: cf. Douglas, C. G.: Die Regulation der Atmung Beim Menschen, Ergebn. d. Physiol., 1914, p. 338.
[2]Scott, R. W.: Am. Jour. Physiol., 1917, xliv, 196.
[3]Hooker, Wilson, and Connett: Ibid., 1917, xliii, 367.
[4]Scott, R. W.: Ibid, 1918, xlvi.
[5]Pike, F. H.: Proc. Am. Physiol. Soc., April, 1919.
[6]Boothby, W. M., and Berry, F. B.: Am. Jour. Physiol., 1915, xxxvii, 433.
[7]Fraser, Lois; Lang, R. S.; and Macleod, J. J. R.: Proc. Am. Physiol. Soc., April, 1919.

—J. J. R. M.

Hemoglobin

THE essential substance in the blood, so far at least as oxygen is concerned, is hemoglobin. This substance is the respiratory material of the body, the substance upon which depends completely the presence of oxygen when it is needed, and in the amounts in which it is needed. Absence of hemoglobin is not compatible with life, and diminution of it produces disease, as is so well known from studies of chlorosis, and other forms of anemia.

If one stops to think of the remarks of Barcroft he will at once be impressed with the meaning of the thing. "In warm-blooded animals, muscle, when working at its full power, uses up its own volume of oxygen in about ten minutes. This oxygen is carried to it by the hemoglobin of the blood—a substance so rich in oxygen that a relatively small quantity of blood satisfies the need of the muscle. Were it not for this pigment some 200 c.c. of fluid would have to be circulated through every gram of muscle in ten minutes of time. To put the matter in another way, blood carries about 40 times as much oxygen as the same volume of plasma. Therefore, to convey as much oxygen around the body as is carried by the blood, would, in the absence of hemoglobin, demand 150 kilos of plasma, or perhaps more. The contents of the vascular system would therefore amount to twice the present weight of the body. The body would, in short, be unable to cope with the weight of its own blood. The whole basis of its economy therefore hinges upon the accidental possibility of the occurrences and proper-ties of hemoglobin."

Since hemoglobin is the essential oxygen carrying substance of the body, loss of any proportion of it or any interference with its function must have the most far-reaching results. For the most part the recognized and appreciated re-sults of hemoglobin loss, in amount or activity, are grouped with the anemias.

Now anemia, the word, literally means without blood, and blood can be lost or reduced in a variety of ways. For instance, there may be interference with the production of the red cells of the blood—the cells which contain the hemo-globin. Hemoglobin itself may not be found in sufficient amount because of fail-ure of the supply of iron in the diet, or a breaking down of the mechanism by which it is formed. Red blood cells may be produced in sufficient numbers to satisfy the needs of the economy, but they may be destroyed by parasites, or by poisonous substances, malaria on the one hand; quinine on the other. In any case, however, the fact of importance in this group of anemias is that there is not enough hemoglobin to satisfy the demand for oxygen by the body.

But besides these hemoglobin anemias, there is probably another group of conditions in which despite a quantitatively sufficient amount of hemoglobin, oxygen is not carried in amounts compatible with health. Such conditions are those in which the hemoglobin is not able to combine sufficient oxygen, even though the supply of that gas is normal. Perhaps the simplest example of such a condition is that due to cold—simple chilling of the body. Other examples, it may be discovered, may be due to abnormal salt concentrations of the plasma, perhaps even to unusual amounts of a single salt. Such conditions are not well defined at the present time because too litttle is known concerning the special effects of salts in the blood. What little is known is that the affinities of hemo-globin for oxygen are profoundly modified by temperature and by the general salt content of the plasma. It is also known that the dilution of the blood has no effect on the oxygen capacity,* i.e., mere plethora does not modify the amount of oxygen the blood can carry. The reaction of the blood is we know of funda-mental importance in modifying the oxygen supply.

Temperature acts in reducing the percentage saturation of hemoglobin, and in increasing the reduction. For instance, Barcroft gives the following figures:

Temperature	16°	24°	32°	38°	49°
Percentage saturation	92	71	37	18	6

A similar experiment, at a much higher oxygen pressure, with a hemoglobin solution made in a different way but also dialyzed, yielded the following results:

Temperature	16°	25°	32°	38°
Percentage saturation (observed)	96	89	77	52
Percentage saturation (calculated)	97	89	74	54

*Barcroft, p. 25 (Burns' figures):

Degree of Dilution of Blood	O-capacity by Ab-sorption Method	O-capacity by Ferri-cyanide Method
Undiluted	17.6%	17.4%
5 times	17.6%	17.5%
7 times	17.8%	17.1%

In bringing about reduction, Barcroft says, at the conclusion of an experiment, that while "at 18° C. 35 minutes were required for the reduction of the hemoglobin from 100 per cent to 94 per cent saturation, at 38° C. it only required 7.5 minutes to reduce it from 94 per cent to 77 per cent."

It appears from these facts that the amount of oxygen which hemoglobin can take up, and the amount and rapidity with which it can give up combined oxygen varies with the temperature of the body, a state of affairs that must have some important significance in fevers.

But, besides the temperature, there is another factor which is essential in regulating the transfer of oxygen; namely, the salt content of the blood. This is what might be expected from the fact that hemoglobin is a colloid, and from what we know of the effects of electrolytes on colloids. From experiments it has been found that potassium salts are partially efficient in causing hemoglobin to absorb oxygen (Macleod, p. 386). In fevers and other conditions associated with loss of water, the salt concentration of the body may be of the greatest import and the mere loss of a seemingly unimportant amount of water may react in greatly reducing the necessary oxidations of the body. Especially may this be true when with the salt effects are united those due to heightened temperature.

Finally there is the factor of acidity—of hydrogen-ion concentration—which has a tremendous influence on the activities of hemoglobin. The effect of increased acidity of the solution is to lessen the effective concentration of the oxygen in the solution which contains the hemoglobin. The concentration of free carbonic acid in the solution, necessary for production of a measurable change in the affinity of hemoglobin for oxygen amounts to something of the order of one part in one hundred million (Barcroft, p. 53), and lactic acid acts in precisely the same way.

These three factors—temperature, electrolytes, and reaction—are of the utmost importance in determining the direction of disease, and they are in no way less important in indicating the direction of therapeusis. A single example of what might happen in the body, with respect to its internal respiration, may be given as follows:

The temperature of the body rises, and because of this, the blood (hemoglobin) is able to combine with less oxygen in the lungs. Because of the increased temperature, metabolism is increased, and the products of metabolism accumulate, and these are not promptly and efficiently removed because of the decreased oxygen in the blood. The products of metabolism are not uncommonly acid, and therefore those remaining in the tissues cause the latter to hold water and to take more water for the circulating fluids. The result of this is that the plasma loses water and its salts become more concentrated, a state of affairs that leads to still further reduction of the oxygen-combining power of the hemoglobin. At the same time the reaction of the blood (the H-ion concentration) is increased and again a more or less serious state of affairs arises, depending upon the degree of the process.

The above verbal scheme is given merely because it is suggestive of what might happen with reference to the hemoglobin alone. If the scheme is useful from the side of treatment it means first, that in fevers water is primarily necessary, and that second, alkalies are valuable. The one makes evaporation from the body possible, and this in addition to radiation, serves to reduce the temperature. At the same time the concentration of the plasma tends to be reduced. The other acts to reduce the available acidity of the blood. Both together tend to act to increase the combining power of hemoglobin for oxygen, and the oxygen in its turn is the fundamental agent in getting rid of waste products of metabolism.

BIBLIOGRAPHY

Barcroft: The Respiratory Function of the Blood, 1914, Cambridge University Press.
Mathews: Physiological Chemistry, New York, 1915, Wm. Wood & Co.
Macleod: Physiology and Biochemistry in Modern Medicine, St. Louis, 1918, C. V. Mosby Co.
Gradwohl and Blaivas: The Newer Methods of Blood and Urine Chemistry, St. Louis, 1917, C. V. Mosby Co.

—*P. G. W.*

The Journal of Laboratory and Clinical Medicine

| Vol. V. | St. Louis, November, 1919 | No. 2 |

ORIGINAL ARTICLES

STUDIES ON IRRITABLE HEART
II. The Etiology of Irritable Heart

By Louis M. Warfield, (Milwaukee) Recently Major, M. C., U. S. Army,
and Fred M. Smith, (Chicago) 1st Lieut. M. C., U. S. Army,
Jefferson Barracks, Mo.

TERMINOLOGY

IN the report of Lewis[1] and his associates, they discussed various terms to describe the group of symptoms known in the British Army as D. A. H., and finally considered "effort syndrome" to be the most satisfactory. Later, Rothschild and Oppenheimer[2] used the term neurocirculatory asthenia, which has recently (MacFarlane)[3] been criticized and neurocirculatory myasthenia has been suggested. It seems to us that Lewis' original name "'effort syndrome" is preferable to the later suggested name.

The condition in question is not a disease as would certainly be indicated by the employment of such names as the last two noted above. It is a group of symptoms brought on only by effort and found in connection with a number of diseases. It is no more a disease than a combination of headache, fever and increased pulse rate. It no more deserves a special suggestive name than such a combination noted above. The characteristic of the group of symptoms is that they are brought out on exertion, which is invariably far less severe than that required to bring out some or all of the symptoms in a normal person. We have found the group of symptoms typically in such widely different diseases as chronic malaria, cirrhosis of the liver, chronic focal infection, hookworm infection, pulmonary tuberculosis (early), exophthalmic goiter, and as a result of severe infection with the streptococcus hemolyticus (empyema), etc. Such being the case it would appear that no better term has yet been suggested than 'effort syndrome." We prefer that term, although in making diagnosis for Surgeon's

Certificates of Disability we employ 'irritable heart," chiefly for the reason that it "gets by" with less correspondence. Hence we have used this heading as a title to our studies.

METHODS

In our studies of the cases presenting the symptoms which Lewis gave as criteria; viz., breathlessness, pain, exhaustion, giddiness and fainting, also less frequently, palpitation, headache, lassitude, coldness of hands and feet, irritability of temper, sleeplessness, we have had the hearty cooperation of the surgeon, Lt. Colonel C. E. Freeman, M. C. We have found early in our studies that in order to classify the men who, on routine examination, revealed tachycardia, we would have to place them under observation. We were given a pavilion ward where we sent the men. One of us was in charge of the hospital, the other the cardiovascular examiner in the examining barracks, hence we had excellent opportunity to observe the cases. Men found with tachycardia by the examiners doing the routine heart and lung examinations were sent to be further examined by Captain R. E. Adkins, the pulmonary examiner, and one of us, the cardiovascular examiner. By this method the cases held up were most carefully examined. All the suspects who could not at once be accepted or rejected were sent to the hospital where they were later examined a number of times at intervals.

In order to obtain uniformity in the history; a form was prepared as follows:

HISTORY FORM

Family History

1. Father or mother alcoholic? Ans.
2. Father or mother nervous? Ans.
3. Father or mother insane? Ans.
4. Father or mother tuberculous? Ans.

Past History

1. How long have you worked? Ans.
2. Just what do you do?
    Sedentary Light Moderate Heavy
3. Have you had to quit a job because too hard?   When?
4. Ever become dizzy or faint at work? at play?   When?
5. Are you short of breath on exertion?
6. Ever had pain over your heart?   When?
7. Ever had palpitation of the heart?
8. Do you sweat or flush easily?
9. Are you subject to headaches? What part of the head?
10. Are you nervous, easily excited?
11. What fevers have you had?
    When each one?
12. When did you *first* notice any trouble?

From the answers to these our history statistics are taken.

The men were exercised by a soldier whom we had schooled in the work, and were observed by one or both of us while exercising. We used Lewis' C[15] and D[30] together with short hikes and shorter periods of double-quick. Some men could not stand the exercise for five minutes without becoming obviously distressed. Others went through the whole series, including the hike. In this way we determined which men would most probably not make good as soldiers, and which men we could conscientiously accept for military service.

ETIOLOGY

During the past two months we have observed 275 cases. Two hundred fifty of these have been classified and form the basis of this report. Of these, 132 were rejected at the examining barracks, 118 were sent to the hospital for observation, further examination, and graded exercise.

DISPOSITION OF CASES AT EXAMINING BARRACKS

61 cases	(45.4%)	diagnosed	hyperthyroidism	rejected
47 "	(35.6%)	"	pulmonary tuberculosis	"
21 "	(15.9%)	"	irritable heart	"
2 "	(1.5%)	"	cirrhosis liver	
1 "	(0.7%)	"	bronchial asthma	

132

DISPOSITION OF CASES OBSERVED IN THE HOSPITAL

33 cases	(27.8%)	considered	normal	accepted
47 "	(39.8%)	diagnosed	pulmonary tuberculosis	rejected
19 "	(16.2%)	"	irritable heart	"
17 "	(14.5%)	"	hyperthyroidism	"
2 "	(1.7%)	"	cirrhosis liver	

118

It will be seen that only 15.9 per cent of the referred cases at the examining barracks were rejected because of irritable heart, and 16.2 per cent (practically the same percentage) were rejected from the cases studied in hospital.

It might be objected that the cases at the examining barracks were not sufficiently studied. In reply it can be said that in such cases at least two examiners could find absolutely nothing even suggesting any abnormalities except the rapid heart, the history, and the poor response to the hopping exercise. Such cases were so evidently unfit that they were rejected at once.

In both series a number of cases were diagnosed pulmonary tuberculosis. Considering the fact that no sputum examinations were made at the barracks and only a few in the hospital, objection might be raised as to the validity of the diagnosis. We can only reply that it is a poor diagnostician who can not make the diagnosis of pulmonary tuberculosis before tubercle bacilli can be found in the sputum. Furthermore, the diagnosis was in every case the result of numerous examinations (in the hospital cases) by several men independently. We feel justified in making this diagnosis in those cases.

Hyperthyroidism was another cause for rejection. Some of these cases were frank exophthalmic goiter. Others showed only certain eye signs, tremor, tachycardia. Some clinicians call such cases exophthalmic goiter although they lack both exophthalmos and goiter. Potentially they are Graves' disease and represent the acute Graves' disease seen after some sudden shock. For we doubt whether ever a normal person develops acute Graves' disease.

Cirrhosis of the liver, chronic malaria and bronchial asthma showed the same effort syndrome and are therefore included in the figures.

Table I shows the similarity of the symptoms in the histories of the so-called "effort syndrome" in all of the cases:

TABLE I

	FAMILY HISTORY			OCCUPATION					PAST HISTORY CASES							
	Alcoholism	Nervousness	Tuberculosis	Sedentary	Light	Moderate	Heavy	Change to Light	Dizziness	Breathlessness	Precordial Pain	Palpitation	Sweating	Headache	Nervousness	Totals
Irritable Heart	8	10	1	1	13	3	0	12	14	17	15	16	16	14	16	17
Pulmonary Tuberculosis	5	28	10	7	27	15	1	18	33	34	30	37	28	22	39	47
Hyperthyroidism	3	10	3	2	12	3	1	6	8	15	12	16	11	9	15	18
EXPRESSED IN PERCENTAGE																
Irritable Heart	47.0	58.8	5.8	5.5	76.5	1.7	0.0	70.5	82.4	100.0	88.2	94.1	94.1	82.4	94.1	17
Pulmonary Tuberculosis	10.6	59.5	21.3	14.9	57.4	31.9	0.2	38.3	70.2	72.3	63.4	78.7	59.5	46.8	83.0	47
Hyperthyroidism	16.6	55.5	16.6	11.1	66.6	16.6	0.5	33.3	44.4	83.3	66.6	88.8	61.1	50.0	83.3	18

It is readily seen that the characteristic symptoms of the "effort syndrome" as described by Lewis and his coworkers are uniformly found in the cases of irritable hearts. Also such symptoms are found in a large percentage of the other two diseases. It is noteworthy that most of the cases were doing light work, practically none heavy work, and many had changed from moderately heavy or heavy work to light work.

A train of symptoms similar in all respects to that of the "effort syndrome" is found in many men who have had serious acute illnesses, particularly streptococcus pneumonia complicated with empyema, scarlet fever, acute rheumatism, etc. We have not had opportunity to follow, for more than a few months, a few such cases, but it has seemed to us that the myocardial damage produced by intense toxemia renders the victims incapable of violent exertion. In a few cases of three to four months' standing no improvement has resulted after graded exercise. Such men have been discharged on a Certificate of Disability.

We analyzed our histories in respect to previous infectious diseases as shown in Table II.

TABLE II

CASE NO.	ILLNESS	YEARS SINCE ILLNESS	TIME ONSET EFFORT SYNDROME (YEARS)
1	Malaria	6	4
2	None	0	2
3	None	0	6
4	Pneumonia	20	11
5	None	0	10
6	Pneumonia	17	12
	Typhoid	12	
7	None	0	1
8	Pneumonia	2	7
	Rheumatism		
9	None	0	1
10	None	0	3
11	Acute bronchitis	4 months	2 months
12	Malaria	10	15+
13	Malaria	12	15+
	Pneumonia	12	
14	Diphtheria	18 and 3	6
15	None	0	9
16	None	0	2

Just half of the 16 cases had no history of serious illnesses. In the other half the connection was not shown definitely. This we feel can be excluded as a major factor in the etiology of these cases.

A striking feature of these cases is the neuropathic element. The members of the psychiatric board diagnosed several of our cases, psychoneurosis, neurasthenia. This neurotic element was early noted and has recently been emphasized particularly by Oppenheimer and Rothschild.[4]

The "effort syndrome" may be the result of some slow chronic poison acting on the nerve cells and muscle cells. The list of diseases in which such symptoms occur after exercise includes all those named at the beginning of this paper. When all means of diagnosis at present at our disposal are exhausted, there yet remains a large group of true irritable hearts, so-called neurocirculatory asthenia, for which no cause can be found. We are thrown back for an inadequate explanation upon the overworked term, "constitutionally defective." There appears to be some very definite weakness or loss of tone in the vasoconstrictor nerves and in the sympathetic nerve ganglia controlling tone in the skeletal muscles. Defects or lesions of these nerve cells would account for all the somatic symptoms. Cotton, Rapport and Lewis[5] concluded from their experiments on controls and irritable hearts that as atropine was identical in its effect, the raised cardiac rate in patients "appears to be conditioned by hyperirritability of some portion of the system which includes the accelerator reflex arc." Further, the hyperirritability of the sympathetic is apparently shown by the experiments of Fraser and Wilson[6] who found the hearts in the patients more susceptible to adrenalin than hearts of normal men.

There is no especial change in blood pressure. There is no change in the complex of the electrocardiogram. The most important change found by Lewis[7] and his associates was the slight but definite intolerance to CO_2 causing exaggerated breathlessness on slight exertion. This was shown to be due to a reduction of "buffer salts" which allowed a slight excess of CO_2 to render the blood more acid than it should be in normal persons, and this caused increased stimulation of the respiratory center.

SUMMARY

We still prefer the name 'irritable heart" for the condition described although we agree that "effort. syndrome" is better when discussing the disease around patients. Neurocirculatory asthenia and neurocirculatory myasthenia are cumbersome terms.

Many diseases and convalescence from many other diseases reveal practically the identical syndrome. However, the cases of true irritable heart have one factor not usually found in other cases showing similar syndrome. That is history dating back years with no definite cause. The victims at times seem to be born with a constitutional inferiority. The least touch of the throttle races the engine. They seem unable to get into gear and carry the load.

Exercise under observation is unquestionably the surest and quickest method of sorting the fit from the unfit. This syndrome is not at all uncommon in men in ordinary life. It does not need gas or high explosive shells to bring it out. These men may be used for certain kinds of limited service, but even the most limited service usually demands occasional work at high pressure, and that is what these men can not do. Altogether, the safest plan is to reject unconditionally all these cases.

BIBLIOGRAPHY

[1]Lewis, Thomas: Medical Research Committee, Special Report Series No. 8, 1917.
[2]Rothschild, M. A., and Oppenheimer, B. S.: Mil. Surgeon, 1918, xlii, 409.
[3]MacFarlane, Andrew: Jour. Am. Med. Assn., 1918, lxxi, 730.
[4]Oppenheimer, B. S., and Rothschild, M. A.: Jour. Am. Med. Assn., 1918, lxx, 1919.
[5]Cotton, T. F., Rapport, D. L., and Lewis, Thomas: Heart, 1916-17, vi, 293.
[6]Quoted by Lewis.
[7]Lewis, Thomas, Cotton, T. F., Barcroft, J., Milroy, T. R., Dufton, D., and Parsons, T. R.: Brit. Med. Jour., Oct. 14, 1916, p. 517.

STUDIES ON IRRITABLE HEART

III. The Value of Exercise in the Diagnosis and the Determination of the Fitness of the Irritable Heart for Military Service

By Louis M. Warfield (Milwaukee) Recently Major, M. C., U. S. Army, and Fred M. Smith (Chicago) 1st Lieut., M. C., U. S. Army, Jefferson Barracks, Mo.

GRADED exercises have been used by Thomas Lewis[1] and his coworkers in England, and by Robey[2] and others in this country as a means of developing those men who broke down in military service with irritable heart to a point where they could again do duty. The Lewis reports are encouraging. However, as was pointed out in a previous communication,[3] he was dealing with a different class of men than those under consideration here. His men had all seen active service at the front. Major Robey, working with men who had failed in their training, reports no improvement with this form of treatment.

It is generally believed that those men who break down in this military training are not benefited by graded exercises. How much overwork at the beginning of the training has to do with the failure of these men is a question which has not been settled. It is evident, however, if graded exercises are of any value in this class of cases, they must be instituted at the time when these men enter service, with an idea of gradually developing them to a point where they can stand the physical strain of the military training. This was one of the objects in undertaking the work. Incidentally, however, the graded exercises, together with careful observation with regard to pulse and temperature, proved to be valuable in finding an organic basis for many of these irritable hearts.

One hundred forty-two men were given graded exercises. Eighty-one of these had just come from civil life and were sent directly from the examining barracks to the hospital before induction into service. They were men in whom we were in doubt as to their ability to do general military service. All had tachycardia and many had subjective symptoms. The remaining sixty-one of the series were either men who were picked up during the examination for overseas service or men who had failed in their military training. In these two groups we had men with irritable hearts who had had no military training, and those who had broken down in service. They were purposely exercised together in order that their response might be compared.

THE EXERCISE

The exercises used were those outlined by Lewis. They consist of the simpler setting-up type, designed to put into play as many of the muscles of the body as possible. They are grouped so that no excess strain is put on the body in going from a lower to a higher grade. For a more complete description of these exercises the reader is referred to the work of Lewis.

They were given by a soldier whom we had schooled to do the work. The response was carefully noted on an outlined form as shown in Tables 1-6. Usually one or both of us were present. Care was taken not to advance the grade of exercise too rapidly. The men were separated into classes, depending upon their response. Those who satisfied us that they had no ill effects from graded exercises were ultimately given, in addition, short hikes of from two to five miles. The period over which the treatment was given varied from a few days to three weeks, depending upon the response and whether an organic basis was found for the irritable heart.

RESULTS OF EXERCISE

One hundred forty-two men were exercised. Forty-four were returned to duty. The remaining ninety-eight were either rejected or recommended for Surgeon's Certificates of Disability.

Those who were returned to duty were men who had been picked up in the examining barracks and sent to hospital for observation of tachycardia. They complained of few or no symptoms. The response to exercise was good with the exception of a few who ultimately developed subjective symptoms. This left us uncertain as to whether more of this class of men would finally complain when greater strain was put upon them. In a large majority of these men the pulse ranged from 90 to 110, and no cause was found for the increased rate.

The ninety-eight which did not, in our minds, qualify for general military service, gave about the same response but varying in degree. A majority of them complained of shortness of breath, feeling of exhaustion, palpitation of the heart, dizziness and precordial pain on exertion, which dated back to civil life. They never improved under the exercise treatment, regardless of whether they came directly from civil life or were already in the army.

These men in our series fall into three large groups: first, those in which no cause could be found for irritable heart; second, irritable heart with toxic or exophthalmic goiter as a basis; and third, irritable heart in which a diagnosis of active pulmonary tuberculosis was made.

In the first group there were twenty-one. The response was uniformly very poor with no improvement. They were men who had never done work which required physical strain. They were exercised and re-exercised for some organic basis for their trouble, but none was ever found. In our minds they were simply constitutionally inferior men.

In the second group there were twenty-five men. Those with true Graves' disease had all of the typical symptoms of the irritable heart, while those in the incipient stage of the disease had many of the symptoms. The response in the former group was very poor and gradually became worse. In the latter group, while the response was better, the toxic symptoms became aggravated.

In the tuberculosis group there were fifty-two men. Symptomatically they could not be distinguished from the irritable heart in which no organic basis was found. The asthenia grew more marked with exercise. As soon as the diagnosis was made the exercise was stopped.

VALUE OF EXERCISE IN DIAGNOSIS

Those men in whom a diagnosis of pulmonary tuberculosis was made were examined at the examining barracks by two different men, one, Captain R. E. Adkins, the tuberculosis examiner. They were regarded as suspicious and sent to the hospital for observation. Here they were given daily exercise, and had temperature and pulse taken every three hours. In a majority of them under exercise definite activity appeared in one or both apices, and the temperature rose. Chart I shows the temperature of a man who had lost weight, had a slight cough, in whom we suspected pulmonary tuberculosis. He had all the symptoms of irritable heart. The curve shows an increase of temperature after ex-

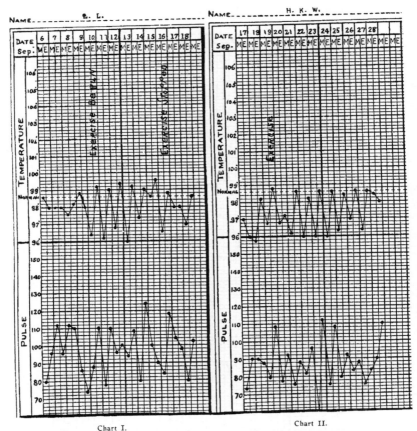

Chart I.   Chart II.

Chart I.—Pulmonary tuberculosis, incipient. Loss of weight, great lassitude, inability to do even light work because of great exhaustion. Slight physical signs at one apex with slight haziness of apex shadow on x-ray plate. Labile pulse. Chart shows effect of exercise on temperature during period of exercise, and extreme lability of pulse.

Chart II.—Irritable heart. Chart showing that exercise did not cause any elevation of temperature although pulse rate was at times raised, even twenty to thirty minutes after exercise when temperature and pulse were recorded.

ercise on five successive days in which he was given this treatment. The physical findings and x-ray justified us in making a diagnosis of active pulmonary tuberculosis. Charts II, III and IV show temperature charts of case of irritable heart, hyperthyroidism and cirrhosis of the liver, and the response to exercise. In neither of these is there any increase of temperature following the exercise.

Those men with true Graves' disease were not difficult to recognize. However, those in the incipient stages were not easy to diagnose. The exercises aggravated the toxic symptoms, and some men while in the ward developed eye signs. No doubt the mental strain of the first few days in an army post was a large factor in bringing out these latent eye signs.

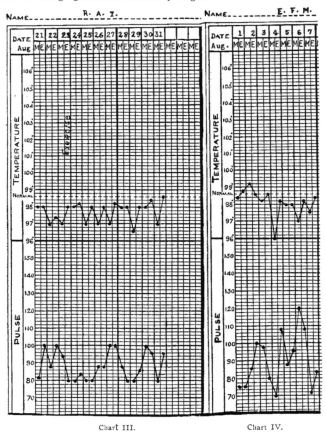

Chart III.   Chart IV.

Chart III.—Hyperthyroidism. Chart showing that exercise had no effect in raising the temperature. All evening temperatures and pulse rates were taken twenty to thirty minutes after the afternoon exercise.

Chart IV.—Cirrhotic liver with syndrome of irritable heart. No rise of temperature following exercise.

CONCLUSIONS

From the result of our studies we feel certain conclusions are justified:

1. The irritable heart is not uncommon among young men in civil life.

TABLE 1

TABLE SHOWING SUCH POOR RESPONSE THAT IT WAS FELT TO BE DETRIMENTAL TO CONTINUE

Name   A. B.   Date   Aug. 16, 1918 R. V.   Age 22

FORM OF EXERCISE	DATE	DYSP.	PRECOR. PAIN	FLUSH-ING	PALP.	GIDDY	EXHAUS.	PULSE	RESP.	B. P.
C15	16	+	+	0	++	+	+	150	40	140-90
C15	17	+	+	0	+	0	+	154	36	148-94

TABLE 2

TABLE SHOWING RESPONSE TO EXERCISE GROWING STEADILY WORSE IN PATIENT WHOSE TEMPERATURE CHART IS SHOWN IN CHART 1.

Name   L. L.   Date   August   R. V.   Age 21

FORM OF EXERCISE	DATE	DYSP.	PRECOR. PAIN	FLUSH-ING	PALP.	GIDDY	EXHAUS.	PULSE	RESP.	B. P.
C15	15	0	0		+	0	0			
C15	16	0	0		+	0	0			
C15	17	0	0		+	+	+			
hike C15	19	+sl	0		+	-:-	+			
hike C15	20	+	+		+	+	0			
hike C15	21	+	+		+	+	+			
hike C15	22	++	+		+	++	++			
hike										

TABLE 3

CASE WITH TACHYCARDIA, DUE TO PULMONARY TUBERCULOSIS. GREW WORSE UNDER EXERCISE. DISCHARGED FROM ARMY.

Name   J. E.   Date   August   R. V.   Age 23

FORM OF EXERCISE	DATE	DYSP.	PRECOR. PAIN	FLUSH-ING	PALP.	GIDDY	EXHAUS.	PULSE	RESP.	B. P.
C15	13	+	0		+	0	+			
run C15	14	+	0		+	0	+			
C15	15	+	+		+	+	0			
run C15	16	+	0		+	+	+			
run C15	17	+	+		+	+	+			
hike C15	19	+	+		+sl	+	+			
hike C15	21	+	0		+sl	+	+			
hike C15	22	+	+		+	+	++			
hike C15	23	++	+		++	++	++			

TABLE 4

TABLE SHOWING POOR RESPONSE TO GRADED EXERCISE IN CASE OF IRRITABLE HEART. DISCHARGED FROM ARMY.

Name   P. C.   Date   August   R. V.   Age 35

FORM OF EXERCISE	DATE	DYSP.	PRECOR. PAIN	FLUSH-ING	PALP.	GIDDY	EXHAUS.	PULSE	RESP.	B. P.
C15 hike	20	+	+	0	+sl	+	0			
C15	26	+	+	0	+	+	0			
C15	28	+	+	0	+	+·	+			
C15	29	+	+	+	+	+	+			
C15	30	+	+	+	+	±	+			

TABLE 5

TABLE SHOWING SIMPLE TACHYCARDIA CASE. GOOD EXERCISE RESPONSE. RETURNED TO DUTY.

Name   G. E. McK.   Date   August   R. V.   Age 25

FORM OF EXERCISE	DATE	DYSP.	PRECOR. PAIN	FLUSH-ING	PALP.	GIDDY	EXHAUS.	PULSE	RESP.	B. P.
C15	20	0	0		+	0	0			
C15	21	+sl	0		+	0	0			
C15 hike	22	0	0		+	0	0			
C15	23	0	0		+	0	0			
C15	26	0	0		+	0	0			
C15	27	0	0		+sl	0	0			
C15	28	0	0		+sl	0	0			
C15	29	0	0		0	0	0			
C15	30	0	0		0	0	0			
C15	31	0	0		0	0	0			

TABLE 6

Table showing case of man who has been doing hard physical labor as log carter in Louisiana and Arkansas from the time he was 15-16 years old. Had never had any difficulty until in July, 1918, after having an attack of bronchitis. Became winded easily, felt exhausted after exercise, and was dizzy. Under graded exercise gained 25 pounds in weight and all symptoms disappear. Was discharged to duty and has had no trouble since.

Name   L. D. G.   Date   August   R. V.   Age 19

FORM OF EXERCISE	DATE	DYSP.	PRECOR. PAIN	FLUSH-ING	PALP.	GIDDY	EXHAUS.	PULSE	RESP.	B. P.
C15	1	+	0	0	0	0	+			
C15	2	+	0	0	0	+	+			
C15	3	+	0	0	0	+	+			
C15	4	+	0	0	0	+	+			
C15	5	+	0	0	0	+	+			
C15	6	+	0	0	0	+	+			
C15	7	+	0	0	0	+	+			
C15	8	+	0	0	0	+	+			
C15	9	0	0	0	0	0	+			
C15	10	0	0	0	0	+sl	+sl			
C15	11	0	0	0	0	0	+sl			
D30	28	+	0		0	0	+sl			
D30	29	0	0		0	0	0			
D30	31	0	0		0	0	0			

2. The syndrome of the irritable heart is only a syndrome and is found in a variety of diseases.

3. Army training should begin with graded exercises, such as the training of college men for athletic sports.

4. Men with incipient irritable hearts are easily broken down by military training.

5. Graded exercise is valuable in sorting the fit from the unfit, but graded exercise is not of therapeutic value for the cases of irritable hearts coming to the army from civil life.

6. Graded exercises are valuable in bringing to light suspected cases of incipient tuberculosis.

7. Graded exercise is also valuable in diagnosing between cases of irritable heart and pulmonary tuberculosis.

8. Cases of irritable heart are not fit for general or limited military service.

NOTE: C-15 of the Lewis exercise is a very light form of setting-up exercise lasting fifteen minutes. The C-15 second part adds a few more movements, none of a violent nature. The D-30 takes thirty minutes to perform, includes the simple movements of the former and adds some rapid leg exercises with upward jumping. One had to be in good condition to go through this series without undue exhaustion. The recovery time, as well as the degree of exhaustion, must be considered.

BIBLIOGRAPHY

[1]Lewis, Thomas: Medical Research Committee, Special Report Series No. 8, 1917.
[2]Robey, W. H. Jr.: Jour. Am. Med. Assn., 1918, lxxi, 525.
[3]Warfield, L. M., and Smith, F. M.: Jour. Am. Med. Assn., 1918, lxxi, 1815.

SOME USES OF NONSPECIFIC PROTEIN THERAPY*

BY WILLIAM BOYD, M.D., WINNIPEG, CANADA

IT is not so many years ago that the word specificity was one to conjure with. When vaccine therapy was first introduced into medical practice under the aegis of Sir A. E. Wright, the importance of specificity was emphasized, almost to the exclusion of other considerations. The specific reaction to bacterial infection or to injection of bacteria was observed and estimated by means of the opsonic index, and solemn warnings were issued against neglect of such precautions. This emphasis on the importance of specific reactions was well justified, but even in the early days it was noted that a nonspecific element was present which could not be ignored. A patient who had been immunized against one type of organism was found, in not a few cases, to have a heightened resistance to some other organism to which he had previously been unduly susceptible. The tendency, however, was to minimize or ignore these cross reactions.

Now the pendulum has made its inevitable swing, and medical literature occupies itself with the importance of nonspecific reactions, a movement which is by no means without its dangers. It is generally admitted, however, that following injection of protein material, bacterial or otherwise, nonspecific reactions occur which are of the greatest importance in therapeutics. These reactions are of much greater intensity and exert a more marked therapeutic effect when the protein substance is given intravenously than when the subcutaneous method is used.

Many explanations have been attempted of this curious effect, but it is probable that several factors are in operation in each case. Following an intravenous injection of foreign protein the phenomena of protein shock which may be observed are rigors, hyperpyrexia, sweating, marked leucocytosis, increased flow of lymph, and rise in both the ferment and antiferment content of the blood serum. Any or all of these may exercise a beneficial effect on the toxic condition of the patient.

Davis and Petersen[1] have shown that protein shock is accompanied by an increased flow of lymph. The antibodies which are present in the blood pass in increased quantity into the lymph, and thus are brought into contact with bacteria which may be lodged in the lymph spaces.

The work of Jobling and Petersen[2] has demonstrated the marked changes in the ferments and antiferments of the blood which follow protein shock. The increase in the ferments—protease and ereptase—is probably a valuable aid in detoxication. The toxins, which are mostly protein-split products, are hydrolyzed by the ferments to lower nontoxic forms, so that a temporary improvement of a few days' duration may be observed. But the bacteria remain unaffected by the ferments, and the symptoms may reappear after a brief interval.

The rise in the antiferment content of the blood is perhaps of greater importance. The antiferment power of the serum is due to the presence of lipoids, in the form of unsaturated fatty acids, whose activity is dependent on their

*From the Department of Pathology of the University of Manitoba and the Winnipeg General Hospital.

colloidal state of dispersion. This, according to Jobling and Petersen, is increased as the result of protein injections, so that adsorption of the lipoids occurs at the surface of the bacteria, with, as a result, the injury or destruction of the latter.

In a recent paper Herrmann[3] has brought out the very important fact that a specific reaction may be brought about by injection of a nonspecific protein. Working with streptococci he was able to show that the specific opsonins and agglutinins in the blood of animals inoculated with streptococci could be greatly increased by the injection of a nonspecific protein, such as ascitic fluid or human serum. The explanation given is that the antigenic power of the streptococci was sufficient to produce an excess of receptors, but not to liberate them from the cells. The second nonspecific stimulus served to bring about their liberation. This is a very helpful conception in interpreting some of the results obtained in clinical work.

The method of protein therapy was first employed with success in the treatment of typhoid fever and arthritis, both acute and chronic. Since its introduction it has been applied to a multiplicity of conditions, in many cases with little rational justification, and it is very important to have some basis on which the cases to be treated may be chosen. In my own work I have found that the most suitable cases are those in which there is a chronic intoxication from some focus of infection which can not be located or removed. The toxins may give rise to arthritis, myositis, neuritis, or iritis, depending on the organ whose resistance is below normal, but if the focus can be attached and the toxins neutralized, benefit will follow.

Infective arthritis is often relieved by protein injections in a manner which can only be described as extraordinary. Some cases, however, respond little or not at all, and unfortunately it is at present impossible to predict which cases will be benefited and which will not. An example of what the treatment may do is afforded by the following case:

The patient, a medical man of middle age, developed an inflammation of the throat, followed some weeks later by arthritis beginning in the ankles and passing to the knees, hips, shoulders, elbows, wrists, and fingers. It was essentially fleeting. A joint would suddenly become swollen, tender, and very painful. In a day or two the symptoms would as suddenly disappear, and the joint return to normal. The inflammation involved the synovial sheaths and fibrous tissues as well as the joints. In the intervals between the attacks, the patient, who had previously enjoyed robust health, felt in poor condition, and suffered from constant tachycardia. Even when lying at rest in bed he could feel his heart thumping against the chest wall. The pulse rate was seldom below 100. At times he broke out into a severe sweat. This state of affairs had lasted for ten weeks. At the time of the first injection the patient was unable to move in bed. He could not lift his head owing to pain in the neck. The hip was very painful, and the wrists and fingers much swollen. The pulse was 120. He was very depressed. An intravenous injection of 50 million typhoid bacilli was followed in 20 minutes by a violent rigor, in which the patient "nearly shook the bed to pieces," was drenched with perspiration, vomited freely, and felt as though he were being asphyxiated. The temperature rose to 103.2°, and there was a leucocytosis of 20,000. When I saw him five hours later I found him sitting up in bed in the highest spirits, without a trace of pain, and able to move his neck and all the joints of his body with perfect freedom. The pulse was 80. A second injection a week later again produced a sensation of choking and asphyxiation suggestion of an anaphylactic phenomenon. Since that time the patient has remained quite well, free from arthritis, tachycardia, and malaise.

The value of protein injections in arthritis is, of course, well recognized. The following case of neuritis serves to show that this treatment may be equally valuable in other forms of toxic inflammation.

The patient, a medical officer in the army, had a severe attack of tonsillitis in January, 1917. This was followed by some stiffness of the joints. In the course of a few weeks the patient developed toxic symptoms, such as malaise, profuse sweats, and attacks of tachycardia. The tonsils were removed two months later; the joints improved, and the patient felt better. In May, 1917, when in France, he fell upon his right hand, bruising it slightly. A month later he slipped and again hurt the same hand, but not at all severely. About a week afterwards he began to feel pain in the region of the injury, radiating down to the little finger and up to the elbow. Later he had attacks of redness, swelling, and tenderness over the hypothenar eminence occurring every seven to ten days with curious periodicity. These inflammatory signs gradually spread up the forearm. The condition was diagnosed by several neurologists and consulting physicians as neuritis, but no treatment was of the slightest use. In October he slightly sprained his ankle, and since then has had attacks of pain and swelling in the ankle about every ten days. In January, 1918, he was given two injections of 50 million typhoid bacilli. The first injection was followed by a feeling of tingling in the right hand, passing down to the little finger. He has remained quite free from subsequent attacks, and the power of the hand, which was much impaired, has fully returned.

These cases are samples, although certainly favorable ones, of what may be done with protein injections in toxic conditions. It will be noticed that both patients showed symptoms of general toxemia, as well as manifestations of a toxin attacking a tissue naturally weak or weakened by injury.

On looking around for other conditions of a similar toxic and focal nature, conditions in which the symptoms were probably produced by the action of toxins manufactured elsewhere than in the apparent seat of the disease, the case of toxic iritis was suggested by Harvey Smith. It is well known that a toxic focus elsewhere may set up an iritis extremely intractable to treatment and which can only be cured by the removal of the focus. The analogy to toxic arthritis was so evident that it was determined to give the method a trial.

The first case chosen was that of a young doctor who had just graduated, but who was unable to work owing to the condition of his eyes, which became so serious that entire loss of sight was threatened. In August, 1916, he first noticed small specks moving in front of the right eye, followed a little later by the appearance of a fine film. There was no pain or inflammation. In the following March the right eye became acutely inflamed and painful, and presented marked ciliary injection and other signs of serious iritis with decemititis. During the summer the eye remained fairly quiet, but in August he had an attack of iridocyclitis, this time in both eyes, following which there was marked impairment of vision. He now began to have a series of attacks which were curiously periodic in character, at first occurring every three weeks, but later at intervals of ten days. During the attacks the pain was very severe, and there was intense photophobia, ciliary congestion and contraction of the pupils.

The patient was under the care of Harvey Smith, who suggested that if ordinary treatment proved unavailing it would be worth while trying the protein injections which had been giving such good results in infective arthritis. The teeth, throat, nasal sinuses, and prostate were all carefully examined and found to be perfectly normal. The tuberculin and Wassermann tests were negative, as also was blood culture. On October 1 the tonsils were removed, but with no beneficial effect. A streptobacillus was found in a catheterized specimen of the urine, and a vaccine was prepared and given, but with no result. The condition of the eyes was steadily becoming worse, and the patient was threatened with complete loss of sight.

On November 26 an attack was due, and the patient on awakening displayed the early symptoms. An injection of 25 million typhoid bacilli was given, with the result that the attack was completely aborted. The usual general reaction was pronounced, accompanied by a leucocytosis of 18,000, but there was no local reaction in the eye—a question which had caused us considerable anxiety—and next day the eyes had returned to what may be called the interval condition. Nine days later a second injection of 50 million was given, and this time the attack was prevented. By this time a marked improvement was to be observed in both eyes, and the ciliary congestion was distinctly less. A series of five injections in all was given, by the end of which time the improvement was so great as to be almost unbelievable. The patient was soon able to discard the dark glasses which he had been wearing for many months, and has remained well up to the time of writing (June, 1919), practicing his profession.

Two other cases of what may be called toxic iritis have been treated in the same manner with satisfactory results, but in neither case was the condition nearly so advanced.

About this time a girl aged eighteen, who suffered from a very severe degree of tuberculous iritis, came under observation. Four months previously a mass of tuberculous glands had been removed from the right side of the neck. The eye condition had been treated for some months, but she was steadily getting worse. When first seen she was unable to distinguish a hand held close to the face. A diagnostic hypodermic injection of 0.5 mg. tuberculin produced a marked ocular reaction, as well as an elevation of temperature of 3 degrees, and a scarlet erythema of the skin around the operation scar in the neck. Six injections of typhoid vaccine were given, at the end of which she was able to read a letter and the time on a watch. Some time after leaving the hospital, however, the tuberculous trouble in the neck again became active, accompanied by a relapse in the eye condition.

The cases thus far treated had been examples of inflammation of the uveal tract. It hardly seemed probable that neuroretinitis would be benefited by the same line of treatment, but when a case presented itself it was decided to give the method a trial.

The patient was an Italian, thirty-two years of age, a cabinet-maker by trade. In January, 1918, he contracted syphilis. He was at once given a vigorous course of treatment, consisting of intravenous injections of salvarsan. In July the sight of the left eye began to fail, and the condition rapidly became worse. In November the right eye became affected, and the patient feared that he was going to become blind. On admission to hospital in January, 1918, the vision in the right eye was found to be $\frac{7}{10}$, but with the left eye he could only count fingers at 18 inches. There was no inflammation of the iris, but in both eyes there was a condition of neuroretinitis with edema of the disc, the condition being much more marked on the left side. It was realized that even a slight focal reaction might be accompanied by disastrous consequences, and the initial injection on January 15 consisted, therefore, of only 5 million bacilli. This produced no effect of any kind. Larger injections were then used, up to 100 million, seven in all being given. Marked improvement in the ophthalmoscopic picture was soon noticed, accompanied by steady improvement in vision. When the treatment was finished, the vision with the right eye was $\frac{10}{10}$, and with the left eye he could count fingers at 8 feet. On admission he was quite unable to read, but on discharge he could do so readily. The improvement certainly greatly exceeded any expectations that had been formed.

The conditions above described have been of the nature of focal toxic infections. There is another condition, bearing no apparent relation to the preceding, in which intravenous injections of proteins have proved of great benefit, namely bronchial asthma. The work of I. C. Walker[4] and others has shown that bronchial asthma is due in the majority of cases to a state of hypersensitiveness to foreign proteins, either animal, vegetable, or bacterial. The most scientific method of treating the disease is to discover which protein—food, pollen, bacteria, etc.—is at fault, and to gradually desensitize the patient to that protein. It has been found, however, that the condition of shock produced by the injection of an indifferent nonspecific protein results in great relief and sometimes complete cure of the asthmatic condition. There is much in common between the shock following intravenous injection of proteins and that characteristic of the anaphylactic condition. It seems probable that in this relationship is to be found the explanation of the desensitizing action of such injections.

The following case is an example of such a result:

A little girl, aged four years, had for the last two years been a martyr to bronchial asthma. The attacks, which occurred every week or two, were of ever-increasing severity, and even in the intervals there was constant wheezing. All kinds of drastic alterations in the diet had been tried, but without success. No relation to foodstuffs could be detected. It was intended to prepare a vaccine from the bronchial secretion, but no sputum could be obtained. An intravenous injection of 25 million typhoid bacilli was accordingly given during one of the paroxysms. The effect was remarkable. After a violent reaction of the usual nature, the child passed from a condition of acute distress to one of complete comfort. The asthma returned in a few days' time, but a second injection was followed by a complete cure. Here again the result greatly exceeded expectations.

Enough has been said to show that remarkable results, interesting to the scientific investigator and gratifying to the patient, may be obtained by the intravenous injection of various protein substances. A note of warning may, however, be sounded in conclusion. No method of great possibilities is safe from abuse, and the danger is especially great in the case of a method so easily applied as that under discussion. If we are to avoid falling into an unreasoning and unjustifiable empiricism, it is essential that we should try to form some mental picture of what is going on within the body, and that we should select the cases for treatment with judgment and discrimination. The criteria in forming such a judgment should apparently be evidence, general as well as local, of toxic absorption. The cases in which the most satisfactory results were obtained have been those showing such general symptoms as malaise, irregular attacks of mild pyrexia, sweating, palpitation, etc. A periodic character in the local attacks has also been noteworthy in the cases giving the best results.

NOTE: After the above work was completed it was found that a paper had appeared by L. Müller and C. Thanner in the *Medizinische Klinik,* Berlin, October 22, 1913 (abstracted in the Jour. Am. Med. Assoc., 1916, lxvii, 2041) on "Treatment of Eye Affections by Parenteral Injection of Nonspecific Protein." These workers used intramuscular injections of milk in a number of cases of iritis, and obtained favorable results. No intravenous injections were given.

BIBLIOGRAPHY

[1]Davis and Petersen: A Comparative Study of Lymph and Serum Ferments During Protein Shock Reaction. Jour. Exper. Med., November, 1917.
[2]Jobling and Petersen: The Nonspecific Factor in the Treatment of Disease, Jour. Am. Med. Assn., 1915, lxv, 515.
[3]Herrmann, S. F.: Liberation of Antibodies on Injection of Foreign Proteins, Jour. Infect. Dis., 1918, xxiii, 457.
[4]Walker, I. C.: The Treatment of Bronchial Asthma with Vaccines, Arch. Int. Med., 1919, xxiii, 220.

THE INCIDENCE OF SYPHILIS AMONG WHITE AND COLORED TROOPS AS INDICATED BY AN ANALYTICAL STUDY OF THE WASSERMANN RESULTS IN OVER TEN THOUSAND TESTS*

By William Levin, Dr.P.H., Parsons, Kans.

Late Captain, Sanitary Corps, U. S. A., Chief of Laboratory Service, U. S. Army Base Hospital, Ft. Riley, Kansas.

THE VENEREAL PROBLEM IN THE ARMY

BY far the greatest problem army authorities had to cope with during the world war was the control and eradication of venereal diseases. From time immemorial each army had its camp followers; their presence was not only tolerated but also encouraged. Venereal diseases were rampant, and their consequences far more destructive and deadly than bullet or shell. With the clearer conception of sex morality, particularly its relationship to health, attempts were made to legislate and control prostitution, and thus remove from the soldier his greatest enemy. The results were encouraging. It remained for the recent world catastrophe to demonstrate that, with proper measures, prostitution with its accompanying venereal diseases, could not only be controlled, but also eradicated. Congress, by creating the five mile zone, and the several organizations as the American Red Cross, Y. M. C. A., Jewish Welfare Board, Knights of Columbus, and the Salvation Army, by their various activities, were the factors in making the American Army the cleanest in the history of the world.

Formerly the army was considered a menace to the health of the civilians; in the present war it was demonstrated that the source of danger was not the soldier but the civilian. "Statistics show that venereal disease is much more prevalent among civilians than among soldiers. It has been positively demonstrated that instead of civilian communities needing protection against soldiers so far as venereal diseases are concerned, the soldier needs protection from civilian communities."[1] In numerous instances soldiers were not permitted to visit cities adjacent to their camps because of the unsanitary conditions existing there. Only when the sanitation of the city approached that of the camp was intercourse between the two allowed. That the civilian communities, not the army camps, were the sources of venereal diseases is well shown by a study of Tables I and II.

TABLE I

ANNUAL RATE PER 1000. VENEREAL DISEASES, U. S. ARMY[2]					
Week Ending	All- Troops in U. S.	Regulars in U. S.	Nat'l Guard, All Camps	Nat'l Army, All Camps	Expeditionary Forces
Mar. 1, 1918	97.1	121.5	53.4	100.6	44.2
Mar. 8, 1918	100.2	67.2	59.1	146.3	48.5
Mar. 15, 1918	90.6	90.4	54.6	109.8	46.0
Mar. 22, 1918	78.5	85.9	39.4	95.3	68.7

*Authority to publish granted by the Surgeon-General's Office, Washington, D. C.

These figures, taken at random for one of the months during mobilization, show that the national army men—drafted from the rank and file of our population—brought in more cases of venereal diseases than existed among the regulars, or the national guards, or the Expeditionary Forces. Sanitary regulations, and measures were the same for all camps, hence it can not be said that all cases of venereal diseases among the national army men originated in the camps. With the cessation of hostilities and the subsequent stoppage of recruiting the venereal rate fell down markedly. Table II gives a striking comparison of the venereal rate at a period when large numbers of recruits were being received at the camps, and at a period when none were being received.

TABLE II

ANNUAL RATE PER 1000. VENEREAL DISEASES: ALL TROOPS IN THE U. S. A.
AUGUST, 1918, AND NOVEMBER-DECEMBER, 1918[2]

For the Week Ending		For the Week Ending	
August 2, 1918	162.4	November 15, 1918	190.72
August 9, 1918	218.3	November 22, 1918	155.66
August 16, 1918	232.2	November 29, 1918	53.53
August ʹ23ʹ 1918	199.8	December 6, 1918	31.00
August 30, 1918	171.3	December 13, 1918	54.65

Thus far statistics have been cited for all the camps. Undoubtedly certain camps had a much higher venereal rate than others, whereas some undoubtedly had a lower venereal rate than the average of all camps. The location of the camps and particularly the states from which they drew their recruits must be given serious consideration in the study of the venereal rate. Camp Funston, Kansas, located geographically in the center of the United States, drew its recruits from an area representing equally well the urban and rural communities, the various strata of society, and the black and white races. With the incorporation of the national army into the U. S. Army men were sent to Camp Funston who represented a majority of the states of the Union. Any conclusions arrived at from data available for Camp Funston would hold true, therefore, not to any particular state or section, but to the country as a whole.

VENEREAL ADMISSIONS

Data for the venereal admissions to the Base Hospital at Fort Riley, Kansas, (which was the Base Hospital for Camp Funston), are available only from August 8, 1918. Unfortunately the figures represent all the venereal diseases, and do not indicate the prevalence of their various forms, such as syphilis, gonorrhea, and chancroid.

TABLE III

VENEREAL ADMISSIONS TO U. S. ARMY BASE HOSPITAL, FT. RILEY, KANS.,
AUGUST 8, 1918 TO MARCH 29, 1919[3]

Disease Contracted	Number of Cases	Per Cent
Before enlistment	987	64.7
After enlistment, but before arrival at camp	155	10.2
After arrival at camp	383	25.1
Total	1525	100.0

It is thus seen that 75 per cent of all venereal cases admitted to the hospital from Camp Funston* were contracted before the soldiers arrived at the camp, 65 per cent of which were contracted before enlistment.

THE WASSERMANN TEST

During the year March, 1918, to March, 1919, I made over ten thousand blood Wassermann tests on troops stationed at Camp Funston, The Medical Officers' Training Camp, and at Fort Riley. Many of these tests were made on syphilitic suspects, either to make or confirm a diagnosis of syphilis. Numerous others were made as routine tests on patients in the hospital, particularly on those to be discharged on a certificate of disability (C. D. D.). A large number of Wassermann tests were also made on men who had no syphilitic lesions or symptoms, nor who gave a history of exposure, such as candidates for commissions, etc. In short, the ten thousand tests represented men from all walks of life, both syphilitic and nonsyphilitic, and both the white and the colored races. A statistical study of· the results of these Wassermann tests would indicate, not only the prevalence of syphilis among the white and colored troops, but would also lead to a fair estimate as to its prevalence among the white and colored civilian population of the same ages.

The Wassermann test is not infallible. Wrong results have been and will be obtained so long as the various workers insist on using their own modifications of the Wassermann and Noguchi methods. So long as there is ununiformity of method will there be differences in the results and in their interpretation. The Wassermann test properly performed is a most valuable aid in the diagnosis and treatment of syphilis; improperly performed it is worse than useless. It is surprising that for such an important test an official method has not yet been adopted.

In the army the methods recommended are those described in Manual No. 6 of the Medical Department,* second edition. Both the antihuman and the antisheep hemolytic systems are allowed. The method used by the writer was essentially that used by laboratory workers in the American Expeditionary Forces. The antisheep hemolytic system was used exclusively.

Early diagnosis and early treatment of syphilis have always been emphasized in the army. A man in the hospital as a patient becomes a noneffective; for the time being he is useless to the army. His return as an effective must, therefore, be made in the shortest possible time; yet, at the same time his medical treatment must be thorough and consistent with his medical need. With that point in view the quicker a diagnosis could be made or verified by the Wassermann test the sooner would the patient be returned to the effective list. The element of time was always a most important factor of the war, equally important in the laboratory as on the field of battle.

TIME OF INACTIVATION OF NATIVE COMPLEMENT

Short cuts in the Wassermann test have been advocated and made by many workers. There is a definite time limit the lessening of which results in inaccuracy. On the other hand certain workers have advocated a time period which

---

*Camp Funston had under its jurisdiction the Fort Riley Post and the Medical Officers' Training Camp.

TABLE IV

COMPLEMENT FIXATION AS INFLUENCED BY VARYING THE PERIOD OF INACTIVATION OF NATIVE COMPLEMENT

SERUM	TIME IN MINUTES	COMPLEMENT FIXATION
1	5	—
	10	—
	15	∓
	30	±
	5	—
	10	
	15	—
	30	∓
9	5	±
	10	+
	15	+
	30	++
11	5	—
	10	∓
	15	∓
	30	+
13	5	++
	10	++
	15	++
	30	++
15	5	—
	10	
	15	—
	30	±
18	5	+
	10	++
	15	++
	30	++
20	5	++
	10	++
	15	++
	30	++
28	5	—
	10	—
	15	∓
	30	±
29	5	—
	10	
	15	—
	30	±
31	5	++
	10	++
	15	++
	30	++
38	5	+
	10	++
	15	++
	30	++

greatly exceeds that used by the majority of laboratory men, which, in my opinion, is not conducive to better results.

By a series of experiments I demonstrated that the period of inactivation of serum need not exceed thirty minutes and should not be less than that, The results are tabulated in Table IV. Small amounts of sera, not exceeding 0.3 c.c. were inactivated at varying periods of five, ten, fifteen,·and thirty minutes. After inactivation the routine test was made on all portions.

Strongly positive reacting sera need be inactivated only a very short period of time. Those sera which contain a little antibody, on the other hand, seem to require a much longer period of inactivation. All sera tested by the writer for syphilitic antibodies, the results of which are given in this paper, were inactivated for thirty minutes.

INCUBATION OF COMPLEMENT

Diversity of opinion is greater on the question of how long an incubation period is necessary for complete fixation of complement. Some authorities consider the ice box incubation method the most delicate and trustworthy. For army purposes this time-consuming method is out of the question. Speed, as well as accuracy, is necessary. Incubation in the water-bath at 37° to 38° C. is used by most workers, and was used in the Wassermann tests performed by me.

From previous experience, as well as from a fairly generally accepted custom, the incubation period decided upon for complement fixation was thirty minutes. With this incubation period it was decided to use 0.1 c.c. serum for the diagnostic test. Experiments demonstrated that this combination gave equal and at times even better fixation than using 0.05 c.c. serum and one hour incubation. This is shown in Table V.

TABLE V

COMPARATIVE RESULTS VARYING THE AMOUNT OF SERUM AND TIME OF INCUBATION

SERUM	30 MINUTES INCUBATION		60 MINUTES INCUBATION	
	0.1 c.c.	0.05 c.c.	0.1 c.c.	0.05 c.c.
39	±	±	±	±
47	++	++	++	++
49	+	—	+	±
50	+	—	+	+
52	++	++	++	++
54	++	++	++	++
57	++	+	++	++
59	++	++	++	++
67	±	—	±	—
68	±	—	±	—
71	++	++	++	++
78	++	++	++	++

Two units of amboceptor and two units of complement were used throughout. The antigen employed for the first 9000 tests was an acetone-insoluble; for the remaining tests a cholesterinized human heart extract. Using both antigens in a series of several hundred sera only a few variations occurred, and in these cases the cholesterinized antigen picked up "plus minus" reactions which were negative with the other antigen. Both antigens checked up very nicely the antisyphilitic treatment given the patients. Unfortunately no data could be gathered to show the percentage of positive Wassermann tests obtained in the various stages of syphilis. Form 97, Medical Department. U. S. Army, sent with the first blood specimen of each patient, requires the following information given: Date of infection, stage of disease, present symptoms, and clinical diagnosis. Many of the forms received at the laboratory show that the medical officers failed to give the required information.

COLLECTION OF SPECIMENS

Blood specimens were obtained according to the method described in the Medical War Manual No. 6.[4] "Paint the area over the veins at the bend of the

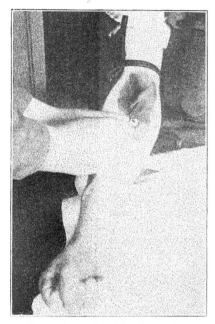

Fig. 1.—Method of obtaining blood specimen.

elbow with tincture of iodine. Apply a tourniquet to the middle of the arm and instruct the patient to extend the arm fully, open and close the hand several times, and then make a fist. The veins will become prominent and can be entered easily.

"Insert a needle of about 20 gauge* (the ordinary Luer syringe needle) into the vein, exercising great care that the needle lies flat and enters the vein almost parallel to the skin surface, thus avoiding passing through the vein.

"As soon as blood flows from the needle tilt the distal (to the patient)

*The 18 gauge was found to be the most serviceable.

end and permit the blood to run into a sterile test tube. The flow of blood can be accelerated by the patient, alternately opening and closing the fist." (Fig. 1.)

Sterility of test tubes for collecting blood specimens was disregarded; emphasis was laid rather on their cleanliness. Thorough soaking in cleaning solution followed by thorough rinsing and drying was insisted upon for all glassware. Tests were run twice weekly, and occasionally oftener when necessary. Only sixteen specimens out of more than ten thousand taken were anti-complementary, the majority of these having been taken at the detention camp during the summer.

COLLECTION OF COMPLEMENT

Collection of complement was made on the night before the "run." At least two and often three or four guinea pigs (depending upon the number of tests to be made) were bled, and the pooled blood after defibrination left in the ice box overnight. On the following morning the blood was centrifuged and the complement drawn off. A dilution of 1-10 was used in the tests. Guinea pigs were bled from the heart. With few exceptions 10 c.c. and even larger amounts of blood were drawn off without much discomfort to the animals. These used pigs, after at least ten days' rest, would be bled again. The mortality among them, using this method of bleeding, was surprisingly low.

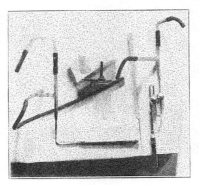

Fig. 2.—Thermoregulators, 37° C. (left) and 56° C. (right). Center: microburner for use with 56° C. Thermoregulator.

INACTIVATING AND INCUBATING BATHS

Inactivation of the sera was accomplished by heating in a water-bath at 56° C. The laboratory was fortunate in having a supply of gasoline—machine gas, which made inactivation and incubation a simple matter. While a student under Dr. F. G. Novy, I learned how to make simple thermoregulators; two of these made from glass tubing available at the Hospital Supply Depot have been in use nearly 15 months, and have given excellent service. (Fig. 2.) A galvanized iron water-bath made large enough to accommodate 20 regulation Wassermann test tube racks (200 sera specimens) was used for incubation. (Fig. 3.) The cost of the inactivating and incubating baths was very low compared to that of commercial water-baths.

An anticomplementary control, besides known negative and positive controls, was run for each serum. The results were read immediately and two hours after the final incubation. The results of the latter reading were those reported.

EXPRESSION OF RESULTS

According to the custom of the Medical Department, U. S. Army, the results of the Wassermann tests are expressed as follows:

++ Diagnostic of syphilis.

  + Not diagnostic unless there is a clear history of symptoms.

  ± Not a diagnostic reaction, but of value in indicating result of treatment.

  — A single negative does not exclude syphilis, particularly in the primary and late stages.

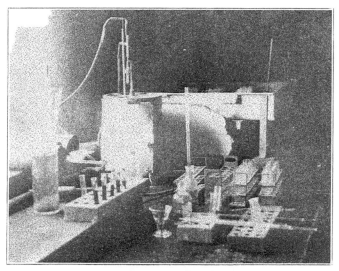

Fig. 3.—Inactivating and incubating baths.

In my opinion this nomenclature does not indicate the results so clearly as the four-plus reactions used in the majority of laboratories. Compared to the four-plus system of recording the army double-plus reaction corresponds with the four-plus; the single-plus with the three- and two-plus; and the plus-minus with the one-plus reaction.[6] Uniformity of expression of results is to be greatly desired, particularly those results indicating the course of treatment.

Simon[6] advocates the use of percentage in designating the amount of complement fixation taking place. "I should therefore propose to designate as a unit such quantity of the syphilitic antibody as requires sixty minutes incubation at from 37° to 40° C. to bring about complete fixation of a standard amount of complement. Such amount of the syphilitic antibody as is capable for fixing the same quantity of complement without any incubation whatsoever I should designate as sixty units and a reaction of the latter type I should term a 100 per cent reaction. I have chosen the above quantity as the standard unit for the reason that when one progressively dilutes a serum that in the usual dilution of 1:5 will give an instantaneous reaction, complete fixation in the highest dilution will require an incubation of sixty minutes."

Whether the syphilitic antibodies met with in the strongest double-plus reactions were insufficient or the technic of the writer faulty—although every step advocated by Simon was scrupulously followed—no instantaneous fixation of complement could be obtained. A certain amount of incubation seemed necessary with all sera. Thus Table VI giving the results on one of many sera tested, showed that 0.0125 c.c. serum which could completely fix complement in fifteen minutes could not, in 0.05 c.c. or 0.1 c.c. amounts fix complement, even to a small degree, instantaneously.

TABLE VI

THE RELATION OF THE INCUBATION PERIOD TO COMPLEMENT FIXATION

TIME OF INCUBATION IN MINUTES	TOTAL SERUM REPRESENTED			
	0.1 c.c.	0.05 c.c.	0.025 c.c.	0.0125 c.c.
0	—	—	—	—
1	—	—	—	—
2.5	±	∓	—	—
5.0	+	±	∓	—
7.5	++	++	+	∓
10	++	++	++	±
12.5	++	++	++	+
15	++	++	++	++
30	++	++	++.	++
60	++	++	++	++

While a numerical system of expression of complement fixation would be preferable to the plus reactions, more work is necessary along that line before coming to any definite conclusions. For the want of anything better the four-plus system, with its wider scope of readings, should be used.

All results given in this paper are in the double-plus system.

RESULTS OF WASSERMANN TESTS

Tables VII to X, inclusive, are the Wassermann results of blood specimens taken from the enlisted personnel only. A "first request" specimen is one taken for the first time in this laboratory. A "second request" specimen is one taken from the same individual the second time in this laboratory, etc.

From an analytical viewpoint the findings on the first request are the most interesting. Out of 6450 white soldiers examined, 680 or 10.5 per cent gave a reaction diagnostic of syphilis; out of 3039 colored soldiers, 558, or 18.3 per cent gave a reaction diagnostic of syphilis. Complete fixation of complement, therefore, was 1.74 times more frequent in the colored than in the white soldiers. A striking coincident is observed in the single-plus reaction, a reaction not considered diagnostic unless there is a clear history of symptoms. Three and three-tenths per cent of the white and 5.8 per cent of the colored soldiers gave the single-plus reaction; this reaction was 1.75 times more frequent in the colored than in the white soldiers. Practically all of those having a plus reac-

TABLE VII
WASSERMANN FINDINGS ON THE FIRST REQUEST

	WHITE		COLORED	
	Number	Per Cent	Number	Per Cent
Negative	5258	81.5	2165	71.2
Double-plus	680	10.5	558	18.3
Single-plus	213	3.3	177	5.8
Plus-minus	299	4.7	139	4.7
Total Examined	6450	100.0	3039	100.0

TABLE VIII
WASSERMANN FINDINGS ON THE SECOND REQUEST

	WHITE		COLORED	
	Number	Per Cent	Number	Per Cent
Negative	422	66.8	201	70.5
Double-plus	101	15.9	54	19.0
Single-plus	53	8.4	14	4.9
Plus-minus	56	8.9	16	5.6
Total Examined	632	100.0	285	100.0

TABLE IX
WASSERMANN FINDINGS ON THE THIRD REQUEST

	WHITE		COLORED	
	Number	Per Cent	Number	Per Cent
Negative	77	61.6	46	73.0
Double-plus	29	23.2	6	9.5
Single-plus	8	6.4	6	9.5
Plus-minus	11	8.8	5	8.0
Total Examined	125	100.0	63	100.0

TABLE X
WASSERMANN FINDINGS ON REQUESTS ABOVE THIRD

	WHITE		COLORED	
	Number	Per Cent	Number	Per Cent
Negative	44	71.0	7	43.7
Double-plus	5	8.1	4	25.0
Single-plus	9	14.5	4	25.0
Plus-minus	4	6.4	1	6.3
Total Examined	62	100.0	16	100.0

tion who were questioned personally by me gave histories of exposure, although
not all admitted symptoms of the disease. The striking similarity in the ratios
of the single-plus and double-plus reactions (1.75 in the former, and 1.74 in the
latter) might indicate that in this particular series of cases the single-plus reaction was also diagnostic of syphilis. With this assumption the percentage of
syphilis among the white soldiers would be 13.8, and among colored soldiers, 24.1.

RESULTS OF WASSERMANN TESTS ON RECRUITS

These figures are approached by results obtained by the examination of recruits suspected of having syphilis. These men had blood specimens taken immediately after going through the camp receiving station, and while still assigned
to temporary units. None of these men had any chance to contract venereal
diseases after their arrival at camp.

TABLE XI

WASSERMANN FINDINGS ON EXAMINATION OF WHITE AND COLORED RECRUITS, SYPHILITIC SUSPECTS

(a) White Recruits	(June-July, 1918)	
Result	Number	Per Cent
Negative	434	79.1
Double-plus	55	10.0
Single-plus	25	4.6
Plus-minus	35	6.3
Total Examined	549	100.0
(b) Colored Recruits	(June-July, 1918)	
Result	Number	Per Cent
Negative	821	73.8
Double-plus	194	17.4
Single-plus	60	5.4
Plus-minus	37	3.4
Total Examined	1112	100.0
(c) Colored Recruits	(October, 1918)	
Result	Number	Per Cent
Negative	143	65.3
Double-plus	39	17.8
Single-plus	15	6.8
Plus-minus	22	10.1
Total Examined	219	100.0

The Wassermann tests on 549 white and on 1331 colored recruits suspected of having syphilis, gave, therefore, practically the same percentage of positive reactions as the much larger number of tests in Table I, which included not only syphilitic suspects, but also known syphilitics, and nonsyphilitics. These results are highly suggestive of the existence of a certain definite percentage of syphilis among the white and colored troops. Leaving the single-plus reaction out of consideration and basing the percentage on the double-plus reaction alone, there would seem to be approximately 10 per cent syphilis among white troops and approximately 18 per cent syphilis among colored troops.

Vedder[7] in a very interesting and instructive article on "The Prevalence of Syphilis in the Army" states that "we may conclude that syphilis is between two and three times more prevalent among colored enlisted men than among white enlisted men." He includes the single-plus reaction in his estimate of the prevalence of syphilis, as shown in Table XII.

Love and Davenport[8] report the rate for syphilis to have been about four times as great in colored as white troops in the army that was mobilized in 1917. Thus they state: "In the army that was mobilized in 1917, the rate for syphilis was about four times as great in colored as white troops, for chancroid four and one-half times, for gonococcus infection two and one-half times. Combining the data of the last ten years the rate for all venereal diseases for colored troops is a little less than double that for whites. The difference between the races in incidence of venereal diseases is probably due partly to a difference in social pressure, partly to a difference in ability to control the sex instinct.

'This greater infection of colored troops with venereal diseases leads to the greater incidence in that race of various complications of those diseases.

TABLE XII

COMPARISON OF FIGURES OBTAINED IN SURVEYS OF WHITE AND COLORED ENLISTED MEN

TROOPS	NUMBER EXAMINED	KNOWN SYPH- ILITICS PER CENT	WASSER- MANN ++ PER CENT	UNDOUBTED SYPHILITICS PER CENT	WASSER- MANN + PER CENT	ESTIMATED PROBABLE SYPHILITICS PER CENT
White	1577	3.44	4.77	8.21	7.87	16.08
Colored	1422	1.08	21.80	22.88	13.11	36.00

Thus, retinitis, iritis, cerebrospinal meningitis, various diseases of the spinal cord—largely, probably, complication of syphilis—are commoner among the colored soldiers. Similarly, arthritis osteomyelitis, endocarditis, nephritis and urethritis—complications of gonorrhea—are two to three times commoner in colored troops than in white."

It would be safe to estimate, from the results given in this paper, the rate for syphilis to be about twice as great in colored as in white troops.

The much larger number of double-plus reactions obtained on the second request (Table VIII), is the consequence primarily of the provocative arsphenamine injection, and secondly, of the failure of certain cases to respond to treatment. Several cases, after most thorough courses of mercury and arsphenamine treatment, persisted in giving double-plus reactions, although their lesions had healed immediately. This was particularly true in four colored patients, as shown in Table X.

EFFICACY OF THE WASSERMANN TEST

The Wassermann test proved to be efficacious in the detection of syphilis where thorough physical examination had utterly failed. Thus out of 515 white candidates for the third officers' training camp, one double-plus reaction was obtained; out of 40 colored candidates one single-plus was obtained. Of the candidates for the fourth officers' training camp, all white, three double-plus and one single-plus reactions were obtained from 206 examined. All of these men had had several physical examinations, and no evidences of syphilis had been found. They had taken the Wassermann test as a matter of routine. Duplicate tests on several of the men giving positive reactions only verified the findings.

PERCENTAGE OF SYPHILIS AMONG OFFICERS AND CIVILIANS

The percentage of syphilis among officers was low. Only one double-plus reaction was obtained from 59 examined. The history of this case is interesting. Lt. C., 51 years old, a medical officer, operated on a patient, about Nov. 3, 1917, for dorsal slit of penis, and infected the index finger of the left hand. A chancre developed at the tip of the finger, but was not recognized as such, being treated for a felon. On January 7, 1918, diagnosis of chancre was made and treatment was begun. The officer at the time of his first Wassermann test at this hospital, on March 22, 1918, had well developed mucous patches. A double-plus reaction was obtained, and with intensive treatment the reaction became negative.

Civilian employees in the Camp gave as high a percentage of double-plus reactions as the colored enlisted personnel. Out of 39 examined, 7 or 18 per cent gave a double-plus reaction, and 1 or 2.5 per cent gave a single-plus reaction. Several of those found syphilitic were employed as cooks.

WASSERMANN TESTS ON SPINAL FLUIDS

The results obtained on Wassermann tests made on spinal fluids indicate that cerebrospinal syphilis was more common among the white than colored soldiers of the Camp Funston command. This is shown in Table XIII.

TABLE XIII

WASSERMANN FINDINGS ON SPINAL FLUIDS

	WHITE		COLORED	
	Number	Per Cent	Number	Per Cent
Negative	87	76.3	36	87.8
Double-plus	20	17.5	4	9.8
Single-plus	3	2.6	0	0.0
Plus-minus	4	3.6	1	2.4
Total Examined	114	100.0	41	100.0

It is of interest to note that in nine cases where the blood Wassermann was negative, 7 double-plus and 2 single-plus reactions were obtained with the spinal fluids. On the other hand six Wassermann tests on spinal fluids were negative where the blood Wassermann gave double-plus reactions. In the latter cases, however, there was clinical doubt as to the presence of cerebrospinal syphilitic symptoms, the spinal fluid Wassermann tests being used as aids in diagnosis.

TOTAL WASSERMANN TESTS FOR THE YEAR

Exclusive of the spinal fluids, 10,782 Wassermann tests were run from March 18, 1918, to March 20, 1919. These tests were practically all made by me personally, being aided by trained enlisted technicians in the routine incidental to this work. All readings (with the exception of those made when on a short leave of absence) were made by me, hence they are all comparable. Table XIV gives the results of all blood Wassermann tests made for the year March 18, 1918, to March 20, 1919.

TABLE XIV

RESULTS OF WASSERMANN TESTS FOR THE YEAR

	WHITE		COLORED	
	Number	Per Cent	Number	Per Cent
Negative	5893	79.9	2420	71.1
Double-plus	827	11.2	622	18.3
Single-plus	287	3.9	201	5.9
Plus-minus	371	5.0	161	4.7
Total Examined	7378	100.0	3404	100.0

DISCUSSION OF RESULTS

It is indeed surprising that practically the same percentages are obtained for the results for the whole year, including officers, civilians, and enlisted men, as are obtained for the results on the first request for the enlisted personnel only. It seems to indicate the existence of a definite percentage of syphilis among the white and colored soldiers. These soldiers, with very few exceptions, were between the ages of twenty-one and thirty-one. At least three fourths, and undoubtedly more, of the syphilis found among the soldiers at Camp Funston were cases existing before their arrival at the camp. Reports from the office of the Surgeon General show that by the enforcement of the regulations suppressing prostitution about the camps, fewer cases of venereal diseases occurred among the soldiers than would have been the case if these men had remained at home. It would not be rash, therefore, to assume that there existed among the civilians of the same ages, i.e., twenty-one to thirty-one years, the same, or a higher percentage of syphilis than found among the soldiers. Assuming the single-plus reaction to be diagnostic of syphilis (and there is every reason to believe in this series it is that), there would be 13.8 per cent syphilitics among the white and 24.1 per cent syphilitics among the colored civilian population, an average of 18.95 per cent. Vedder in his survey of syphilis in the army concludes, "that among the (white) young men in civil life between the ages of 20 and 30, and of the general class belonging to the occupations mentioned, the percentage of syphilis may be estimated at at least 16.77 per cent, and there is a good reason for believing that it is fully 20 per cent." Vedder named 98 occupations, representative practically of every stratum of society.

CONCLUSIONS

1. Wassermann tests made for a year at the U. S. Army Base Hospital, Fort Riley, Kansas, indicated the existence of a definite percentage of syphilis among the white and colored troops.

2. Based on the double-plus reactions alone, there were 10.5 per cent syphilitics among the white and 18.3 per cent syphilitics among the colored soldiers.

3. Considering the single-plus reactions in this series also diagnostic, the percentage of syphilitics was 13.8 for the white and 24.1 for the colored soldiers.

4. Estimate is made that the same and probably higher percentages of syphilitics exist among the white and colored civilians of the ages 21 to 31.

Acknowledgment is made of the loyal and highly efficient service of the enlisted technicians who aided in this work, particularly that of Private First Class, Theodore C. Buck.

BIBLIOGRAPHY

[1]Vaughan, V. C.: The Selective Service Act and Its Lessons, Jour. Lab. and Clin. Med., 1919, iv, 511.
[2]Compiled from telegraphic reports, Surgeon-General's Office.
[3]Compiled from weekly reports, Urologist, U. S. Army Base Hospital, Fort Riley, Kansas.
[4]Medical War Manual No. 6. Laboratory Methods of the U. S. Army. Second edition, 1919.
[5]Craig, Charles F.: The Technic of the Complement Fixation Test for Syphilis, Am. Jour. Syph., 1917, i, No. 4.
[6]Simon, Charles E.: The So-called Doubtful or Partial Wassermann Reactions, Jour. Am. Med. Assn., 1919, lxxii, No. 21, p. 1535.
[7]Vedder, Edward B.: The Prevalence of Syphilis in the Army, Bull. 8, June, 1915, Surgeon-General's Office.
[8]Love, A. G., and Davenport, C. V.: A Comparison of White and Colored Troops in Respect to Incidence of Disease, Proc. Nat. Acad. Sc., 5, No. 3, March, 1919.

A STUDY OF THE TONICITY OF THE SPHINCTER AT THE DUODENAL END OF THE COMMON BILE DUCT

(*With Special Reference to Animals Without a Gall Bladder*)

By F. C. Mann, M.D., Rochester, Minn.*

PREVIOUS work on the function of the gall bladder has shown that cholecystectomy is usually followed by dilatation of all the extrahepatic ducts. This dilatation is dependent on an intact sphincter at the end of the common bile duct. This would seem to imply that there is some relation between the action of the sphincter and that of the gall bladder, a possibility which has been used by Oddi and Meltzer in explaining the cause of some of the diseases of the biliary tract. In a study of the anatomy of the sphincter, no difference was found in species of animals with a gall bladder as compared to those without one.[3] A comparable study of its physiology was therefore made.

The physiologic action of the sphincter at the duodenal end of the common bile duct has been studied, though only in the dog and the cat, by Oddi, Archibald, and Rost; although only the two former investigators measured the tone of the sphincter. Oddi found that the sphincter in the dog withstood a pressure of about 50 mm. mercury, or an equivalent of 675 mm. of water. Archibald found that the sphincter in this same species withstood a pressure as high as 600 mm. of water. Both investigators found that mechanical or chemical irritation throws the sphincter into a spasm.

A series of observations on the physiologic action of the sphincter has been made in our laboratory; a complete report will be made later. The present article deals only with a comparison of the tone of the sphincter in species with a gall bladder as compared with those without one. We had access for this research to only two species in which the gall bladder was lacking, the rat and pocket gopher (G. bursarius).† For controls, the dog, cat, goat, rabbit, striped gopher (C. tridecemlineatus), and guinea pig were used.

The method of estimating the tone of the sphincter was simple. The animal was lightly etherized; in a few experiments urethan was used, a cannula was carefully placed in the common bile duct (in the species without a gall bladder in the hepatic duct), as far as practicable from the duodenum with its point directed toward the duodenum. A T-tube was attached to the cannula and one arm of the tube was arranged so that it could be connected to a syringe; the other arm was connected to a straight glass tube. This T-tube was about 50 cm. in length and had an internal bore of approximately 2.5 cm. The glass tube was graduated in millimeters. Great care was taken to keep the duodenum protected during the operative procedures.

The tone of the sphincter was estimated by two methods: First, an aqueous eosin solution was passed slowly and cautiously into the tube until the point at

*Section on Experimental Surgery. Mayo Foundation. Rochester, Minn.

†These experiments were completed in 1917, but publication was delayed because of attempts to obtain data from a larger number of s, eries lacking a gall bladder. The pigeon and horse were used, but technical difficulties caused failure.

which it began to flow into the intestine was reached. The findings were recorded. Second, the solution was passed quickly into the tube to a high pressure and the point noted at which it ceased to flow into the intestine. In both instances the length of the column of water, after the fluid became stationary, was taken as a measure, expressed in millimeters, of the tone of the sphincter. The specific gravity

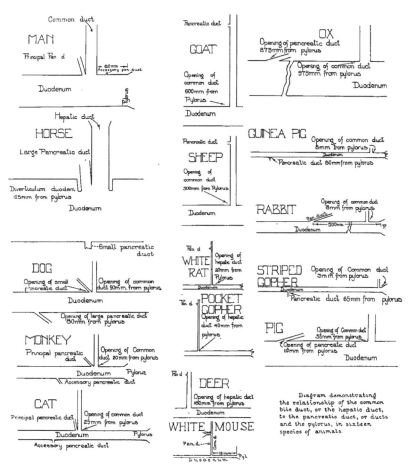

Diagram demonstrating the relationship of the common bile duct, or the hepatic duct, to the pancreatic duct, or ducts and the pylorus, in sixteen species of animals.

of the eosin solution was but slightly greater than that of distilled water and, since the study was a comparative one, this difference was ignored. The solution was either at body or room temperature. Care was taken to have the system free from air before beginning observation. It is obvious that this method does not give absolutely the correct measure of the tone of the sphincter as there are many complicating factors and sources of error. The major portion of the errors may be attributed to two causes: First, the pressure taken as the measure of the duct might be due to other factors, such as friction, etc., thus making the reading greater than it should be. Second, the anesthetic and operative manipulation might decrease the muscle tone, tending to make the measured pressure less than the pressure of the duct really was. As a matter of fact both of these factors were found to be sources of error, but they were in the main obviated so that an approximate reading could be made. The amount that the reading was complicated by resistance to outflow other than that produced by the tone of the sphincter was determined by taking another reading after deep etherization, bleeding, and formalin injections into the duct and after the death of the animal. It was thus determined that the residual pressure was practically a measure of the tone of the sphincter in large ducts, as in the dog and goat: in the smaller animals, a correction of 10 per cent might occasionally have to be made. The part the anesthetic played in complicating the experiment was studied by using ether, urethan, and, in the case of the dog, the development of a method of studying the action of the sphincter in an unanesthetized animal. From the results of the control methods, it seemed that the anesthetic as administered did not offer a very great source of error. The operative manipulations also produced changes, either an increase or a decrease in the tone of the sphincter. Peristalsis was also considered, because peristaltic waves affect the outflow from the common bile duct.

The pressure which seemed to measure the tone of the sphincter was found to vary considerably in the different species and different individual animals. However, the sphincter in each species of animal possessing a gall bladder, except the guinea pig, withstood a minimum pressure of 100 mm. water; sometimes the pressure was much greater, very rarely it was less. In the guinea pig, the pressure withstood was rarely more than 75 mm. and frequently considerably lower; this seemed to be due to the fact that as the common bile duct is very short in this species, the trauma incident to the insertion of the cannula was great. In a very few animals of other species the sphincter did not seem to have any tone.

The pocket gopher and rat were the only suitable species without a gall bladder obtainable for investigation of the tone of the sphincter. The results of a large number of experiments are the same; in no instance was any pressure, or at the most only a very slight pressure, usually not more than 30 mm., maintained by the sphincter. In most cases, all the fluid passed into the duodenum, leaving only a very slight residual pressure.

As I have stated, it was very difficult because of many complicating errors to evaluate the results in this investigation. In the dog and cat, which had been studied by previous investigators, our results did not show that the sphincter withstood so great a pressure as that recorded by others. On the other hand some evidence of a sphincteric tone was found in each species with a gall bladder. Even in the guinea pig there was definite evidence of this action. No such evidence was obtained in the two animals lacking a gall bladder, the rat and the pocket gopher, although many experiments were performed. When the mass of data from a large series of experiments is considered, this distinction between the two groups of species becomes very clear.

SUMMARY

The tone of the sphincter at the duodenal end of the common bile duct was studied in species of animals possessing a gall bladder and in two species in which the gall bladder is lacking. It was found that the tone of the sphincter under the experimental conditions studied varied considerably in the different animals and various species. In each species possessing a gall bladder, however, the sphincter was usually able to withstand a minimum pressure of from 75 to 100 mm. water. In the species lacking a gall bladder, the sphincter would not withstand pressure, or only pressures of less than 30 mm. water. While anatomic studies have shown that a sphincter is present in each species lacking a gall bladder, the sphincter does not seem to functionate appreciably.

BIBLIOGRAPHY

¹Archibald, E.: Does Cholecystenterostomy Divert the Flow of Bile from the Common Duct? Canad. Med. Assn. Jour., July, 1912, ii, 557-562.
The Experimental Production of Pancreatitis in Animals as the Result of the Resistance of the Common Duct Sphincter, Surg. Gynec. and Obst., June, 1919, xxviii, 529-545.
²Judd, E. S., and Mann, F. C.: The Effect of Removal of the Gall Bladder, An Experimental Study, Surg., Gynec. and Obst., April, 1917, xxiv, 437-442.
³Mann, F. C.: A Comparative Study of the Anatomy of the Sphincter at the Duodenal End of the Common Bile Duct with Special Reference to Species of Animals without a Gall Bladder. (In manuscript.)
⁴Meltzer, S. J.: The Disturbance of the Law of Contrary Innervation as a Pathogenetic Factor in the Diseases of the Bile Ducts and the Gall Bladder. Am. Jour. Med. Sc., April, 1917, cliii, 469-477.
⁵Oddi, R.: D'une disposition à sphincter spéciale de l'ouverture du canal cholédoque, Arch. ital. de biol., 1887, viii, 317-322. Sulla tonicità dello sfintere del coledoco, Arch. per le sc. med., xii, 333-339, 1888.
⁶Rost, F.: Die funktionelle Bedeutung der Gallenblase. Experimentelle und anatomische Untersuchungen nach Cholecystektomie, Mittl. a. d. Grenzgeb. d. Med. u. Chir., xxvi, 710-770, 1913.

FURTHER STUDIES IN PLASMOGENESIS[1]

BY ALPHONSO L. HERRERA,[2] MEXICO CITY, MEXICO

I N a previous article[3] I showed that many of the morphologic characteristics of living cells can be mimicked through the action of the vapors of hydrofluoric acid upon glass. Similar forms (as shown in 21, 15, 33 and 39 of Fig. 1) may be obtained by allowing the acid to act upon a dry potassium silicate. Such products, however, become very hard. To obtain moist preparations, I have followed the old technic of Harting. A crystallizing dish, 18 cm. in diameter, is filled with 250 c.c. of colloid silica.[4] The colloid may be made by dialysis or by an easier and more rapid process which I have worked out. It consists in dissolving gelatinous silica, newly precipitated and well washed, in a solution of ammonia water of a density of 26°, the silica being added until all the ammonia

¹Translated from the Spanish by Dario Gutiérrez-Laserna of Bogotá, Colombia, S. A.
²Director of Laboratories and the Study of Biology in the Museum of Natural History of Mexico.
³Herrera, A. L.: Some Studies in Plasmogenesis, Jour. Lab. Clin. Med., 1919, iv, 479.
⁴A solution of sodium silicate of a density of 1.020 may be used instead of the colloid silica since the latter is difficult to prepare though it yields better results.

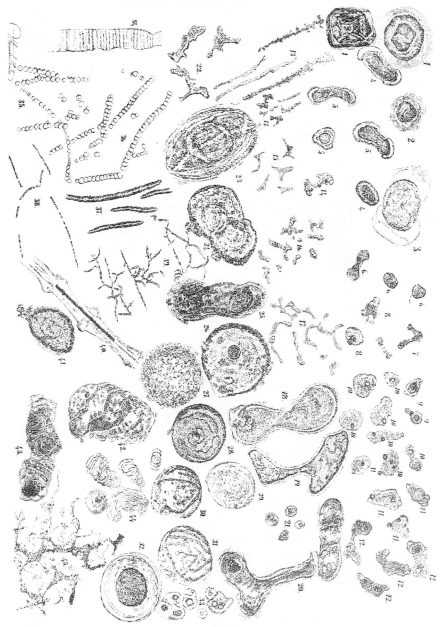

Fig. 1.

is driven off and the mixture has attained a density of not less than 1.032.[5] There are now placed in the crystallizing dish (see Fig. 2) and opposite each other and close to its walls 0.10 to 0.20 centigrams of crystallized potassium bifluoride and 5 gm. powdered, anhydrous calcium chloride.[6] The vessel is covered and kept at a temperature of 15° C. At the end of 24 hours there may be seen in the silica coagulated by the calcium chloride numerous structures which mimic nucleated amebæ (14, 16, 17, 6 to 12, 13, 18, 19, 20, 22 of Fig. 1), often in a state of subdivision (18); nucleated cells (23 to 29); nuclear spiremes (30 and 31); granular nuclei arranged in rows (40) or irregularly (41); egg-like structures (32); and granular or honeycomb structures reminiscent of protoplasm (45).

If alcohol is added to the mixture, complex spirals result (as shown in 42, 43, and 44 of Fig. 1). None of these structures appear if the original silica

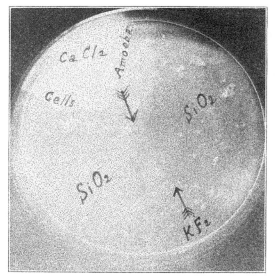

Fig. 2.

solution is too acid or too alkaline or if the reacting substances are impure. The structures do not affect polarized light, they resist acetic acid, alcohol and xylol and can be stained with dyes and fixed in Canada balsam.

These experiments show how easily the structures characteristic of protoplasm may be imitated and with nothing but inorganic materials. That fluorine derivatives should be so effective is important because Gautier has demonstrated the presence of fluorine in all organisms and has emphasized its rôle in the fix-

[5]The solution must contain from at least 3 to 5 percent of the solid silica. The finished solution, if of a density below 1.017, does not yield the structures about to be described.

[6]To delay rate of diffusion it is well to use a solution of calcium chloride in a porous cup. Or sea water may be employed which contains the chlorides of calcium and magnesium. The latter form is interesting since it is believed that life originated through meeting of sea water with the sweet waters of the land containing silica.

ation of phosphorus. The question, therefore, again presents itself whether fluorine may not in fact represent the morphologic basis of the cell, either in combination with silicon or with organic atomic complexes. It is of interest in this connection that there exist more than a hundred organic compounds of fluorine and a great many of silicon. The fact that egg-albumin does not yield these various morphologic structures as readily as do the colloid silicates seems to me to argue against the protein theory of the origin of living matter.

EXPLANATION OF RESULTS

After contact, following slow diffusion, the potassium bifluoride and the silica unite to form a fluosilicate which decomposes the calcium chloride giving origin to diffusion figures and spherocrystals. Two forces are active, first, the centrifugal one of diffusion (which tries to separate and enlarge the forms), and second, the centripetal one of crystallization (which tends to give short forms). If equilibrium prevails, ovules are produced. When the silica is coagulated, precipitation membranes are formed which, when they enclose a crystal of potassium or calcium fluosilicate, may yield osmotic sacs. In 34 and 39 of Fig. 1 there seems to have occurred a peculiar secondary infiltration of some kind in combination with the two forces mentioned. The addition of alcohol makes for more active diffusion figures which may then give rise to spirals (42 to 44). The advantages of the whole method depend upon the fact that the fluosilicates yield simultaneously a colloid (calcium silicate) and a erystalloid (calcium fluoride) which in combination yield ultramicroscopic granules.

CONCLUSIONS

The described experimental procedure is the best thus far known for the production of forms which imitate amebæ, cells in the process of subdivision, structures simulating protoplasm, etc. A gradual hardening of the structures, or their degeneration to crystals, may be avoided by using a sufficiently high concentration of the silica. This factor is of more influence than that of mere chemical composition.

As previously emphasized, no such "protoplasmic" structures are obtainable if eggwhite is used, which fact I think argues against the organic theory of the origin of living matter. Fluorine, it seems to me, might, because of its affinity for silica, be an element of great morphogenetic importance and the inorganic bridge over which the production of organic materials be attained. Fluorine and silicon are certainly the elements which serve best for the imitation of the living forms; and these forms show the slow, ameboid movements of their biologic counterparts.

SEX ATTRACTION*

By Victor C. Vaughan, M.D., Ann Arbor, Mich.

IN many of the lower forms of life there is no sex. The bacillus elongates, divides transversely, and two individuals come from one. Which is the parent and which is offspring? There is no such thing as parenthood and no such relationship as father, mother, son or daughter. The unicellular organism is potentially immortal, and given suitable conditions it might continue to multiply by fission indefinitely and eternally. As multicellular organisms develop, differentiation in structure and function begins. Certain cells are set apart to perform certain definite functions which are essential to the welfare of the whole. In the unicellular organism, all the functions of life are executed by the one cell. It feeds, absorbs, assimilates and eliminates. It maintains itself and procreates for the future. Evidently such forms of life are capable of only a limited development. The higher multicellular organism is limited in its development only by the extent to which differentiation in structure and function can go. This determines the possible evolution of the species. As the scale of existence rises, differentiation becomes more complex and the limits beyond which evolution can not go are extended. In this way sex has been developed. Reproductive organs are developed, and the extent to which this is done determines the position of the species in the scale of existence. At one point in the evolution of life the male and female reproductive organs are found in the same individual. Evidently the evolution of a species provided with this form of reproduction is limited, consequently differentiation proceeds and results in the production of male and female. Certain individuals become responsible for only the male elements essential to procreation, while other individuals are assigned the task of supplying the female elements. Thus, it happens that in the higher plants and animals there are males and females; and the most perfect product of evolution, the genus homo, consists of man and woman. In this genus there is the most perfect development of the sex function. In no other species is the exercise of the sex function so completely under the control of the individuals who possess it. In plant fertilization it is dependent wholly upon the season. Even in the higher animals sexual desire lies dormant the greater part of the time, and asserts itself only as a cyclic physiologic process. Furthermore, there are some good reasons for believing that this holds good to some extent among primitive peoples. It seems that the sexual appetite has grown with the evolution of the race. It has been stated by certain travelers among primitive peoples that lapses from chastity among their women are less common than among us. I do not vouch for the truth of these statements, neither am I in a position to deny them. It certainly is true that in no other species is the reproductive act so under the control of those who participate in it as in the case of man. To some this may seem an unpleasant and even a terrifying statement, but I think when properly understood, it is a most cherishing and hopeful condition. It places the responsibility where it belongs. It makes the par-

* A lecture before the Michigan State Normal School, August, 1919.

ent responsible for the child. In this lies the possibility of the unlimited improvement of the race. It clothes parenthood with a sacred obligation which no man or
woman worthy to assume this function can ignore. It shows that the creature,
man, has been raised by the process of evolution until he has become a coworker
with the creator in the uplift of the race, and that the future of our kind is largely
within man's power to make or to mar, to illume or to darken, to fill with the joy
of life or with the regret of having been born.

I wish to recall a statement I made concerning the unicellular organism that
multiplies by fission. I stated that this organism is potentially immortal. The
same is true of man. The difference between the two is not so great as at first
seems. Man consists of two kinds of cells, the somatic and the reproductive.
The former constitute what we know as the man, but all his somatic cells are out-
growths from the reproductive cells and serve the individual through this short
life. His brain, muscle, liver, stomach, bones etc., are ephemeral. His immortal
part is the reproductive cell. This possesses the potentiality of eternal life, and
it goes on from generation to generation. Life is continuous. The somatic cells
constitute the temporary abiding place of the reproductive cells, and the latter are
influenced by the former, more or less, in each generation. In this way the character of the parent is transmitted. Men are mortal, but man is immortal. The
individual dies, but the race continues. Each individual is a part of the whole,
and the perfection of the whole depends upon the soundness of the individual.
We may have our different views concerning individual immortality; but as to the
continuance of the race, there can be no discussion; and each generation has been,
and will continue to be, what preceding generations have made it. Even those
who do not directly participate in the continuance of the race have much to do
with shaping its destiny by the influence they have on those of the direct line.
There is therefore no one to whom this is not a matter of vital concern.

I have spoken of the differentiation which has led to the development of the
sexes in man. It may be well to inquire as to how far this has gone in our species.
How different are men and women? To what extent has the development of sex
affected the whole structure? We need not be surprised if we learn that the
evolution of so important a function as this has led to differences more or less
marked in every part of the body, and that these differences have touched the
finest and most delicate mechanism of life, even the intellectual and moral being.
On this point we can not speak at present with absolute certainty. This is a
problem with which science is at present busy, but we can say that it is probable
that delicate, but appreciable and even measurable, differences between the male
and female exist in every cell of our bodies. This is a matter which is giving the
educator, the psychologist, and the physician much concern, and one upon which
no one is yet prepared to speak with absolute certainty. While this is true, there
are certain things which seem to be quite definitely demonstrated and upon which
I propose to touch. While the sex function has been developed primarily for
the purpose of procreation, it has come to be a mighty factor in the development
of the character and well-being of the individual. No man can escape the fact
that he is male, and no woman that she is female. This recognition of structural
and functional differences does not imply inferiority in either. The sexual glands
elaborate an internal secretion which permeates every tissue, modifies every func-

tion, and colors our most secret being. Children are practically neuter, but with
the development of the reproductive glands, the rate and manner of growth
change according to the sex. Remove these glands before puberty and the neuter
state or infantilism persists. Any man or woman may go through life with the
average health, doing good work, either physical or mental, bearing himself hon-
orably and treating others justly and kindly without once indulging in the procreative act. Absolute continence is compatible with health, efficiency, and happiness, but disease of the sexual glands is incompatible with any and all of these.
No young woman is under any compunction to accept the rake. The spinster
state is perfectly respectable and is compatible with a long, happy, and useful life;
while she who weds the young man who has been sowing his wild oats is likely
to go to the operating table within a short time, and to spend the rest of her life
in regret. I have touched upon this point in order to make it plain that sexual
health is essential to the well-being of the individual, as well as to the betterment
of the race.

The differentiation which has been necessary in the development of the sexes
in the genus homo has made one the complement to the other. From this, sex
attraction results. By sex attraction I mean the pleasure and the mutual satisfaction that come to two persons of opposite sexes when brought into association.
It may be quite apart from the function of reproduction. Under normal conditions the mother has a warmer spot in her heart for her sons than for her
daughters, while with the father this is reversed. In the children affection follows like lines. The normal big brother would lay down his life for his sister, be
she older or younger than he, while he would be unwilling to make so great a
sacrifice for his brother. Under normal conditions there is much more pleasure
experienced in rendering a service to one of the opposite, than to one of the same,
sex. Likewise, there is greater appreciation of a service rendered when the
doer is of the opposite sex. Words of approbation fall upon more eager ears
when they come from the lips of the opposite sex. This theme might be amplified
indefinitely, but I do not think that any one will question the all-pervading influence of sex—for good or ill. It follows us through the daily routine and becomes an important factor in every decision. It quickens our ambitions, modifies
and often determines our conduct, and weaves the delicate structure of our
dreams. It is a potent agent in either direction. . It may fill the cup of life with
a nectar fit for the gods, or it may drop into the sweet drink a poison which destroys body, mind, and soul. It may lift to the highest heaven or it may cast into
the deepest hell.

We who are engaged in the education of the young should always bear in
mind both the good and the ill that may come to those under our care from sex
attraction. We should not ignore its existence, because it is a biologic function.
It develops in the youth of both sexes at the period of adolescence with some degree of suddenness, and they as a rule are quite unconscious of its significance
and wholly ignorant of its potency, and especially of the harm it may do them.
Its influence is widely different in individuals. In those of good ancestry and
under favorable environment the effects are favorable, and the girl and boy
flower into womanhood and manhood; but in those of defective parentage or
living under untoward conditions, the results may be most disastrous. The steps

of many a girl are turned into downward paths at this period of development. Especially is this true of those who are weak mentally. Prostitution is largely recruited from those of this class, and thoughtful educators are recognizing the fact that many of our schools are not free from these dangers. Being a male, I am inclined to make a special plea for the girls. My deepest sympathy is with them in a most trying period of their development, at a time when they most need wise counsel and help. The girl blooming into womanhood feels this natural and persuasive desire to attract those of the opposite sex, and in her ignorance she falls at least a half willing victim to the lust of some villainous male. She dresses and deports herself under the influence of this potent and subconscious force, and in doing so she risks her all, quite unconscious of the existence of the pit into which she is to fall. It might be said that parents are to blame for this condition. Mothers should caution and protect their daughters. So they should, but many mothers are ignorant, and from a sense of prudery, it is not considered a proper thing for even a mother to speak to her daughter about matters pertaining to sex. Moreover, however wise the precepts of the home, there is the example set at school. Other girls do this and mother belongs to a past generation. She is not supposed to know how girls of the present day should deport themselves. That the behavior of the girls in many of our high schools invites disaster can not be denied. Unpleasant facts have bared themselves to the eyes of teachers and the public, and a task lies before us which we can not shirk. A friend of mine, an observant and intelligent physician in one of the larger cities of the middle West told me some years ago that the street in front of one of the high schools of his city was converted into a peacock alley every noon hour when the weather permitted. The young lady students dressed to attract men and deported themselves with the plain intention of inviting address from the rakes who came to see the parade. A shocking condition of sexual degeneracy came to light in the high school of a smaller city in the Northwest about the same time, and there is undeniable evidence that this is not the only place where such things have occurred. The school is not the only place where the impulse to attract the opposite sex leads the girl astray; but we are teachers, and are especially interested in the school problem. Before proceeding I wish to state that I am not a pessimist, and I do not wish to appear as an alarmist. I believe that the world is better on the whole than it has ever been, and I am aware of the fact that in all ages girls by the thousands have gone astray, but we want the world to hasten its pace toward perfection, and because an evil condition is as old as the world is no reason that it should continue, but all the more reason why we, recognizing it as evil, should cast it out.

What may be done to save the school girl from the dangers of sex attraction? It is well to recognize at the outset that the problem is a complex one, and there is no ready-made and safe way of solving it. Those who undertake to handle it must be tactful and resourceful. Stern commands and prohibitions are likely to fall on deaf ears or to awaken an antagonism which surely means defeat. The experience of the past has shown that even locks, bars, and prison walls are not effective means in attempts to save the silly girl who wishes to throw herself into the arms of some rake. Should the parent be consulted and warned? The answer to this must be determined by the individual case. It is sad, but true, that some mothers encourage their daughters in their attempts to attract the opposite sex. They are proud to have their daughters admired and are not inquisitive concerning the character of the admirer. I think that much may be done, especially by female teachers, in discouraging flashy dressing. Plain, neat, clean, inexpensive dress best becomes the school girl. Both in dress and in deportment the female teacher should be a model to the girls under her charge. I believe that instruction, by the proper person, in the fundamental biologic facts of sex should be given to the girls in all our high schools. I doubt seriously the wisdom of attempting this in the lower grades. When girls reach the age of puberty they should know themselves and the dangers to which they are quite sure to be exposed. They should know the fundamental facts of anatomy, physiology, and hygiene, and the application of these to themselves. They should be instructed how to keep themselves healthy and free from contamination. They should be told that the men whom they are likely to attract by artificial means are exactly the ones whom they should avoid. Ignorance on these points has been tried for centuries, and it has been demonstrated that the results have been disastrous. Let us try knowledge. The truth, properly stated, can hurt no one. Talks upon these subjects can be given to girls by either male or female teachers without embarrassment to either speaker or audience, and with profit to the latter. This statement is not made on theoretical grounds, but it has been tested in our normal schools and universities. There are in this audience teachers who have demonstrated this. I think it best that the lectures dealing with this subject of sex should be a part of a course in general hygiene. In my lectures to the girls at the university I have followed the following general plan: The general anatomy of the female pelvis; the location of the ovaries, fallopian tubes, uterus, and vagina, and the function of each. I have dwelt upon the internal secretion of the ovaries and its great influence upon the health, development, and well-being of the individual. I have attempted to show that healthy secretions can come only from healthy organs. Then I have gone without hesitancy into the diseases which damage these organs. This has been done by others, and by some much better than I have done it. I have never known of a girl bearing herself less modestly on account of this knowledge, and many have testified to its value to them. If such instruction can be given to the girls in our normal schools and universities, why should it not be given to their sisters in the high school? Indeed, this has been done, and is now being done, in more than one high school in this state. The great majority of girls have no education beyond the high school. Some say that the trouble begins in the lower grades, and if this instruction does not reach these, it fails in its purpose. I am painfully aware of the fact that there is much sexual nastiness among both girls and boys in our ward schools. Every physician knows this, but to my mind, this is quite apart from the question of teaching sex hygiene. It is another problem, and it is to be solved by stricter attention to the children, especially in the retiring rooms. Parents also can do much in improving this most undesirable condition.

I do not suppose that instruction in sex hygiene is going to save all the girls. There are thousands of children, even in this country, growing up under conditions, outside of their school life, which render it impossible for them to develop into good citizens. This is quite as impossible as it is for tropical fruits to grow in arctic regions. A few years ago, in Ann Arbor, within a stone's throw of one of the university buildings there lived a woman and her two daughters, the elder no more than sixteen, and all three were prostitutes. That like conditions exist elsewhere there can be no reason to doubt. This family was detected by our efficient probation officer, who, unlike most of those filling this office, is not blind. We boast of our civilization, but there are still many among us who would be stoned to death should they attempt to live in a tribe of savages.

There are sexual perverts among girls as well as boys. The majority of these come from bad stock, are weak intellectually, belong to the alarmingly large class of morons, and constitute a menace to the betterment of the race. When bad environment is added to bad heredity, girls of this class are well-nigh incorrigible. Many of them have pretty, doll-like faces, and are highly attractive to the foolish and over-susceptible of the opposite sex. Instruction will be largely wasted on these, because they are devoid of the mentality necessary to receive it. Unfortunately there are some of these in most of our large schools, and they present a most difficult problem. I believe that in the medical inspection of schools, which has already demonstrated its great usefulness, mental as well as physical tests should be applied to all, and the defective should be assigned to special schools, supplied with experts in dealing with delinquents. This task should be assigned to most tactful and experienced men and women, because it is liable to meet with a storm of protest which in many instances is sure to render its execution impossible.

In the teaching of sex hygiene the boy needs to be handled quite differently from the girl. In sex approach under natural conditions the male is the aggressor. This is physiologic, and it should be understood by both sexes. It has been said with bitterness by women that man is ready to defend a woman's virtue against every other man but himself. There is truth in this saying, and it has a physiologic basis which is often woefully abused by the man. It is man's nature to demand, and it is woman's natural inclination, under certain conditions, to yield. In the sex relationship, under normal conditions, the male is masterful and the woman despises the man who is not. Failure to understand and appreciate this fact will rob the teaching of sex hygiene of half its influence on boys. Boys should be plainly told all about the effects of gonorrhea and syphilis, but don't try to frighten them with the great injury that may come to them personally from these diseases. To the average normal boy the element of personal danger is an incentive to find out for himself. Appeal to his chivalry. Tell him that if he acquires syphilis he becomes a walking culture of most virulent organisms, that mucous patches will develop on his tongue and cheeks, and that his mother or sister can not kiss him without danger of infection, that he poisons every cup from which he drinks and that he becomes a source of danger to those who are dearest to him; that he can never love a pure girl without polluting her with a most loathsome disease, and that he is unfit for parenthood and ceases to be a man in any proper sense. Then go on and awaken his chivalry for the girl whom he may seduce by surprise; tell how the girls trusts and how unmanly it is to betray a trust. I am in the habit of saying to the boys in my classes: "I have lectured to you on heredity. I have shown that you and I are what our ancestors have made us: while I have been giving these talks each of you has been wondering what kind of ancestors he has. Change your point of view; project yourself some years into the future. Then some boy will be wondering what kind of ancestors he had. He will be thinking of you, and it may be that thirty or fifty years from now some young man will be carried to the insane asylum a hopeless and helpless paretic because you, his father or grandfather, got drunk and acquired syphilis." Boys who do not see the force and justness of this argument are by nature bad.

There are boys who seem beyond the reach of any argument. A young man entered this university last fall, and as he afterwards admitted, went fresh from the lectures on venereal diseases to a house of prostitution in Detroit and acquired syphilis. He spent a part of the second semester in University Hospital where he served as an object lesson in the clinics. The idea that prostitution should be permitted in any city or anywhere is a relic of the past of which we should free ourselves. The existence of houses of prostitution renders it all too easy for young men to do themselves irreparable harm. An efficient and honest police force can free any city from every form of this vice. That there is an awakened conscience in this matter is shown by the enactment and enforcement of the Mann law, by the attention now being given to the low wages of girls and by the efforts being made in our cities to suppress this form of vice. What would we think of a city which would permit centers of smallpox infection to exist within their limits. Smallpox is mild in its effects upon the individual and negligible in its disastrous and far-reaching effect upon the community compared with the great pox, syphilis. The former may scar the faces of many and kill a few, while the latter fills insane asylums with its wretched victims, scatters its virus among the innocent, and blights future generations with its withering curses. I have spoken of the parade of silly school girls on the streets of a western city, but let me tell you of a condition which recently existed in one of our large eastern cities. This story was told me by a physician resident of that place. There is a school for boys of from fourteen to sixteen years. This physician thought of placing his son in this school, and preparatory to doing so he made an investigation of the conditions surrounding it. He found that prostitutes gathered about this school as the hour of closing approached, for the purpose of captivating the boys. Think of the painted harlot who waits at the gate of the school to personally conduct the innocent boys through the gates of hell. Think of this condition and ask yourself how far are we yet from true civilization. There is, so far as I know, but one country in the world which makes legal provision for the punishment of the female seducer, and that is the country which we are taught to regard as the most licentious—France. Every large city and many smaller ones permit vampires to lure unwary youths into gilded dens of infamy. Some one should organize a society for the protection of our sons.

We should deal with the venereal diseases as we do with other infectious diseases. Those who contract them should be reported, as we do with smallpox, and then segregated, not in houses of prostitution, but in hospitals. I believe in the segregation of prostitutes both male and female, but not in places where the disease may be disseminated, but where this is impossible. Please do not misunderstand me on this point. I would not deal harshly with any unfortunate. It is not within the province of the medical man to do so. I would not damn any one for making a mistake, especially a mistake dependent upon a frailty so common to man as this. To contract a venereal disease is not a crime; it is a misfortune, a sad misfortune, and one which unfortunately is not always remediable. To infeet another with a venereal disease is a crime, a moral if not a legal one. In this state it is a statutory crime, and one open to serious punishment. We have been harsh and unreasonable in our judgments at least with unfortunates of this class. We have said no one contracts these diseases without committing a deadly sin and he deserves whatever punishment his transgression may bring. We forget the thousands of innocent wives who become infected. We forget the tens of thousands of crippled children who come into the world under a fearful handicap. We refuse to instruct our children as to the dangers that lie in wait for them. The campaign against the venereal diseases must be a humane and just one. We must not set ourselves as "holier than thou," and treat the erring daughter or the wayward son as outcasts. Had I a daughter and she wanted to marry a man whom I knew to be syphilitic, I would investigate the young man. If he were a confirmed roue, I would, of course, never consent. Had he made a mistake through ignorance and was otherwise worthy, I would say, when you are thoroughly cured, I shall give my consent. Some of my professional colleagues have denounced my views on this point as immoral, but I have practiced medicine long enough to know that in the majority of instances, not in all, the venereal diseases are curable and constitute no permanent bar to parenthood. Besides, this is the common experience of all who have had to deal with these diseases. The treatment is long and the mental torture is great, greater than any one save the physician and the victim can imagine. Provided that a complete and unquestionable cure can be secured, and science can now accurately determine this, the question of permitting marriage then becomes strictly a moral one, and I could never find it within my heart to lastingly condemn any one for a mistake. I do not believe in unpardonable sins.

It is said by some that the teaching of sex hygiene can have no effect upon the young, because love is never reasonable and consists wholly of sentiment and feeling. What is true in this statement is largely due to the cloak of ignorance with which we have clothed the sex instinct. Did the young woman know the fearful pollution which the rake brings with him and seeks to transmit to her, she would see all of this and would from the moment of introduction loathe him, notwithstanding his handsome face, manly form, and deferential bearing. Remove the double standard of virtue as applied to men and women and the young woman would look upon the young man who has been sowing his wild oats as she now regards those of her own sex whom he has debauched. Our sons and daughters are what their ancestors, including ourselves, have made them, modified more or less by their environment, for which we are responsible. They see through our eyes or those which we have given them, and if we place riches and social position above clean living, they are likely to do the same. Besides, our children are what we are, not what we pretend to be. Clothing the ass in the lion's skin does not affect the progeny of the former. The devil may wear the livery of heaven, but his sons are devils still. The libertine may hide his vices, but he must not swear at fate when his children are not equally successful in concealing them.

Possibly I am placing too much emphasis on heredity and too little on environment. I am ready to plead guilty to the latter. Environment is a most potent factor in the sex question. Proper association of the sexes is probably the strongest force in the uplift of the race. I desire that my sons should be much in the company of women. Who can measure the power for good that woman has over man? This is quite apart from the reproductive function. The admiration of a good man can hurt no woman, neither is this any reason why the admiration of a good man should be limited to one woman, or vice versa. Good comradeship between the sexes is beneficial to both. I feel quite sure that coeducation, with its disadvantages which are plainly evident, is better than the exclusive form, but this is too big a theme to go into now.

Among certain classes sex association is so intimate that ill naturally, and we might say, necessarily, results. This is a matter of sanitary housing, which has not received the degree of attention it deserves.

Sex attraction, like all other biologic functions, has its abnormal phases and manifestations. All these are interesting, and some are serious in their consequences. In some people it seems wholly wanting. This is of no racial importance, and affects the life of the individual only, or at most concerns only a few intimate associates. A much more serious abnormality is sex antagonism. This is a diseased state, and until recently it has been observed only in sporadic form. There is occasionally a woman-hating man, or a man-hating woman. Recently this disease has become a most alarming epidemic in England, greatly to the inconvenience of the normal of both sexes. It is to be hoped that this disease may not become pandemic. It certainly should be kept out of this country, even if it be necessary to resort to strict quarantine.

There is another perversion of the fuction of sex attraction and this is known as sex-infatuation or intoxication. It is an acute, self-limited disease, which runs a short but violent course. The disease is characterized by illusions and hallucinations in which the victim talks about his affinity or soul mate, and other jargon unintelligible to those in the normal state.

Sex-infatuation is a mirage to which the parties hasten madly, to find themselves overwhelmed by a dust storm.

Sex attraction is the fountain of perpetual youth, long sought by the individual, long possessed by the race. The drinking of its waters endows the race with life eternal, renews each succeeding generation, and will ultimately develop the better man.

I wish to emphasize the fact that while the central purpose in the development of sex attraction is reproduction, this is by no means all. Before there is reproduction there should be something worthy of being produced. The silly moron girl who will entwine her affections about the first man who will permit it is not the type which should be reproduced, neither is the vicious, immoral boy. Our efforts should be directed to the extinction of both of these. He who wastes his substance in riotous use of the reproductive function, whether it be outside or inside of the legal enactments, procreates a kind which does not bless, but curses the race. Said a childless man to me a few days ago: "John Doe's manly sons fill me with regret that I am not a father, while Richard Roe's worthless progeny banish all this regret."

LABORATORY METHODS

A NEW DOUBLE-WAY SYRINGE FOR USE IN INTRAVENOUS MEDICATION, TRANSFUSION, AND ASPIRATION

By H. O. Ruh, A.B., M.D., Cleveland, Ohio

NOT infrequently a syringe is needed in which it is possible to fill the barrel and eject the contents, or vice versa, without removing the syringe from the system in which it is connected. A large number of devices are employed at the present time for the purpose of administering fluids intravenously. The gravity system, in the past, has been one of the methods most largely used and at the present time, the three-way stopcock method is used quite extensively. Both of these methods have a number of objections. To meet these and supply a simple apparatus the syringe described below has been devised.

The essential requirements for a satisfactory apparatus are: accurate measurement of the amount of the fluid injected or withdrawn, control of the rate of injection or withdrawal of the fluid, ease of cleaning, sterilizing and manipulation of the apparatus, and finally simplicity.

In the intravenous administration of therapeutic sera, or drugs, or in case fluid is to be withdrawn from a cavity by negative pressure, as in thoracentesis or in the collection of a large amount of blood from a vein in a short time, the syringe here described works very satisfactorily.

The apparatus is best understood by reference to the accompanying illustration. The barrel is the same as in all glass syringes, but the plunger has a bore running throughout its entire length, while at the upper end it is so drawn out that a rubber tubing can be securely attached. This is shown in Fig. I.

The operation of the apparatus for the introduction of a fluid is as follows: The needle is inserted into the vein and a few drops of blood are allowed to escape. The bottle C having previously been filled with the fluid to be injected, the plunger is held in place and the fluid allowed to fill the tubing proximal to the syringe, the bore of the plunger, and the tube distal to the syringe. After a few drops of the fluid have escaped, the tubing is attached to the needle by the adapter at D. If no pressure is exerted on the tubing at A or B the fluid will run through the syringe into the vein by gravity. This result is generally not desired at the beginning of an injection of sera, or of blood, as the first 10 to 15 c.c. should take at least ten minutes. Therefore after the syringe system (rubber tubing and bore of plunger) is filled with the fluid, pressure is applied at A and the adapter at D is placed in the needle. Now pressure is made at B and released at A, and immediately the barrel of the syringe is filled by the fluid.

Care should always be taken that the chain guard is in place so that the piston is not forced completely out of the barrel. The syringe being filled, pressure is exerted at *A* and released at *B* and the fluid injected as slowly as desired. By repeated fillings any number of slow injections can be given. When enough is given slowly, pressure is released at both *A* and *B* and the fluid will flow by gravity through the plunger and into the vein.

The operation for the aspiration of blood under aseptic precautions or for the withdrawal of exudates or transudates is very simple. The same apparatus

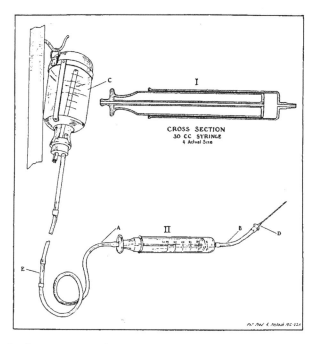

CROSS SECTION
30 CC SYRINGE
¼ Actual Size

as shown in Fig. II is used. The plunger is pushed into the syringe as far as it will go, and the needle introduced into the vein. Pressure is now made at *A* and the plunger pulled out. When the syringe is filled, pressure is released at *A* and applied at *B* and the plunger pushed in, which ejects the fluid or blood into the container at *C*. Provided the apparatus has been sterile, there is no chance of contamination of the fluid. The alternate pressure at *A* and *B* can be applied by digital pressure on the tubing or by the use of pinchcocks.

A DEVICE FOR CENTRIFUGALIZATION AT LOW TEMPERATURES*

By WILLIAM H. WELKER, CHICAGO, ILL.

IN an investigation on hemoglobin it was desired to separate and wash the crystals of this substance by means of centrifugalization at a temperature of about 0° C. It is necessary that this low temperature be maintained while the hemoglobin crystals are being washed with dilute alcohol (25 per cent). If the temperature rises appreciably above 0° C. the hemoglobin is changed from a crystalline to an amorphous substance. For the purpose of this centrifugalization a pair of brass supports was constructed. These supports *(B)* were built to hold 100 c.c. metal tubes *(A)* and to fit snugly inside of 500 c.c. cups *(C)*. The tubes and cups are the regular form of equipment for the larger sizes of the International Equipment Company's centrifuges.

In the construction of the supports, it is important that they should be approximately of the same weight and that their centers of mass should be located

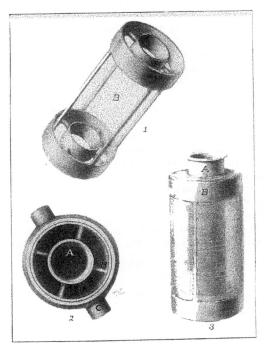

Fig. 1.—Support; Fig. 2.—Apparatus assembled; Fig. 3.—Support with tube and cylinder of ice.

*From the Laboratory of Physiological Chemistry, College of Medicine, University of Illinois, Chicago, Illinois.

at approximately the same point. Unless account is taken of these two considerations there is danger that there will be an inequality in the arm length in the case of the two cups making the pair. This inequality in arm length is liable to damage the machine when operated, because of the unbalanced forces that are developed.

The support and tube are placed into the large cup, the space between the tube and the large cup is filled with water and the outfit subjected to a temperature sufficiently low to congeal the water. This makes possible centrifugalization with a cylinder of ice surrounding the tube containing the substance affected by higher temperature. Depending upon outside conditions, it is possible to operate the machine at a speed of from 1500 to 2000 revolutions for three to five minutes before all the ice is melted.

For the illustrations, I am indebted to Mr. Tom Jones, artist in the Department of Anatomy.

A NEW METHOD FOR THE PRESERVATION OF SPECIMENS

By James S. Platzker, 1st Lt. San. C., U. S. A.

PATHOLOGISTS have long sought a method to preserve histologic and pathologic sections that would not only be well preserved, but also in a condition that would make it handy for demonstrators to pass around to a group of students during a lecture. The method described below is very inexpensive and requires but little skill in performing it. The finished specimen is often only $1\frac{1}{2}$ x 1 x $\frac{1}{2}$ inches in size, and if kept in a cool place during the warm weather, the specimen will keep in an excellent condition for a long time.

The procedure to fix and preserve the specimen is as follows: the gross specimen is fixed in physiologic salt solution containing 10 per cent formaldehyde solution for twenty-four to seventy-two hours, depending upon the size of the specimen. Twenty-four hours is a sufficient length of time to fix a kidney or a spleen, but a heart, breast, uterus, etc., require fixation for about two days longer. After fixing, the specimen is washed for a minute under running tap water and then blotted with a towel. The desired section is then cut from the specimen (a convenient size is $5 \times 8 \times 0.5$ c.m.) and is dehydrated as follows: for 30 minutes in 80 per cent ethyl alcohol, then for 30 minutes in 95 per cent ethyl alcohol. The specimen is then placed into a preserving fluid made as follows:

Potassium acetate	75 grams
Natrium nitrate	25 grams
Glycerine	75 c.c.
Aqua dist. add to	1000 c.c.

The box in which the specimen is preserved is made in the following manner: two (2) pieces of window glass (with as few scratches thereon as possible) are cut, with a diamond pencil or a glass cutter, two centimeters longer and two centimeters wider than the section to be preserved in the box made of the glass plates just mentioned. After cutting the glass plates they are washed with soap and water (the glass must not be cleaned with anything that would tend to scratch its surface) and then dried.

Paraffin wax (with high melting point gives best results) is melted in an agate pot or a porcelain dish and is permitted to cool to a moderately warm temperature. One of the glass plates previously cut is lowered (¼ inch) into the warm paraffin and is quickly withdrawn, the other three sides of the plate are treated in the same manner and the process is repeated until the walls of paraffin formed on the four sides of the plate are a little higher than the thickness of the specimen to be embedded therein. Each time the plate is withdrawn from the melted wax, the cooling of the paraffin may be hastened by blowing (with mouth) on the newly formed layer. Fig. 1 shows a glass plate with the paraffin walls. In order to facilitate the sealing of the paraffin box it is advisable (after the paraffin walls are hardened) to warm the second glass plate over a Bunsen flame, then place it over the paraffin walls, in order to make them all even, then quickly slip off before hardening to the second plate. A spatule should

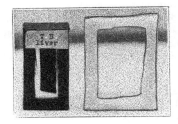

Fig. 1.   Fig. 2.

also be warmed and run over the lower part of the hardened paraffin walls to seal any openings.

The paraffin walled glass is then put into a dish containing freshly filtered preserving fluid as described above. The fluid should be at least ten centimeters above the surface of the walled glass. The section in the preserving fluid, mentioned above, is transferred into the paraffin walled specimen box. The section is moved about in the box several times in order to free it from the air bubbles that may be present underneath it. The paraffin can easily be removed from the glass plate used to smoothen the paraffin walls with a little xylol. The glass plate is then dried and warmed over a Bunsen flame (it is best to hold the glass with two pairs of forceps, one pair in each hand) and then quickly placed over the paraffin walls, holding it first at an angle of about 40 degrees to the specimen box, then lowering it quickly but steadily, taking care to expel all the air bubbles. As soon as the plate rests on the surface of the four paraffin walls, a little pressure (with a block of wood) is put on the glass cover, by so doing, the warm glass is aided to melt a little more wax, which in a few seconds will adhere to the glass cover and make an air-tight and waterproof compartment for the embedded section. The specimen box is then taken out, a little more wax, cooled to a semisolid form, is placed on the sides of the specimen box (with a spatule) to fill some uneven cavities. A warm blade of a knife may then be employed to smoothen the paraffin sides. Specks of wax on the glass may be removed with a little xylol.

To improve the appearance of the specimen box, I use black picture binding. Fig. 2 shows a mounted and framed specimen embedded in June, 1915, at the Kings County Hospital laboratories of the city of New York. The color of the specimen today is the same as when embedded, four years ago.

A SIMPLE LABORATORY SHAKER*

By E. J. WARNICK, CLEVELAND, OHIO

WE have found a shaker made according to the following specifications to be extremely serviceable for general laboratory use.

A box which is made to hold bottles, test tubes, etc., is suspended by the mainspring taken from an alarm clock, cut into lengths five inches long, and fastened to the ends of the box and to the base of the platform of the apparatus. This box is attached by a rod to an eccentric wheel of a low-speed, one-twenty-fifth-horse-power motor.

This shaker is practically noiseless and can be made by any laboratory technician.

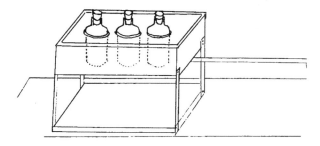

QUICK METHOD FOR MAKING SMALL INNER TUBES FOR DUNHAM'S FERMENTATION TUBES†

By PRIVATE EARL M. TAYLOR, M.D., BASE HOSPITAL, LE MANS, FRANCE

WHEN a large number of fermentation cultures must be run as routine day after day, the quantity of culture medium used becomes an important factor. To conserve culture media it is necessary to have small tubes so that a medium-sized outer tube can be used.

*From the Research Laboratory, Medical Service, Lakeside Hospital.
†Published by permission of the Surgeon-General's Office, Washington, D. C.

METHOD OF MAKING FERMENTATION TUBES

Apparatus.—Blow torch or Bunsen burner, several lengths of the desired size of glass tubing, file, and a pair of large laboratory shears.

Method.—Use a piece of glass tubing of the desired diameter. At a point 2 inches from the end heat in a Bunsen flame. When soft enough cut off with a pair of scissors without removing from the flame. Seal the cut ends by holding in the flame long enough to round off the ends slightly but not long enough to permit the tube to bend. Next move the tube along 4 inches and repeat the process at this point. Continue until the tube has been cut into as many 4-inch pieces as the length permits. After cooling, cut each 4-inch piece in two in the middle by means of a file.

This method makes a better-shaped tube and the process is more rapid than by drawing out the ends. The tubes very seldom, if ever, leak as the pinching done by the shears in the cutting seals the ends at the same time.

The Journal of
Laboratory and Clinical
Medicine

Vol. V. NOVEMBER, 1919 No. 2

Editor-in-Chief: VICTOR C. VAUGHAN, M.D.
Ann Arbor, Mich.

ASSOCIATE EDITORS

DENNIS E. JACKSON, M.D. - -	CINCINNATI
HANS ZINSSER, M.D. - - -	NEW YORK
PAUL G. WOOLLEY, M.D. - -	CINCINNATI
FREDERICK P. GAY, M.D. -	- BERKELEY, CAL.
J. J. R. MACLEOD, M.B. - - -	TORONTO
ROY G. PEARCE, M.D. - -	- CLEVELAND
W. C. MACCARTY, M.D. -	ROCHESTER, MINN.
GERALD B. WEBB, M.D. -	COLORADO SPRINGS
E. E. SOUTHARD, M.D. - - -	- BOSTON
WARREN T. VAUGHAN, M.D. -	. BOSTON

EDITORIALS

Streptococcus Immunity and Immunization

IN a review in this JOURNAL last year[1] the possibilities of specific prevention and therapy in streptococcus infections was rather thoroughly discussed. As we saw at that time, there is very little evidence in human or animal pathology which would lead us to suppose that recovery from streptococcus infections leads to any considerable or durable degree of acquired immunity. A survey of the experimental work that has been done in producing active immunity against streptococcus infections by means of vaccines, and particularly the possibility of its application in human beings, shows it to be practically negligible. On the other hand, extensive studies have been made on the properties of the serum of animals that have been artificially immunized against streptococci. The curative effect of such immune sera is, however, extremely problematical, although certain definite claims have been made for it ever since the initial work of Marmorek on the subject. We may still confess to a justifiable skepticism as to whether there is any streptococcus immune serum that has been proved of practical therapeutic value.

The first favorable experimental results in the hands of Marmorek[2] depended on the fact that he treated septicemias in rabbits by means of an immune sera obtained by immunizing rabbits with the same single strain of streptococcus, and one of the most reasonable and justifiable explanations of our failure to get more uniformly encouraging results has been that we have failed to comply with the requirements of strict specificity implied in his experiments. In other words, it has been pretty generally admitted that there are a number of different streptococci concerned in human infections, and although it may be true that the organisms of certain large groups of streptococci are particularly concerned with some type or types of human infection, we have no certainty that any particular variety of the streptococcus is definitely correlated with any disease process. Any particular strain of streptococcus that is concerned in any particular instance of disease must obviously be combated by its own specific antiserum, as has been done in the case of pneumococcus infections. It is furthermore suggested by Marmorek's work and borne out by subsequent observations that it might be better to treat human infections with the serum of animals that had been immunized by "humanized" strains of streptococci, that is to say, strains of the organisms grown on human blood or tissue medium or recently isolated from human beings.

Progress has been made in recent years and months in the determination of the actual types of streptococci concerned in disease processes. We learned some years ago to differentiate between the viridans group and the hemolytic group by their growth on a blood medium. It is further known that the viridans group of streptococci is more particularly concerned with subacute processes and the hemolytic organisms with the acute and more virulent diseases. It seemed evident from the preliminary work on biologic and immunologic classification that there were certain further facts of importance in reference to these two organisms. On immunologic grounds the viridans streptococcus is apparently more heterogeneous, and until a short time ago, it was supposed that the hemolytic varieties were homogeneous. It was known, however, that hemolytic streptococci may be separated by their fermentative reactions on culture media into some eight or more groups (Holman[3]).

In the last year two very important contributions have been made to the classification of the hemolytic streptococci which still further complicates the problem of active and passive immunity in streptococcus infections. Havens and Hamilton,[4] Havens,[5] and Dochez, Avery and Lancefield[6] have shown by protective and agglutination experiments that the hemolytic organisms belonging to a single variety of Holman's classification, namely, the Streptococcus pyogenes group, are again separable into three or more immunologic types. As their experiments show, any therapy against any one of these types, to be successful, must depend on the utilization of a corresponding antiserum. It is evident, then, that we have only just arrived at a point where we are able to intelligently test experimentally, and later perhaps to apply practically, serum therapy in streptococcus infections. This application will further depend on some rapid method of type differentiation of the particular streptococcus concerned in each individual instance of disease.

BIBLIOGRAPHY

[1]Gay, F. P.: Recent Aspects of Streptococcus Infection, Jour. Lab. and Clin. Med., September, 1918, iii, 3.
[2]Marmorek, A.: Le Streptocoque et le serum antistreptococcique, Ann. Pasteur, 1895.
[3]Holman, W. L.: The Classification of Streptococci, Jour. Med. Research, 1916, xxxiv, 377.
[4]Havens, L. C., and Hamilton, C. D.: Hemolytic Streptococci, Jour. Am. Med. Assn., 1919, lxxii, No. 4; January 25, p. 272.
[5]Havens, L. C.: A Biologic Classification of Hemolytic Streptococci, Jour. Infect. Dis., 1919, xxv, 315.
[6]Dochez, A. R.; Avery, O. T.; and Lancefield, R. C.: Jour. Exper. Med., 1919, xxx, No. 3, p. 179.

—F. P. G.

The Cause of Resolution and Crisis in Pneumonia

THE true explanation of these two most characteristic phenomena of lobar pneumonia is a question which has always interested and has baffled the medical profession. We are well acquainted with the anatomic condition of a consolidated lung, and know that the physiologic process of resolution consists of resorption of the exudate through the alveolar walls, together with the elimination of considerable quantities by coughing. We are accustomed to explain the essential process as digestion by proteolytic enzymes produced in the breaking down of leucocytes. Further than that our theories do not take us. The explanation of the occasional true cases of delayed resolution is still to be sought.

Concerning the phenomenon of crisis, there are in general two schools, neither possessing any large volume of data to reinforce their hypotheses. On the one hand there is the feeling that crisis in pneumonia is in some way intimately associated with the phenomena of immunity and that by the seventh day of the disease, or later, an immunity is suddenly established and critical fall in temperature and convalescence follow. On the other hand, there are those who explain the phenomenon as a result of the biologic activity of the infecting organism itself.

The recent work of Lord[1] and of Lord and Nye[2] sheds a clear light on the problem, and suggests new methods of approach. Lord ground up the substance of pneumonic lungs in the stages of gray hepatization and of red-gray hepatization, and after purification and sterilization incubated a saline suspension of the substance on the surface of Loeffler's blood serum medium. The different specimens of medium were acidified in graded strengths up from neutral,—from a hydrogen-ion concentration of 7.3 up to one of 3.1. He found that there was present in the pneumonic cellular material a proteolytic enzyme which was active in an acidity of P_H 7.3 to P_H 6.7, in other words in a low acidity. In more acid concentration the enzyme ceased to erode the surface of the coagulated blood serum. Further results on peptone with determination of amino acid and total nitrogen amounts in varying concentrations of acid indicated the presence of a proteolytic enzyme which splits peptone to amino acids. The enzyme is most active in higher acid concentration than is the first proteolytic enzyme mentioned, (P_H 6.3 to 5.2), but is operative over a wide range up from slightly on the alkaline side of neutral (P_H 8.0 to 4.8).

In the course of pneumonia these ferments or enzymes are liberated as we have before assumed by the breaking down of cellular elements of the exudate. The first, capable of digesting fibrin, is active in weakly alkaline and weakly acid solutions, and as the hydrogen-ion concentration of the exudate gradually increases, it ceases to act, but the enzyme capable of splitting peptone to amino acids continues its work, increasing in activity as the acidity increases, up to its optimum point. By the action of these two enzymes the resorption of the exudate is rendered possible.

But do we know that acidity of the exudate actually does increase? Pneumococcus in glucose broth medium grows rapidly, producing as a result increasing amounts of acid. Growth continues abundant up until a hydrogen-ion concentration of 6.8 has been reached. In a concentration of 5.1 the pneumococcus lives but a few hours. (Lord and Nye). This figure of 5.1 corresponds well with the figure of 5.0 found by Avery and Cullen. The range of optimum activity of the peptone splitting organism is from P_H 6.3 to 5.2, the higher acidity of which, (5.2), corresponds in an interesting way with that of cessation of viability of the pneumococcus (5.1).

We can then visualize the digestion of the pneumonic exudate, increasing as the acidity increases, and reaching a maximum at about the time when the infecting organism is killed by its own products. This period would correspond to the time of crisis in the clinical history.

Such an hypothesis which is suggested by Lord and Nye is attractive, but probably is not the complete explanation. Immunologic processes are probably also at work, as is shown particularly by the results of serum therapy. Further it remains to be proved that *in vivo* there does actually exist this progressive increase in acidity,—that the body has no mechanism for removing it or neutralizing it in the exudate. It is interesting to conjecture on this hypothesis whether delayed resolution may be due to insufficiency of ferment or to its insufficient activation.

BIBLIOGRAPHY

[1]Lord, F. T.: Jour. Exper. Med., xxx, No. 4, p. 379.
[2]Lord, F. T., and Nye, R. N.: Ibid., p. 389.
[3]Avery and Cullen: Ibid.

—W. T. V.

Fever

THE temperature of the body is regulated by radiation, conduction, and evaporation. As the heat production of the body increases, heat elimination by all three methods increases, but the percentage of loss by evaporation becomes most important. In order that this may be true the body must have an available supply of free water. Krehl and Matthes found that during fever an increase of heat elimination by radiation and conduction as well as by evaporation, the loss by evaporation was not sufficient to maintain a temperature equilibrium as in a healthy body. This failure of evaporation to compensate for the loss of heat which can not take place through radiation and conduction would indicate that something hinders the evaporation of water in fever. Either the total supply of water runs out, or the water becomes more firmly bound in the tissues and less available for evaporation.

Emphasis of the foregoing statements was given during certain experiments by Woodyatt and Sansum. They observed in dogs and man that fever occurred when, under the influence of intravenous injections of glucose, the rate of sugar injection was sufficiently in excess of the tolerance limit to produce a marked glycosuria with its concomitant diuresis; when the rate of water administration was less than the rate of diuresis, and when these conditions were sustained until the animal or man had lost a certain weight by dehydration. Chills also occurred after the temperature had begun to rise. Both chills and fever subsided when water was administered.

The obvious explanation was that the body lost so much water by diuresis and primary evaporation that none was finally available for heat dissipation and that therefore evaporation was interfered with. In other words the body had lost its "free" water. This free water might be lost in two ways, i.e., by elimination, or by physico-chemical fixation in the tissues. At any rate the observations were the starting point of a series of new experiments undertaken by Balcar, Sansum, and Woodyatt.[1]

The experiments showed that the body temperature could be driven readily to 111° F., while in one instance the temperature rose to 126.6° F. Fevers of 111° F. were produced by common salt and by lactose as well as by glucose. They also showed that sugar is able to cause fever by its mere presence in the body under certain circumstances, but that no amount of sugar which can be introduced easily will cause fever unless the water reserve of the body is low. Finally sugar fever was produced in dogs, rendered poikilothermic by cutting the cervical cord, a result which demonstrates that the fever had no connection with a nervous heat-regulating mechanism.

The series of experiments demonstrates that the production of fever is dependent upon the water of the animal body. The production of high temperature depends upon checking of evaporation from the body. One method of affecting this is to remove water from the body to such an extent that not enough remains to carry off the excess heat, and this is what salt and sugar solutions accomplish. In certain circumstances these substances may at the same time make water unavailable by causing it to become fixed in the tissues.

The writers refer to the so-called "inanition fever" of infants, which is readily counteracted by water. "Inanition fever" is a thirst fever. "Salt fever" is the same, and water stops it. They conclude that the fever symptom, which appears in the infectious diseases, proteose intoxication, and all febrile diseases except insolation and the like, may mean a deficit of free water in the body. They suggest that in these diseases the deficit of free water is the result of an abnormal tendency on the part of the colloids of the body to bind water, and so to increase the "fixed" water and reduce the "free" water. If this is what happens then the tissues would be swollen and the secretions concentrated—as they are. It would account for the thirst of fever patients and for the sudden release of water in the form of urine and perspiration at a crisis. Also if all this be true one could completely abate a fever by the use of water. Only experi-

[1]Balcar, Sansum and Woodyatt: Fever and the Water Reserve of the Body, Arch. Int. Med., 1919, xxiv, 116.

ments can tell whether the administration of the necessary water can be accomplished without danger. Up to the present time but few experiments have been made. In three pneumonia patients the temperatures were brought to normal by mere water administration. The work is proceeding. The water treatment of fevers it should be noted in passing is not new. It is being used by many practitioners everywhere—men who have not the time or inclination to write. But a consideration of this physico-chemical theory of fever will be of great value in stimulating experimental work, and of still greater value in opening the minds of the myopic group of physicians, who, everywhere are afraid of water and sodium chloride, except as external applications.

—*P. G. W.*

Tonsils and Streptococci

THE experiences of the war have placed all the necessary emphasis upon the occurrence of pathogenic microorganisms in the throats of human beings. In every cantonment the flora of the tonsillar and postnasal areas has been studied, and the results tabulated. At Camp Devens, Spooner showed that practically 100 per cent of the normal persons from whom cultures were made, harbored streptococci, and that from 62 to 71 per cent of the officers and nurses in the Base Hospital showed organisms of the hemolytic type. The following table shows the incidence of hemolytic streptococci in apparently normal persons according to various workers.

	Normal Persons
Spooner	62-71 %
Guming, Sprunt, and Lynch	6 %
Nichols	75 %
Opie, Freeman, and Blake	22.4%
Blandon, Burhaus, and Hunter	90 %
Smillie	50 %
Ruediger	59 %

These figures are sufficiently striking to indicate the wide distribution of the organisms which when the proper opportunities are offered enter the blood stream and produce the most various lesions, from mere transient myositis to rheumatic fever, acute endocarditis, myocarditis, pneumonia, and empyema.

In order to gain still more information regarding the presence of these streptococci, and to discover how they were affected by surgical procedures, Tongs* has studied the distribution of them with special reference to their occurrence after tonsillectomy. Of 100 cultures made from the throat, 67 showed the presence of hemolytic streptococci; of the nasal cultures only 5 per cent were positive. Of the 100 cases, 39 were school children sent for examination by their schools, and 80 per cent of them were positive. Of 61 average individuals in this series, 57 per cent showed hemolytic streptococci on cultures. The higher percentage in children seemed to be due to the presence of tonsillar hypertrophy.

In his studies on hypertrophied tonsils Tongs studied 125 pairs of excised organs. Before tonsillectomy an ordinary throat culture was made. in which case there were 64 positive results. After tonsillectomy the tonsils were dropped into

---

*Tongs: Jour. Am. Med. Assn., 1919, lxxiii, 1050.

25 per cent silver nitrate and kept for 5 minutes, after which the contents of the crypts were examined. In this case the cultures were positive in 83 per cent of the cases.

These figures are striking enough, but when taken into consideration with the conditions after operation, they are startling. Tongs examined 342 persons to learn whether hemolytic streptococci are as frequently present after tonsillectomy as before. Of this number 17 (0.05 per cent) throat cultures and 10 (0.03 per cent) nasal cultures were positive. In 5 of the positive throat cases, remnants of tonsillar tissue were found.

Finally in order to learn whether hemolytic streptococci may be present or absent regularly in throats with tonsils removed from tonsillectomized persons previously known to be carriers, and eleven tonsillectomized persons previously known to be noncarriers were studied. In the latter group every examination was negative; in the former (carriers) two were positive on each examination, one was positive once out of three times, and one, twice out of three times.

This work points distinctly to the fact that tonsils are a very common breeding place for hemolytic streptococci, and that in a large number of cases the throat may be completely freed from these organisms by tonsillectomy. The fact that an excised tonsil may be soaked in 25 per cent silver nitrate for five minutes and may still furnish a culture of streptococci from its crypts, shows how futile are the usual treatments by applications for anything except superficial cleansing.

—*P. G. W.*

"The Effects of the English Hunger Blockade on the German Children"

SUCH was the heading of an editorial in the *Deutsche Medizinische Wochenschrift,* in which definite figures are quoted concerning the results of food shortage in Germany during the war. The figures are chiefly those of Siegmund Schultze head of the Berlin juvenile court. As early as the autumn of 1915, the effects of the food shortage, or as the Germans prefer to call it,—the English hunger blockade,—were felt in the larger cities. Mortality rates in 1917 were 2.4 per cent higher than in 1913, among nursing infants; 49.3 per cent higher among children from 2 to 6 years of age; and 55 per cent higher among school children (6 to 15 years). The mortality increase among schoolchildren was greater than that for any other age. Fifty thousand more small and schoolchildren died in 1917 than in 1913.

In Berlin alone deaths from pulmonary tuberculosis increased as follows:

Age	1915	1916	1917
4 to 5 years	20 deaths	35 deaths	47 deaths
6 to 10 "	38 "	55 "	55 "
11 to 15 "	53 "	94 "	133 "
16 to 20	296	316	494

Fatal gastro-intestinal cases increased to a similar extent:

Age	1915	1917
2 to 3 years	13 deaths	31 deaths
4 to 5 "	10 "	36 "
6 to 10 "	5 "	23 "
11 to 15	1	3

Siegmund Schultze has collected similar figures from many other large German cities.

Even greater increases were obtained for morbidity than for mortality rates. In Breslau, the tuberculosis hospital which had in the last year of peace cared for 8692 cases, in 1917 housed 20,669 patients.

Under circumstances such as these, the tremendous fall in birth rate is considered to be almost fortunate. It is computed that between 1914 and 1919, in Prussia alone, the births decreased by 2,555,010. In 1917, 603,496 living children were born, as contrasted with 1,192,081, the average annual births for 1910-1913.

The infant mortality showed the lowest increase, but the mortality of nursing infants would naturally decrease, with decreasing birth rate, so that, had the birth rate been as high as usual, the infant mortality figures would have been much greater.

Following the exposition of these figures, the German editorial proceeds to place entire and unstinted blame for the existing conditions, upon the allies, more especially upon the English, and in particular upon President Wilson and Lloyd George, who it is claimed were repeatedly given copies of the above figures by Siegmund Schultze, himself. The high officials among the allies therefore had, we are informed, not a vague notion of child mortality in Germany, but a comprehensive knowledge. "These irrefutable figures stand as a severe impeachment, and, in spite of all denial by the Entente will tell their frightful story throughout all time; and this impeachment is especially heavy because the Entente did know of the effects of the hunger blockade."

In the same editorial and on the same page, appear the following sentences, which we find difficult to reconcile with the foregoing bit of rhetoric:

"Only a few of the initiated (Germans) knew the entire extent of this untold suffering; the truth was withheld from the people by a, perhaps very short sighted, censor."

"Furthermore the author (Siegmund Schultze) was repeatedly prohibited by the military authorities and by the censor from disclosing these facts."

"There stand also many German doctors who have by no means covered themselves with glory, in that they misled the people with beautifully colored descriptions, and sought to paint a false picture for the enemy."

We find no suggestion in the editorial that another contributory cause of the food shortage might be the unexpected failure to utilize all of the French crops after the capture of Paris. —*W. T. V.*

An Appeal for Human Embryological Material

In 1906 I observed certain malformations of the human shoulder-blade, and in contributions to current literature I have given them the collective name— "the scaphoid type of scapula," and pointed out some of its hereditary, clinical and anatomical significance.

Probably the most important observation connected with this type of scapula in man is its age incidence, that is to say, it occurs with great frequency among the young and with relative infrequency among the old. There appear to be two possible explanations of this fact:

Either *A*. One form of shoulder-blade changes into the other during development and growth; or *B*. Many of the possessors of the scaphoid type of scapula are the poorly adaptable, the peculiarly vulnerable, the unduly disease susceptible—the inherently weakened of the race.

I have attempted to answer these questions by seeking evidence in various directions and one of the most important of these has been a study of intrauterine development of shoulder-blades. My investigations in this direction have been limited by the material at my disposal, which has been inadequate for a definite solution of this phase of the problem. I am, therefore, appealing to physicians for fetuses in any and all stages of human development.

It is desired that the material, as soon as possible after delivery, be immersed in ten per cent formalin in a sealed container, and be forwarded to my address; charges collect. Due acknowledgment will be made to those forwarding material.

—*Wm. W. Graves, M.D., 727 Metropolitan Building, St. Louis, Mo.*

The Journal of
Laboratory and Clinical
Medicine

| Vol. V. | St. Louis, December, 1919 | No. 3 |

ORIGINAL ARTICLES

APPLICATIONS OF THE PRAGMATIC METHOD TO PSYCHIATRY*

By E. E. Southard, M.D., Boston, Mass.

*W*HAT *difference would it practically make to anyone if this notion rather than that notion were true?* If no practical difference whatever can be traced, then the alternatives mean practically the same thing, and all dispute is idle": such is one of the briefest formulations that Professor William James ever made of the pragmatic method. Again, there can be "no difference in abstract truth that doesn't express itself in a difference in concrete fact, and in conduct consequent upon the fact, imposed on somebody."

That the pragmatic method, altogether aside from any philosophic implications, must have very important relations to medicine would nowadays be denied by no man. In fact, the whole attitude of the medical man to medicine would not suffer if it should receive the designation "pragmatic." The very founder of the idea of pragmatism, Charles Peirce, used to speak of it as the "laboratory habit of mind." Pragmatism in medicine must have especially close relations with treatment and prognosis. This can be clearly seen from one of the better and longer statements of the nature of pragmatism as given by James in Baldwin's *Dictionary of Philosophy and Psychology*: Pragmatism is "the doctrine that the whole meaning of a conception expresses itself in practical consequences, couse-quences either in the shape of conduct to be recommended or in that of experiences to be expected, if the conception be true; which consequences would be different if it were untrue, and must be different from the consequences by which the meaning of other conceptions is in turn expressed. If a second conception should not appear to have other consequences, then it must really be only the first conception under a different name. In methodology it is certain that to trace and compare their respective consequences is an admirable way of establishing the differing meanings of different conceptions."

*Read in abstract at the Thirty-fourth Annual Meeting of the Association of American Physicians, Eleventh Triennial Session of the Congress of American Physicians and Surgeons, Atlantic City, June, 1919.

It is my object in the present paper to apply pragmatic principles to some problems of psychiatry.

1. PSYCHIATRY AND CLINICAL NEUROLOGY

In the first place, does psychiatry exist as distinct from neurology? It can be pointed out that the research basis of psychiatry and of clinical neurology is a unit, namely, theoretical neuropathology, considered in both structural and functional aspects. Let us, however, apply the pragmatic method. Is psychiatry only clinical neurology under a different name? The moment we trace and compare the respective consequences of these two ideas, we perceive that clinical neurology leads to a quite different effect upon the patient from that to be expected when psychiatry approaches him. Psychiatrists and clinical neurologists have had no identical education as clinicians, and they have not the same outlook. This is a practical situation which has pragmatic consequences. It is simply a pious wish when we state that clinical neurologists and psychiatrists are all really nothing but neuropsychiatrists. Perhaps they ought to be and perhaps they soon will be, but they are not. It makes a great deal of difference to the patient whether he is approached by a psychiatrist or by a clinical neurologist.

I have elsewhere gone into more detail upon this matter, referring especially to the different points of view, e.g., toward mild cases of schizophrenia (dementia precox) and cyclothymia (manic-depressive psychoses), maintained by neurologist and psychiatrist respectively. I will not here discuss the point further.

Clinical neurology and psychiatry are pragmatic entities, for they have different consequences when their points of view are applied to the victims of disease.

2. THE SO-CALLED "UNITY OF INSANITY"

Turning to the subject matter of psychiatry, the largest question hangs upon whether we define mental diseases as a unit or as a set of entities. English writers, among them some of the more subtle, such as Charles Mercier, have for years plumped for the unitarian view. One must have a certain respect for any Anglo-Saxon view of the topic, seeing that it no doubt has a certain relevance and practical applicability. However, I think the progress of psychiatry proves, not only that mental diseases can be analytically split up into logical entities, but that these logical units have pragmatic value. At the same time that a thinker like Mercier insists upon the "unity of insanity," he also insists upon grades of responsibility in medicolegal cases and claims to be one of the earliest to have made this distinction. In fine, Mercier lugs in at the finish what we practically want in the matter of subdivisions within psychiatry. If we look more narrowly at other British authors, we find that they often dispose of the unity question in mental diseases by throwing into the field of "nervous" diseases everything which does not handily fit a preconceived legal definition of insanity. This again may comport with Anglo-Saxon notions of practicality and may have a certain relevance from the standpoint of law courts. But assuredly we do not get on very measurably in psychiatric research, if we simply redistribute our material to suit some nonmedical criterion, such as some standard of the practical responsibility of mental cases.

It seems to me that the progress of psychopathic hospitals, in the few places in the world where they have been rigorously tried out, shows beyond cavil that psychiatry is an art dealing with numerous entities. Possibly (according to a rough enumeration from popular systematic works) there may be between eighty and one hundred of these practical entities.

The pragmatic question is, what difference does it make to the patient whether he is said to be affiliated with one or the other of these entities? I am not sure that I can prove that there is a different "conduct to be recommended" or different "experience to be expected" (to use James' phrases) for all of these eighty-odd entities. But I am entirely sure that it makes a great difference to the patient whether he is to be placed in one of ten or a dozen major groups of these entities. Perhaps I entirely miss the point of the British contentions for the unity of insanity; but I really can not see that their viewpoint has a leg to stand upon when we contemplate the present nosological situation. It certainly makes a great deal of difference to the patient, as well as to the social unit in which he lives, whether we regard the patient as a victim of neurosyphilis or whether we regard him as a victim of alcoholic psychosis. Now, possibly the English authors would wish to exclude the victim of neurosyphilis and of alcoholic mental disease from the realm of insanity altogether. Very well,—let this happen. We should then at best attain a conception of the unity of insanity only by greatly diminishing its contents, as ordinarily conceived. But would any author deny that it makes a great deal of difference to the patient whether he is a victim of psychoneurosis cr of some depression falling in the group termed by Kraepelin manic-depressive psychosis (which I think might as a group better be termed the cyclothymic group)? Now again, if the unitarian wishes to diminish the field of insanity by cutting off the psychoneuroses, so be it. Again we shall attain unity by a Procrustean process. The psychiatrist will give up any insight he may have into the psychoneurotic and hand his patient forthwith over to the clinical neurologist. Yet the research basis for the understanding of psychoneuroses is no doubt identical for both the psychiatrist and the clinical neurologist. Again the pragmatic method should be applied. If it is true that it is going to make a great difference to the patient whether he is regarded psychiatrically or neurologically, then we must decide that there are real differences under discussion.

Parceling out the psychoneuroses and the cyclothymias to the neurologists and the psychiatrists, respectively, may seem logically the right thing to do. Pragmatically I believe it will have, not only practical, but evil consequences if we execute this partition.

3. DIAGNOSIS BY ORDERLY EXCLUSION

Dismissing the question of the unity of insanity, I wish to approach a few other pragmatic questions in psychiatry and to hang them upon the order concept. Last year I advocated before the Association in a paper *"Diagnosis per Exclusionem in Ordine*: General and Psychiatric Remarks" the application of the principle of order in psychiatric diagnosis, and called attention to the existence of eleven major groups of entities which seemed to me to have practical value. Of course I was aware that the principle could be applied to many other branches of medicine, and I am glad to say that in correspondence with Dr. Richard C. Cabot, we have together concluded that the principle might very effectively be installed at an early date in many of the specialties, if not in the whole of medicine. As Dr. Cabot has said to me, if one gets hold of a *list* of things it is manifest that said list may be turned into a *sequence* or order and that this sequence or order may have practical value. I shall not here repeat the considerations of the above-mentioned paper, at least to any extent; but I wish to claim that the application of the order concept is an example of pragmatic method. It makes a difference to the patient both in "conduct to be recommended" and "experience to be expected" whether we approach him diagnostically in an orderly fashion.

4. NEUROSYPHILIS AND GENERAL PARESIS

It has in the past made a good deal of practical difference to many psychopathic patients that they have not been primarily considered as possibly victims of neurosyphilis. Time was when the Wassermann serum reaction was taken only in cases in which one suspected general paresis. Nowadays so protean have been proved to be the forms of neurosyphilis that for practical purposes no mental patient can fail to be thought possibly syphilitic. That hypothesis must be disposed of one way or the other.

But if neurosyphilitic, what form of neurosyphilis is in play? It makes a great deal of difference to the patient whether we set up the hypothesis that he has general paresis (with all the evil prognostic connotations of that entity) or whether we limit our initial idea to his being merely neurosyphilitic. An application of the pragmatic method to the orderly diagnosis of the subentities of the neurosyphilitic group would make us consider at some point the *nonparetic* forms of neurosyphilis. We should, in the pragmatic interest of the patient, keep our diagnostic ideas in solution at the level of undifferentiated neurosyphilis rather than leap to the diagnosis "general paresis." We have practically seen a great deal of evil happen to patients by reason of these premature leaps to the diagnosis "general paresis," on the basis of a few clinical similarities to the entity as described in books. There is, therefore, much scope for the application of pragmatic method in the field of neurosyphilis.

5. DIAGNOSTIC PRECESSION OF "FOCAL" VERSUS "SYMPTOMATIC" CASES

To facilitate the rest of my discussion I will here reproduce the eleven groups of mental disease from my paper on *"Diagnosis per Exclusionem in Ordine."*

Mental Disease Groups (Orders)

I. Syphilitic	Syphilopsychoses.
II. Feeble-minded	Hypophrenoses.
III. Epileptic	Epileptoses.
IV. Alcoholic, drug, poison	Pharmacopsychoses.
V. Focal brain ("organic," arteriosclerotic)	Encephalopsychoses.
VI. Bodily disease ("symptomatic")	Somatopsychoses.
VII. Senescent, senile	Geriopsychoses.
VIII. Dementia precox, paraphrenic	Schizophrenoses.
IX. Manic-depressive, cyclothymic	Cyclothymoses.
X. Hysteric, psychasthenic, neurasthenic	Psychoneuroses.
XI. Psychopathic, paranoiac, et al	Psychopathoses.

Why is Group V of the Encephalopsychoses placed prior to Group VI, the Somatopsychoses? Logically, it might well seem that we should approach, in the process of diagnosis, the somatic diseases that give rise to mental symptoms prior to the focal brain diseases that produce mental symptoms. But logic is not practice. In the general hospital clinics, where somatic diseases, nonnervous in nature, are habitually approached logically prior to the nervous and mental diseases, we have not found much progress in psychiatry or much grasp of the psychiatric point of view. Mental cases will for many years to come in our hospital practice, devolve more seriously upon the attention of neurologists and psychiatrists than they will upon the attention of internists. If a man has mental disease and if one has excluded the great groups of syphilis, feeble-mindedness, epilepsy, and alcoholism (with all their practical social implications), then one naturally desires to clear up other large brain aspects of this mental case. Although we are in possession of numerous data to show that mental symptoms may be merely symptomatic of bodily (nonneural) diseases, yet there is no doubt that the nervous system exerts in some ways a prior claim on the attention. Perhaps the practical answer would be that in internists' clinics, the order of logical consideration should be reversed and Group VI placed before Group V, whereas in psychiatric clinics the order might remain as stated. Let me insist at this point on something which is logically clear, but practically not always envisaged. *This system of orderly exclusion in diagnosis has nothing whatever to do with the practical order in which data are collected.* It is a plan to be put into effect *after the data are all in hand.* It does not matter whether the data about the pupils or the reflexes are chronologically collected before the data concerning bodily infection. The question is one of logical, not of chronological, priority. In the end, however, I am willing to acknowledge that the question, whether the encephalic or the nonneural somatic conditions should be diagnostically placed in the order I recommend, is an open question. The question can be answered in the long run only pragmatically.

6. DIAGNOSTIC PRECESSION OF SCHIZOPHRENIC VERSUS CYCLOTHYMIC CASES

One other example may be offered looking in the same direction. I have placed the schizophrenoses (dementia precox, etc.,) in Group VIII, ahead of the cyclothymoses (manic-depressive, etc.), Group IX. Now it might be pointed out that as manic depressive phenomena are more nearly normal than schizophrenic phenomena, it should be well to consider the patient normal before we consider him abnormal. Let the patient be regarded as innocent of mental symptoms before he is regarded as guilty of such. Well, the pragmatic answer to this question is that it appears to have important practical consequences whether we consider a patient schizophrenic logically prior to our considering him cyclothymic. A group of schizophrenic symptoms is much more convincing as to a patient's being a victim of the disease schizophrenia than is a group of cyclothymic symptoms convincing as to his being a victim of cyclothymic disease. Just in virtue of the quasi-normality of the ups and downs in mood of the manic-depressive does it transpire that practically every form of mental disease is capable of showing these ups and downs in mood. By consequence if we fix our minds upon cyclothymic phenomena, we are rather inclined to premature fixation of our minds upon the diagnosis of the entity manic-depressive psychosis. Seeing cyclothymoid symptoms, we rush to the idea of the cyclothymic entity. In short a group of schizophrenic symptoms is much more "pathognomonic" than a group of cyclothymic symptoms. It was upon this pragmatic basis that Group VIII was placed before Group IX.

Why should we place the psychoneuroses in a Group X, following the schizophrenias and cyclothymias? I am bound to admit that this placement was an exceedingly practical one. We have in psychopathic hospital practice seen so many cases in which the diagnosis 'nervous prostration" has been affixed to a patient who was really a mild example of schizophrenia or of cyclothymia (and this much to the therapeutic detriment of the cases in question) that it seemed wise to relegate the psychoneuroses to a subsequent position in the diagnostic list for orderly exclusion.

7. PLACEMENT OF INVOLUTION-MELANCHOLIA

Another example of the application of the pragmatic method is in the question of involution-melancholia. Controversy rages as to whether the involution-melancholias belong in the senile group (in my own arrangement, Group VII, the Geriopsychoses) or whether they belong in the cyclothymic (manic-depressive group) Group IX of the above list. Logically there might be some argument for placing the involution-melancholias among the senile and presenile conditions. The very *term* involution suggests this. However, it seems to me that we must grant that we know next to nothing (and pragmatically I should say absolutely nothing) about the etiology and genesis of involution melancholia. No doubt there is a darkling idea that involution melancholia is somehow an endocrine affair. We know nothing about the etiology and genesis of manic-depressive psychoses. But here the pragmatic method allows us to employ even our ignorance to advantage. There is not the slightest doubt that to place a case in the senile or presenile sub-groups of the Geriopsychoses is to give the case an evil prognosis with respect to tissue destruction and degeneration, perhaps unjustly and harmfully.

To place the involution-melancholias in the senile-senescent group is to cause certain experiences to be expected. Now, practically, we know that such experiences are not always to be expected in involution-melancholia, in short that clinical deterioration is not always found to suggest brain tissue degeneration. Pragmatically speaking, therefore, it seems to me that the reply as to the placement of the involution-melancholias is unconditionally to place them in the cyclothymic group, as compared with the senile-senescent group — and this despite our dense ignorance of the nature of involution-melancholia.

SUMMARY

1. Psychiatry should more and more adopt the 'Laboratory habit of mind," become more and more pragmatic, and bring itself in line with the rest of medicine.

2. Seven applications of the pragmatic method to psychiatry are offered:

(a) It makes a difference to the patient whether he is seen by a psychiatrist or by a clinical neurologist: There is thus for the moment a real difference between psychiatry and clinical neurology, though the future may destroy that difference and produce "neuropsychiatry."

(b) It makes a difference to the patient whether we take "insanity" as a unit or as a collection of entities: The pragmatic rule decides in favor of a pluralistic view of mental diseases.

(c) The principle of *orderly* exclusion in the diagnosis of complicated cases is of pragmatic value.

(d) Especially is this true of the diagnostic field of neurosyphilis, where it is important to maintain the *non*paretic hypothesis as long as possible in the interest of the patient's therapy.

(e) Opinions might differ as to the advisability of entertaining the hypothesis of focal brain disease before or after the hypothesis of somatic (non-neural) disease in a given case: The pragmatic rule might decide one way for general hospital clinics and the other way for mental clinics.

(f) Schizophrenia should be eliminated before cyclothymia on the pragmatic basis, for a group of schizophrenic symptoms is much more decisive for dementia precox than a group of cyclothymic symptoms is decisive for manic-depressive psychosis.

(g) The pragmatic method decides that in the face of complete ignorance of its true nature, involution-melancholia is better placed in the cyclothymic (manic-depressive) group than in the senile-senescent group, if it is to be placed in either group.

THE RELATION OF GLYCOGEN TO THE PATHOLOGIC CHANGES IN PANCREATIC DIABETES*

By Dwight M. Ervin, A.B., Cincinnati, Ohio

IN a previous article evidence was given that the pancreatic diabetic state is a condition in which little or no glycogen is formed from the ingested glucose. In order to make clear the argument following in this article, we will restate our former conclusion—"the pancreatic state of diabetes is a condition where, by failure of the pancreatic internal secretion, glucose is not rapidly enough built into glycogen. By failure to synthesize glucose into glycogen and so remove the glucose from the blood, there results a hyperglycemia and glycosuria." This absence of glycogen in the tissues I shall offer evidences for in this article, accounts for the associated pathologic changes of diabetes such as fatty degeneration and acetonuria.

The importance of glycogen in the prevention of fatty changes of the liver and tissues has been recognized before (Rosenfeld;[1] Graham[2, 3, 4, 5]). In the work of these two observers it was found that the fatty degeneration following such poisonings as mercury, chloroform, was largely prevented by the previously administered diet rich in carbohydrates. Both, in their explanation of the beneficial effect of carbohydrate, came to the conclusion that it was a faulty oxidation of fats when carbohydrates were not being burned. I believe that it is not a question of oxidation directly, but one depending upon the hydrophilic property of glycogen.

Still other observers have called attention to the fatty change when glycogen had disappeared from the cell (Starling,[6] Stolibno). So marked was this fatty degeneration in the absence of glycogen that there was formulated a belief that glycogen and fat existed in a cell only in an *inverse ratio* to each other. Why this was apparently so is easily explained upon the colloidal properties of glycogen and the difficulty in staining fat in a highly dispersed form as it exists in an emulsified state.

GLYCOGEN AND EMULSION

M. H. Fischer[7] has expressed the view that the fat of the tissue is held in an emulsified state by means of proteins; and that the power to emulsify fat is dependent upon the hydrophilic nature of the colloid (protein). We may add that glycogen also is a hydrophilic colloid and as such has a better emulsifying power for the services of the biological kingdom because it is capable of holding more oil or fat than protein, and is more resistant to acids, alkalies and salts. In a system with protein and fat, such as a protein-glycogen-fat emulsion, its stabilizing properties are still noticeable by making the complete system more stable. This is shown by the following experiments with three types of emulsions:

*From the Pathologic Department of the University of Cincinnati.

A.		B.		C.	
Casein	2 gm.	Casein	1 gm.	Glycogen	2 gm.
N		Glycogen	1 gm.	N	
— Sodium Carb.	20 c.c.	N		— Sodium Carb.	20 c.c.
20		— Sodium Carb.	20 c.c.	20	
Oil (cotton seed)	30 c.c.	20		Oil (cotton seed)	30 c.c.
		Oil (cotton seed)	30 c.c.		

In the proportions given above, the emulsion A (protein fat) is a firm mixture; B (protein-glycogen-fat) rather a liquid; and C (glycogen fat) is a liquid. The pure emulsions, though made with the yellow cotton-seed oil, are pure white in color.

EMULSIFIED FATS AND STAINS

M. H. Fischer[7] has called attention to the fact that when fat is finely dispersed as in the emulsion state it does not show the stains, scarlet red and sudan iii. Not only does the fat not respond to the stains, but glycogen, which stains red with iodine (a method used to indicate the presence of glycogen), does not stain when in the emulsified state. An emulsion similar to C (glycogen-oil) was made, but in place of cotton-seed oil, an oil that stained a deep cherry with iodine was used. This emulsion could not be stained in any manner with iodine; neither the glycogen nor the oil would show the red stain of iodine. Oil was then taken and stained a deep cherry red with iodine and then emulsified by glycogen. The resulting emulsion was as though no iodine had been added, a pure white.

It is this failure of fat to stain in the fine dispersion of an emulsion that has led to the belief of the *inverse ratio* of glycogen and fat in tissues. When glycogen is present the emulsion state is normal and the fat (there in large quantities) does not stain; but as the glycogen disappears from the cells the fat is permitted to coalesce into such sized particles as are capable of showing the stains. The stains do not show an accumulation of fat, as Stolibno, in observing phosphorus poisoning, said, "there is an increase in the fat content of the liver formed at the expense of the carbohydrate constituents of the cell, for with the increase of fat there is a relative decrease in glycogen;" but the stains do show a breaking emulsion with coalescing of the fat particle because the glycogen, a stabilizing agent against acids and salts when there, is being hydrolyzed out. It is this breaking of the emulsion, protein-glycogen-fat, by the hydrolysis of glycogen, that stains and lends an apparent inverse ratio presence of fat and glycogen. Rosenfeld[10] found that the fat chemically estimated in fatty degenerated livers was actually less than normal.

GLYCOGEN AS AN EMULSIFYING AGENT

The amount of oil that an emulsifying agent will hold may be taken at the point where the oil characters begin to appear, such as a greasy feel or a yellowish cast of color to the emulsion. This is at the point that M. H. Fischer[9] calls the change from the protein-oil to the oil-protein emulsion. In the former the protein is considered as the dispersion system, and the oil the dispersed; in the second, the oil has become the dispersion means and the protein the dispersed. A comparison between a protein type and a glycogen type of emulsifying agent shows a marked difference in the oil holding properties of the two.

In the type of an emulsion where protein is used as the dispersing means, less oil is held than in one where glycogen is used. In A, 2 gm. of protein, 20 c.c. of N/20 sodium carbonate, the oil began to appear as the external phase when 50 c.c. of oil were added: but in C, 2 gm. of glycogen, we were able to add before the oil began to appear as the external phase, as much as 90 c.c. of oil.

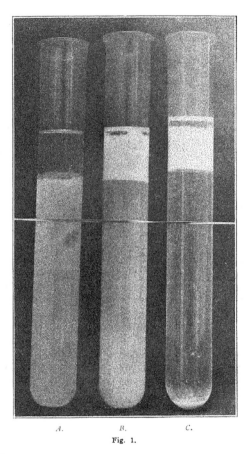

A.   B.   C.

Fig. 1.

The addition of glycogen to a protein oil emulsion raises the quantity of oil that may be emulsified.

GLYCOGEN AND ACIDS

The stability of an emulsion depends upon the relative values of oil, water, and hydrophilic colloid. If the ability of the colloid to hold water be changed, as by dehydration (by acids, alkalies or salts) so that the combined water becomes separated, it permits the coalescing of the fat and a breaking of the emulsion.

The breaking of the three types of emulsions by acids depends upon the presence of glycogen in the system. Glycogen as a stabilizing agent in the emulsion adds to the system a strong element of resistance to acids. The protein-fat system is readily broken by the addition of strong acid but the glycogen fat is with great difficulty broken. Fig. 1 shows the behavior of the three types of emulsion (see above, A, B, C). A has had added to it just sufficient hydrochloric acid to cause its breaking. B has had twice the same amount as A, and C has had four times the amount of hydrochloric acid. The emulsion A is completely separated into protein, water and fat. B has been changed very little, while C continues to hold its emulsion form. The addition of glycogen gives to the emulsion a stabilizing power against the breaking by acids.

It is this stabilization by glycogen that in the body serves to prevent fatty degeneration, or dissolution of the cell, as long as glycogen is present, but when the glycogen is hydrolyzed by acids, the protein-fat cell breaks easily into edematous protein and free fat, which we interpret as fatty degeneration.

GLYCOGEN IN DISEASE

Bearing in mind the two important properties, resistance to acids, salts, etc., and emulsifying power, given to an emulsion by glycogen, we find an easy and unstrained explanation of the relation of fat and glycogen in disease.

Rosenfeld[11] observed several points of considerable interest bearing upon such an interpretation as I have given. (1) Various poisons, phosphorus, arsenic, mercury, chloroform, produce always a fatty liver, and in every instance such a liver is glycogen-free. This condition is also true in pancreatic extirpation. (2) Carbohydrates, when fed, prevent a fatty liver. He explained this upon the belief that fats are burned with difficulty without a simultaneous oxidation of carbohydrate, and that in these cases oxidation is seriously lowered. Lusk,[12] however, found the metabolism increased in phosphorus poisoning.

What I believe takes place is that acids formed through the action of the poisoning, hydrolyze the glycogen (as witnessed by hyperglycemia and glycosuria), then causes a separation of the protein-fat emulsion or system that remains. While glycogen is present, the system protein-glycogen-fat is broken by acid only with difficulty, and glycogen is maintained in the system by carbohydrate feeding. I would add here that glycogen is maintained in the system or cell only when the equation glucose = glycogen takes place in a medium of right reaction and such a reaction can not be acid. Graham[13, 14, 15] observed the protective value of glycogen against fatty degeneration of the liver.

In the treatment of poisonings such as from mercury, chloroform, etc., the patient should first be alkalinized to make it possible for the reaction to go from glucose to glycogen, then fed carbohydrates in plenty to furnish glucose from which to build a protein-glycogen-fat system that is stable.

FATTY DEGENERATION IN DIABETES

There is little difference between the foregoing fat pathology in the poisonings and in diabetes. In the poisonings the glycogen is hydrolyzed from the pro-

tein-glycogen-fat system, leaving the easily separated protein-fat, while in diabetes there is little glycogen formed, and therefore the emulsion of the diabetes
is always a protein-fat emulsion. Consequently feeding alkalies and carbohydrates
is of only small value because of the failure to form glycogen from glucose—a
reaction which depends upon the internal secretion of the pancreas and is at
fault in pancreatic diabetes.

HYPERGLYCEMIA

In all acute fevers, typhoid, pneumonia, etc., Heger[16] found a hyperglycemia.
In death after such fever we find the organs have all undergone a fatty degen-

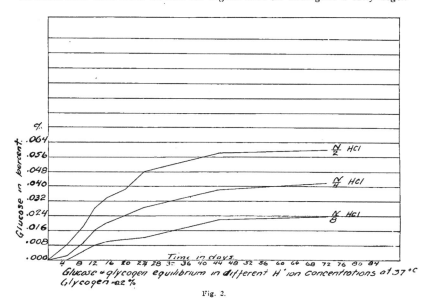

Glucose + glycogen equilibrium in different H⁺ ion concentrations at 37 °C
Glycogen = .02 %

Fig. 2.

eration. In nephritis, Hopkins and Cole[17] found a hyperglycemia. Williams and
Humphreys[18] in 80 cases found the blood sugar high in proportion to the gravity
of the disease, and in the state of coma the blood sugar rose as high as in diabetes.
These conditions, I believe, follow the same law as in mercury and similar poisonings; i.e., it is the result of the catalytic power of the hydrogen ion to shift the
equilibrium point between glycogen and glucose.

As the hydrogen ion increases in effective concentration, the reaction shifts
towards the glucose side. The shifting may take place to such an extent that
the glucose will rise high enough to reach the kidney level. Glycosuria is found
in fevers and nephritis. The shifting of the equilibrium of glucose from glycogen by the catalytic power of the hydrogen ion is almost in a direct proportion
to the increase of the concentration of the ion.[19] In mercury and chloroform the
shifting is only more severe toward glucose, but otherwise the chemical law in

the poisonings and in the fevers is one and the same law. In nephritis and the fevers, fatty degeneration is always present and glycogen is absent. The shifting of the glycogen towards glucose, gives an increase of glucose concentration to the cell, and as the glycogen disappears, the protein-fat system remaining is separated easily by the acids, and gives likewise an increase of fat to the cell. It is the increase of fat and glucose concentration that gives the increase in metabolism. Fig. 2 gives the rate of hydrolysis of glycogen and the different equilibriums of glycogen-glucose in different concentrations of the hydrogen ion.

The pathology associated with diabetes, fatty degeneration and acetonuria has the same underlying cause. Chemical and physicochemical laws govern, as in mercury, phosphorus, chloroform, starvation, nephritis and the fevers. It is the emulsification and stabilizing characteristic of glycogen in the protein-glycogen fat emulsion.

ACETONURIA

An acetonuria is merely the indication of what is taking place in the liver and other tissues. It is the rapid separation of the fat held in the protein-fat emulsion of the body and an overwhelming load of fat delivered to the cell. In mercury, and chloroform, there is a sudden and rapid hydrolysis of the glycogen (a shifting of the glycogen-glucose equilibrium until the glucose concentration in the blood rises high enough to pass through the kidney). This leaves the easily separated protein-fat system which is then broken rapidly by acids with the liberation of a large concentration of fat. It is this increase of glucose and fat upon the cell that gives the increased metabolism found by Lusk. It is another evidence of the law of Guldberg and Wagge that the velocity of a reaction is proportional to their masses. But there is a limit to the oxidizing power of the cell, and the whole of the fat molecule is not burned completely. By this we do not mean that as the molecule of fat reaches the stage of the acetone molecule it is no longer burned, for it is, and a deal is got rid of by the body in that manner; but that in the burning of a large amount of fat, a high concentration of acetone (oxybutyric acid and aceto-acetic acid) is developed and accordingly diffuses through the kidney before it is burned and we detect it. Acetonuria is in reality not a failure in oxidation as we have been accustomed to believe, but an oxidation of too great a load of fat permitting a formation of a high enough concentration of intermediate compound, e.g., acetone, etc., that while a portion is burned completely to CO_2, another portion passes out through the kidney.

Such a condition must manifestly develop where the fat concentration to the cell becomes extremely high. This extreme concentration of fat to the cell may be brought about by either a rapid liberation of the fat already emulsified in the body or by a failure to emulsify the fat of a meal. The first condition is that of starvation, mercury, phosphorus and such poisons, nephritis and fevers; the second is that of diabetes. In this last disease, glycogen is not synthesized and stable emulsions are not formed. When too little glycogen is formed as in carbohydrate starvation with fat feeding, the rate of emulsification is too low and the fat reaches the cell in large quantities. Zeller[20] observed when only 5 per cent of the diet of fat and carbohydrate was carbohydrate, acetone bodies appeared in abundance. Fat is normally regulated in its concentration to the cell by emulsification in the system protein-glycogen-fat, and by the nicety of the dissolution of this system it reaches the cells in the concentration best suited to their need.

LIPEMIA

The condition of lipemia is another inevitable result from the condition of fat in the system of protein-glycogen-fat. After the taking of a heavy fat meal there will appear in the blood, fat sufficient to produce turbidity.[21] Bloor[22] gives a table of the rise in the blood fat after a fat meal.

24 hrs. after food	0.6 % fat
3¼ hrs, after 100 c.c. olive oil	0.73% fat
6¼ hrs. after 100 c.c. olive oil	1.20% fat
8 hrs. after 100 c.c. olive oil	.87% fat

And Lusk[23] calls attention to the fact that the curve of metabolism after a fat meal runs closely parallel to the rise of fat in the blood as found by Bloor. The temporary lipemia found by Bloor is a result of the slow emulsification of fat, while the lipemia of diabetes is the failure to emulsify the fat even at a slow rate. The lipemia of a diabetic will disappear with the elimination of fat in the diet. This change of concentration of the food stuffs to the cell is likewise the cause of the change in the respiratory quotient.

Lusk,[24] and Joslin and Benedict[25] found in diabetes and in phosphorus poisoning that while metabolism had increased the respiratory quotient had become lower than 1.0. Voit[26] modified the law of Guldberg and Wagge and applied it to biology. The rate of oxidation of the cell is increased by an increase of concentration of food to the cell. In phosphorus poisoning and in diabetes we have an increase of food to the cell—in the former, because in the shifting of the equilibrium of glycogen towards glucose, the concentration of the latter is increased. Likewise with the dissolution of the cell by removal of glycogen, the rate of fat liberation is increased. In diabetes the concentration of glucose is high because it is not emulsified. This increase of concentration of food to the cells gives the increase in metabolism. The change of the respiratory quotient is a change in the respective concentrations of fat and glucose to the cell. In the normal person burning carbohydrates the respiratory quotient is 1.0 because the concentration of fats, soaps, and amino acids in proportion to the glucose is relatively low. But as the concentration of fat rises, the respiratory quotient drops and approaches that of fat alone, 0.72. When a mixture of glucose and fat is burned, the quotient must be somewhere between 1.0 and 0.72. If the glucose is high in relation to the fat, the quotient will be close to 1.0 and if low in relation to fat, the quotient is nearer 0.72. In diabetes the quotient can be raised only slightly by the feeding of carbohydrate because the fat concentration can not be lowered by its storage. In sugar starvation the quotient is low because the fat is increased by the dissolution of the protein-glycogen-fat system. When glucose is fed, the system is rebuilt and the fat concentration lowered. But in diabetes there is no appreciable storage of fat by emulsification, and the feeding of carbohydrates can have but little effect. Similarly whenever the normal concentrations of glucose, soap (fats) or amino acids are altered about or in the cell the relative oxidation is changed and with it the respiratory quotient.

SUMMARY

Glycogen is a stabilizing colloid in the cell and as such prevents the breaking of the emulsion or fatty degeneration by its resistance to acids, salts, etc.

Glycogen is hydrolyzed by acids, and when hydrolyzed, there is left a protein-fat emulsion that is but poorly resistant against acids.

In diabetes no glycogen is formed, the fat is only slightly emulsified, permitting a high concentration of the fats or soaps to reach the cell and a consequent limited oxidation with the production of the acetone bodies.

The equilibrium of glycogen with glucose is shifted towards the glucose side by the presence of the hydrogen ion, which is the explanation of the high blood sugars in fevers, mercury and phosphorus poisoning, and nephritis.

BIBLIOGRAPHY

[1]Rosenfeld: Fettbildung Ergbn. d. Physiol., 1903, ii, 1-30.
[2]Graham: Jour. Exper. Med., 1915, xxi, p. 185.
[3]Graham: Jour. Exper. Med., 1915, xxii, 49.
[4]Graham: Jour. Biol. Chem. Prac., 1915, xx, 25.
[5]Graham: Jour. Am. Med. Assn., 1917, lxix, 166.
[6]Starling.
[7]Fischer, M. H., and Hooker, M. O.: Fats and Fattv Degeneration, New York, 1917, p. 61.
[8, 9]Idem., p. 62.
[10]Rosenfeld: Ergebn. der Physiol., Abt. 1, 1902 (11) 651; ibid., 1903 (2) 50.
[11]Rosenfeld: Berl. klin. Wchnschr., 1906, pp. 978-981.
[12]Lusk: Science of Nutrition, 1917, p. 491.
[13]Graham: Jour. Exper. Med., 1915, xxii, 49.
[14]Graham: Jour. Biol. Chem. Proc., 1915, xx, 25.
[15]Graham: Jour. Am. Med. Assn., 1917, lxix, 166.
[16]Heger: Deutsch. med. Wchnschr., 1911-1917.
[17]Hopkins: Am. Jour. Med. Sc., 1915, cxlix, 254.
[18]Humphreys and Williams: Arch. Int. Med., 1919, xxiii, 5.
[19]Arrhenins: Ztschr. phys. Chem., 1889, iv, 226.
[20]Zeller: Arch: f. Physiol., 1914, p. 213.
[21]Neisser and Braunning: Ztschr. Jour. Exper. Path. u. Ther., 1907, iv, 747.
[22]Bloor: Jour. Biol. Chem., 1914, xix, 1.
[23]Murlin and Lusk: Jour. Biol. Chem., 1915, xxii, 15.
[24]Lusk: The Science of Nutrition, 1917, p. 492, Ibid., p. 474.
[25]Benedict and Joslin: Metabolism in Diabetes Mellitus, 1910. Metabolism in Severe Diabetes, 1912.
[26]Voit: Physiologie des Hoffwechsels, 1881.

PATHOLOGY OF INFLUENZA-PNEUMONIA*

By ORVILLE J. WALKER, M.D., YOUNGSTOWN, OHIO

First Lieutenant, M. C., U. S. Army, Camp Sherman, Chillicothe, Ohio

T HE pandemic of acute respiratory disease which swept over the world during 1918 has already furnished a voluminous literature in the shape of reports from numerous sections where it occurred. In reviewing this literature one is impressed with the fact that though the various reports differ in certain minor details, they are remarkably similar in essential points. In spite of the enormous amount of work done by numerous observers in widely separated sections of the country, there has curiously enough been little added to our knowledge of these conditions. The specific etiologic agent of influenza has not been determined to the satisfaction of every one. At a recent meeting of the American Public Health Association, after a thorough and searching effort on the part of some of the ablest men of that eminent gathering, the conclusion reached was that "the microorganism or virus primarily responsible for this disease has not yet been identified."[1]

Pneumonia, the most constant complication of influenza and the most prolific cause of the terrible mortality which accompanied it, has been studied by a great many workers and all are agreed that, although lesions resembling both lobar and bronchopneumonia have been met with, these conditions are not absolutely typical of true lobar or bronchopneumonia. Evidently we are concerned with a peculiar type of pulmonary lesion. No one has yet attempted an exact description and classification of influenza-pneumonia as an entity. This paper is therefore written in an effort to add something to the sum total of the records of the pandemic in the form of a report of the pneumonia occurring at Camp Sherman, Ohio; and in the second place to attempt a logical and orderly classification of the conditions met with, together with our ideas of why they assumed the peculiar and particular character which they did. These conclusions have been reached chiefly through a careful study of the first one hundred postmortems held on cases dying at this camp during the epidemic period, from September 16 to November 15. In all more than 150 cases were examined postmortem, but only the first 100 were selected for careful scrutiny and study as a basis for this report. Helpful suggestions were also derived in the elaboration of these views by a careful review of the reports of similar conditions occurring throughout this country.

During the period from September 16 to November 15, 1918,† there occurred 9,380 cases of influenza at Camp Sherman. Of this number, 7,776 were admitted to the Base Hospital. The incidence of pneumonia from influenza in this camp was 2,827, or 30.13 per cent of all influenza cases. Of the total number of pneumonia cases treated in this hospital, 2,181 cases were admitted as such, while only 646,(8.3 per cent) cases developed from the 7,776 cases of influenza treated in the hospital. The number of deaths occurring from influenza and pneumonia during the period mentioned was 1,091, a mortality in our pneu-

*Published by permission of the Surgeon-General's Office, Washington, D. C.
†Official Report to Surgeon-General's Office.

monias of 38.59 per cent; or as a result of all the influenza occurring in the camp, a mortality of 11.63 per cent.

It is questionable whether the term "influenza" should be used in connection with our latest pandemic and applied to the pneumonia following it. However, the designation has been so universally applied in this connection that it would hardly avail to substitute another term for it. Obviously, however, if this name be accepted denoting the disease complex occurring during the epidemic, Pfeiffer's organism, also called Bacillus influenzæ, should not retain that name or be associated as the causative agent of the disease until definitely proved as such.

There seems to be a great diversity of opinion among observers in regard to the exact type of pneumonia occurring as a complication of influenza. Some speak of the lesion as a bronchopneumonia which in severe cases developed a conglomerate character simulating lobar pneumonia. McCallum[2] suggests that while these pneumonias are characteristic interstitial broncho in type, the rapid growth of virulent organisms was such that it spread rapidly producing a widespread homogeneous consolidation, owing to the filling of the alveoli with leucocytic exudate loaded with organisms. Nuzum[3] speaks of it as a massive, confluent, pseudolobar pneumonia. Symmers[4] calls attention to the similarity between influenza-pneumonia and Bubonic plague pneumonia. That all are tacitly agreed that we are not dealing with a typical broncho- or a typical lobar pneumonia, is evidenced by the fact that practically every one refers to the pulmonary condition following influenza as either broncho *type* or lobar *type* of pneumonia.

The pulmonary lesion under discussion differs from true lobar pneumonia in that (1) during the stage of red hepatization the cut surface of the involved lung is never dry, but moist and viscid; (2) there is no abrupt transit between the area of consolidation and the surrounding tissue, but rather the whole lobe, and often even the whole of both organs, is involved with a patchy process of smaller or larger areas; (3) the process is not limited as in typical lobar pneumonia to an exudation within the alveoli, but extends itself to the interstitial tissue including blood vessels, lymphatics, and bronchial tubes, resulting in great damage to all these structures, and ending not in resolution but in extensive organization and pulmonary fibrosis; (4) the presence, in many cases, of enormous numbers of large mononuclear wandering cells in the earlier stages of involvement.

It is an interesting fact to note the similarity that exists between influenza and influenza-pneumonia, on the one hand, and such exanthemata as typhoid, measles, purpura hemorrhagica, and certain chemical poisonings, such as benzol, menthol, sulphanol, and so forth, on the other. All show a blood picture varying from a slight reduction in the total leucocyte count, to even a severe leucopenia. McCallum[5] and others have noted the similarity existing between the pneumonias occurring as a complication of measles and of influenza. Typhoid pneumonia and the postinfluenzal pneumonias are similar, in that the large mononuclear wandering cell, or endothelial leucocyte, which is characteristic of typhoid lesions is found conspicuously in the latter condition.

Of the one hundred cases selected for study, necropsies of the first twenty were performed by Wheeler,[6] and the gross findings reported by him. As this series included some of the earliest cases dying as the result of influenza, they were of peculiar interest for the purposes of this study. Careful microscopic study was made in all these cases by the author.

In the diagnosis of our pneumonias an attempt was made to group them after the fashion generally used in reports coming from other army camps, i.e., 1, acute pulmonary edema; 2 bronchopneumonia, (a), interstitial type, (b), lobular type; 3, lobar pneumonia type. Table I shows the incidence, distribution and stages found.

PULMONARY EDEMA

A number of writers have described this as the very earliest pulmonary lesion causing death in influenza cases. Friedlander, et al.,[6] described such a condition as seen at this camp, and called it "acute inflammatory pulmonary edema."

TABLE I

DISTRIBUTION AND STAGE OF PROCESSES OCCURRING IN ONE HUNDRED AUTOPSIES ON INFLUENZA-PNEUMONIA

CONDITIONS	TYPE PNEUMONIA						
	BRONCHO-INTERSTITIAL	BRONCHO-LOBULAR	BRONCHO-LOBULAR AND INTERSTITIAL	LOBAR (ALONE)	LOBAR AND BRONCHO-INTERSTITIAL	LOBAR AND BRONCHO-LOBULAR	LOBAR, BRONCHO-INTERSTITIAL AND BRONCHO-LOBULAR
Cases	34	33	12	12	2	5	2
Right side alone	4	5	0	3	0	1	0
Left side alone	2	3	0	2	0	0	0
Bilateral	28	25	12	7	2	4	2
Lower lobes involved	34	25	12	10	2	3	2
Upper lobes involved	31	22	12	9	2	4	2
Middle lobe involved	22	10	8	6	0	4	0
Congestion and edema	7	8	3	5	1	2	0
Red hepatization	20	10	7	5	2	1	1
Gray hepatization	12	9	1	7	2	3	2
Organization	12	6	3	0	0	0	0
Abscess	6	4	0	3	0	1	0
Resolution	0	0	0	0	0	0	1

Lyons[7] described a similar condition under the term, "Hemorrhagic Pneumonitis." Brem, et al.,[8] referred to the condition as "acute hemorrhagic edema."

At the autopsy table one was impressed by the marked cyanosis of the skin, particularly about the face, neck, and fingers. The mouth and nares frequently contained a brownish or reddish, bloody fluid.

The thoracic cavities nearly always contained a definite increase of fluid on the involved sides. This varied considerably in amount from a few c.c. to 1000 c.c. Its color varied from a light brownish-yellow to a dark red, while in character it was serous to serosanguineous.

The visceral pleura generally presented a smooth, glistening appearance, which was, however, rather constantly broken by groups of tiny, petechial, hemorrhagic extravasations beneath the pleura. The spots varied in size from pin-point to 8 or 10 mm. in diameter, and were in shape generally round, but sometimes irregular. Frequently they conglomerated to form large irregular-shaped areas. They were seen anywhere on the visceral surface, but most frequently on the diaphragmatic and interlobar surfaces, and about the hilus of the lung.

The lungs varied in color, depending upon the degree of involvement, from a deep red through grayish-blue to a light pinkish-gray in the congested areas. The lesions varied depending upon the extent of the process from tiny patchy areas of hemorrhage to large conglomerate areas involving the greater part of a lobe. These areas were increased in consistency, did not crepitate, and pitted on pressure. In no instance was an entire lobe involved by the hemorrhage, air-containing tissue being found in every case on close inspection. These areas were usually found about the periphery of the lobes, or, in cases of interstitial and lobular involvement, between the areas of hemorrhage. Such areas were noted on the surface as nonresilient, emphysematous tissue standing out above the darker, more doughy, hemorrhagic areas. As a result of this air-containing tissue scattered throughout the organ, such a lung when placed in water would float, or at least only partially sink, depending upon the degree of involvement. If, however, a piece of hemorrhagic tissue were cut out from the surrounding organ, it would sink in water. These lungs were large, distended, showing no tendency to collapse, and often showing depression marks of the ribs on their surface. The order of frequency of involvement of the lobes was right lower, left lower, right upper, left upper, and right middle (see Table I). Usually the posterior portion of the lobe was involved, while the anterior portion was frequently free from hemorrhage and congestion, but quite emphysematous. Often, the posterior portions of both upper and lower lobes were involved about equally, while the anterior portions were free. In many instances, the posterior pyramidal portion of the middle lobe was the only part of that lobe involved. Not uncommonly, the posterior portion of both lungs was included in the process.

On section of the lungs, there was an immediate pouring out of dark, bloody, frothy, fluid exudate. The amount of fluid welling from the cut surfaces of the lungs without any undue pressure being exerted on the tissue was often enormous, measuring as much as 200 c.c. in some cases. On scraping away the fluid exudate from the surface, irregular dark-red areas of hemorrhage were seen mottling the whole surface, interspersed with lighter, pinkish-gray areas of the intervening, uninvolved lung tissue. The darker areas were dull, firm, and doughy, with smooth or finely granular surfaces, and varied in size from tiny, scarcely visible specks to large, conglomerate masses occupying the greater part of the lobe. Often, the hemorrhagic areas were limited to a single or a few lobules, and their lobular outline could be distinctly followed. The smaller bronchi stood out above the surrounding surface, their mucous membrane being swollen and edematous. There appeared to be a distinct thickening of their walls, with a consequent narrowing of their lumens. They contained a thin, frothy, blood-tinged fluid, little mucus, and no pus. The trachea and larger bronchi presented much the same appearance as the smaller ones seen on the surface, their mucous membrane being swollen and edematous, and in color, varying from pale pink to a deep, purplish-red.

Microscopically, the lung tissue in the involved areas presented intense congestion and engorgement of the interalveolar capillaries and lymphatics, with extravasation of blood serum and red blood cells into the neighboring alveoli. In fact, the air sacs in these areas were often tensely distended with blood serum and cells. Close to the lining membrane of the alveoli and ducti alveolares a very thin layer of fibrin was seen, in many instances, the only fibrin present. Underneath this, the epithelial lining of the walls was often in a state of necrosis, appearing as a thin, hyaline membrane. Again, air sacs irregularly distributed throughout the hemorrhagic areas were filled with fibrin network, which enmeshed the cellular elements. The walls of the interstitial capillaries and even the larger vessels constantly showed a similar hyaline membrane in which the outline of the individual endothelial cells could no longer be discerned. The hemorrhagic areas were usually sharply delineated from the noninvolved lung tissue. In t he latter areas the air sacs were widely dilated, with thin walls, which, in some instances, were even ruptured. In other areas bordering on the hemorrhagic areas, the lung tissue was in a state of collapse, whole lobules or groups of lobules often being involved. Microorganisms were conspicuous by their absence in these lungs, unless perhaps an occasional organism might be seen in or near the bronchi.

BRONCHOPNEUMONIA TYPE

Both the interstitial and lobular types of bronchopneumonia so ably described by McCallum[9] in cases of pneumonia following measles were met with numerous times. (See Table I.) All stages and degrees of involvement were seen, and did not differ materially from the lesion noted by McCallum. We were, however, very forcibly impressed by the finding of the pneumococcus Types III and IV in culture, and in tissue section from these lungs, as the only organism present, nearly as often as the Streptococcus hemolyticus. (See Table II.) Again, mixed infections of Streptococcus hemolyticus and pneumococcus were found. This is contrary to McCallum's statement that this type of lesion is typical of the hemolytic streptococcus invasion. Thomas[10] mentions finding the pneumococcus Type IV in five such cases at autopsy at Camp Meade. Blanton and Irons,[11] in a report of pneumonias at Camp Custer, state, "Strange as it may seem, there was no difference to be made out in the nature of the process caused by streptococcus, pneumococcus, or influenza bacillus." In a later article, McCallum[3] reports Pfeiffer's organism of influenza as the etiologic agent in the interstitial type of bronchopneumonia. Obviously, we can not therefore accept these types of pneumonia as typical of the invasion of the hemolytic streptococcus. McCallum[2] reports cases of pneumonia resembling closely the lobar pneumonia produced by the pneumococcus occurring in association with typical peribronchial and interstitial changes. From these nothing but the hemolytic streptococcus was isolated. Attention is called to Table II which shows the incidence of the hemolytic streptococcus and pneumococcus in lobar and bronchopneumonia. In fact, it is doubtful whether the type of bacteria isolated from pulmonary tissue in pneumonia is of any value in making a differential diagnosis between broncho- and lobar pneumonia, and it certainly is not between interstitial and lobular types of bronchopneumonia.

INTERSTITIAL BRONCHOPNEUMONIA

Interstitial bronchopneumonia, first described by Kaufman, and first noted in this country by Mathers,[12] was met with in our series thirty-four times as the only type of lesion. The lobular type of bronchopneumonia, referred to by Cole and McCallum[9] in connection with their studies on pneumonia following measles, occurred in our series thirty-three times. These two types occurred together, often in the same lobe, twelve times.

In the earlier cases diagnosed as interstitial bronchopneumonia, the lungs

TABLE II

ORGANISMS AND TYPES OF LESIONS IN ONE HUNDRED CASES OF INFLUENZA-PNEUMONIA

TYPE OF PNEUMONIA	HEMOLYTIC STREPTOCOCCUS	PNEUMOCOCCUS TYPE IV	PNEUMOCOCCUS TYPE III	PNEUMOCOCCUS TYPE II	HEMOLYTIC STREPTOCOCCUS AND PNEUMOCOCCUS TYPE IV	HEMOLYTIC STREPTOCOCCUS AND PNEUMOCOCCUS TYPE III	HEMOLYTIC STREPTOCOCCUS AND STAPHYLOCOCCUS	PNEUMOCOCCUS TYPE IV AND PFEIFFER'S BACILLUS	PNEUMOCOCCUS TYPE IV AND STAPHYLOCOCCUS	NON-HEMOLYTIC STREPTOCOCCUS AND PNEUMOCOCCUS TYPE IV	STERILE
Lobar	3	4			2	1					2
Broncho-Interstitial	12	9	2		4	1	2	1	1	1	1
Broncho-Lobular	11	9	2	1	2	1		2	1		4
Broncho-Lobular and Interstitial	3	2		1	2						
Lobar and Broncho-Interstitial	1	1									
Lobar and Broncho-Lobular	2	1			2						
Lobar, Broncho-Lobular and Interstitial		2									

were found to be distended as in the state of full inspiration. Pleural surfaces were frequently smooth and glistening, but usually covered with a thin, finely granular fibrin. On section, the surface of the lung was moist and covered with a yellowish-brown or brownish-red viscid material. Pulmonary tissue was a light grayish-pink color, uniformly dotted with areas two to five millimeters in diameter of yellowish-gray appearance, like disseminated, conglomerate tubercles. These areas were usually surrounded by halos of dark red-colored tissue, and on pressure a tiny drop of pus was expressed from the center of each area. Frequent patchy areas of pulmonary collapse were to be noted. Hyperemia of this lung tissue was very striking.

Microscopically, the bronchioles and infundibuli were filled with polymorphonuclear cells and the invading organisms. These corresponded to the miliary, opaque, yellow spots above noted. Closely hugging the walls of the ducti alveolares and alveoli was a hyaline membrane which was composed of the coagulated necrotic cells of the mucosa. Fibrin in a thin layer frequently covered this process. In these areas, interalveolar tissue was quite swollen, and capillary vessels thrombosed, their adventitia replaced by a thin, hyaline membrane of necrotic tissue. The lymphatics were plugged with cells. Adjacent alveoli were frequently filled with blood and a few leucocytes. In some places, the process was so limited to the immediate vicinity of the bronchioles that it was designated "acute bronchiolitis."[13]

In somewhat older cases, the cut surface of the lung was dryer and covered with numerous, tiny, firm, projecting nodules, evidently a further process of the one just described. The cross sections of the pus-filled bronchioles gave to the lung surface an appearance not unlike that of miliary tuberculosis. The lung tissue immediately surrounding these miliary foci was consolidated. These areas of consolidation were, if anything, perhaps larger than the areas noted in the previous stage, and, in many instances, had become confluent, forming irregular patchy areas of consolidation through coalescence of the original peribronchial areas. Areas supplied by the involved bronchioles were collapsed and airless. Consolidated areas in the vicinity of the involved bronchi were sometimes surrounded by alveoli in a state of extreme congestion not unlike that seen in the stage of engorgement in lobar pneumonia. The intervening tissue, often collapsed, showed a viscid edema throughout its whole extent.

Microscopically, the bronchioles and infundibuli were seen to be most intensely affected, forming the center of the picture. Their lumen was tightly packed with polymorphonuclear leucocytes, mononuclear wandering cells, and desquamated epithelium. The walls of the bronchi were largely stripped of their lining epithelium. The bronchi together with the tissue immediately surrounding them were intensely swollen, due to infiltration with polymorphonuclear and mononuclear leucocytes, new-formed connective tissue cells, and serum. The infiltration extended to the walls of the adjacent alveoli with consequent thickening of the interalveolar tissue. The alveoli also contained a dense exudate consisting of desquamated flakes from the necrotic mucous lining, polymorphonuclear leucocytes, mononuclear wandering cells, and, in many instances, fibrin plugs. The walls of the sacs were lined with mononuclear cells among which mitotic figures were commonly seen. About the periphery of this process, the exudate was replaced by fluid which was dense and viscid. Organisms were found in the lumen of the bronchi and in the alveolar exudate, but were found most abundantly in the lymphatic channels of this region. The lymphatics were plugged with the infiltrating leucocytes and organisms. Blood vessels were thrombosed, their adventitial tissue being frequently in an advanced state of necrosis, more often infiltrated with leucocytes, lymphoid in nature. In older cases, the exudate in the alveoli and bronchi was found in a process of organization.

LOBULAR BRONCHOPNEUMONIA

In cases diagnosed as lobular bronchopneumonia, the lungs were extremely voluminous and did not collapse when the chest was opened. The pleural surface was frequently mottled with patchy areas of dark bluish-red color, often covered with thin, finely granular fibrin in the very earliest cases. These areas were depressed below the grayish-white colored, intervening surface, or rather the latter were bulging over the consolidated area by reason of the compensatory nouresilient emphysema. On palpation, these areas were felt throughout the entire organ as nodular masses varying considerably in size. On the cut surface, islands of dark red consolidated lung showed against a paler background of nonelastic, emphysematous pulmonary tissue. These islands appeared as irregular-shaped areas several centimeters in width, sometimes perhaps including only a single lobule, more often a group of several. Their dark red-colored, finely granular, elevated surface was in marked contrast to the intervening grayish-red, crepitating, air-containing, partially collapsed lung tissue. The surface of these lungs was exceedingly moist, the consolidated areas being bathed in large quantities of a viscid, yellowish-red fluid, while the surrounding tissue was covered with a bright-red, frothy fluid. Frequently, these areas were dotted with tiny, yellowish-gray foci not unlike those areas noted in interstitial type. In a somewhat later stage of this type, the process just described, corresponding to the stage of red hepatization in lobar pneumonia, had apparently changed in character to one resembling in many respects the stage of gray hepatization. The cut surface was brownish-gray to grayish-white in color, had lost its finely granular appearance, and was at first dry or nearly so, being covered later with a brownish-red to yellowish-gray sticky, mucopurulent fluid.

Microscopically, the bronchi and bronchioles were found filled with purulent exudate very similar to that seen in interstitial type. The alveoli were tightly packed with leucocytes and fibrin, in some instances, and many organisms. Necrosis of the alveolar walls was constantly seen. The interstitial tissue was swollen and edematous with serum, infiltrating leucocytes, and thrombosed capillaries. The alveolar capillaries were occluded by hyaline, fibrinous thrombi. A little later organization was found to have taken place, the whole area being a mass of granulations. In many cases the granulating tissue was interrupted by areas of coagulated, opaque, yellow, necrotic tissue. These abscesses varied in size from tiny, pinhead areas to abscessed cavities several centimeters in diameter.

LOBAR TYPE OF PNEUMONIA

Twelve cases were met with which were termed lobar *type* of pneumonia. These cases presented larger or smaller areas of distinct consolidation, varying in color depending upon the age of involvement from a dark reddish-brown or brownish-gray to a light gray. In no instance was an entire lobe involved.

Early cases of this pseudolobar process resembled the stage of red hepatization seen in true lobar pneumonia. Pleural surfaces had lost their normal gloss and were covered with a thin, finely granular fibrinous layer, and frequently with subpleural petechia. The involved areas were dense, firm, heavy, airless, and sank in water. These lungs were in size, that of the organ at full inspiration, often with depression marks of the overlying ribs on their surface. On section, the bronchi were reddened with swollen, edematous mucosa, and plugged with a mucosanguineous material. The surface was moist, finely granular, deep red or brownish-red in color. Scraping produced a reddish, sticky fluid. The consolidated area stood out in sharp contrast to the remainder of the lung substance which collapsed, allowing its air content to escape. This latter portion crepitated and oozed a bright red, frothy fluid. Commonly these large areas of deep red consolidation were dotted with numerous miliary, grayish-yellow foci similar to those noted in the interstitial lobular types. Later cases differed from the earlier in having thicker, fibrinous coats on their surfaces, and a yellowish-gray to purplish-gray color. The cut surface was bathed in a slimy, sticky, mucopurulent fluid.

Microscopically, in the earlier cases, the air sacs were filled with red blood cells, a few white blood cells about the periphery, and, in some cases, considerable fibrin; also many mononuclear wandering cells. Red blood cells often had lost their hemoglobin and were mere shadows. About the walls of the infundibuli and alveoli was constantly found an irregular, hyaline membrane, in which the outline of the individual epithelial cells was lost. Blood vessels and lymphatics were thrombosed and distended with hyaline, coagulated serum, and necrotic cellular debris. Later cases showed the alveoli to be densely packed with polymorphonuclear and endothelial cells, together with partially degenerated red blood cells and coagulated serum. Fibrin was sometimes present and sometimes absent. Many bacteria were found, both in the alveoli and in the interstitial lymphatics. The necrotic epithelium lining of the air sacs and bronchi was largely desquamated and broken up into flaky pieces. The interstitial capillaries and lymphatics were packed with polymorphonuclear and mononuclear wandering cells and bacteria.

ORGANIZATION

Organization has been mentioned by numerous workers as a rather constant feature of influenza-pneumonia, and this has been our experience. Organization in these cases has not differed greatly from that occasionally seen following other types of pneumonia. It has occurred irrespective of the type of pneumonia involved. Resolution occurred only exceptionally in late cases coming to post, and in these it was either incomplete, or entirely lacking. The organized lobe remained more or less completely distended as in the stage of exudation, was heavy, and did not crush easily, being almost as resilient as live rubber. The cut surface was smooth, not granular, and of a moist, glassy appearance. Its color was grayish or reddish-gray, often dotted with yellow, due to alveoli or bronchi still filled with leucocytes; or the young vascular granulations which had replaced the affected bronchi and alveoli immediately adjacent might account in some cases for the small tubercle-like bodies which were seen in gross examination of the lung. The granulating areas varied in size, depending upon the extent of the pneumonic involvement, from areas about the bronchi and vessels, with consequent thickening of the interalveolar tissue, to large areas several centimeters in diameter. The process began with the appearance of the fibroblasts in the interstitial tissue between the air sacs, and in the smaller bronchi and bronchioles. Lymphatic canals were at times found converted into solid vascularized cords of connective tissue. In such areas, the most beautiful, hyaline, fibrous thrombi filled the capillaries of the alveolar walls. From the interstitial areas, fibrosis spread through the alveolar walls, into the air sacs, filling these with granulations consisting of embryonic connective tissue and numerous new-formed capillary blood vessels, gradually replacing the fibrin and purulent material in the sacs. During this invasion some of the alveoli still remained filled with purulent material, some often containing large numbers of endothelial cells filled with fat droplets, giving the cut surface the appearance of miliary tuberculosis or tiny miliary abscess formation. In areas of collapsed lung tissue, fibrosis also fused the walls of the collapsed alveoli. In some instances, the combination of atelectasis and organization so completely transformed the lung that one could almost be excused for not recognizing it as pulmonary tissue. As the organized tissue became older, it was found to be infiltrated with numerous plasma cells. There was evidently an attempt at aeration of this healed lung tissue, for, frequently, numerous air spaces, more or less round in shape, were seen lined with epithelial cells and having wide bands of fibrous tissue between them. Still later, such scar tissue evidently contracted, compressing and drawing these new-formed alveoli, as well as the air sacs on the edge of the lesion, into grotesque-shaped, gland-like cavities lined with cubical epithelium. Frequently, the lung tissue was reduced to a dense fibrous mass with few or no epithelial elements left. Again the fibrosis occurred in the form of broad bands, or as isolated islands dotting throughout the entire organ. In some cases it was limited to thickening about the bronchi, together with an overgrowth which accentuated the fibrous trabeculæ. The fibrin deposit on the pleural surfaces was likewise organized, forming a thin or enormously thick, velvety layer of granulations on the pleura. Later, this became organized into a tough, leathery coat which bound the visceral and parietal surfaces together, either over large areas or as fibrous bands. Frequently, such thick, tough, fibrous walls inclosed empyema cavities, preventing inflation of lung tissue, and collapse and healing of the empyema cavity.

All gradations of the above-described pneumonic types and stages were met with. Not infrequently, interstitial, lobular, and lobar types were found in the same case; at times even side by side in the same lobe. Often different parts of a lobe would show different stages of the process, as the acute, hemorrhagic extravasation in one part and pneumonic process in another; or a given part may have progressed to the stage of organization, while another part of a different lobe was still in an earlier stage. Although, in the cases dying within a few hours of acute hemorrhagic edema, this was frequently the predominating lesion, in every instance a careful search demonstrated at least a beginning pneumonic process in some part of the organ.

PLEURAL EFFUSIONS AND EMPYEMA

Pleural effusion occurred in our series in 87 per cent of the cases. Table III shows the character and distribution of these findings. The character of the fluid found in the pleural cavities depended largely upon the age of the pneumonic condition. In the very earliest cases, termed "acute hemorrhagic edema," the pleural surfaces were constantly smooth and glistening, with a greater or less degree of subpleural, hemorrhagic extravasation as described under that condition. In these cases, the fluid was either serous or serosanguineous in character, and varied in amounts from a few c.c. to 1000 c.c. They occurred ten times on the left side, nine times on the right, and six times bilateral. In the earliest pneumonic conditions described as 'broncho or lobar type" the pleural surfaces were covered with a fibrinous exudate, sometimes over the

TABLE III

CHARACTER AND DISTRIBUTION OF PLEURAL CONDITIONS OCCURRING IN 87 PER CENT OF NECROPSIES ON INFLUEN$_2$A-PNEUMONIA

TYPE	LEFT	RIGHT	BILATERAL	TOTAL
Serous	4	3	4	11
Serosanguineous	6	6	2	14
Serofibrinous	6	4	8	18
Fibrinopurulent	15	11	8	34
Purulent	5	3	0	8
Fibrinous	10	11	14	35
Fibrous Adhesions	11	11	9	31
POCKETS				
Apical	3	0	0	3
Mediastinal	2	2	3	7
Diaphragmatic	1	0	0	1
Interlobar	1	2	0	3

area involved alone, often over considerable of the adjacent pleura. In the very earliest cases, this appeared as a very thin, scarcely discernible clouding of the pleura, or a little later as a thin, finely granular, ground-glass appearing surface; or in the older cases by spongy, light, creamy-yellow fibrinous layer up to three centimeters in thickness. The character of the fluid in these cases varied, depending upon the age from a serofibrinous, fibrinopurulent to a thick purulent material. The fibrin appeared in the serofibrinous fluid as flaky or coarsely granular particles. These fluids occurred most frequently on the left side, and bilateral only sixteen times. Walled off pockets were discovered in a number of instances, occurring most frequently in the following order: mediastinal, seven times; apical, three times; interlobar, three times; and diaphragmatic, once. Thirty-five cases showed a dry, fibrinous involvement of the pleura without any increase in fluid content of the cavity. Thirty-one of the hundred cases presented fibrous adhesions of varying extent, including fibrous bands between visceral and parietal pleura, fibrous obliteration of interlobar fissures to adhesions between parts of or entire surfaces such as the diaphragmatic, mediastinal or pericardial. Thirteen cases showed no discernible pleural change other than a few petechial hemorrhagic areas, on either diaphragmatic, interlobar or mediastinal surfaces. Empyema was not diagnosed unless the fluid was serofibrinous, fibrinopurulent or purulent. Fluids of this character were found sixty times. In cases of excessive fluid, large portions of the lung, frequently an entire lobe, were found collapsed, due probably to the pressure of the fluid. These lungs were dark reddish-black in color, the consistency of live rubber, smooth and velvety on pleural and cut surfaces, in some instances showing pneumonic consolidation, nodular and even conglomerate in type; more often showing no consolidation at all. The cut surface of this tissue was dry, smooth and velvety, with bronchi often standing out above the surrounding surface as thickened tubes filled with thick, brownish or purulent exudate.

CONDITIONS OTHER THAN PNEUMONIA

Following is a list of conditions other than pneumonia found at autopsy:

Respiratory conditions other than Pneumonia
Bronchitis
Acute catarrhal 44
Suppurative 56

Pulmonary tuberculosis	8
Pulmonary collapse	12
Pulmonary infarct	1
Circulatory conditions	
Pericarditis, acute	
Serous	35
Serosanguineous	2
Serofibrinous	18
Fibrinopurulent	10
Myocarditis, acute	48
Myocarditis, chronic fibrous	5
Myocardial congestion	23
Acute cardiac dilatation	84
Endocarditis, acute vegetative	6
Valvular nodules	45
Lymph Gland conditions	
Adenitis, acute, simple	
Peribronchial	69
Mediastinal	61
Axillary	8
Inguinal	1
Mesenteric	5
Calcified peribronchial	8
Tuberculous, peribronchial (caseation)	11
Abdominal conditions	
Peritonitis, acute	
Serous	1
Serofibrinous	4
Fibrinopurulent	1
Liver	
Passive congestion	4
Acute congestion	67
Acute cholecystitis	2
Chronic cholecystitis	14
Hepatic cirrhosis	2
Perihepatitis, chronic fibrous	18
Acute hepatitis (focal necrosis)	28
Hepatic tuberculosis	2
Hepatic infarct	1
Spleen	
Acute splenitis, hemorrhagic	29
Splenitis, subacute	2
Chronic interstitial splenitis	1
Acute congestion	56
Perisplenitis, chronic, fibrous	9
Splenitis, tuberculous	2
Splenic infarction	7
Supernumerary spleen	9
Pancreas	
Acute congestion	47
Stomach and Intestines	
Acute congestion	62
Acute gastritis	1
Intestinal adhesions	
Intestinal obstruction	

Appendix
    Appendicitis, acute   1
    Appendicitis, chronic   36
Genitourinary conditions
    Kidneys
        Nephritis, acute, glomerulo-tubular   52
        Nephritis, chronic diffuse   3
        Renal tuberculosis   1
        Amyloid degeneration   2
        Renal infarct, anemic   3
        Acute congestion   74
    Acute suppurative pyelitis   9
    Cystitis, purulent   1
Skin and Subcutaneous tissue conditions
    Skin
        Vesicular dermatitis   15
        Pustular dermatitis   2
        Jaundice   25
    Emphysema
        Subcutaneous   3
        Mediastinal   14
    Abscess, subcutaneous   3
    Rupture of rectus abdominis muscles   6
Head
    Brain
        Abscess   1
        Cerebral congestion   3
        Cerebral embolism   3
    Ear
        Otitis media purulenta
        Mastoiditis, purulenta   .
    Edema of right orbit   1
    Pyorrhea alveolaris   7
    Subconjunctival hemorrhage   1

The condition of the trachea and larger bronchi very closely simulated that noted in the smaller bronchi and bronchioles. The mucous membrane was nearly always marked by hyperemia, extremely swollen, and deep purplish-red in color. In earlier cases the hyperemic, swollen condition was usually not so marked, and in some the mucosa had nearly a normal pinkish-gray appearance altered only with hemorrhagic petechia, similar to those on the pleural surfaces of the lungs. The content of these tubes was always large in amount, varying in character from a reddish or pinkish, frothy fluid in the earlier cases to a thick, mucopurulent substance in the later cases. In the later there was a partial or complete necrosis of the mucous membrane, while the contents consisted of a comparatively dry exudate composed of polymorphonuclear leucocytes and mononuclear wandering cells, much mucus and varying amounts of fibrin, all in a more or less complete state of disintegration.

Pericarditis was a very frequent finding, occurring fifty-five times, and usually associated with pleural effusions large in amount. Amounts varied from 30 c.c. to 600 c.c. Fluid up to 25 c.c. was considered normal, unless of a pathologic character. Suppurative pericarditis was seen most frequently in late cases associated with empyema or general sepsis. In the serous type the fatty tissue underneath the pericardium was usually found to be quite edematous.

The right heart showed evidence of acute dilatation in some degree in 84 per cent of cases. This varied from moderate dilatation in which the right auricle and ventricle were filled with thick, tenacious, black and white clot, to perfectly enormous dilatation of the right heart in which the right auriculo-ventricular orifice measured 16 cm. from cut edge to edge. In these hearts the myocardium on the right was usually flabby and toneless, while that on the left was firm and contracted with little or no blood clot in the cavities. In the earlier cases the myocardium presented a picture of extreme congestion. Later, there was definite evidence of acute inflammatory change with cloudy swelling and granular degeneration, fragmentation, and even polymorphonuclear infiltration. These hearts varied greatly in size, the average weight being 344.5 grams. The largest heart, 589 grams, was found in a case of interstititial bronchopneumonia involving practically 90 per cent of both lungs. The smallest, weight 200 grams, occurred in a case of broncho-interstitial type pneumonia of nineteen days' duration complicated by pulmonary tuberculosis with abscess formation, and amyloid degeneration of the kidney. The valves of the heart frequently presented a glassy, nodular condition along their free borders about the insertions of the chorda tendinæ. This was attributed to the condition of generalized edema about the heart. Fatty degeneration of the aorta was observed in 35 per cent of cases. This was most marked in the older cases and occurred most frequently at the base of the aorta about the openings to the coronary vessels. It occurred here in the form of irregular-shaped plaques raised slightly above the surrounding surface. These plaques measured from 3 mm. to 8 mm. in diameter. Occasionally, similar plaques were found on the arch of the aorta about the openings to the neck vessels. Along the descending aorta the degenerative process assumed the form of fatty streaks lying parallel to the longitudinal axis of the vessel, and most marked about the openings of the intercostal arteries. In only two cases was the aorta involved below the diaphragm. In two cases the fatty degeneration had progressed to an atheromatous state.

Lymph nodes about the hilus and in the mediastinum were usually in an acute inflammatory state, except in the very earlier cases of hemorrhagic edema. In these cases, the picture under the microscope was that of intense engorgement of the lymphatics. In the older cases, however, nodes were enlarged, soft and gelatinous, with glassy edematous appearance on their cut surfaces.

The average weight of the liver was 1805 grams. The largest weighed 2772 grams, and occurred in a case showing an intense congestion of the organ, with widely dilated central and intralobular veins. The liver cells about the central veins showed extreme fatty degeneration and vacuolization. The smallest weighed 906 grams and occurred in a case of interstitial bronchopneumonia and pulmonary tuberculosis. The liver was very generally involved with miliary type of tuberculosis, showing typical tubercle formation with caseation necrosis. The liver cells were extensively involved with fatty degeneration and infiltration, and there was a marked lymphocytic infiltration throughout the entire organ, more particularly noticeable about the vessels. Two rather distinct types of liver involvement were noted in connection with influenza-pneumonia. The one was termed an acute congestion, and was noted 67 times in our series. This was manifested by enlargement of the entire organ, with a tense capsule, and a purplish-blue surface. The cut surface bulged over the edge of the capsule and was usually a light to dark reddish-brown color. Considerable blood dripped from the cut surface. Microscopically, all blood vessels, afferent and efferent, but more particularly the central veins and intralobular capillaries, were found to be widely dilated.

The second type of liver was usually not so markedly enlarged, and was of a light bluish-gray color, frequently mottled on the surface by pale yellow, irregular-shaped areas. The cut surface of these livers was less bloody, did not bulge over capsule, and was of a light yellowish-brown color, sometimes uniformly so, sometimes distributed in the form of irregular sized and shaped areas throughout the organ. Microscopically, there was found to be quite a marked fatty degeneration of the liver cells, frequently including only a narrow zone about the central vein, often however, involving the entire, or greater portion of the lobule. These yellowish livers were frequently associated with jaundice, but not constantly so. These cases were termed "acute hepatitis," twenty-eight in all being found. Four cases of typical nutmeg liver, or passive congestion, were seen.

Conditions most frequently seen in the spleen coincidently with influenza-pneumonia were acute congestion and acute hemorrhagic splenitis. The cases termed "acute congestion" occurred 56 times, and were manifested by an increase in size, at times enormously so, tense consistency, dark red color, eversion of cut edge, and soft friable pulp substance. The prominent Malpighian bodies and trabeculations were noteworthy. Microscopically, sinuses were seen to be intensely engorged with blood, and the Malpighian bodies swollen and edematous.

In acute hemorrhagic splenitis, the organ was comparatively pale, only slightly or moderately increased in size, and frequently marked on the surface with light grayish-pink, soft areas. On section, the cut surface was either uniformly a light grayish-pink color, soft, and friable, or else presented numerous areas of this appearance several centimeters in diameter and irregular in outline. The Malpighian corpuscles and trabeculations were indistinctly seen or entirely obliterated. Microscopically, this splenic tissue was seen to consist of an extravasation of blood elements into the splenic substance, sometimes involving and destroying even the Malpighian bodies. These areas sometimes were minute in size; again, including a large part of splenic tissue. In some instances the red cells were in remarkably fresh state; again, they were decidedly degenerated and the area infiltrated with polymorphonuclear and large mononuclear wandering cells. Definite splenic infarcts were noted in 7 per cent of the cases. The average weight of these spleens was 170 grams. The largest was 673 grams, occurring in a case of interstitial bronchopneumonia, and was a combination of the congestion and acute splenitis types. The smallest weighed 30 grams, and occurred in a case of combined broncho- and lobar types of pneumonia. This was noted as an acute hemorrhagic splenitis.

Acute congestive condition of the kidneys was noted 74 times. Acute nephritis of a glomerulo-tubular type was diagnosed 52 times. These kidneys were swollen, showing eversion of their cut edge, the color of the latter being either an intense purplish-red, or grayish-white. Hemorrhagic extravasations were not infrequent. Cloudy swelling and granular degeneration of glomerular and tubular epithelium was marked, and, in many instances, desquamation of tubular epithelium was quite extensive. Right kidneys in these cases averaged 169 grams in weight, the largest weighing 315 grams, and occurring in a case of bronchopneumonia, the kidney condition being diagnosed acute glomerulo-tubular nephritis. The smallest right kidney weighed 84 grams, and was found in a case of broncho-interstitial pneumonia. The kidney was an infantile lobulated type. The left kidneys averaged 161.1 grams in weight. The largest, weighing 348 grams, was seen in a case of interstitial bronchopneumonia with intense renal congestion. The smallest left kidney weighed 60 grams, and occurred in a case of interstitial bronchopneumonia. No lesion could be determined in this kidney other than slight amount of congestion.

Emphysema was noted with striking regularity in cases denoted hemorrhagic edema, and the various types of pneumonia. Quite constantly this was present as a compensatory condition in those parts of the lung tissue not involved by the hemorrhage. In fourteen instances, it was found in the loose aureolar tissue of the mediastinum, and, in three instances, had extravasated to the subcutaneous tissue over the front of the chest and neck. In one case this had become so extensive as to extend over the entire face and neck, down the arms to the hands, over the thorax and abdomen, into the scrotum and over the upper half of both thighs. Clark and Synnott[14] reported twenty such cases occurring in influenza-pneumonia. Brenn, et al.,[8] reported two cases of subcutaneous emphysema found in thirty necropsies done on influenza cases.

A peculiar condition was noted on the skin surface of a number of these cases which was termed a "vesicular dermatitis." It was characterized by tiny, pinhead, water-clear blisters of the epidermis. So thin were these vesicles that they could be rubbed off in passing the hand over the skin surface. They gave one the impression of tiny drops of water resting on the body. They occurred most commonly over the chest and abdomen, but, in some instances, were found over the shoulders and upper arms, neck, and upper thighs. Application of irritant substances to the skin surface was ruled out as a causative factor. Consultation with dermatologists resulted in the conclusion that this was a form of toxic dermatitis. In two instances, the vesicular condition had become pustular. Jaundice was noticed twenty-five times and varied anywhere from a slight icteric condition of the conjunctivæ to a generalized deep saffron yellow. In some instances, this could be accounted for by a condition of acute toxic hepatitis, but, in other cases, no liver disturbance could be found.

Rupture of the rectus muscle occurred so frequently as to attract attention. The separation usually occurred midway between the symphysis pubis and umbilicus, but one case was found where it occurred between the ensiform and umbilicus. In one case it was complete, but usually only involved a few fibers. In four cases the rupture was bilateral. It was usually accompanied by large hematoma underneath the sheath of the rectus. The hemorrhage frequently had dissected downward in front of the bladder. Microscopically, the muscle fibers showed granular degeneration, cloudy swelling, and fragmentation. In later cases, the hematoma and muscle fibers were profusely infiltrated with polymorphonuclear leucocytes and mononuclear wandering cells. Frequently, they were localized into definite abscesses.

BACTERIOLOGY

Table IV shows the incidence of the various organisms occurring in our pneumonias. The table is the result of the autopsy examination of the lung, spleen, kidney, pleural and pericardial fluids, and heart's blood. Blocks of tissue were taken from the lung, spleen and kidney after searing the surface

TABLE IV

POSTMORTEM CULTURES FROM ONE HUNDRED CASES OF INFLUEN₂A-PNEUMONIA

ORGANISM	LUNG	SPLEEN	KIDNEY	PLEURAL FLUID	PERICARDIAL FLUID	HEART'S BLOOD
Pneumococcus Type II	1	0	2	1	1	2
Pneumococcus Type III	7	1	1	2	2	2
Pneumococcus Type IV	50	19	8	26	40	42
Streptococcus Hemolyticus	45	35	0	23	35	36
Pfeiffer's Bacillus	4	0	0	5	0	0
Staphylococcus	2	0	0	0	0	0
Nonhemolytic Streptococcus	1	0	0	0	0	0

with a red-hot spatula. These tissue blocks were macerated in sterile salt solution and planted on blood agar plates and plain broth. Smears also were made from this macerated tissue and stained by Giemsa's and Gram's method. Sections from these various tissues were also stained by Goodpasture's modification of the Gram-Weigert method, which we have found a most excellent stain for demonstrating bacteria in tissue. Pfeiffer's organism is stained very readily by this method. Pleural and pericardial fluids and heart's blood were cultured in plain broth.

Table II is a summary of the organisms occurring in the various types of pneumonia. It is to be noted that hemolytic streptococcus was found alone three times, and hemolytic streptococcus and staphylococcus twice, and pneumococcus Type IV occurring four times. A mixed infection of hemolytic streptococcus and pneumococcus Type IV occurred two times, while the combination of hemolytic streptococcus and pneumococcus Type III occurred once. In interstitial bronchopneumonia type, hemolytic streptococcus was found as the only organism in twelve cases, pneumococcus Type IV in nine cases, and pneumococcus Type III in two cases. Combinations of hemolytic streptococcus and pneumococcus occurred five times, and hemolytic streptococcus and staphylococcus twice, and pneumococcus and Pfeiffer's bacillus once, and pneumococcus and staphylococcus once. In the lobular type of bronchopneumonia, hemolytic streptococcus was the predominating organism eleven times, pneumococcus Type IV nine times, pneumococcus Type III two times, pneumococcus Type II once, hemolytic streptococcus and pneumococcus three times, pneumococcus and Pfeiffer's bacillus two times, and pneumococcus and staphylococcus once.

INFLUENZA-PNEUMONIA AS AN ENTITY

As a result of our studies in influenza-pneumonia, I wish to present the following conception and classification of the condition. Influenza-pneumonia may be defined as a primary, acute, hemorrhagic lesion, interstitial, nodular, or massive in extent, arising from a pulmonary capillary phlebitis with disseminated capillary necrosis due to some toxic agent and resulting in a secondary purulent pneumonia with healing by organization. Primarily and essentially, the pulmonary injury in influenza is an acute hemorrhagic and serous condition, evidently the result of some toxic agent,[13] chemical in nature, whether organic or inorganic it is impossible to say. It is not inconceivable that such toxic agent should emanate from a part remote from the lungs themselves. For example, Pfeiffer's bacillus or some other as yet unidentified organism, localized in the nose or throat, might eliminate a toxin so virulent as to account for the condition under discussion. It is a known fact that toxins eliminated by such organisms as the diphtheria or tetanus bacillus cause disastrous injury in parts of the body remote from the point of localization of the organism. In influenza, the acute hyperemia of the conjunctiva and the intense lividity of the pharynx described as a red fringe, or crescent bordering the hard palate, with minute hemorrhages and a papulovesicular rash in the livid mucosa has been referred to by many observers.[15] One who has seen many of these cases is struck by the fact that there is a decided and severe disturbance in the character of the blood and the circulatory system in general. That such a toxic agent has not only altered the character of the blood, but has affected all tissues that it bathes is reflected in the finding of generalized conditions throughout the whole body. A definite hemoglobinemia has been noted. Hemorrhagic extravasations are found in practically every organ throughout the body, including the musculature. The condition might be compared to that seen in purpura hemorrhagica of a severe type. That the lungs were so severely affected is not surprising when we think of the vulnerability of their anatomic structure to any toxic agent carried in the blood stream. The lung with its delicate network of capillary vessels surrounding the alveoli forms the most susceptible organ of the body for attack. The thrombosis and adventitial necrosis of the pulmonary vessels has been noted above in the descriptions of the lung conditions. Lyons[7] has suggested that the location of the hemorrhage largely in the posterior parts of the lungs—all lobes—is connected with posture as in hypostatic congestion. When we remember the extreme early prostration of these cases and the fact that they are most frequently found "flat on their backs," this suggestion becomes most plausible. On the other hand, it is conceivable that the toxic agent should have reached the lung parenchyma by way of the respiratory tract either in a liquid or gaseous state. The constant finding of necrosis of the lining epithelium of the infundibular and alveolar walls in all types of pneumonia has been noted in our descriptions of these conditions. Goodpasture[13] succinctly states this viewpoint as follows: "The pulmonary injury and reaction being so acute and often widespread, and the fact that in certain very early cases, bacteria of any kind are so scarce or not found at all, make us feel, notwithstanding the demonstration of influenza bacilli in pure culture in the lungs in all but one instance, that at this stage organisms are as yet comparatively few within the alveoli, and their primary injury is due to a very potent toxic substance elaborated in and disseminated through the larger air passages."*

We consider this primary lesion a serous and hemorrhagic pneumonitis, of toxic origin, starting as a phlebitis of the pulmonary capillaries. The pneumonitis results in the production of multiple infarcts of various sizes throughout the lung. Beginning with the circulatory system, we note an intense engorgement of all the vessels, large and small, but particularly the interalveolar capillaries, arterioles and venules. Vessel walls are intensely swollen and edematous, the adventitia being frequently in a state of necrosis as noted before. In places these have ruptured, filling the neighboring air sacs with erythrocytes and serum. In some instances, this hemorrhagic extravasation is confined largely to the interstitial tissue and to small areas two or three millimeters in diameter about the bronchioles and infundibuli. In other cases, sometimes in other parts of the same organ, even sometimes within the same lobe, are seen areas of hemorrhagic extravasation larger in extent involving an entire, or several lobules. In still other cases, the involvement has become massive, either through conglomeration of-the previously described lesions, or because of the severity of the process, and generalized lack of resistance on the part of the lung. In other words, this primary influenzal lesion may be interstitial, nodular, or massive in distribution. Presumably these types of lesions are determined by the amount and virulence of the toxic agent on the one hand, and the resistance of the tissue on the other hand. Possibly the only reason why the entire five lobes do not become uniformly involved in some cases is that death necessarily occurs from lack of air before so complete an involvement can take place. At any rate, it is surprising how extensive the process became in some instances before death intervened. Curiously enough, a careful study of these very earliest lesions fails to discover the presence of any organism in the hemorrhagic areas, either by culture or by tissue sections. The rather sharp differentiation between the areas of hemorrhagic extravasation and the uninvolved tissue is also notably in favor of this conception. Obviously, the interstitial and nodular types have not been seen in this stage except in connection with the conglomerate types, as they alone would hardly be extensive enough to cause death. In any event, these types of hemorrhagic lesion form an excellent foundation for the secondary pneumonic lesion.

Thus the condition of multiple pulmonary infarction, interstitial, nodular, or conglomerate in type forms the starting point, out of which grows the secondary stage of influenza-pneumonia. The injured pulmonary vessels accompanying the bronchi and bronchioles down to their final ramifications and surrounding the alveoli with a delicate network of capillaries make the whole bronchial tree a point of markedly lowered resistance to any pathogenic organism which might gain access to the respiratory tract, or to those bacteria normally present there. The areas consisting of clotted blood and serum form a most excellent medium for the rapid growth of any organism that should gain access to it. Very likely these organisms are planted through the respiratory tract. That this is probable is evidenced also by the fact that the more common organisms found normally in

*While this paper was in the course of preparation LeCount (Jour. Am. Med. Assn., lxvii, No. 21, p. 1519) called attention to the "disseminated necrosis" of the pulmonary capillaries of the lung in influenza-pneumonia noted above, and concluded from his studies that the evidence was in favor of this condition being prodromal to the hemorrhage rather than secondary to the pneumonia. This is in keeping with the above conception of the pneumonia lesion.

the nose and throats of individuals have been the ones most frequently concerned in the so-called secondary influenza-pneumonias. The diversity of the organisms found in the pneumonias occurring in various sections of this country is an additional argument in favor of this conception. Seemingly, the organism, or organisms, predominantly present in the nose and throat of individuals in any particular section of the country is the organism predominantly found in cultures and tissue sections from the lungs of pneumonias in that section. Thus from one community Pfeiffer's bacillus[16] has been found in the majority of instances (as high as 82.6 per cent of lung cultures), while in others, pneumococcus type III or IV, hemolytic streptococcus,[7] Streptococcus viridans, staphylococcus, micrococcus catarrhalis, or Friedländer's bacillus[16] have been found predominating. That this is so, and that recognized reliable workers have made such reports from different sections of the country increases the strength of the foregoing statement.

It is also conceivable that some at least of these pneumonias derived their secondary invaders by way of the blood stream. Positive blood cultures have been frequently obtained from these cases. Ritchie and Goehrings[17] found that in cases of marked prostration, septicemia was very common, and that the more common bacterial inhabitants of the body, such as staphylococcus, streptococcus, etc., were the most common invaders. Oberndorfer[18] has defined influenza as a bacteremia.

Obviously, the type of the secondary pneumonia would largely be determined in the beginning, at least, by the type of the primary condition, i.e., interstitial, nodular, or conglomerate. In the very earliest cases of invasion the areas of infarction are seen to be in a process of invasion by the polymorphonuclear leucocyte, and the large mononuclear wandering cell on the one hand, and the secondary invading organism on the other hand. Red blood cells are in a process of disintegration, in many instances, having lost their hemoglobin, and appearing as mere shadows. Still later they have lost even their shadowy outline. This corresponds roughly to the stage of red hepatization mentioned in the lobular and lobar types previously described. Somewhat later, the lesions are characterized by a mass of polymorphonuclear and endothelial cells, together with a yellowish-gray, sometimes mucoid, fluid. This corresponds to the stage of gray hepatization, and is simply a purulent stage of this secondary pneumonia. All types, interstitial, nodular, and massive, pass through these stages, differing only one from the other in extent of the lesion. True, there is an extension in many instances of this secondary pneumonia beyond the limits of the primary infarction, due to the activity of the secondary process. In these cases, the former uninvolved area becomes intensely congested about the periphery of the hemorrhagic area, and gradually passes through the stages of engorgement, red and gray hepatization.

Mention already has been made of the extensive damage done to the lung tissue and the resulting organization. Coincidently with the beginning of organization, there is a walling off of the various purulent areas by the more resistant tissue with the formation of abscesses varying in size from the miliary foci seen in the interstitial type to areas several centimeters in diameter seen in the nodular and conglomerate types. As organization proceeds, these abscess areas are replaced by granulations rarely persisting as pulmonary abscess cavities. The areas not primarily involved in the hemorrhagic process, but secondarily invaded as extension from the primary foci, are more prone to undergo typical resolution, the damage to the lung tissue seemingly having not been as destructive here.

Following is a schematic outline of the classification and conception of influenza-pneumonia as just discussed:

	Division as to causative agent	Types with respect to extent	Stages in point of time
INFLUENZA-PNEUMONIA	I. Primary (some unknown toxic agent)	a. Interstitial and peribronchial b. Nodular or lobular c. Massive or conglomerate	1. Serous 2. Hemorrhagic
	II. Secondary (the predominating organism occurring in the nose and throat of the individuals of a given section)	a. Interstitial b. Nodular c. Massive	1. Purulent infiltration (hemorrhagic) 2. Abscess formation 3. Organization

CONCLUSIONS

The pneumococcus and hemolytic streptococcus were the most frequent secondary invaders found in the lungs at autopsy in the pneumonias at Camp Sherman. Pfeiffer's bacillus was found in only 4 per cent of the cases.

Interstitial and lobular bronchopneumonia can not be regarded as typical lesions resulting from the invasion by the hemolytic streptococcus. The pneumococcus was found to be the only invader just as frequently as the hemolytic streptococcus in these types of pneumonias. In fact, it is doubtful whether the type of organism isolated from pulmonary tissue in pneumonia is of any great value in determining the type of pneumonia present, for the type of organism concerned and the type of lesion in the lung are decidedly variable at different times even at the same station.

Influenza-pneumonia is primarily an acute, hemorrhagic lesion, interstitial, nodular, or massive in extent, rising from a pulmonary capillary phlebitis with disseminated capillary necrosis due to some toxic agent and resulting in a secondary purulent pneumonia with healing by organization.

That organism or organisms predominately present in nose or throat in the individuals in any particular section of the country is the organism most commouly found in cultures and tissue sections from the lungs of secondary pneumonias in that region.

Empyema and pericarditis are frequent complications.

BIBLIOGRAPHY

[1]Report of Special Committee of the American Public Health Association, Jour. Am. Med. Assn., lxxi, No. 25, p. 2068.
[2]McCallum, W. G.: Pathology of Epidemic Streptococcal Bronchopneumonia in Army Camps, Jour. Am. Med. Assn., lxxi, No. 9, p. 704.

[3]Nuzum, John W., et al.: Pandemic of Influenza and Pneumonia in a Large Civil Hospital, Jour. Am. Med. Assn., lxxi, No. 19, p. 1562.
[4]Symmers, Douglas: Pathological Similarity between Pneumonia of Bubonic and Pandemic Influenza, Jour. Am. Med. Assn., Nov. 2, 1918, p. 1482.
[5]McCallum, W. G.: Pathology of Pneumonia Following Influenza, Jour. Am. Med. Assn., lxxii, No. 10, p. 720.
[6]Friedländer, McCord, Sladen, and Wheeler: The Epidemic of Influenza at Camp Sherman, Ohio. Jour. Am. Med. Assn., lxxi, No. 20, p. 1652.
[7]Lyons, M. W.: Gross Pathology of Epidemic Influenza at Walter Reed General Hospital Jour. Am. Med. Assn., lxxii, No. 13, p. 924.
[8]Brem, Walter V., Bolling, George E., and Caspar, Irving J.: Pandemic Influenza and Secondary Pneumonia at Camp Fremont, Jour. Am. Med. Assn., lxxi, No. 26, p. 2138.
[9]Cole, Rufus and McCallum, W. G.: Pneumonia at a Base Hospital, Jour. Am. Med. Assn., Apr. 20, 1918, p. 1146.
[10]Thomas. Henry M.: Pneumonia at Camp Meade, Md., Jour. Am. Med. Assn., lxxi, No. 16, p. 1307.
[11]Blanton, W. B., and Irons, E. E.: A Recent Epidemic of Acute Respiratory Infection at Camp Custer, Mich., Jour. Am. Med. Assn., lxxi, No. 24, p. 1988.
[12]Mathers: Tr. Chicago Path. Soc., April 1, 1916.
[13]Goodpasture, Ernest W.: Broncho-Pneumonia Due to Hemolytic Streptococcus Following Influenza, Jour. Am. Med. Assn., lxxii, No. 10, p. 724.
[14]Clark, E. C., and Synnott, M. J.: Influenza-Pneumonia Cases Showing Gas in Fascial Tissues, Am. Jour. Med. Sc., Feb., 1919, p. 219.
[15]Alexander: Berl. klin. Wchnschr., 1918, No. 38, abstr.
Deutsch. med. Wchnschr., 1918, xliv, 1171.
Bloomfield and Harrop: Bull. Johns Hopkins Hosp., 1919, xxx, 1.
[16]Keegan, J. J.: The Prevailing Pandemic of Influenza, Jour. Am. Med. Assn., lxxi, No. 13, p. 2068.
[17]Ritchie and Goehrings: Jour. Med. Research, 1918, xxxviii, 421.
[18]Oberndorfer: München. med. Wchnschr., 1918, lxv, 810.

THE CHOICE OF SERA IN THE TREATMENT OF MENINGOCOCCUS SEPSIS*

By M. B. Cohen, M.D., Ashland, Ohio

THE epidemics of meningococcus sepsis which have occurred in army cantonments have necessitated an intensive study of meningitis therapy.

Following the success obtained in the treatment of this disease by Flexner and Jobling by the intraspinal injection of immune·serum, a number of observers have noticed variations in the therapeutic result following the use of different sera. These differences were explained on the basis of the existence of various serologically different strains of the meningococcus.

Studies by the Royal Army Medical Corps in England, the Pasteur Institute in France, and the Rockefeller Institute in the United States have shown that the group of meningococcus bacteria is a heterogeneous one, and that there are at least four strains or varieties that can be separated by serologic methods. Though each group of workers claims to include in its classification the serologic types of the others, it is, at the present time, impossible to state the exact relationship between these various classifications.

The various commercial polyvalent antimeningococcic sera are made from a number of strains of meningococcus isolated from the spinal fluids of cases of meningitis, and are supposed to contain immune bodies for the four main groups. In spite of the polyvalency of the sera, however, many cases have not responded properly to serum treatment. Clinicians have been in the habit of changing sera when proper results were not obtained, as their experience had shown that the change was frequently associated with clinical improvement. This experience has led them to condemn the sera of some manufacturers as unreliable.

Some clinicians have suggested that the agglutination titer of the various commercial sera in stock be determined for the organism isolated from the patient. Until the present, however, such tests have been impractical, because of the difficulties in isolating and cultivating the meningococcus in sufficient amount with such rapidity that a report could be sent to the clinician within forty-eight hours after the patient's admission to the hospital.

That such growth can be obtained in less than twenty-four hours, by smearing the spinal fluid on any suitably enriched medium, such as blood agar or sheep serum agar, has been recently demonstrated by the author and Fleming.†

As most sera are at present tested for potency by agglutination reactions against known strains, and as this method is reasonably rapid and is less subject to error than the other available serologic procedures, the agglutination reaction was selected as an index of potency of a serum against the organism isolated from the spinal fluid of the patient.

Each available commercial serum was tested in dilutions of 1-50; 1-100; 1-200; 1-400; 1-800; and 1-1600 with a suspension of meningococcus isolated

*From the Department of Pathology and Surgery of the Ashland Clinic.
†Jour. Infect. Dis., 1918, xxiii, 337.

from each patient as described above. Controls of saline suspension and horse serum were included in each series. The following protocol serves to illustrate the method and result.

AGGLUTINATION OF MENINGOCOCCUS STRAIN No. 101 ISOLATED AT PARTIAL TENSION ON BLOOD AGAR. SUSPENSION MADE FROM 18 HOUR CULTURE AT 37° C. AGGLUTINATION CARRIED OUT AT 55° C. FOR 18 HOURS

COMMERCIAL SERUM	1-50	1-100	1-200	1-400	1-800	1-1600	1-50 HORSE	SALINE
A	** **	** **	**	*	–	–	–	–
B	** **	** *	*	–	–	–	–	–
C	**	*	–	–	–	–	–	–
D	** **	** **	** **	** *	*	–	–	–
E	** *	**	*	–	–	–	–	–

*Positive. –Negative.

From the foregoing protocol it is evident that Serum D would be the best to employ for the case in question, whereas Serum C would be considered the least reliable.

When a new patient was admitted to the meningitis ward, the laboratory was notified. While waiting for the arrival of the bacteriologist, the clinician made a lumbar puncture and collected a specimen of spinal fluid. The bacteriologist, upon his arrival, removed 10 to 20 c.c. of blood from the median basilic vein for a blood culture, and immediately returned to the laboratory with both specimens. The clinician used his own judgment as to treatment based on a preliminary bacteriologic report, using any available serum, until he received a report from the laboratory on the agglutination titer of the various sera available against the strain isolated from the case in question. He would then choose the serum which had the highest titer for further treatment of the patient.

The procedure described above has been found by actual test to be practical and very satisfactory. It requires for its success the full cooperation between the clinical and laboratory services.

LABORATORY METHODS

ABOUT A NEW STOMACH EXAMINER, BASED ON THE HYDRAULIC PRINCIPLE

By Dr. Komanosuke Togami, Igakuhakushi, Fukuoka, Japan

TO OBTAIN the stomach fluid, the expression method is considerably employed. This method is successful in cases in which the stomach secretion is abundant, but is often a failure in those with diminished secretion or pronounced atony. Apart from this, it requires a long time to take the stomach contents, and sometimes it causes a damage of the mucus of the stomach. Therefore it is necessary to apply the negative pressure to obtain the contents of the stomach, in every case of the stomach examination. For this purpose we have Boas' bulb and the Potain's apparatus. The former shows sometimes insufficiency of the negative pressure, while the latter is very circumstantial and may cause at times serious damage of the mucus of the stomach, by producing heedlessly unnecessary negative pressure.

I have lately designed a new aspirating apparatus, by which the negative pressure produced at once automatically by water pressure, and the variation of the pressure can be measured by a manometer at every moment. The procedure is very simple and one can aspirate the stomach contents safely and quickly. Moreover the apparatus can be applied for several important examinations of the stomach, as shown in the following.

In the first place it will be necessary to give a description of the construction of this apparatus and make some remarks upon the hydraulic principle employed.

A closed vessel A and an open vessel B are placed in a row, and the closed vessel A, having a capacity of about 3000 c.c., provided at the lower part with a discharge pipe K and a cock K', and fitted at the upper part with a bent pipe (a), which is divided in three branches R, U and V (Fig. 1). The upper branch R is connected with the air gauge E, and the other two with the closed vessels C and D, arranged on the lower stage. The closed vessel C is fitted at the lower part with a discharge pipe F and a cock F' and provided at the upper part with a connecting pipe M which connects the closed vessels C and D. The closed vessel D is fitted at the lower part with a discharge pipe H and a cock H' and provided at the upper part with a joint pipe P. The open vessel B, having a capacity of about 4000 c.c., is provided at the lower part with a discharge pipe G and a cock G' this being connected in a T-shape with a connecting pipe Q of an elevating vessel J, and the communicating pipe Q is fitted with a cock Q', and its further end is connected with a cock N' of a communicating pipe N.

By opening K', after closing K', F', H' and the upper cocks of A, C, D and the pipe P, the water in the closed vessel A will run down through the discharge pipe K. With the lowering of the water level in the vessel A, the air in the vessel C and D will increase its volume. According to Mariotte's law the pressure is reciprocal to the volume and with an increase of the volume of the air the pressure of the air will be gradually reduced. When the sum of the pressure of the air in the vessel A and of the water in the vessel A and the pipe K is equal to atmospheric pressure, the water will no longer run out through the discharge pipe K, and the water level will remain constant. On the other hand, the diminution of the air pressure in the vessel C and D can be read by the difference of the levels of the mercury of the air gauge, and to produce a greater negative pres-

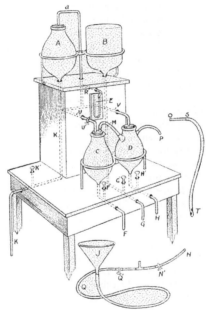

Fig. 1.

sure, it will be necessary either to raise the closed vessel A to a higher position or to lengthen the discharge pipe K, in order to increase the height of the water column.

PREPARATIONS FOR OPERATIONS

Before performing operations the following points should be noted.

1. The closed vessel A and the open vessel B should be filled with water.

2. The upper parts of all closed vessels A, C, D and the cocks K', F', G' and H' should be closed air-tight.

3. In case of lavage, the lotion should be poured into the open vessel B in place of water. If one operates only for the aspiration of the gastric fluid, it is not necessary to fill the vessel B with water.

OPERATIONS

1. The aspiration of the gastric contents.

After connecting P and S, the tube T should be introduced into the stomach, and the cock K' opened. The water in the vessel A will run down through the discharge pipe K and there arise a negative pressure in the closed vessels C and D, which is read by the manometer. When there is fluid in the stomach, it will be at once drawn up into the closed vessel D, going further into the closed vessel C, in case the vessel is full of liquid through the pipe M. After taking the stomach contents, P and O should be separated and the tube drawn out from the stomach. When we open the cocks H' and F', the stomach contents in the vessels C and D can be taken in a receptacle for the examination.

To take the fluid out of the stomach, the expression method is considerably employed, but in certain pathologic conditions, especially when the fluid is deficient, it is very often a failure, even when the stomach contains little fluid, for example, in cases of marked atony. In cases of ulcer, there is possible danger of damaging the mucus of the stomach when it is carried out irrespective of the pathologic conditions of the organ. Very frequently we meet with cases of ulcer, in which there is no special evidence pointing to ulcer. Sometimes the clinical significance is quite latent and the recent bleeding may be frequently overlooked. Therefore it is an important fact to obtain the stomach contents with the utmost care in every case, by means of the safest and the most exact method. By this apparatus the operation can be carried out very quickly and successfully in every case, with less chance of damaging the mucus of the stomach.

2. The aspiration of gas or gases in the stomach. Close the cock U', and connect the pipes F and G by means of a piece of glass tubing. After filling the vessels C and D with water, close F' and G', and connect P and the stomach tube S. Then the tube will be introduced in the stomach and the cock H' opened. With the lowering of the water level in the vessel D, the gas in the stomach will be collected in the vessel D. When the vessel D is filled with gas, the cock H' should be closed and the cock F' opened. Then the gas will be obtained in the vessels C and D. The volume of the gas under the normal atmospheric pressure may be estimated by the following two ways:

(A) Supposing that

X = The volume of the stomach gas under the normal atmospheric pressure D.

V = The volume of the stomach gas under the negative pressure P. Then we have the following equation.

$$DX = PV \qquad \therefore \; X = \frac{VP}{D}$$

(B) After we take the stomach gas in the closed vessel D, the joint pipe P should be closed and the pipes G and H connected by means of a piece of glass tubing.

By opening the cocks G' and H' the water in the open vessel B will run down in the vessel D, and the pressure in the vessel D will gradually increase. At the instant when the pressure in the vessel D is equal to that of the external atmospheric pressure, the cocks G' and H' should be immediately closed. Then the volume of the stomach gas under the external atmospheric pressure may be read by the scale of the vessel D.

3. Volumetric measurement of the gas in the stomach. In this operation the stomach gas will be aspired in the closed vessels C and D, containing no water. Only by the lowering of the water level in the vessel A the amount of the stomach gas may be measured by the following two ways.

Before the operation, the joint pipe P and the stomach tube S should be connected. After we introduce the tube in the stomach, the cock K' should be opened. A negative pressure will be produced in the closed vessels C and D

(A) Suppose

$X =$ The volume of the stomach gas under the normal pressure D.

$V =$ The volume of the air in the vessel (C and D) and pipes, connected with the vessels, under the normal pressure D.

$V' =$ The volume of water, run out through the discharge pipe K.

We have the following equation.

$$(V + V')P = (V + X)D$$
$$PV + PV' = DV + DX$$
$$X = \frac{P}{D}(V + V') - V$$

(B) After the stomach gas is all taken in the closed vessel D, the cock K' and the joint pipe P should be closed. Then connect the pipes G and H, and open the cocks G' and H'.

The water in the vessel B will run down in the vessel D, and the low pressure in the vessel D will gradually become normal. The quantity of the water to change the negative pressure P to the normal atmospheric pressure D can be readily read by the scale of the vessel D.

Supposing

$V =$ The volume of the air in the vessels (C and D) and pipes, connected with the vessels.

$V' =$ The volume of the water to produce the negative pressure P in the closed vessel D.

$V'' =$ The volume of the water to change the negative pressure P to the normal atmospheric pressure D.

$X =$ The volume of the stomach gas under the normal atmospheric pressure D.

According to the law of Mariott we have the following equation:

$$X + V = V + V' - V'' \qquad X = V' - V''$$

In the first place it will be necessary to give a description of the construction

4. Estimation of the capacity of the stomach. Connect the joint pipe P and the stomach tube S; introduce the tube in the stomach; connect G and F. Close th cock U'; open the cocks G' and F', the water in the open vessel B will run down into the closed vessel C, going further into the vessel D, in case vessel C is full

of water, through the pipe M. Thus the air in the closed vessels C and D will be forced into the stomach, and the stomach will be distended. The resulting pressure in the stomach may be read by the manometer, and the volume of the air, forced into the stomach, by the scale of the blood vessels C and D. From the relation of the quantity of the air, forced into the stomach and the resulting intragastric pressure we can estimate the capacity of the stomach very easily and correctly. Preceding the maximum distention of the stomach, a gradual increase of the intragastric pressure will be noted in cases of normal muscular tone of the stomach. In cases of atony of the pressure increase, preceding the maximum distention, lasts a short time, or is not so considerable as in cases of the normal muscular tone. Therefore a careful observation of the variation of the intragastric pressure will afford a significance for the diagnosis of atony of the stomach.

There are two methods of gas inflation of the stomach, namely, air inflation and carbonic acid inflation. The former is to distend the stomach by pumping the air in the stomach by means of a double bulb, after the introduction of the tube into the stomach. The latter consists in administering internally tartaric acid and sodium bicarbonate to produce the gas in the stomach. These two inflation methods are employed to render the stomach visible to inspection for the diagnosis of the dilatation or gastroptosis. But at times there may be escape of gas or air through pylorus and a distention of the intestines may occur, which may be a hindrance for the determination of the margin or the position of the stomach. It would be more difficult or impossible to get correct findings, when there is an ascites or tympanites of marked degree. By using the new apparatus for the examination, the capacity of the stomach could be estimated far more exactly and quickly than by the inflation methods, by reading the variation of the intragastric pressure, though there may be a slight escape of gas through pylorus, and neither ascites nor tympanites would be an obstacle for the examination. This new method will also tell the degree of the extragastric pressure upon the stomach, which is caused by the ascites or the gas in the intestines.

5. Lavage. Introduce the tube in the stomach, and connect the pipe G and the T-shape. By opening the cock G' the lotion in the open vessel B will run down in the elevating vessel J. When one elevates funnel J higher than the patient, the lotion in the funnel will enter the stomach of the patient through the stomach tube. Before the funnel is empty, one quickly lowers it below the level of the stomach to allow the washings to siphon out into a receptable. As soon as the lotion all runs out, the cock G' should be opened, to make the lotion run down to the funnel, as before. Thus, repeating the procedure the lavage can be quickly performed, without the trouble of pouring the lotion by the hand of the operator. This procedure should be repeated until the return becomes quite clear. When the lavage is over, one should separate the pipe N and the stomach tube and connect the stomach tube with the joint pipe P. By opening the cock K' the remnant of the lotion in the stomach can be completely sucked up in the vessel D. Thus the patient will feel no discomfort in the stomach after lavage, which may be caused very often by the remnant of the lotion in the stomach. Patients who are accustomed to lavage can perform it very easily without any assistance.

In practice there will arise at times an emergency, by which a simpler and transportable form of this apparatus is necessary. For this purpose, I have designed one, based upon the same hydraulic principle. This apparatus can be operated by the bed of the patient, with very little assistance from others. One who understands the principle and the procedure of the original apparatus could employ this simple one in any operation. Further remarks and description about it would be perhaps unnecessary, but I will mention here, in addition, some remarks for the sake of better understanding.

The vessels B and D are arranged in a case, as Fig. 2 shows. The closed vessel A, having a capacity of about 600 c.c., is provided at the upper part with a bent pipe C, connected with pipe F, which is divided into two branches R and V The branch R is attached to the air gauge E and the other branch V connected

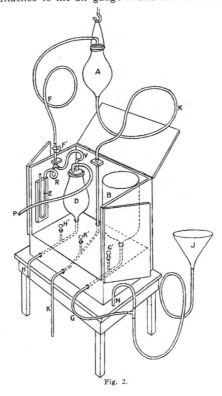

Fig. 2.

with the closed vessel D. The vessel A is fitted at the lower part with the discharge pipe K with a cock K'. The closed vessel D is fitted at the upper part with a joint pipe P. The upper part M of the vessel D is closed with a rubber stopper.

The open vessel B, having a capacity of about 4000 c.c., is provided at the lower part with a discharge pipe G with a cock G', which communicates with a connecting tube N, attached to a funnel J.

This apparatus can be operated in the same manner, mentioned already. Before any operation the following points should be noted. Close H', K', G'.

The vessel A should be filled with fresh water, the vessel B with a suitable lotion. Close the upper part of the vessel A, open the cock F'. One can hold the vessel A in any height to produce a suitable pressure, because the air pressure in the vessel D depends upon the height of the water level of the vessel A.

1. The aspiration of the gastric contents. Connect the pipe P and the tube in the mouth. Open the cock K'.

With the lowering of the water level in the closed vessel A, the air pressure in the closed vessel D would be reduced, which is shown by the air gauge E. The gastric fluid can be sucked up completely in the closed vessel D.

2. The aspiration of the gas or gases in the stomach. Fill the vessel D with water. Close the cock F', connect the pipe P with the tube in the mouth. Open the cock H'.

. With the lowering of the water level in the vessel D the gas or gases in the stomach will be sucked up in the vessel D. According to the same means, mentioned above, the volume of the stomach gas can be estimated.

3. Volumetric measurement of the gas in the stomach. Connect the joint pipe P with the tube in the mouth. Open the cock K'

With the lowering of the water level in the vessel A a negative pressure will be produced in the vessel D and the gas or gases in the stomach will be forced in the vessel D. After the same way which I have mentioned already, the volume of the stomach gas can be estimated.

4. Estimation of the stomach capacity. Connect the joint pipe P with the tube in the mouth. Fill the vessel A with water. Open the upper part of the vessel A. Close the cock F'

When we open the cock K', after connecting pipes H and K, the water in the vessel A will run down to the vessel D and the air in the vessel D will be forced into the stomach. The air gauge will show the variation of the pressure in the closed vessel D, which is equal to that of the intragastric pressure.

5. Lavage. The lotion should be poured into the open vessel B. Connect the pipe N with the tube in the mouth. Open the cock G'. When we hold the funnel below the position of the patient, the lotion will run down to it. By elevating the funnel, the content in it will run down in the stomach, the washings flowing out of the stomach again when the funnel is lowered below the patient's stomach. The procedure will be repeated until the gastric fluid returns clear. After lavage the pipe P and the tube should be connected. By opening the cock K' the remnant of the washings in the stomach can be sucked up in the vessel D.

PREFORMED AMMONIA IN THE SPINAL FLUID*

By P. F. Morse, M.D., and E.S. Crump, M.D., Detroit, Mich.

THE determination of the various nitrogen partitions in the spinal fluid for clinical purposes seems to have been largely neglected. Kahn[1] showed that with certain modifications Folin's direct Nesslerization methods were applicable to the spinal fluid, and gives tables showing the value of the various partitions. He found the total nitrogen to be 17.5 mg. to 31.25 mg., the nonprotein nitrogen 14.0 to 33.63 mg., and the urea nitrogen 6.31 to 21.62 mg. per 100 c.c. of spinal fluid. The wide variation in each of these series is interesting and the fact that the nonprotein nitrogen of one series slightly exceeds the highest total nitrogen value in the other makes the wide variation all the more apparent. Two years ago we tried the direct Nesslerization of spinal fluid by adding Nessler's reagent directly to the fresh spinal fluid and noting the depth of brown color which developed. We satisfied ourselves that in cases of acidosis and uremia the preformed ammonia was increased. On account of difficulties with the technic Nessler's solution was given up for the time for nitrogen determinations and the Kjeldahl method resumed for blood work. No more spinal fluids were tested until Folin's[2] new system for blood analysis was published, when direct Nesslerization methods were again resumed with satisfying results. No doubt a complete study of spinal fluid nitrogen partitions would be of clinical value, and we have carried this far enough to find that these determinations can be made with great simplicity using the reagents employed in the system of Folin referred to above. Kahn believed that the calcium present in the spinal fluid prevented successful Nesslerization and added alkali and filtered to prevent this. We find it much simpler to add a small crystal of potassium oxalate and centrifugate after solution has taken place. The total nitrogen can then be determined very simply, using 2 c.c. of spinal fluid and one c.c. of the sulphuric phosphoric digestion mixture.

At this time we wish to present an extremely simple method for the determination of excess preformed ammonia in the spinal fluid. As far as we have gone this increase has run parallel to blood nitrogen retention wherever the latter could be determined, and we have found this simple test to be of great value for quickly determining the cause of coma. After a little practice a close approximation of the blood nitrogen can be estimated from the depth of color developed.

The test is performed as follows:

To an appropriate quantity (2 c.c.) of spinal fluid, an equal quantity of Nessler's reagent is added. In normal persons and in conditions not tending to acidosis or nitrogen retention, scarcely any brown color develops. A cloudy greenish gray precipitate gradually forms and the fluid turns a dirty pale green color. When there is acidosis or nitrogen retention from

*From Buhl Memorial Laboratory, Harper Hospital, Detroit. Mich.

CASE	ALBUMIN IN URINE	BLOOD PRESSURE	CELL COUNT	GLOB.	SPINAL FLUID WASS.	BLOOD NON-COAG. N.	CLIN. DIAG.	NESSLER-IZATION OF SPINAL FLUID
1						98	Uremia: Prostatic Hypertrophy	++++
2						30	Cerebrospinal Lues	neg.
3						32	Normal person	neg.
4						75	Chr. Nephritis. Uremia	++++
						38	Brain abscess	neg.
6	+++	230	1	neg.	neg.	63	Chr. Nephritis with hypertension	++++
7			20	+	++++		Cerebrospinal Lues	neg.
8						35	Subacute Pancreatitis with exacerbations	+
9			700	+			Mastoiditis with brain abscess.	±
10			450	+			"	neg.
11			Pus	+			10 hours before death	+
12	++++	160				35	Chr. focal Nephritis	±
13			6	+	++		Cerebrospinal Lues (?)	neg.
14		118	370	+	neg.		Otitis Media Brain abscess	neg.
15	++++		Pus	+			Pneumococcus Purulent Encephalitis. Rt. convexity following frontal sinusitis. Autopsy	neg.
16			4	+	blood		Syphilis, Brain (Gumma) Autopsy	neg.
17			18	.	+++	60	Tabes Dorsalis	+++
18								+++
19			16	+	+++		Cerebrospinal Lues	neg.
20			40	+	+++		General Paresis	neg.
21			10	+	+++		Cerebrospinal Lues	neg.
22			6	neg.			?	neg.
23	neg.	148	3	neg.	blood +++ S. F. neg.		Syph. Endarteritis	neg.
24			40	+			Tabes with Gastric Crisis	neg.
25					neg.		Gastric Ulcer	neg.
26							Non-Syph. Chorioretinitis	neg.
27				.				++++

any cause, a deep brown color develops immediately, the depth of color depending upon the amount of ammonia present in the spinal fluid. Only one precaution is necessary. The fluid must be free from contaminating bacteria. These form ammonia and give false readings. Sterile spinal fluids well corked give good reactions even when several days old. The reaction is read immediately (within thirty seconds). In general, cases of acidosis associated with infection, and terminal stages of meningitis, develop less color than cases of uremia with nitrogen retention.

We have tried several substances for standard tubes to assist in reading the reaction. Appropriate mixture of Bismark brown with triple strength Lugol's solution will give a color which exactly matches Nesslerized nitrogen standards even in the Duboscq colorimeter. The color gradually fades, however. Tubes of different strength picramic acid can be used for rough comparison as pointed out by Egerer and Ford.[3] Inasmuch as a considerable cloudiness develops upon the addition of Nessler's reagent to spinal fluid, we think that for practical clinical purposes standards are not necessary, and we estimate the depth of color reading from negative to four-plus. The table which follows shows the results in 28 consecutive examinations. The data was taken from the routine laboratory card and is not always complete in all details.

The accompanying table requires no analysis to show that cases of nitrogen retention give a strong reaction for ammonia in the spinal fluid. Cases 1, 4, 6, and 17 demonstrate this. Cases included with a bracket are successive examinations on different spinal fluid samples from the same patient. Samples 9, 10, and 11 are from a child with brain abscess and general meningitis from a mastoid, in whom a certain degree of acidosis presumably developed. The weak reaction given by No. 8. was also due to acidosis. The specimen was removed when the patient was unconscious and having a convulsion. Recurrent attacks of vomiting followed by unconsciousness and convulsions associated with deep jaundice occurred intermittently over a period of two weeks after a gall bladder drainage. The patient finally recovered completely.

The case from which specimens 17 and 18 were removed is especially instructive. No kidney insufficiency had been detected. The man had all the signs and symptoms of tabes, including a Charcot joint. After we obtained a strong ammonia reaction on two different occasions, the blood nitrogen examination was made with the result that 60 mg. per 100 c.c. was found. The ammonia increase in the spinal fluid and the nitrogen retention thus pointed to the additional factor of kidney insufficiency. Specimen 27 was a spinal fluid from an unknown source which had been allowed to stand around the laboratory until heavily contaminated by bacterial growth. The ammonia reaction obtained was probably due to this. Case 12 with a heavy urinary albumin and a blood pressure of 160 shows a blood nitrogen of 35 and a doubtful spinal fluid ammonia reaction. These findings are correlated and are common in acute exacerbations of focal nephritis where parts of the kidney are acutely affected, leading to the urinary findings of nephritis without clinical or laboratory evidence of nitrogen retention or, in other words of lowered kidney function. In these cases there is enough normal or functionally normal kidney parenchyma still left to carry on the function.

The Nessler's solution which we use is made according to Folin's[1] directions as follows: "Transfer 150 gm. of potassium iodide and 110 gm. iodine to a 500 c.c. Florence flask with 100 c.c. of water and an excess of metallic mercury (140-150 gm.) Shake the flask continuously and vigorously for 7 to 15 minutes or until the dissolved iodine has nearly disappeared. The solution becomes quite hot. When the red iodine solution has begun to become visibly pale, though still red, cool in running water and continue the shaking until the reddish color of the iodine has been replaced by the greenish color of the double iodide. This whole operation does not take more than 15 minutes. Now separate the surplus mercury by decantation and washing with liberal quantities of distilled water. Dilute the solution and washings to a volume of two liters. If cooling is begun in time, the resulting reagent is clear enough for immediate dilution with 10 per cent alkali and water and the finished solution can at once be used for Nesslerizations."

For use 75 c.c. of the above stock solution are added to 75 c.c. of water and 350 c.c. of 10 per cent NaOH. The NaOH must vary but little from 10 per cent. We make up a 60 per cent solution of NaOH as Folin advises, allow the sediment to settle out and pipette off the supernatant fluid and dilute it to 10 per cent. It must be titrated against standard acid and the strength adjusted to exactly 10 per cent if it is to be used for the nitrogen determinations according to Folin's method.

We report this simple laboratory test at this time because it can be done so easily and quickly by anyone without special apparatus and with reagents obtainable anywhere. Complete data regarding all the nitrogen partitions in the spinal fluid might add still more clinical information, but this simple test for preformed ammonia in the spinal fluid we have found clinically helpful. We have not yet had an opportunity to test the reaction in diabetic coma.

BIBLIOGRAPHY

[1]Kahn: Jour. Biol. Chem., xxviii, 203.
[2]Folin and Wu: Jour. Biol. Chem., xxxviii, 81.
[3]Egerer and Ford: Jour. Lab. and Clin. Med., iv, 439.

The Journal of Laboratory and Clinical Medicine

Vol. V.   DECEMBER, 1919   No. 3

Editor-in-Chief: VICTOR C. VAUGHAN, M.D.
Ann Arbor, Mich.

ASSOCIATE EDITORS

DENNIS E. JACKSON, M.D.	CINCINNATI
HANS ZINSSER, M.D.	NEW YORK
PAUL G. WOOLLEY, M.D.	CINCINNATI
FREDERICK P. GAY, M.D.	BERKELEY, CAL.
J. J. R. MACLEOD, M.B.	TORONTO
ROY G. PEARCE, M.D.	CLEVELAND
W. C. MACCARTY, M.D.	ROCHESTER, MINN.
GERALD B. WEBB, M.D.	COLORADO SPRINGS
E. E. SOUTHARD, M.D.	BOSTON
WARREN T. VAUGHAN, M.D.	BOSTON

EDITORIALS

Bilharziasis in the Light of Modern Experimental Treatment With Antimonial Compounds

SINCE the days when "Mineptah's soul, like a bird, suddenly flew up to heaven to exist forever in the bark of the sun," thereby entrusting the salvation of ancient Egypt to his distinguished son Rameses II, the humble servants of the Pharaohs and their successors have suffered from an ailment known as the ĀĀĀ disease. This affliction Phister[1] has supposed was none other than that of Bilharziasis, whose true etiology remained a mystery from the time of Rameses (and perhaps very much earlier) until it was finally worked out in the year 1852. Thus, now for over half a century the true exciting organism of this disease, i. e., the Schistosoma hematobium (Bilharz) has been well known. But notwithstanding the prolonged period during which man has suffered from this tropical, or semi-tropical, disease, many of the most fundamental questions regarding it have been answered only in the most recent times, or else still remain unanswered.

The parasite which causes bilharziasis belongs to the extensive group of organisms known as trematodes, or fluke worms. The fluke worms are usually flattened organisms, somewhat tongue-shaped, and provided with powerful suckers and occasionally hooklets. In man there are four different clinical classes of trematode diseases (distomatosis, distomiasis) which may be regarded as typical, in the sense that in these four instances the infection of man by certain trematodes is more or less normal in the life cycle of the parasite under consideration. These cases include (1) pulmonary distomiasis, with cerebral or other infection as secondary; (2) hepatic distomiasis, with splenic or intestinal infection as secondary; (3) intestinal distomiasis, and (4) a venal distomiasis, while in a few rare instances (5) an ophthalmic distomiasis, which may be an accidental secondary form of hepatic distomatosis, has been described.

A point of very marked interest in reference to recent discoveries, is the fact that the parasites in question, *except the blood flukes* (which cause bilharziasis) are hermaphrodites. The life cycle of the trematodes is quite complicated and may involve one or more generations which live outside of man. The parasites may require an intermediate host, or in some cases, direct infection may perhaps occur. Blood fluke disease in man may be due to either of two distinct organisms, the African blood fluke (Schistosoma hematobium or S. mansoni) or the Asiatic blood fluke (S. japonicum). The latter organism, which has been known only since 1904, is found in Japan, China, and the Philippines. The African blood fluke is found chiefly in Africa and the adjacent islands, but extends to Persia, Arabia, India, rarely to Panama, Cuba and Porto Rico and occasionally elsewhere, including the United States.

The sexes are distinct in these blood flukes, but the female, which is longer but much smaller in diameter than the male, is carried in a gynecophorous groove running along the ventral surface of the male. The eggs of the African fluke are oval, 135 to 160μ long by 55 to 66μ broad and are provided with a terminal (Bilharzia hematobia) or lateral, subterminal (Bilharzia mansoni) spine, but not with an operculum. The eggs of the S. japonicum are 60 to 90 by 30 to 50μ, and are not provided with the terminal or subterminal spine, nor with an operculum. The young S. hematobium and mansoni worms live in the veins of the liver; in the portal vein there are but few young paired individuals, but in the veins of the intestine and bladder wall paired flukes are numerous. Oviposition begins while the parasites wander from the portal vein to the pelvis, and eggs are deposited in various organs. The ova increase in size as they work their way through the tissue, into the lumen of the intestine or bladder. During this process a ciliated embryo (miracidium) is developed, and this organism escapes from the egg shell when it comes into water. But the eggs apparently do not hatch out so long as they remain in undiluted urine. In 1915 Leiper[2] worked out the complete cycle of development and life history of the bilharzial worms. He found the noneyed, bifid-tailed cercariæ characteristic of the genus in two genera of snails, Bullinus contortus and Planorbis boissyi. These snails were shown to harbor two different species—Bilharzia hematobia (terminal spined ova) and Bilharzia mansoni (lateral spined ova). Recently Fairley[3] has demonstrated that bilharzial parasites and their ova exert a deleterious influence on the tissues of their definite host, man, mainly by the production of toxins, and not merely mechanically. These toxins call into action cellulo-humeral responses which neutralize or limit their activity. As a result immune bodies, including complement-fixing substances, are produced, and a complement-fixation test for bilharziasis has accordingly been devised by Fairley.[3] As antigen an alcoholic extract of the infected livers of snails (P. boissyi) was employed. Positive complement-fixation was obtained in a high percentage of cases in man as well as in experimentally infected monkeys. The praetical application of this test, Fairley considers, will facilitate the diagnosis of bilharziasis in the early stages of the disease before localizing symptoms have developed, and also in estimating the effect of the intravenous administration of drugs on the adult parasites.

It has long been supposed that the clinical symptoms of the disease are not due so much to the presence of the adult worms as to that of their ova which are liable to obstruct vessels and give rise to important pathologic developments. Lodged, for example, in the small veins of the vesical plexus, an inflammation of the bladder and rupture of the occluded vessel with the appearance of blood in the urine are apt to result; or if in the wall of the lower bowel, proctitis or colitis with dysenteric hemorrhages. The vesical symptoms are not infrequently marked, pain and tenderness in the hypogastrium, a burning pain in the urethra, especially on micturition, difficulty of micturition, sometimes evidence of prostatic swelling, with urine containing blood, pus and mucus as well as the ova of the parasite. Sometimes the inflammatory disturbances may extend along the ureter to the pelvis of the kidney and the latter organ itself, inducing the symptoms of a more or less grave nephritis. Occasionally from passage of the ova into the liver or lungs symptoms referable to these organs may also be met. Fatal results are to be apprehended after a variable period of such symptoms, with secondary anemia, debility and exhaustion.

In Japan and China the Schistosoma japonicum has been met in cats and in man, and has been believed to be responsible for an endemic affection known in Japan as Katayama, which is characterized by enlargement of the liver and spleen, disturbances of the appetite, diarrhea (the dejecta often containing blood and mucus), and in severe cases anemia, fever, ascites, and edemas, and occasionally death from exhaustion. The parasite inhabits especially the arterial side of the portal system. It is somewhat smaller than the African fluke, and the male is distinguished by his nontuberculated integument. The ovum has no spine, is regularly oval, perfectly smooth, and with a much thinner shell. The ova are deposited mainly in the mucosa and submucosa of the large and small intestine, especially the former. From here they escape with the feces. The life history of these flukes outside the human body is still obscure.

Notwithstanding the prolonged lapse of centuries during which man has suffered from bilharziasis, still nothing but palliative treatment has been known until the present time. The story of the recent accomplishments in the management of the African blood fluke disease constitutes one of the brightest pages in the history of medicine. In 1918 Christopherson[4] introduced the use of tartar emetic by intravenous injection for the treatment of these patients. He was led to try this form of medication by reason of the encouraging results which had followed the use of antimonyl tartrate in such diseases as oriental sore, internal leishmaniasis and naso-oral leishmaniasis (espundia) as found in the Sudan.

The method used by Christopherson consisted in giving a course of injections on alternate days for a period of 15 to 30 days, commencing with ½ grain dissolved in 6 mils of distilled water and increasing by ½ grain up to 2 grains and continuing this dosage until a total of 25 or 30 grains had been given. This amount Christopherson considers to be the required killing dose, notwithstanding that all the symptoms of the disease often completely disappear after the first few injections. This method was introduced by Christopherson at the Khartoum Hospital in May, 1917, and was found to be equally effective in curing both rectal and vesical cases. By September, 1918, he had treated 13 cases of the disease with apparently complete cure in all instances, but with relapse in from one to eight months in three cases. As a result of his experiences he considered that potassium antimonyl tartrate is a definite cure for bilharziasis, and that the intravenous injection of the drug kills the Schistosomum bematobium in the blood and tissues and renders it harmless. If the dosage be too small to completely destroy all the organisms, still their activities will be suspended or considerably interfered with. As a matter of interest here it may be noted that McDonough has reported that he had made some use of tartar emetic before Christopherson published his experiments, and Major Strong of the Australian Medical Service with one or two of his colleagues had also used tartar emetic in small doses at week intervals as early as 1916. But no one felt convinced of the possibility of curing the disease, nor had any one the courage to adopt the truly heroic dosage which is necessary to affect the bilharzia worm and its ovum.

In order to follow the course and rapidity of the drug's action in curing the disease, Innes[5] has studied the change in the length of time required for ova which have been freshly passed in the urine to hatch out when the urine is diluted with water. Thus in one case before treatment ova (which were numerous in the urine) hatched out in ten minutes on the addition of water. On Nov. 5, one-half grain of tartar emetic was given, on Nov. 7, one grain, on Nov. 9, one and one-half grains and on Nov. 11, two grains. On these last two days the ova hatched in 15 minutes. Thereafter 2 grains were given every second day until Nov. 27. On Nov. 13 the ova hatched in half an hour; on Nov. 15 in one hour; on Nov. 17 in one and one-fourth hours; on Nov. 19 the ova hatched, but movements were very sluggish; on Nov. 21 the ova did not hatch in three hours, as was true also on Nov. 23. On Nov. 25 there were a few ova, and on Nov. 27 none. The patient was discharged on Nov. 28. When examined again on Jan. 12, 1919, the urine was quite clear, but contained a few black ova, which did not hatch. This case also illustrates another point which has been emphasized by Christopherson,[6] namely, that dead ova may be discharged by a patient for many months (up to two years) after the parent worms may be considered to be dead (that is, after completion of the course of injections).

That the embryos in the tissues are attacked and killed is a matter of the greatest importance, for thus the patient ceases to be a carrier of the disease and the ova discharged can no longer infect the various species of fresh water molluscs (such as Bullinus dybowski, B. innesi, B. contortus and Planorbus bois-syi) which act as intermediate hosts for bilharziasis in Egypt. The fact that antimony given to a bilharzia patient kills the parent worms in the patient means benefit to one human being, but the fact that antimony also sterilizes the ova which have been deposited by the parent worms before death in the bladder and rectum, renders the effect of antimony a hundred fold greater, for the benefit extends possibly to hundreds who might be infected by the patient, and this goes on all the time the ova are being eliminated. Thus a direct frontal attack on bilharzia as an endemic disease is possible, and it seems probable that by this prophylactic action of the drug, bilharzia may be practically banished from such countries as Egypt.

The dangers attendant upon the administration of such large quantities of antimony are by no means to be underestimated, and fatal results[7] in connection with the use of the drug have already been reported. The double salt [K(SbO)$C_4H_4O_6$] is not readily dissociated, and it is therefore much less corrosive than the antimony chloride. Other compounds of antimony will in all probability be found to be useful in the disease, and by analogy with the complex organic compounds of the closely related arsenic, we may expect that some of these bodies may be more effective, and in all probability, much safer than tartar emetic itself. Already Caronia[8] as early as 1916, experimenting with antimonyl preparations in external kala-azar and leishmaniasis, has employed acetyl-p-aminophenyl stibiate of sodium which he preferred on account of its greater efficacy, easy absorption and less toxicity. And Sir Leonard Rogers[9] has used colloid antimony sulphide and sodium antimonyl tartrate.

Toxic symptoms[10] following the injection of the drug are very common but usually not serious. Among these may be mentioned cough and pharyngeal irritation, stiffness of the neck and shoulder muscles, nausea. vomiting, diarrhea, headache, pyrexia, vertigo, body pains, general pruritus and loss of weight. In some cases, of course, if the extent of the treatment has been insufficient there will be a relapse with hematuria, etc. Of the complications resulting from the injections themselves one may get a marked depression with vertigo, weakness, coughing, dyspnea, etc., if the solution is injected too rapidly. Phlebitis may occur in the injected vein, and if any of the solution escapes into the surrounding tissues a severe, inflammatory reaction with probable necrosis and sloughing is prone to be produced. This reaction is much more severe than usually occurs under similar circumstances with arsphenamine. This has, of course, long been known as the result of injections of antimony in trypanosomiasis, etc.

In cases in which the treatment is too intensive or prolonged, there is the constant danger that symptoms of chronic antimony poisoning may occur. In ordinary circumstances cases of chronic poisoning with antimony are rare and difficult to diagnose. Headache, giddiness, drowsiness, confusion and indistinct sight appear, and the patient complains of anorexia, heaviness, discomfort or pain in the stomach region, and diarrhea is liable to be marked. Pustular eruptions may develop, and general weakness, albuminuria, exhaustion and final collapse mark the severer stages of the intoxication. Albuminuria in a patient, unless caused by the disease, therefore, demands caution in the administration of the drug. When taken by stomach the minimum fatal dose of tartar emetic is very variable, as the greater amount of the substance is usually removed by vomiting. Recovery has occurred after very large quantities, but in other instances one-tenth of a gram (2 grains) has caused death. Acute poisoning with antimony resembles very closely that produced by arsenic and is characterized by excessive perspiration, salivation, nausea and vomiting, profuse, watery diarrhea, great muscular weakness, and finally collapse. When large quantities are injected intravenously or subcutaneously vomiting and purging occur because the metal is excreted into the stomach and intestines and here acts as a severe local irritant. In chronic poisoning there may be ulceration in the small intestine, especially around the lymphatic follicles and Peyer's patches, and extensive fatty infiltration of the internal organs occurs. In an animal with chronic antimony poisoning we have seen an intense icterus which permeated every tissue of the body. This was perhaps largely secondary to fatty infiltration of the liver.

Regarding prophylaxis against bilharzia Elgood and Cherry[11] have made some interesting suggestions. These authors believe that infection generally occurs from coming in contact with, or using the water contained in the small irrigating channels in the fields, or in small pools, and not as a rule, from the large open canals or from the Nile itself. The reason for this seems to be that the snails from which the cercariæ are derived are found in great numbers along the small water channels or pools, but are much less often found along the larger bodies of water. And the authors suggest that destruction of these snails by ducks, such as the Pekin, Muscovy or Indian Runner might be of great assistance in limiting the spread of the disease. And by way of experimentation this means of destroying the snails might first be tried out on a small scale by supplying a good number of ducks to a limited section all of which was supplied by water derived from a single small canal and its branches.

As mentioned above trematode infections are due to a variety of different organisms, and in view of the splendid results obtained with tartar emetic in the case of the African blood fluke disease, the question naturally arises as to whether or not antimony compounds might be used in other fluke infections also. But as pointed out above, all these other trematodes are hermaphroditic except the blood flukes. It will be a matter of interest to see what the later history of these other varieties of distoma infections may be.

In conclusion it is interesting to note that antimony has long borne a most vacillating reputation in the history of medicine. Raised to great prominence in the 16th century by Paracelsus, in 1604 John Thölde, who wrote under the pseudonym of the mythical fifteenth century monk, Basil Valentine, published his "Triumphant Chariot of Antimony," which popularized the metal with the medical profession for centuries. Tartar emetic was first described by Adrian Mynsicht in 1631, and in 1657 Louis XIV was cured of typhoid fever by antimony. Notwithstanding numerous deaths produced both accidentally and otherwise by the administration of antimony, John Huxham was able in 1755 to win the Copley medal for his essay on antimony. At one period graduates in medicine of the University of Heidelberg were required to take an oath never to use it, because of the injury which its very extensive employment was believed to cause. In recent years, at Cushny's suggestion, various investigators have used injections of antimony-sodium tartrate successfully in the treatment of experimental and human trypanosomiasis. And the latest use of antimony as applied to the treatment of bilharziasis bids fair to be the most lasting of all.

BIBLIOGRAPHY

1Garrison, F. H.: An Introduction to the History of Medicine, 1917, Philadelphia, p. 47.
Pfister, Edwin: Evidence from the Ebers Papyrus which dates back to about (1550 B.C.) the time of Rameses II. See Sudhoff's Arch., 1912-13, vi, pp. 12-20.
2Leiper: Report on the Results of the Bilharzia Mission to Egypt, Jour. Royal Army Med. Corps, 1915, July-Sept.
3Fairley: Jour. Royal Army Med. Corps, 1919, June, p. 449. Lancet, London, 1919, 1, 1016.
4Christopherson, J. B.: Lancet, London, 1918, ii, p. 325; ibid., 1919, i, 1021. Brit. Med. Jour., Dec. 14, 1918.
5Innes, Arthur: Brit. Med. Jour., Sept. 13, 1919, p. 340.
6Christopherson. J. B.: Brit. Med. Jour., Oct. 18, 1919, p. 494. Lancet, London, Aug. 16, 1919, p. 298.
7Knowles: Indian Jour. Med. Research, 1918, p. 548.
Archibald and Innes: Jour. Trop. Med. and Hyg., 1919, p. 53.
8Lancet, London, Sept. 6, 1919, p. 457.
9Rogers, L.: Lancet, London, 1919, i, 505.
10Taylor, F. E.: Lancet, London, Aug. 9, 1919, p. 246.
11Elgood and Cherry: Lancet, London, Oct. 11, 1919, ii, p. 636.
12Low, G. C., and Newham, H. B. G.: Lancet, London, Oct. 11, 1919, p. 633.
13Cawston, F. G.: British Medical Journal, 1919, Sept. 20, p. 380.
14Wiley, C. J.: Brit. Med. Jour., 1918, ii, 716.

—D. E. J.

The Spread of Bacterial Infection*

TOPLEY treats this broad, interesting, and important subject in the Goulstonian Lectures for the current year. He starts out by saying: "The subject may be approached from at least three sides, the epidemiological, the bacteriological and the biometrical. The first and the third may perhaps be regarded as identical, but the statistics of the epidemiologist, who is concerned mainly with the historical and geographical aspects of his subject, differ so widely from those mathematical methods more recently evolved that biometrics has developed a technic which it seems better to regard as belonging to a separate branch of biological science. While it is with the bacteriological aspect of the question that I am here mainly concerned, yet it is impossible to consider one side of the problem alone without losing all sense of proportion."

There are, so far as we know no new epidemic diseases. All have afflicted mankind through all historical time. They flare up, manifest great activity, and then subside and may apparently at least, wholly disappear from wide geographical areas for variable periods of time. An explanation of why the specific virus remains dormant for certain periods and when and how it exists during these periods is highly desirable, as is also a knowledge of the stimuli which awaken it into renewed activity. So far as we know no disease-inducing virus can continue to multiply and live, at least through generations on inorganic matter. A few, like the plague bacillus, may thrive on certain lower animals, but there is no evidence that this is true of the causal agents of most infectious diseases. Even in those diseases common to man and beast, like tuberculosis, the strains

*Lancet, July 5, 12-19, 1919.

have been confined to the animal species so long and so continuously that they have acquired characteristics sufficiently marked to render their differentiation easy and certain.

Topley is inclined to conclude that during the interepidemic period the virus continues its existence as a harmless parasite in man. He says: "The first difficulty with which we were faced in forming any theory of the spread of bacterial infection, which should conform to the known facts of epidemiology, was to find some explanation of the perpetuation of the virus during interepidemic periods. The bacteriological data which have accumulated, especially during the last twenty years, have shown that the causative agents of specific diseases are to be found in apparently normal persons who give no history of having been in contact with the disease in question as well as in contact with actual cases of the disease. Moreover, the organisms in question have been shown, in certain cases, to persist for long periods of time in or upon the tissues of their hosts, and we must always remember that the difficulty of bacteriologic technic is likely to lead to a serious underestimate. Clinical and epidemiological investigations have yielded confirmatory evidence, and we are thus left with a conception of the virus of a given disease being distributed fairly widely throughout the world as an apparently harmless parasite on the human host, but taking on during epidemic periods a new and sinister role, only to relapse again into comparative quiescence as the epidemic subsides."

He explains the rise of the epidemic wave as follows: "There are at least three possible explanations—an increase in the power of the parasite to produce disease, a decrease in the resistance of the host, and some attraction in the surrounding circumstances which favor the transference of parasites from case to case without any alteration of the pathogenicity of the one or in the resistance of the other. The third of these hypotheses may, I think, be disregarded. That alterations in environment may be the determining cause in initiating an outbreak of bacterial disease is probable enough; but they will almost certainly act through the variations which they bring about in the other two factors. The whole of bacteriological knowledge is clearly against the occurrence of a considerable epidemic in which the pathogenicity of the parasite and the resistance of the host remain constant. Again, while we may well believe a lowered resistance of a certain number of the host-species to be an important factor in the initiation of the process, yet we can not believe that it is the whole story. The widespread ravages of many epidemics would seem altogether to preclude such an explanation. We seem forced therefore to the conclusion that an increase in the pathogenicity of the specific parasite is an essential factor in the rise of epidemics, excluding from this category small sporadic outbreaks which may be due to the introduction of a fully virulent parasite by a healthy carrier in some other way."

In regard to the decline of the epidemic, Topley thinks that this may be due to a decrease in the virulence of the bacterium, increased resistance of the host or to changed environmental conditions, resulting in lessened opportunities for the transference of the parasite. He rejects the possibility of the termination of an epidemic by the exhaustion of susceptible material. On this point we wish to dissent. That epidemics of measles and mumps are often terminated only by the exhaustion of susceptible material we believe to be fully demonstrated by experience with those infections in some of our camps. The history of measles at Camp Wheeler seems to be best explained in this way; in fact, no other explanation occurs to us.

—V. C. V.

Food Poisoning

PERHAPS it is true that since the beginning of the great war the number of cases of food poisoning, especially those due to preserved and canned foods has increased. If one can judge anything from the number of serious studies in scientific journals this is probably true. If one can judge from the number of instances cited in the daily press it is certainly true. Nevertheless this truth has not been established by scientific investigation. What has happened is that investigators have turned seriously to work to determine how much infection of canned foods exists, what proportion of canned food is spoiled and the causes of the spoiling, and what the causes of the deterioration of the food are due to. Because, during the war, the amount of home canning and preserving increased tremendously, it would be of value to know the number of cases of sickness and death caused by eating home products as compared with factory products. This we do not know except by inference.

The most pretentious work on the bacteriology of canned foods is that of Weinzirl[1] who by way of introduction calls attention to the fact that the annual consumption of canned foods probably totals 250,000,000 cases. Weinzirl undertook to determine the organisms present in canned foods both in commercial and in spoiled samples. His series includes specimens of spoiled canned food, including fruits, vegetables, meat and milk; experimental packs chiefly vegetables and sardines; and commercial canned foods purchased in the market and received from packers in every part of the United States. In all 1,018 samples were studied. In spoiled and in underprocessed food spore-bearing and non-spore-bearing bacteria were found. In spoiled sardines the colon group prevailed. Swelling of fruits and vegetables is caused by yeasts and anerobic bacteria, most commonly B. welchii. In commercial canned foods microorganisms (all spore-formers) were found in 23 per cent of the samples. In no instance were members of the paratyphoid-enteritidis group found nor was B. botulinus ever isolated. In other words no food poisoning organisms were found. The conclusion from this work seems to be that the ordinary commercial canned foods are safe.

It is to be borne in mind that Weinzirl made no intensive study of putrid food, because it was presumed such food would never be consumed. This presumption is taken exception to by Thomas, Edmonson and Giltner who have made a study of a series of poisonings due to canned asparagus[2] which was definitely spoiled and which had an offensive odor. In this case the asparagus was preserved by the cold-pack method with single sterilization. Of the five persons who ate of this, four died within 36 hours. From the material B. botulinus was isolated. The organism isolated resisted heating to 100° C. for one hour, and resisted autoclaving at 10 pounds pressure for 15 minutes. The toxin was destroyed by heating for ten minutes at 70-73° C. The organisms can live and multiply at 12° C., in foods (cheese and peas).

B. botulinus is a spore-bearing, heat-resisting anerobe, which produces a powerful toxin. Fortunately it is not a very common contaminator of food. It is one which can probably be completely eliminated from foods by careful selection of the materials to be canned and by careful attention to the canning apparatus. If the utensils are scrupulously clean, and only fresh, sound, clean fruits and vegetables are used, and treated by the best processes little if any danger will exist.

It is probably true that most cases of food poisoning are due to food which has been "set aside to be used up." In such food unless it is kept very cold, fermentation may occur with the production of toxic chemical substances (ptomaines). Opportunities for this are present always, particularly perhaps in fish. Hunter and Thomas[3] found 224 out of 530 cans of salmon to contain spores of a particular organism but found no evidence that it caused changes in the material after it was canned. Obst[4] found that anerobic spore-formers were abundant in the sardine canneries, that they were not killed by commercial process and that it was only necessary to incubate a few cans at 37° C. to obtain one or more "swells."

All these facts taken together serve to emphasize the warning to avoid spoiled food of any sort, but particularly spoiled canned food. Most canned food is perfectly safe. Any can that is "swelled" should be discarded and destroyed, and canned food, especially canned fish, should be used immediately after it is opened, and not allowed to remain for many hours before it is eaten.

But the recent cases of food poisoning that have created much excitement; i.e., the Canton, Ohio, and the Detroit, Michigan, cases were not due to home preserved food nor were they due to fish or to food left open. They followed eating canned ripe olives. In these cases not only were the disease-producing organisms found in the cans from which the food had been taken, but they were also isolated from the contents of unopened cases, and were, apparently, B. botulinus. The offending product was that produced by a single firm of manufacturers and its sale has been stopped and all possible of the stock on hand in several states has been seized and condemned. It is probable that an investigation of the factory will be undertaken.

BIBLIOGRAPHY

[1]Weinzirl: Jour. Med. Research, 1919, xxxix, 349.
[2]Thomas, Edmonson and Giltner: Jour. Am. Med. Assn., 1919, lxxiii, 907.
[3]Hunter and Thomas: Jour. Indust. and Engin. Chem., 1919, xi, 655.
[4]Obst: Jour. Infect. Dis., 1919, xxiv, 158.

—*P. G. W.*

Constitutional Visceroptosis

IN CONTRAST to diseases manifested by pathology in the organs above the diaphragm and which are for the most part easily detected and diagnosed by the simpler methods of examination, pathological processes of the gastro-intestinal tract are often obscure and frequently difficult of accurate diagnosis. Even renal disease has, following the application of the various functional tests, become susceptible to more accurate qualitative and quantitative determination than are some of the equally common conditions found in the abdomen. The use of the roentgen ray has aided greatly in the study of gastrointestinal disease, and particularly those conditions having as a basis of prominent symptom, either abnormal position or abnormal motor function of the abdominal viscera. The advent of detailed x-ray examination of the intestinal tract has added considerably to our knowledge of constitutional visceroptosis with its concomitant neuraesthenic and other symptoms,—a condition which the busy practitioner is called on almost daily to remedy.

This constitutional or primary condition must first be differentiated from secondary ptosis, due to weakness of the musculature of the abdominal wall. The latter is most frequently seen in women who have borne children and is evidenced by a loose, pendulous abdomen. The primary form on the other hand is often, in fact usually, found in thin individuals with flat or even scaphoid abdomen. Secondary ptosis, according to Keith and Sherrington, may depend for its existence on the absence of integrity of the reflex nervous arcs between the peritoneal nerves and the abdominal muscles. In their opinion muscle tone of the abdominal wall results from afferent stimuli from the sympathetic nervous system including the Pacinian bodies and neuromuscular terminations in the intestines. Weakness of this mesenteric plexus reflex may produce the disease. On the other hand it may be due to inherent weakness of the muscles themselves. Severing of the abdominal muscles of an upright cadaver results in a severe degree of ptosis with the external signs as described and a marked dropping of the abdominal viscera. In secondary ptosis the prolapse of the organs is due to lessened support and not to lengthening of the mesenteric and ligamentous attachments.

Primary or functional splanchnoptosis is based on a developmental abnormality, chiefly a lengthening of these attachments, and is usually associated with certain other developmental deviations. Keith describes a quasi-inflammatory process in the peritoneum that takes place normally between the third and fifth months of embryonic development and which results in fixation of the mesenteries to the tissues near the spinal column, of the ascending colon to the perirenal tissue, of the back of the cecum to the abdominal wall, and of the terminal ileum in the iliac fossa. This he considers a necessary expedient preliminary to assuming the upright posture and one which prevents later twists and kinks.

Failure of or diminished intensity of this adhesive process would result in looser peritoneal and longer ligamentous attachments. These and the frequently accompanying long, narrow chest, acute intercostal angle, and narrow upper abdominal aperture, all combine to produce the familiar visceroptosis with prolapse of the stomach, liver, kidneys, cecum, transverse colon and colic flexures. Naturally in many instances the picture as described is not complete.

It is important to emphasize the fact that the developmental deviation is rarely, if ever, limited to this peritoneal process, but is accompanied by other more generalized changes, particularly in the skeletal form. Ansell, in classifying the various degrees and types of visceroptosis as seen by the roentgenologist, suggests that individuals be classed in four groups. These he describes as the *hypersthenic habitus*, the *sthenic*, conforming to the average or normal build, the *hyposthenic*, and finally the *asthenic* habitus.

The individual corresponding to the first type is characterized by massiveness of build, wide intercostal angle, a short, broad and deep thorax, a long abdomen with relatively narrow pelvis, and showing on roentgen examination transverse heart, short, broad lungs with narrow upper lobes, and a digestive system high in the abdomen and of quite marked tonus. The stomach is small, steer-horned in form, and transversely placed. Gastric peristalsis and motility are rapid and the stomach emptied in three to three and one-half hours. It is characterized as hypertonic. The small intestine does not rest in the pelvic basin, the cecum is high in the right iliac fossa and the colic flexures are high, particularly the splenic flexure, which is often on a level with the fundus of the stomach. The transverse colon is on a level with the umbilicus and presents haustra which are small and numerous. The sigmoid flexure is short. Barium meal residue, twenty-four hours after ingestion, is either small or entirely absent.

At the opposite extreme, the asthenic habitus is described as of frail and slender build with long, narrow, flat chest, relatively wide pelvis, and narrow intercostal angle. By x-ray the heart is vertical, the lung shadows are long, narrower at the base, and broader at the apices. The greater curvature of the stomach rests in the true pelvis, and the small intestines are in the true pelvis. The colon is low and usually spastic, although sometimes atonic, and presents haustra which are few and large. The stomach empties in six hours and is described as atonic. There is usually considerable twenty-four hour barium residue in the colon. The two intermediary stages are gradations between these extremes. The sthenic habitus is characterized radiographically by the orthotonic type of stomach which may be tubular, bulbous or fish-hook in shape and which empties itself as a rule within three and a half or four and a half hours. Hyposthenic individuals present general physical characteristics approaching more nearly the asthenic type. In them the stomach is hypotonic, fish-hook in shape, the lesser curvature lies below the interiliac crest and the pylorus is at the umbilicus. Peristalsis and motility are poor and the stomach usually does not empty itself in less than five or six hours. The small intestine is a pelvic organ and the cecum is low and towards the midline.

Ansell emphasizes the statement that only the asthenic type is usually considered as needing remedial therapy, whereas frequently the hyposthenic needs it as badly. Even a few with sthenic habitus are improved by similar treatment. He also calls attention to the fact that at times the stomach may be in good position and of good tonus, but the colon markedly prolapsed. This would illustrate the importance of always making a complete roentgen examination. He also touches on the differential diagnosis from ulcer, appendiceal and gall bladder inflammation.

Concerning treatment a few words may be said. Various procedures are recommended from physical exercise at one end to pure mental therapy at the other. The former seeks two results,—first, by exercise and a more evenly balanced daily routine to alleviate the constipation and, second, to strengthen the abdominal and thoracic musculature. The theory concerning the latter is that with more powerful chest muscles and better physical carriage the intercostal angle becomes widened. This increased flaring of the lower rib margins with the resulting increase in size of the upper abdominal aperture will result in a raising of the various abdominal organs from their prolapsed position. The ligaments are not shortened, but their upper attachments are raised and spread apart. The mechanism may be likened to the raising of the sliding cylinder on an umbrella stick, the steel supports representing the ligaments, and the umbrella when closed corresponding to a narrow intercostal angle, or when opened to a wide angle. However, it is uncertain to what extent muscle training can alter skeletal conformation.

Psychotherapy alone in certain cases undoubtedly does good. This type of individual is usually rather nervous and at times markedly so. Food of proper quality and character, sufficient healthy exercise of any sort, and ample opportunity for mental employment are the three essential conditions of therapy, to which should be added additional details strictly according to the exigencies of the individual case. Perhaps no two cases will be treated in the same manner. The fundamental process is quite similar in all, but the individual reaction is different. These reactions must be studied and treated accordingly. As a rule drugs are to be avoided, although at the beginning of the treatment, when it is highly important that the physician gain the complete confidence of the patient, their use is at times justified. At other times much better results are obtained by avoiding all drugs from the start. Often a patient who has been for years on a very closely restricted diet, when placed immediately on a large and varied diet, will after considerable misgivings discover that it is true that he can eat practically whatever he pleases. McClure reports very satisfactory results with this method.

In short, after ruling out other organic disease and after applying the basic principles enumerated, each case must be treated according to its own merits.

BIBLIOGRAPHY

Keith, Sir Arthur: Lancet, London, 1915, ii, 371.
Grace and Overend: Lancet, London, 1915, i.
Ansell, P. L.: Am. Jour. Roentgenology, vi, 459.
McClure, C. W.: Bost. Med. and Surg. Jour., 1919, clxxxi, 399.

—*W. T. V.*

Army Base Hospitals to be Held Intact

IN accordance with the wishes of the military authorities and as part of the peace program of the American Red Cross, Base Hospitals organized by the Red Cross for the Army, and which saw war service, will be held intact against future emergencies. War may never again visit this country, it is true, but there are the great disasters of peace—floods, earthquakes, epidemics—which might require immediate facilities, such as only could be supplied by a carefully organized and equipped system of base hospitals, which the Red Cross has as a legacy from its war experience.

These fifty base hospitals are located at important points through the country and their personnel recruited from the staffs of the hospitals in their vicinity. As a result of their war service, the doctors and nurses are incomparably well fitted to undertake such emergency tasks, and virtually, in all cases are being kept enrolled for duty when needed.

The army is cooperating with the Red Cross by providing each base hospital with a unit of equipment in accordance with military standards, stored in a government storehouse as near as possible to the city in which the base hospital is situated. Red Cross Chapters, also, are assisting in the reorganization of the base hospitals for peace times, and will cooperate when base hospitals may be called for emergency service.

A Caucasian Medical School

THE gift of supplies and equipment for the new City Hospital at Ekaterinodar, in southern Russia, by the American Red Cross, has served as a stimulus to the establishment of a first class medical school in the Caucasus.

The hospital, which occupies the former "gymnasium," or high school building, is complete with wards containing 350 beds, laboratories and three operating rooms, and is one of the most modern buildings in the country. It covers a ground area of about five acres, is constructed of red brick and sandstone, and faces the park of the Cathedral. To the right of the main entrance is a bronze tablet, inscribed: "This Hospital Was Established Through the Generosity of the People of the United States of America by the American Red Cross, 1919."

The equipping of the hospital was effected with medicines, instruments and supplies landed from a Red Cross ship at Novorossick, which were installed under the direction of Dr. J. J. Szymanski of Passaic, N. J.

The staff has some of the best professors and surgeons of Petrograd and Moscow, who fled to the Cossack State at the beginning of the Bolshevist regime. Professor Alexiensky, formerly of the University of Moscow, will be chief surgeon. The school will therefore have the benefit of some of the finest medical and surgical talent in Russia.

The Journal of
Laboratory and Clinical
Medicine

Vol. V.   St. Louis, January, 1920   No. 4

ORIGINAL ARTICLES

THE RELATION OF THE COMMON BILE DUCT TO THE PANCREATIC DUCT IN COMMON DOMESTIC AND LABORATORY ANIMALS

By F. C. Mann, M.D.; J. P. Foster, V.M.D.; and S. D. Brimhall, V.M.D.
Rochester, Minn.

THE relation of the common bile duct to the pancreatic duct is of some importance from the physiologic standpoint and of great importance from the pathologic standpoint. In studying the function of the gall bladder it seemed desirable to know whether there is any particular relationship of the common bile duct to the pancreatic duct in species of animals with a gall bladder as compared with species without a gall bladder.

There have been a few general and some special studies made on the relationship of these two ducts.[2, 3, 4, 6, 8, 9, 10, 11] No attempt seems to have been made to obtain data with regard to the function of the gall bladder or the cause of pancreatitis by a study of this phase of comparative anatomy.

We made a comparative study of the relationship of these two ducts in species of animals that can be used for research purposes. A few species not commonly employed in laboratories were added for comparison. In each species several dissections were made, and both fresh and fixed material were employed. An attempt was made to group the species with reference to the relationship of the two ducts. On this basis all the species studied can be included in three groups.

Group 1.—This is the simplest group and contains the species in which both ducts enter the duodenum by separate openings. The animals investigated in this group were the ox, the pig, the rabbit,* the guinea pig, and the striped gopher (C. tridemlineatus).

---

*This species, as well as some of the others in Group 1 might have been included in Group 2, but as a functionating duct is very rarely found entering with the bile duct, the species was placed in Group 1.

Group 2.—This group, to which man belongs, is probably the best known; it contains those species in which the two ducts are distinct, but have a common entrance into the duodenum. Each species in this group, either regularly or occasionally, has a second or accessory pancreatic duct opening at some distance

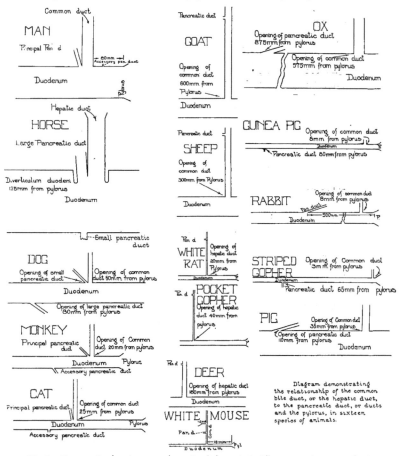

Fig. 1.—Diagram showing the exact size and relations of the bile duct to the pancreatic duct and the pylorus. The column on the left hand side contains those species included in Group 2; the column on the right side contains those species included in Group 1, while in the middle column are the species in Group 3.

from the common opening of the two ducts; in some instances this second duct is the major one. The species examined in this group were the horse, the monkey (M. rhesus), the dog, and the cat.

Group 3.—In this interesting group are the species in which the pancreatic duct empties directly into the common bile duct, usually at quite a distance from the opening of the latter into the duodenum. The animals studied in this group were the goat, the sheep, the deer, the mouse, the rat, and the pocket gopher (G. bursarius).

We have not been able to find any reason why the various species should fall into these groups when they are classified on the basis of the relationship of the two ducts. No other common factor was found in the species in any of the groups. Some very general statements may, however, be made:

The majority of the species noted in Group 1 belong to the rodentia and have some general traits in common. No closer comparison can be made. The only carnivora studied fall in Group 2, but animals of the group as a whole have nothing in common. In Group 3 the goat, the sheep, and the deer are closely related in some of their life habits, but have nothing in common with the remaining species of that group.

The important points to consider in the relationship of the comparative anatomy of these ducts to their comparative physiology and pathology are: (1) the presence or absence of a gall bladder, (2) the relation of the point of entrance of the duct to the pylorus, and (3) the presence or absence of a tendency to develop pancreatitis.

Four of the species studied and grouped in our classification do not possess a gall bladder. One of these, the horse, belongs to Group 2, and the other three, the deer, the rat, and the pocket gopher belong to Group 3. All the species included in Group 1 have a gall bladder. It is quite possible that if a larger number of species had been studied, one without a gall bladder, in which the two ducts open separately, might have been found. We have not been able to find mention of such a species; the nearest approach to this was in the horse, in which the ducts are quite distinct but have a common opening. It is interesting to note that in most of the species in which a gall bladder is absent, the pancreatic duct empties directly into the common bile duct. Probably much importance should not be attached to this, however, because other species in which the gall bladder is well developed also have the same anatomic structure. (Compare the deer, goat, and sheep).

One of the most interesting interactions in the body is that between acid and alkali at the pylorus. From the standpoint of comparative anatomy the important point is a consideration of the relation of the pylorus to the entrance of the biliary and pancreatic ducts. A review of our data shows that the species can not be grouped with reference to this relationship.

No comprehensive comparative study of pancreatitis seems ever to have been made; our knowledge of the disease has been secured by the study of the condition in man. The usual explanation for the cause of pancreatitis in man, particularly of the acute form, is that it is due to the injection of bile into the pancreatic duct following the pathologic transformation of the two ducts into a closed system.[1, 7] According to this hypothesis one would anticipate, from our data on the comparative anatomy of the two ducts, that some species of animals (those of Group 3 that possess a gall bladder) would have pancreatitis quite frequently, and that other species (those in Group 1) would very rarely have this disease. We have been unable to obtain any data to substantiate this. The extensive experiences of two of us (Foster and Brimhall) in inspecting carcases in the packing plants show that pancreatitis in the species observed and at the ages at which the animals are slaughtered is exceedingly rare. The experiences of one of us (Mann) with pancreatitis in laboratory animals are identical with those of Foster and Brimhall. The results of a large series of necropsies on dogs, goats, cats, rabbits, and guinea pigs show that pancreatitis must be very rare in these species. In our laboratory, spontaneous pancreatitis has been observed only in dogs, and but in a very few instances in this species.[5] These data seem to show that pancreatitis is not common in the species of animals included in our study, or that it is not present at the ages at which the animals come to necropsy. Also there does not seem to be a relationship of the comparative anatomy of the biliary and pancreatic ducts to pancreatitis.

SUMMARY

A comparative study of the relationships of the common bile duct to the pancreatic duct was made in fifteen species, which represented mainly the common domestic and laboratory animals. It was found that each of the species could be included in one of three groups. No reasons for the relationship of the two ducts in the different groups were found. It was noted that there was no definite connection between the presence or absence of the gall bladder and the relationship of the two ducts, although of the four species in the series of animals that did not possess a gall bladder, three belonged to one group.

BIBLIOGRAPHY

[1]Archibald, E.: The Experimental Production of Pancreatitis in Animals as the Result of the Resistance of the Common Duct Sphincter, Surg., Gynec. and Obst., 1919, xxviii, 529-545.
[2]Baldwin, W. M.: The Pancreatic Ducts in Man Together with a Study of the Microscopical Structure of the Minor Duodenal Papilla, Anat. Rec., 1911, v, 197-225.
[3]Gage, S. H.: The Ampulla of Vater and the Pancreatic Ducts in the Domestic Cat (Felis domestica), Am. Quart. Micr. Jour., 1878-79, I, 123; 169.
[4]Heuer, G. J.: The Pancreatic Ducts in the Cat, Johns Hopkins Hosp. Bull., 1906, xvii, 106-111.
[5]Mann, F. C., and Brimhall, S. D.: Pathologic Conditions Noted in Laboratory Animals, Jour. Am. Vet. Med. Assn., 1917, lii, 195-204.
[6]Milne, E. H.: Lecons sur la physiologie et l'anatomie conparée de l'homme et des animaux, Paris, Masson, 1859, vi, 507.
[7]Opie, E. L.: Disease of the Pancreas, Its Cause and Nature, Philadelphia, Lippincott, 1910, 387 pp.
[8]Oppel, A.: Lehrbuch der vergleichenden mikroskopischen Anatomie der Wirbeltiere, Jena, Fischer, 1900, iii, 1180 pp.
[9]Owen, R.: Comparative Anatomy and Physiology of Vertebrates, London, Longmans, 1868, iii, 492-500.
[10]Revell, D. G.: The Pancreatic Ducts in the Dog, Am. Jour. Anat., 1901-02, i, 443-457.
[11]Van Balen Blanken, G. C.: Bijdrage tot de kennis der anatomie van pancreas en lymphaatstelsel der primaten, Amsterdam, N. V. Drukkerij "de Nieuwe Tijd," 1912, 65 pp.

A SECOND MODEL ILLUSTRATING SOME PHASES OF KIDNEY SECRETION*

By Martin H. Fischer, M.D., Cincinnati, Ohio

I. INTRODUCTION

I HAVE recently made use of a principle first discovered by Thomas Graham and of another emphasized chiefly by Maly which, in connection with various observations of my own, make easy the laboratory demonstration of certain physiologic and pathologic facts regarding secretion in general, or urinary secretion in particular, which are ordinarily assumed to be inexplicable in simple physicochemical terms, and, for the understanding of which, the vague, "vital" forces of protoplasm are too often called into action. It is still a source of wonder to many biologic workers that a neutral or alkaline kidney parenchyma can be the mother of an acid urine; that the kidney assiduously "protects" the living animal from being overwhelmed by acid or alkali; that various constituents characteristic of urine are found here in a different proportion from that of these same substances in the kidney parenchyma or in the blood flowing through this; etc. It is to the further analysis of the nature of these allegedly strange biologic facts and to their easy demonstration in class room that the remarks of this paper are addressed. As the following shows, the entire biologic fabric is readily reproducible from the simple strands furnished by the concepts of modern colloid chemistry.

II. NOTES ON GRAHAM'S DIALYSIS EXPERIMENTS

Thomas Graham[1] showed many years ago that when any readily hydrolyzable salt, like ferric chloride, is put into a sac (like parchment) which is permeable to molecularly dispersed substances (crystalloids), but impermeable to more grossly dispersed ones (colloids) and the whole is then hung into water, as shown in Fig. 1 (is subjected, in other words, to dialysis) the following changes occur: Because of the hydrolysis of the ferric chloride, ferric hydroxide and hydrochloric acid are produced. Since the hydrochloric acid is highly diffusible, it at once begins to escape through the parchment membrane into the surrounding bath of water. Ferric hydroxide remains behind.

The example here chosen is, of course, not an isolated one. It is characteristic in general of all the hydrolyzable salts. This dialysis method was, in fact, used by Graham for the production of many different kinds of nondiffusing "colloids" from the pure solutions of what were originally only molecularly dispersed and highly diffusible salts.

A quantitative study of the *chemical* changes which occur in the experiment just described has been made by S. E. Linder and H. Picton.[2] This shows that the proportion of iron to hydrochloric acid steadily increases within the diffusion thimble while it as steadily decreases in the water surrounding the thimble. In other words, the amount of ferric hydroxide increases progressively within the

*From the Eichberg Laboratory of Physiology in the University of Cincinnati.

thimble, while the amount of the hydrochloric acid increases without. Iron finally ceases to come out from the internal liquid. The reason for all this is found in the fact that the originally diffusible iron chloride gradually goes over into a "colloid" iron hydroxide which can no longer pass through the parchment membrane since it contains no holes large enough to let such supermolecular aggregates through.

A quantitative study of the *physical* changes of the thimble contents in this dialysis experiment has been made by N. Sahlbom.[3] By subjecting the solution of iron contained within the diffusion capsule to "capillary analysis" (in which are utilized the principles first discovered by John Uri Lloyd[4] and Friedrich Goppels-

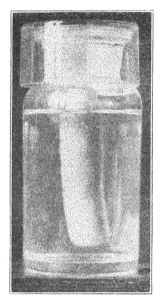

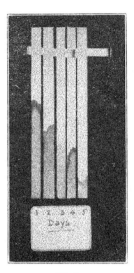

Fig. 1.   Fig. 2.

roeder[5]) the gradual replacement of the originally highly diffusible iron salt by a nondiffusing colloid one can easily be made a matter of ocular demonstration. If strips of filter paper are simply dipped into the liquid contents of the diffusion thimble on successive days, it is found that, on the first day, both the dispersion medium (water) and the dispersed substance (iron salt) ascend the paper as shown in the first strip of Fig. 2. However, as the change in the thimble contents progresses, the dispersion medium is still found to ascend the paper, but there is a progressive reduction in the height to which the iron salt will go. In the final stages of the experiment (after the dialysis has been continued for several days) the colloid ferric hydroxide scarcely diffuses at all, coming to rest almost immediately above the surface of the liquid into which the filter paper has been dipped, as shown in the right hand strip in Fig. 2.

This whole experiment may be readily repeated for demonstration purposes in the following fashion: An ordinary parchment paper diffusion thimble (one capable of holding 20 c.c. or more) is filled to near its top with a $\frac{1}{5}$ molar (about 5 per cent) solution of ferric chloride ($FeCl_3.6\ H_2O$). The thimble with its contents is then suspended in a larger bottle or Erlenmeyer flask as shown in Fig. 1, enough distilled water being poured into the container to bring its level up to the level of the ferric chloride in the thimble. The distilled water must, naturally, be changed two or more times daily in order to get rid of the products of diffusion.

The acid nature of the wash water is readily demonstrated by adding to it some indicator like methyl red. The presence of iron in it is betrayed by the slightly yellowish tinge observable in the first few hours or days of the experiment. If desired, the iron may be demonstrated quantitatively by adding to a given

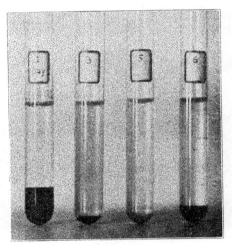

Fig. 3.

amount of wash water a solution of potassium ferrocyanide. While originally a heavy precipitate is obtained as shown in the left hand tube of Fig. 3, it becomes progressively less until, at the end of four or five days, it disappears entirely. This is shown in the tube marked 5 in Fig. 3. If, now, when the loss of iron has dropped to this zero point, some hydrochloric acid is added to the contents of the diffusion thimble, the iron reappears in the surrounding water as shown in the right hand tube of Fig. 3.

The change to the electronegative ferric hydroxide within the diffusion thimble may be followed by dipping strips of filter paper into the diffusion thimble from day to day and noticing the height to which the color ascends. In the first days the iron salt and the water rise together to a great height, but later (after four to ten days) the water still rises, but the now colloid iron comes to rest just over the surface of the liquid as shown in Fig. 2.

III. THE ANALOGY BETWEEN GRAHAM'S EXPERIMENT AND CERTAIN BIOLOGIC FACTS

It is important to point out next the analogies which exist between this simple experiment and certain facts of kidney function. If we will call the contents of the diffusion capsule "kidney parenchyma" and the water surrounding the capsule "urine"—the entirely secondary importance of the diffusion capsule will be pointed out later—the following facts will at once become apparent.

It is obvious, first of all, that there is always derived from the thimble contents a secretion more acid than the medium from which it comes, just as there escapes from the kidney a urine more acid than the tissues themselves. In the later stages of the diffusion experiment an acid secretion is obtained not merely from a medium which is less acid, but from one which is actually "alkaline." The fact that the ferric hydroxide no longer ascends the filter paper means just

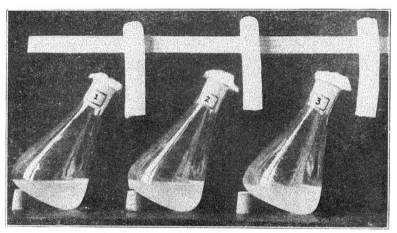

Fig. 4.

this. It is, in other words, an electronegative (alkaline) colloid. But the analogy to kidney physiology and pathology goes further. Ferric hydroxide, except in low concentrations, is a definitely "gelatinous" colloid. Even in the concentrations employed in these experiments it is not an ordinary hydrophobic or "suspension" colloid, but shows distinctly hydrophilic properties. As is now well known, it is this hydrophilic type of colloid which constitutes the bulk of what is termed protoplasm. The "alkaline" ferric hydroxide is, in other words, the analogue of the normal "electronegative" colloids which make up kidney parenchyma.

It is in the later stages of Graham's experiment when an acid secretion of molecularly dispersed substances containing no iron is being derived from a hydrophilic colloidally dispersed matrix that we have the parallel of what happens in kidney and urine under physiologic conditions. The hydrated ferric hydroxide in the presence of traces of salts does not "dissolve" in water (just as no albumin dissolves out of the kidney to appear in normal urine). But if the acid content of the ferric hydroxide is slightly increased, the colloid "dissolves" more easily, shows increased diffusibility and becomes readily miscible with water. In the case of Graham's experiment the iron now diffuses through the parchment capsule and appears in the "urine." This is analogous to what happens in the kidney under pathologic circumstances, as in nephritis. Under the influence of the abnormal production or accumulation of acids (or of similarly acting substances like alkalies, amines, pyridin and urea) in the kidney parenchyma, this not only swells, but shows an increased tendency to diffuse and an increased miscibility with water, and this explains why the material of the colloid matrix, in other words, albumin, begins to appear in the liquid which bathes the parenchyma. The urine, in other words, from which under normal circumstances albumin is absent, now contains such. Accompanying such change, however, there is an increase in the titration or hydrogen-ion acidity of the urine expressive of the increased acid content of the kidney parenchyma. In similar fashion, in Graham's experiment there is a loss of iron during the first hours and while the acid content of thimble mixture and external fluid is high, to become less and less as the more rapid loss of acid allows the iron to change to a hydroxide and to a nondiffusible form. The renewed addition of acid to the colloid iron hydroxide within the thimble again increases the solubility and diffusibility of the iron and at once this manifests itself by a renewed appearance of this metal in the wash water about the diffusion thimble.

The diffusion capsule, it must be clearly kept in mind, is of entirely secondary importance. Even if it were absent, the same results would be obtained, for the parchment thimble only manages in mechanical fashion to keep together the iron solution. Separation through diffusion is the same whether such diffusion is "free" or partially hampered through a colloid membrane.

In the case of a normal kidney the parenchyma itself (the protoplasm of the cells) behaves like the parchment thimble. In nephritis such colloid structures are destroyed and the kidney mixes with the urine just as the noncolloid iron salt would mix with the water, were no parchment thimble present.

IV. VERIFICATION OF THESE PRINCIPLES IN THE CASE OF A SALT-PROTEIN (GELATIN) MIXTURE

In order to show that an entirely analogous behavior is observable if a protein is used instead of an iron salt, the following experiment with gelatin was devised. Gelatin shows, like other proteins, an increasing tendency to liquefy or "dissolve" (an increased degree of dispersion and an increased tendency to diffuse) in the presence of sodium phosphate as the acid or alkaline content of the phosphate mixture is increased from a given low point.[6] The Erlenmeyer flasks of Fig. 4 contained the following gelatin-phosphate-water mixtures:

(1) 50 c.c. 2% gelatin + 3 c.c. 1/1 m NaH_2PO_4 + 4 c.c. 1/1 n H_3PO_4 + 43 c.c. H_2O
(2) 50 c.c. 2% gelatin + 3 c.c. 1/1 m NaH_2PO_4 + 3 c.c. 1/1 n H_3PO_4 + 44 c.c. H_2O
(3) 50 c.c. 2% gelatin + 3 c.c. 1/1 m NaH_2PO_4 + 2 c.c. 1/1 n H_3PO_4 + 45 c.c. H_2O

As shown in our previous observations on this gelatin, these mixtures are just liquid to decidedly liquid at 21° C., a fact readily manifest in the photograph.

These liquid mixtures were poured into ordinary parchment diffusion capsules and dialyzed against distilled water for a number of days. On the fourth day of the dialysis the gelatin in the diffusion thimble of 3 had become semisolid, while that in the remaining thimbles was still liquid. On the fifth day the gelatin from the third mixture was solid, that in the second semisolid, while that in the first was still liquid. At the end of ten days all were solid.*

To understand what has happened it is only necessary to call to mind Richard Maly's[7] classical observations on diffusion. In order to get a physicochemical counterpart of the production of a secretion (like gastric juice or urine) more acid than its source (the glandular parenchyma or the blood) he studied the separation which occurs when free diffusion or diffusion through a parchment membrane is permitted a mixture of acid with an acid salt or one of an acid salt with a neutral salt, etc. Generally speaking, the more acid constituents of such a mixture leave it first, leaving behind the more neutral compounds. It is this principle which is utilized in the experiment described above. From a phosphate mixture containing phosphoric acid, the phosphoric acid diffuses out sooner than the acid phosphate; while from the acid phosphate itself an acid fraction diffuses out leaving behind disodium phosphate. As this occurs, the previously liquid gelatin becomes more and more viscid until, as neutrality is approached, the mixture becomes solid.

The experiment shows in reverse order the state which characterizes the kidney in nephritis and normally. As often emphasized before,[8] albuminuria represents a "solution" of the previously insoluble kidney and is brought about through an accumulation in the kidney parenchyma of materials like acids (alkalies, amines, pyridin or urea). The continuance of the kidney in its normal solid state is dependent upon the maintenance in this structure of a reaction more nearly neutral. In the experiment described above this "normal" state of the kidney is represented by the solid gelatin in the diffusion capsule at the end of the experiment; the nephritic state, by the liquid gelatin readily miscible with water with which the experiment was started. While the urine of the carnivora is for most of each day and normally more acid than the kidney parenchyma or the blood, this acidity is greatly increased under the pathologic circumstances which are associated with "nephritis." These facts, too, may be readily observed in the described experiment.

The more acid nature of the "secretion" in the experiment described above as compared with that of the "parenchyma" (the gelatin mixture) may be observed at any stage of the diffusion by adding some indicator like methyl red or litmus to the capsule contents and to the wash water surrounding the capsule. While I hold that there are serious objections to be raised against the application of indicator methods to definitely colloid systems and to the interpretations which are ordinarily made of such findings[9] it is nevertheless true that the acidity of the wash water about the gelatin always seems decidedly higher than that of the thimble contents. With the progress of the experiment the absolute acidity of the wash water gradually falls. While originally, for example, methyl red is turned

*To reduce liability to infection with liquefying organisms it is well to make up the gelatin mixtures in sterile form, to soak the diffusion capsules in boiling distilled water before use and to keep the diffusion flasks stoppered with sterile cotton plugs.

violently red, this indicator shows only a reddish brown color when diffusion has
been allowed to progress for several days.

BIBLIOGRAPHY

[1]Thomas Graham: Quoted by Wolfgang Ostwald, Handbook of Colloid Chemistry, translated by Martin H. Fischer, ed. 2, Philadelphia, 1919, p. 233.
[2]Linder, S. E., and Picton, H.: Trans. Chem. Soc., London, 1905, 1909.
[3]Sahlbom, N.: Kolloidchem. Beihefte, 1910. ii, 79.
[4]Lloyd, John Uri: Proc. Am. Pharmaceut. Assn., 1884, xxxii, 410, where references to
 even earlier studies by him on "capillary analysis" may be found.
[5]Goppelsroeder, Friedrich: Capillaranalyse, Basel, 1901, where references to his earlier
 papers may be found.
[6]Fischer, Martin H.: Science, 1917, xlvi, 189.
 Fischer, Martin H., and Coffman, Ward, D.: Jour. Am. Chem. Soc., 1918, xl, 303.
[7]Maly, Richard: Zeitschr. f. physiol. Chem., 1877, i, 174.
[8]Fischer, Martin H.: Oedema and Nephritis, ed. 2, New York, 1915, p. 484, where references to the earlier papers, may be found.
[9]Fischer, Martin H.: Science, 1919, xlix, 615; Chem. Engineer, 1919, xxvii, 271.

A REPORT OF FIVE CASES OF POISONING BY NICOTINE

By William D. McNally, A.B., Chicago, Ill.

DEATH by nicotine poisoning is very infrequent, which is all the more remarkable when we consider the large quantity of tobacco consumed each
day. Nicotine is a liquid alkaloid and is the chief poisonous basic principle in
tobacco, existing in all parts of the plant, but principally in the leaves which contain from 0.6 to 8.0 per cent, the larger proportion being found in the less es-
teemed varieties. One cigar contains a quantity of nicotine which would prove
fatal to two persons if directly injected into the circulation. Witthaus[1] reports
that he was able to find references to only six instances of poisoning by the alkaloid nicotine in the human subject, all of which were fatal. One of these cases,
Affaire-Bocarmé, is of special interest as it was here that Stas first used his
process for the separation of alkaloids from organic mixtures.

The literature contains many references to tobacco poisoning where tobacco
had been swallowed with suicidal intent, accidental poisonings, as in tobacco
enemata in the treatment of constipation and pinworms, the use of too much
snuff, external applications of leaves to wounds and the use of tobacco powder
sprinkled on the skin for favus, Weidanz[2] reporting the death of one child and
the serious illness of two others, from this last source. Less severe poisonings
have been noted by nearly every one upon beginning the use of tobacco, where
the peripheral and nauseant actions predominate. Even chronic smokers often
experience ill effects and pain from smoking. Husemann[3] cites a case seen by
Hellwig of two brothers who died after continuous smoking of seventeen and
eighteen German pipefuls of tobacco. Sonnenschein (quoted by Weidanz[2]) relates the cases of two suicides in which death took place in three and five minutes
respectively after swallowing one to two ounces of tobacco. Merriam[4] alludes
to an instance of death in a child from the incautious employment of a strong
decoction of tobacco, as a lotion for ringworm of the scalp. A man[5] died three

hours after using a tobacco decoction for the cure of an eruptive disease. Grahl[6] of Hamburg relates a case where an ounce of tobacco was boiled in water fifteen minutes and the infusion was administered by the advice of a female quack. The individual was seized in two minutes with vomiting, violent convulsions, and stertorous breathing and died in three-quarters of an hour. After using an infusion of two ounces of tobacco in mistake for two drams, a woman[7] died immediately. M. Travagot[8] records a case where two ounces and one dram were used in place of a dram and a half for an injection in a man affected with ascarides. Death occurred in eighteen minutes. In another case[9] a man died in one hour after an enema of two drams of tobacco in eight ounces of boiling water. A dram is reported as having caused death in one case[10] in a few hours after injection and the same amount to have caused death in thirty-five minutes.[11] Reynolds[12] reports a singular case of nicotine poisoning in which tobacco had been accidentally dropped into food warming on the stove. The food was given twice to a baby five months old, the baby became cyanotic, vomited twice, extremities were cold and clammy to the touch, pulse weak and irregular. Death occurred 13½ hours after the first feeding. In the majority of the cases reported, death was caused by infusions of tobacco. Feil[13] reports a case of a woman, 52 years of age who took an insecticide containing 12 per cent nicotine in mistake for cascara, dying in twenty minutes.

Death occurred in nearly all of the cases of nicotine poisoning within a few minutes to a few hours, although I find record of one instance in which death did not occur for two days after the drinking of wine in which Spanish snuff had been placed by a practical joker, causing the death of the French poet Santeul.[14] In another instance where death did not occur in a few hours, a child,[15] age three, used for an hour an old pipe for blowing soap bubbles. Symptoms of poisoning developed and the child died on the third day.

During the last two years in Cook County, Illinois, five cases of poisoning have occurred from taking by mistake for whiskey, insecticides containing nicotine. The free alkaloid is a colorless oily liquid which rapidly becomes brown in color, closely resembling whiskey in appearance, which accounts for its accidental consumption. The first three poisonings occurred in men employed in green houses who drank the insecticide and as the organs were not analyzed, I will briefly state the circumstances:

CASE 1.—A man drank an unknown quantity of liquid containing 44.84 per cent nicotine. The concentrated solution of the insecticide was kept in a cognac bottle, a small portion of which was diluted in a large volume of water for spraying lettuce and radishes. A similar bottle containing liquor was kept on the shelf alongside the insecticide. The man took one swallow of the liquid, realizing immediately his mistake, ran 75 feet to the house, raised a bottle of milk to his lips, dropping dead before he was able to take a drink of the milk.

CASE 2.—Under the influence of liquor, a man went to the kitchen of his home and drank an unknown quantity of insecticide containing 43.24 per cent nicotine from a whiskey flask, causing death in a few minutes.

CASE 3.—The circumstances are very similar to that of Case No. 2, although the man was not intoxicated. The insecticide was not analyzed, but from the minutes of the coroner's inquest it was learned that the insecticide contained nicotine and was used for spraying plants.

CASES 4 AND 5 occurred on Nov. 7, 1918, at Morton Grove Illinois. Two men, celebrating the first report of the armistice, visited the home of a mutual friend, who was asked to give them a drink of liquor. Three bottles of beer were opened, the host then recalled that he had a bottle of whiskey in the pantry, which he produced and poured out three whiskey glasses full. The capacity of the glasses was 90 c.c. and were said to have been two-thirds filled with the fluid from the whiskey flask. The two visitors drank about half of the portion given to them, one making the remark "what funny tasting booze." Both men had a sensation of choking, dropped to the floor gasping for air, became cyanotic, dying within five minutes. Neither of the men vomited. One of them had a frothy mucus coming from his mouth and nose and had urinated and defecated. The host claimed he drank some of his liquor and immediately produced emesis by drinking a large quantity of salt and water.

A postmortem examination upon the bodies, Cases 4 and 5, made three hours after death showed an intense hyperemia of all of the organs. The stomach was highly congested in both men, having the odor of alcohol. Upon opening the thoracic and abdominal cavities, there was no distinct odor of nicotine. The head was not posted. The stomachs were removed for chemical examination.

The stomach and content of E. N., weighed 345 grams. A volatile distillate of 200 grams of stomach and content showed the presence of 0.4465 grams of nicotine, making a total of 0.7702 grams in the organ.

The stomach and content of F. P. weighed 659 grams. From 115 grams I recovered 0.8673 grams of nicotine, a total of 4.9609 grams.

The whiskey flask from which the nicotine was obtained, contained a light brown colored liquid, of a strong alkaline reaction with the characteristic odor of stale tobacco smoke or odor from an old pipe. A volatile distillate gave 39.84 per cent of nicotine using the silicotungstic method.

The nicotine was identified in the distillates from the stomachs and flask by chemical and physiologic tests. The most delicate test is that of the silicotungstic acid method. At a dilution of 1 in 300,000 of nicotine in the presence of one-tenth of one per cent of hydrochloric acid, an opalescence appears almost immediately. Upon standing, a definite crystalline form will appear (Bertrand and Javillier[16]). Silicotungstic acid does not form such insoluble precipitates with all alkaloids.[17] Conine, for instance, which is of interest in this connection for the reason that it is also volatile with steam, yields no precipitate with silicotungstic acid at dilutions greater than 1 in 5,000.

Gold chloride produces a yellow or brown, amorphous precipitate in neutral solutions of nicotine salts, which is nearly insoluble in acetic or hydrochloric acid, but readily soluble in caustic alkalies. A cloudiness appears slowly at a dilution of 1 in 10,000.

Picric acid throws down an amorphous precipitate of nicotine picrate, which rapidly changes to a mass of crystalline tufts. The picric acid must be added in great excess, if the test is made in small capillary tubes, the nicotine can be detected microscopically in dilutions of 1 in 25,000.

Platinic chloride in strong solutions of the alkaloid or its salts produces a yellowish amorphous precipitate, which on standing becomes crystalline. With more dilute solutions up to 1 in 5000, the precipitate appears more slowly and is crystalline.

Mercuric chloride gives a white precipitate with the free alkaloid, which is at first white and curdy, becoming crystalline upon standing. The precipitate can be obtained in dilutions, 1 in 3000, dissolves in a solution of ammonium chloride from which it is redeposited. The precipitate is soluble in hydrochloric or acetic acid.

Roussin's reaction is the least delicate of the tests used for nicotine. If an ethereal solution of iodine be added to a solution of nicotine in ether, a brownish precipitate is produced in solutions of 1 in 100, which is converted into long, needle-shaped crystals after standing for some hours. Nicotine reacts energetically with epichlorhydrin when heated to 120, giving a deep red product; in concentrated solutions the reaction is violent. In one-half of a c.c. of a 1 in 500 solution in alcohol is boiled with 2 c.c. epichlorhydrin, a distinct red color is obtained. A lesser quantity may be detected by boiling the mixture for a longer time.

Nicotine produces a cloudiness or precipitates with the general alkaloidal reagents. Tannic acid gives a white precipitate soluble in warm hydrochloric and reappears as the solution cools. Its delicacy, according to Wormley[18] is 1 in 10,000. Phosphomolybdic acid produces a cloudiness up to 1 in 40,000 in acid solution. Waguer's reagent in an acid solution gives a reddish brown precipitate 1 in 250.000 (Wormley). Mayers' reagent in a neutral solution of the alkaloid gives a white amorphous resinous precipitate in dilutions 1 in 15,000 (Dragendorff).

Conine gives negative results with Roussin's reaction, gold and platinic chlorides in dilution over 1 in 100, silicotungstic acid in dilutions greater than 1 in 5000, and Schindelmeiser's reaction. The odor of the distillate with nicotine is so characteristic that it would hardly be confused with the mousy odor of conine.

Physiologic Tests.—If 1 c.c. of 1 in 1000 solution be injected into a 30 gram frog, in about eight minutes a peculiar position will be assumed, the forelegs will be pressed backwards against the sides and the hind legs will be drawn up so that the thighs stand at right angles to the frog's body and the legs will become fixed so that the feet rest upon the back. If the legs are pulled out, they will immediately resume the above position when released. There will be slight muscular spasms in the hind legs. The respiration is first accelerated, then becomes slow. Using this method 1 c.c. of a 1 in 500 solution (made from a 38.94 per cent solution of nicotine) the above described symptoms were obtained. With an injection of ½ c.c. of the original solution from the flask (38.94 per cent nicotine), a severe clonic convulsion was caused, followed by an immobility of the position noted above from the injection of a weaker solution. The respiration was arrested without an acceleration, the heart continuing to beat. The frog is very susceptible to the action of nicotine, and as no elaborate apparatus is required to elicit the above reaction, the unknown drug should be first tried on the frog.

During the examination of the stomach and content of E. N., it was noted that the distillation had to be continued until a thousand or more c.c. of distillate were collected, before obtaining a negative test with silicotungstic acid. When a portion of the distillate is titrated with standard acid, using iodoeosin as an indicator, the results obtained were uniformly higher than by the gravimetric silicotungstic acid method. In this laboratory I have adopted the following method for the determination of nicotine in organs; 100 grams of macerated tissue are placed in a Kjeldahl distilling flask and a sufficient amount of water and caustic soda is added to make the solution strongly alkaline. A few small pieces of pumice are placed in the distilling flask and the distillation carried on with a rapid current of steam through a condenser and an adapter, into 15 c.c. of dilute hydrochloric acid (1 to 4) in a large flask. When the distillation is well started, apply heat to distillation flask to reduce the volume of the liquid and hasten distillation. The distillation is continued until a few cubic centimeters of the distillate collected from the condenser, after the removal of the adapter, shows no cloud or opalescence when treated with a drop of silicotungstic acid solution, followed by a drop of hydrochloric acid. The distillate is made up to a definite volume and filtered through a large dry filter paper. A portion of the filtrate should be tested with methyl orange, to be certain that the solution is acid. From a standard burette an aliquot portion is withdrawn into a beaker, adding for each 100 c.c. of liquid, 3 c.c. of dilute hydrochloric acid (1 to 4) adding 1 c.c. of a 12 per cent solution of silicotungstic acid for each 0.01 gram of nicotine supposed to be present. Stir thoroughly and let stand for eighteen hours. The crystalline precipitate is filtered onto a quantitative filter paper and washed with cold water containing 1 c.c. of concentrated hydrochloric acid per liter. A portion of the filtrate should be tested with a few drops of nicotine distillate to prove excess of silicotungstic acid. Wash the precipitate several times until no more opalescence appears when a few cubic centimeters of fresh filtrate is tested with a few drops of the nicotine distillate. The wet paper and precipitate is transferred to a weighed platinum crucible, drying carefully and finally burning off the carbon at as low a temperature as possible; the crucible is then ignited over the full heat of a Bunsen burner, followed by the heat of a blast lamp for five minutes. Cool in a desiccator; the weight of the residue multipled by 0.114 gives the weight of nicotine in the aliquot taken for precipitation.

BIBLIOGRAPHY

[1]Witthaus and Becker: Medical Jurisprudence, Forensic Medicine and Toxicology, ed. 2, iv, 1003.
[2]Weidanz: Heilkunde, Berlin., 1907, pp. 333-390.
[3]Husemann: Handbuch der Toxicologie, 1862, p. 481.
[4]Merriam: London Med. Gaz., 1839-40, i, 561.
[5]Jour. de Chimie Med., 1830, p. 329.
[6]Grahl: Hufel Ard's Jour. d. Prak. Heilk., lxxi, iv, 100.
[7]Jour. de Chimie Med., iii, 23.
[8]Travagot: Gaz. med. de Paris, Nov. 28, 1840; or Edinburgh Med. and Surg. Jour., 1841. lv, 558.
[9]Edinburgh Med. and Surg. Jour., 1813, ix, 159.
[10]Aceta Helvetica, 1762, v, 330.
[11]Jour. de Chimie Med., 1839, p. 328.
[12]Reynolds: Jour. Am. Med. Assn., 1914, lxii, 1723.
[13]Feil: Cleveland Med. Jour., 1916, xv, 174.
[14]Fontanelle, Julia: Jour. de Chimie Med., 1836, ii, 652.
[15]Pharm. Jour., 1877, p. 377.
[16]Bertrand and Javillier: Bull. d. Sc. Pharmacol., January, 1909, xvi, No. 1, pp. 7-14.
[17]Javillier: Bull. d. Sc. Pharmacol., June, 1910, xvii, No. 6. pp. 315-320.
[18]Wormley: Micro-Chem. of Poisons, ed. 2, p. 442.

ECTOPIC ADENOMYOMA OF UTERINE TYPE (A REPORT OF 10 CASES)

By Arthur E. Mahle, M.D., and Wm. Carpenter MacCarty, M.D.,
Rochester, Minn.

IT is evident, regardless of the amount of literature which has been written on the subject, that the importance of adenomyoma has not been recognized either clinically or surgically.

Adenomyomas of the uterus and tubes and those extending into the broad ligament were described before 1894 by Babes, Breus, Diesterweg, and others. In 1896 von Recklinghausen's complete work, "Die Adenòmyome und Cyst-adenomyome der Uterus und Tubenwandung" appeared. Adenomyomas of the round ligament, ovarian ligament, rectovaginal septum, and ovary[14] were reported in the latter part of the nineteenth century. So-called adenomyomas occur also in the stomach and intestines, and have been described in the kidney and gall bladder. In the latter cases, the glandular elements resemble those of the tissue in which they are found.

Cullen, in 1908, in his book, *Adenomyoma of the Uterus,* published a review of 83 cases of adenomyoma occurring in 1283 cases of fibromyomas of the uterus; about 5.7 per cent of all the cases. In 1919, MacCarty and Blackman reported a total of 211 cases of adenomyoma in 3398 fibromyomas of the uterus; 6.43 per cent of all the cases.

In 1916, Cullen published his comprehensive work, *The Umbilicus and Its Diseases,* in which he collected all the cases of adenomyoma of the umbilicus reported up to that time, thirteen in number. In his opinion, it was doubtful whether four of.these cases should be included in the group.

The 10 cases herewith reported were extrauterine and extratubal tumors, diagnosed at the time of operation as adenomyomas. These growths contained glandular portions resembling typical uterine mucosa, surrounded by a fibrous connective tissue, and smooth muscle stroma, the latter in varying amounts. The distribution of the tumors was as follows: Umbilicus 1, abdominal wall, 2, sigmoid 1, groin 2, and rectovaginal septum 4.

ADENOMYOMA OF THE UMBILICUS

CASE 1.—This patient, aged forty-two, had been married for twenty-three years, during which time she had been pregnant four times, the last pregnancy occurring thirteen years before. She had noticed a growth in the "navel" four years before, but it had disappeared until several months before examination. At this time she noticed a hard, bluish tumor, which seemed to be growing larger, "broke open", and discharged a bloody serous fluid. The tumor became quite painful at the time of menstruation.

On examination, the enlargement was found, as described, with bluish areas beneath an intact epidermis, and, clinically, it was considered a "suspicious tumor." Excision of the tumor was followed by a Mayo operation for umbilical hernia. The tumor had no connection with the peritoneum or any abdominal viscus. (Plate I, Fig. 2. Plate II, Figs. 1 and 2.)

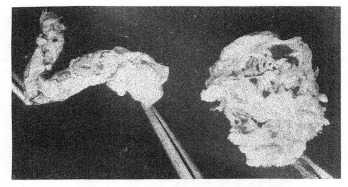

Fig. 1.—(Case 2, 251296.) Adenomyoma of tube and abdominal wall. The thickened portion of tube (adenomyoma, Plate II, Fig. 3) was adherent to adenomyoma of abdominal wall. (Plate II, Fig. 4.)

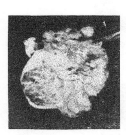

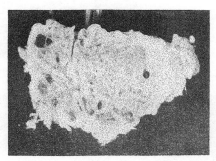

Fig. 2.   Fig. 3.

Fig. 2.—(Case 1, 261880.) Adenomyoma of the umbilicus cut in cross sections, showing small cystic areas filled with dark brown pigment.

Fig. 3.—(Case 3, 177844.) Adenomyoma of the abdominal wall with white fibrous bands of connective tissue extending through substance of tumor with cystic areas filled with dark brown pigment.

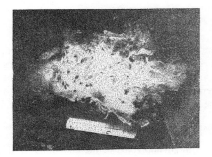

Fig. 4.—(Case 5, 109474.) Adenomyoma of the groin.

PLATE I.

Some patients in the cases of adenomyoma of the umbilicus reported by Cullen gave a history of enlargement of the tumor at the time of menstruation, and one patient noticed a bloody, serous discharge which occurred during catamenia. This author because of the very close resemblance, pathologically, of these tumors, to adenomyoma of the uterus, believes them to have originated from misplaced uterine mucosa or from remnants of Müller's ducts. Goddard, in 1909, expressed the same opinion. While this may be correct, we believe that

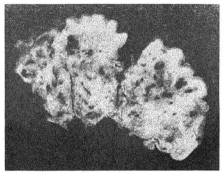

Fig. 5.—(Case 8, 29640.)   Adenomyoma of the rectovaginal septum with epithelium intact over tumor mass.

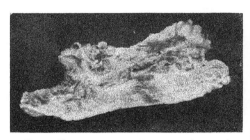

Fig. 6.—(Case 6, 281149.)   Adenomyoma of the groin.

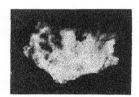

Fig. 7.—(Case 10, 277751.)   Adenomyoma of the rectovaginal septum with small cystic areas filled with dark brown pigment.

PLATE I.

up to the present time no conclusive evidence has been offered, and that the real origin of these tumors is not positively known. Of the cases which have been reported previously, all have been cured by simple excision of the tumor. Our patient, who was operated on quite recently, has been relieved of all symptoms, but not sufficient time has elapsed to assure a permanent cure.

ADENOMYOMA OF THE ABDOMINAL WALL

The two patients with adenomyoma of the abdominal wall had been operated on elsewhere for retroversion of the uterus, for which one had an internal shortening of the round ligaments, and the other a ventral suspension.

CASE 2.—This patient, aged thirty, complained of a tender lump, of two years' duration, in the lower abdominal wall, under a previous laparotomy scar. The lump was painful at the time of menstruation.

On examination a palpable mass, 3 cm. in diameter, was found beneath the lower end of a median laparotomy scar; this was hard, nodular and painful to touch. It was apparently not attached to the uterus, and, clinically, was thought to be a fibrous tumor in a previous laparotomy wound.

At operation, the mass was removed; it extended through the abdominal muscles, and was attached to the left tube about 4 cm. from the uterine horn. (Plate I, Fig. 1, Plate II, Figs. 3, 4, 5 and 6.)

CASE 3.—This patient, aged forty-six, had had a ventral suspension performed several years before and had been pregnant nine times, the last pregnancy occurring ten years before. She complained of lumps in the abdominal wall, which she had noticed for the last year. These lumps had not grown noticeably larger, but were always painful following menstruation.

On examination, a mass was found in the suprapubic region, apparently in the abdominal wall, movable with it, and possibly connected with the fundus of the uterus. Clinically, it was thought to be a fibrous growth, attached to the abdominal wall on a previously ventro-suspended uterus.

At operation, the fundus of the uterus was found attached to the abdominal wall. The tumor, 8 cm. in diameter, was situated to the right of the midline, and extended down to the right side of the uterus. It was solid, with glandular, cystic areas filled with black pigment. Because of its extension into the retroperitoneal tissue, and apparent inoperability, only a piece of tissue 6 cm. in diameter was excised for diagnosis. (Plate I, Fig. 3. Plate II, Fig. 7.)

In the cases of adenomyoma of the abdominal wall it was not possible to trace a direct continuity of uterine endometrium to the adenomyoma. Cullen, however, has shown that in many adenomyomas of the uterus, this relationship between the endometrium and the adenomyoma could be demonstrated. In Case 2, the adenomyoma of the tube was adherent to the abdominal wall, and from the similarity of the pathologic picture of the two tumors, one is led to believe that the adenomyoma of the abdominal wall arose from that of the tube. In Case 3, the anatomic relationship to the uterus was established, but their pathologic relationship was not microscopically demonstrated. It is therefore impossible to say definitely that the adenomyoma arose from the uterine endometrium.

ADENOMYOMA OF THE SIGMOID

CASE 4.—The adenomyoma of the sigmoid occurred in a patient, aged thirty-one, who had been married eleven years and pregnant once. She had had an appendectomy, salpingectomy, and partial oophorectomy performed elsewhere. At that time she was told that she had a tumor of the lower bowel which would become a cancer. She presented herself at the clinic because of this tumor. X-ray of the colon, and a proctosigmoidoscopic examination proved negative.

At operation a tumor mass was found encircling the sigmoid, involving a segment of the bowel 4 cm. in length. The sigmoid and the bladder were adherent to a mass around the uterus. Twelve centimeters of sigmoid were removed as well as "tarry" cysts of both ovaries. (Plate III, Figs. 3 and 4.)

Since the mass in this case was not removed and its true pathologic condition was not known, only the anatomic relation between the uterus and the sigmoid was established. Leitch, however, reports a similar case of an adenomyoma

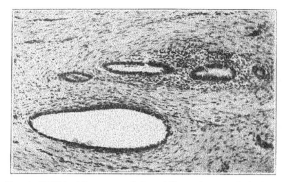

Fig. 1.—(Case 1, 261880.) Adenomyoma of the umbilicus. A group of glands are surrounded by a cellular stroma resembling a typical adenomyoma of the uterus.

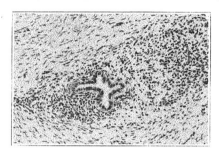

Fig. 2.—(Case 1, 261880.) Same as Fig. 1.

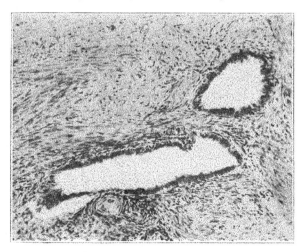

Fig. 3.—(Case 2, 251296.) Adenomyoma of the tube.

PLATE II.

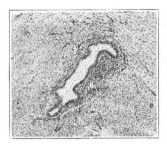

Fig. 4.

Fig. 4.—(Case 2, 251296.) Adenomyoma of the abdominal wall, showing gland lying in a cellular stroma.

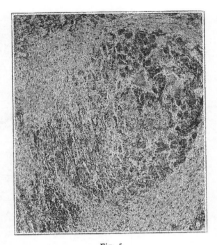

Fig. 5.

Fig. 5.—(Case 2, 251296.) Adenomyoma of the abdominal wall, showing areas of old hemorrhage around striated muscle fibers.

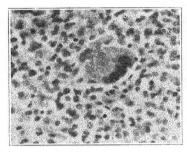

Fig. 6.

Fig. 6.—(Case 2, 251296.) A foreign body giant-cell absorbing old hemorrhage, surrounded by endothelial cells containing old blood pigment.

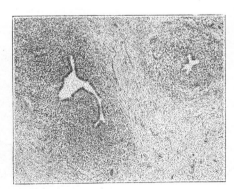

Fig. 7.

Fig. 7.—(Case 3, 177844.) Adenomyoma of abdominal wall.

Fig. 8.

Fig. 8.—(Case 5, 109474.) Adenomyoma of the groin. Note typical uterine gland surrounded by cellular stroma as seen in uterine endometrium.

PLATE II.

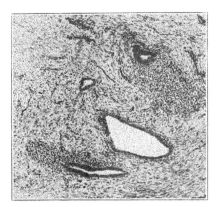

Fig. 1.—(Case 6, 281149.) Adenomyoma of the groin.

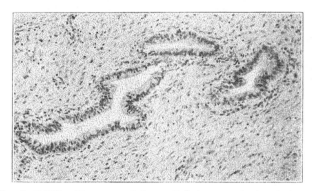

Fig. 2.—(Case 7, 144034.) Adenomyoma of the rectoVaginal septum, showing glands surrounded by smooth muscle.

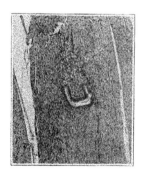

Fig. 3.—(Case 4, 250372.) Adenomyoma of the sigmoid.

PLATE III.

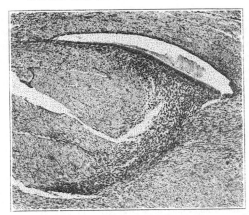

Fig. 4.—(Case 4, 250372.) Adenomyoma of the sigmoid, showing cellular stroma invading muscle fibers. Note old blood and serum in lumen of the gland.

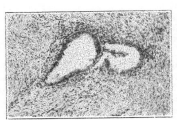

Fig. 5.—(Case 10, 277751.) Adenomyoma of the rectovaginal septum.

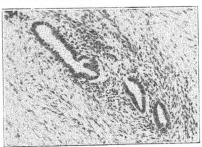

Fig. 6.—(Case 9, 101953.) Adenomyoma of the rectovaginal septum.

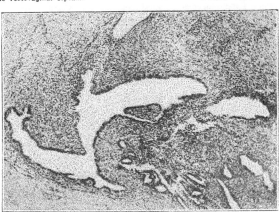

Fig. 7.—(Case 8, 29640.) Adenomyoma of the rectovaginal septum, showing a small cavity surrounded by a cellular stroma containing small glands.

PLATE III.

of the sigmoid, in which this viscus was attached, to the posterior wall of the uterus. Specimens from the uterus and the sigmoid showed the same pathologic picture. The simple facts in these 2 cases lead us to believe that the adeno-myomatous tissue invaded the sigmoid from the adenomyoma of the uterus. In neither case was the mucosa of the sigmoid involved, thus indicating that these growths infiltrate from the outer bowel wall and grow between muscle fibers and into the loose connective tissue of the serosa and submucosa.

ADENOMYOMA OF THE GROIN

Cases 5 and 6 were classified as adenomyoma of the groin, although in Case 6, the tumor was located in the lower right abdomen beneath a scar due to an appendectomy.

CASE 5.—This patient who had been married eight years, but had never been pregnant, had come to the clinic five years before because of sterility. At that time her examination was negative, except for several small nodules which were felt behind the uterus. She returned four years later, complaining of a large gland in the right inguinal space which she had noticed only a short time, and which at the time of menstruation became larger and tender.

On examination, a tumor mass was found, fairly hard and tender to touch, presumably a gland, 4 cm. in diameter, in the right inguinal group of lymphatic glands.

This patient returned 1 year later. The gland had enlarged, and she complained of some pain in the back and lower abdomen. Since nothing further was found on examination than had been noted on former visits, it was decided to excise completely the tumor in the groin. The tumor was diagnosed pathologically as adenomyoma. (Plate I, Fig. 4. Plate II, Fig. 8.)

CASE 6.—This patient, aged fifty, single, had had an appendiceal abscess drained twenty-five years before. She complained of a palpable tumor, a right inguinal hernia, and a thickening of the appendiceal scar. Four years before she had noticed in this scar two small lumps, slowly increasing in size, which became painful at the time of menstruation.

On examination, some induration of the appendectomy scar was noticed, as well as a right inguinal hernia and a large pelvic tumor, presumably a fibromyomatous uterus.

At operation, the fibromyomatous uterus was removed and the inguinal hernia re-paired from within. Later, under local anesthesia, the appendectomy scar was dissected out. The specimen appeared as an indurated mass resembling a keloid, but underneath were cystic areas filled with brown fluid. This tissue, which extended down to the femoral ring, was diagnosed pathologically as adenomyoma. (Plate I, Fig. 6.)

Those adenomyomas of the groin, which have been reported in the literature, were, in most instances, connected with the round ligament.[4] The tumors in our cases showed no relation to this structure, but were situated lateral to it and, at operation, no association could be established, either to the round ligament or any structure closely related to the uterus.

ADENOMYOMA OF THE RECTOVAGINAL SEPTUM

Cases 7, 8, 9, and 10 of adenomyomas of the rectovaginal septum comprise the entire number observed in the Mayo Clinic during a period of ten years. Since so much has been written concerning such tumors, we shall not describe our cases in detail, but consider them in a group. The importance of the condition should, however, be emphasized.

CASES 6 to 10.—The average age of these patients was thirty-seven, ranging from thirty-three to forty-five. Two patients were married, one of them was sterile, the other had been pregnant three times. Menstruation in each was regular with no intermenstrual bleeding. Two had had previous gynecologic operations elsewhere, one a myomectomy and a ventral suspension, and one a vaginal hysterectomy for hemorrhage and a cervix suspicious of malignancy.

One patient only came for examination because of symptoms traceable to the tumor, which were pain in the rectum at the time of menstruation and difficulty in defecation. In all the other cases the adenomyomas of the rectovaginal septum were found in the course of routine physical examination; all showed a tumor situated in the rectovaginal septum, varying in size from 0.5 to 3 cm. in diameter. No case showed an involvement of the rectal or vaginal mucosa. Only one had a polypoid tumor formation raising the vaginal mucous membrane on the posterior vaginal wall. The diagnosis of adenomyoma was not made clinically in any case.

The postoperative results are of interest, in that the patient with definite symptoms from the tumor, complained, three years later, of a pain in the vagina associated with a greenish-yellow discharge. This patient had been treated with radium with questionable results. The other patients have no subsequent history of note. (Plate I, Figs. 5 and 7. Plate III, Figs. 2, 5, 6, and 7.)

Pathologically, extrauterine adenomyomas are identical in appearance regardless of where they are found. They differ grossly from adenomyoma of the uterus, in that the cystic areas are larger and the contents darker brown. (Plate I, Figs. 1 to 7.) Grossly, the tumors are solid, fibrous, and of a light gray color. Here and there, white bands extend into the tumor substance, while between these bands are areas, dark brown to almost black, varying in size from the head of a pin to cystic areas 1 cm. or more in diameter. On pressure, a dark brown fluid exudes from the larger cystic areas.

Microscopically, the stroma consists of fibrous connective tissue and smooth muscle fibers, the latter in varying amounts. Within the stroma are gland spaces lined with cylindrical epithelium. Some glands are surrounded by a very cellular stroma, the cells of which are regular with round or oval nuclei resting in a very fine reticulum, while other glands are immediately surrounded by smooth muscle or connective tissue. In some portions of the tumor substance there is marked evidence of recent and old hemorrhage. In the latter areas are clumps of endothelial cells filled with old blood pigment and in one of these areas a typical foreign body giant cell is seen enclosing a mass of blood pigment. The adenomatous portions of these tumors with their cellular stroma are identical with uterine endometrium. (Plates II and III.)

Clinically, these tumors give no consistent group of symptoms on which an accurate diagnosis can be made. However, their location and their slow growth, extending over a period of years, suggest benign tumors. Further, the occasional relation to the time of menstruation, of pain or swelling of the tumor, or less frequently a bloody discharge should be very suggestive of adenomyoma.

Surgically, adenomyomas, regardless of their remarkable infiltrative characteristics, should be differentiated from malignancy. Especially is this true of tumors in the pelvis, adherent to the sigmoid or the abdominal wall or other structures. Adenomyomas may be recognized grossly in most cases by the fibrous stroma which contains cystic areas filled with a bloody, dark brown, or serous fluid.

The pathologist should distinguish adenomyoma from carcinoma by the regularity of gland structure with normal differentiated epithelial cells without mitoses, and, in most tumors, by the characteristic stroma surrounding the glands. He should also recognize that they are benign tumors, that they grow by invasion, and do not metastasize.

It is also of interest that in our series of cases the true nature of the growth was not suspected before operation. Two were diagnosed malignant, one questionably malignant, and the others were left to be diagnosed pathologically at the time of operation.

All cases occurred in patients between the ages of twenty-nine and fifty. Pregnancy apparently had no influence, for six of the cases occurred in nulliparous women.

Of the 10 patients, 6 gave a history of symptoms directly referable to the tumor. One stated that a tumor mass was found during operation, elsewhere, for other symptoms of which the patient complained at that time. The remaining 3 patients had adenomyomas of the rectovaginal septum which were so small that they were giving no trouble. In these cases, the symptoms, when they were noted in the history, were enlargement, pain in the rectum or vagina at the time of menstruation, or a vaginal discharge.

Our knowledge of the origin of these tumors at present is only theoretical. von Recklinghausen thought they arose from the Wolffian body or duct. Ivanoff, and later Aschoff, according to Lockyer, suggested their origin from the epithelium of the peritoneum of the different regions in which these tumors are found. Cullen believes them to be from remnants of Müller's ducts or misplaced uterine endometrium. No doubt more extensive work on the embryology of the genitourinary tract will solve this interesting problem.

BIBLIOGRAPHY

[1]Aschoff, L.: Cystisches Adenofibrom der Leistengegend, Monatschr. f. Geburtsh. u. Gynäk., 1899, ix, 25-41. Cited by Lockyer.

[2]Babes, V.: Über epitheliale Geschwülste in Uterusmyomen, Allg. Wien. med. Ztg., 1882, xxvii, 36-48.

[3]Breus, C.: Über wahre epithelführende Cystenbildung in Uterusmyomen, Wien, 1894, 36 pp.

[4]Cullen, T. S.: Adenomyoma of the Round Ligament, Bull. Johns Hopkins Hosp., May-June, 1896, vii, 112-114.

[5]Cullen, T. S.: Adenomyoma of the Uterus, 1908, Philadelphia, W. B. Saunders Co., 270 pp.

[6]Cullen, T. S.: Embryology, Anatomy, and Diseases of the Umbilicus, together with Diseases of the Urachus, 1916, Philadelphia, W. B. Saunders Co., 680 pp.

[7]Diesterweg, A.: Ein Fall von Cystofibroma uteri verum, Ztschr. f. Geburtsh. u. Gynäk., 1883, ix, 191, 234,

[8]Goddard, S. W.: Two Umbilical Tumors of Probable Uterine Origin, Surg., Gynec. and Obst., 1909, ix, 249-252.

[9]Ivanoff, N. S.: Drüsiges cystenhaltiges Uterusfibromyom compliciert durch Sarcom und Carcinom, Monatschr. f. Geburtsh. u. Gynäk., 1898, vii, 295-300. Cited by Lockyer.

[10]Leitch, A.: Migratory Adenomyomata of the Uterus, Proc. Roy. Soc. Med., vii., Pt. ii, Obst. and Gynec. Sec., pp. 393-398, Oct. 9, 1913.

[11]Lockyer, C.: Fibroids and Allied Tumors, New York, Macmillan, 1918, 603 pp.

[12]MacCarty, W. C., and Blackman, R. H.: The Frequency of Adenomyoma of the Uterus, Ann. Surg., February, 1919, lxix, 135-137.

[13]v. Recklinghausen, F. D.: Die Adenomyome und Cystadenome der Uterus und Tubenwandung; ihre Abkünft von Resten des Wolff'schen Körpers, 1896, Berlin, Hirschwald, 247 pp. Cited by Lockyer.

[14]Russell, W. W.: Aberrant Portions of the Müllerian Duct Found in an Ovary, Bull. Johns Hopkins Hosp., 1899, x, 8-10.

THE IMPORTANCE OF BIOLOGIC CLASSIFICATIONS IN EPIDEMIOLOGY

By L. C. Havens, M.D., Iowa City, Iowa

TO the epidermiologist the prime factor of importance in the study of patho-genic bacteria is their mode of transmission from one person to another. Epidemiology is concerned primarily with the study of the sources of infection and means of transmission of the diseases due to these organisms with the purpose of increasing knowledge of methods for their prevention. The following consid-erations are set forth to show the practical necessity, in epidemiologic work, of a biologic classification of the microorganisms which cause disease.

A morphologic classification into Coccaceæ Bacteriaceæ and Spirillaceæ is, of course, fundamental. A morphologic study furnishes a practical basis for nomenclature and comparison. However, such a grouping is no more than fun-damental. We know that there are a goodly number of species of streptococci or of the bacilli of the colon-typhoid group, for example, that can not be differ-erentiated morphologically but that can be shown to be unlike by their cultural characteristics, that is, they produce different appearances in their growth on artificial media, their ability to split sugars and the higher alcohols varies, and thus we have a further means of identification.

These two methods, the study of cultural and morphologic characteristics, together with tinctorial properties, have, until recently, been our only means for the recognition of bacteria, and much progress has been accomplished by their use. With a few striking exceptions, all the bacterial causes of disease have been determined by these methods and in a number of instances, a potent therapeutic agent has been obtained.

In spite of this progress, there is still much that is unknown and this is especially true from an epidemiologic standpoint. Former methods for the classi-fication of bacteria have disregarded the reactions which they arouse in their natural host, the animal body. The study of the measures used by the body to resist infection has progressed rapidly from empirical observations to the status of a separate science. From the observations that many diseases leave the in-dividual resistant to a second attack has developed the science of immunology. One of the well-known basic principles of immunology is that immune reactions are as a rule, highly specific, that is, each race or "strain" of bacteria stimulates the production of antibodies when injected into the body, either naturally or artificially, and furthermore these antibodies are specific for a small group; other groups, although morphologically and culturally identical, being often not in-cluded in the antibody formation.

It is rational, then, to expect that a biologic classification would bring out many points of interest in relation to epidemiologic studies of disease. That this may be so is shown by the increased knowledge of the epidemiology of pneu-monia following the discovery that the pneumococcus, instead of being one species, was composed of several distinct biologic types, which, nevertheless, are identical culturally.

Pneumonia was formerly considered an endemic disease, the causative organism being supposedly universally carried in the secretions of the nose and throat and that consequently it was useless to attempt any preventive measures. The main hope of decreasing the incidence of pneumonia lay in increasing individual resistance to the disease by hygienic measures, while attempts to increase resistance by prophylactic vaccination met with failure. It also seemed that pneumonia was an exception to the infectious diseases in that it failed to confer an immunity of any duration, since second and third attacks were common.

Since the discovery of the biologic types of the pneumococcus[1] it has become evident that pneumonia is a true epidemic disease, that the organisms carried universally in normal mouths are commonly some of the less virulent strains of Type IV and that if a person is found to harbor one of the more virulent types it is usually because he has been in contact with a case of pneumonia of that type. That this is not always the case has been shown by a survey at an army camp[2] and a routine examination of surgical cases before operation[3] where carriers of the more virulent types were found. We know that an epidemic of pneumonia due to one type may occur coincidently with an epidemic of a second type. In other words, the epidemiologist is aided in tracing the sources of infection. We know, furthermore, than an attack of pneumonia confers an appreciable immunity of considerable duration and that further attacks are due to other types of the pneumococcus against which no immunity has been produced. Finally experiences in the army[4] in the last year have shown that prophylactic inoculation against pneumonia may be efficient by the inclusion of representatives of all groups in the vaccine.

Another group of organisms which was supposed to be a unit from morphologic and cultural evidence is the meningococci. Formerly the serum treatment of meningitis was followed by many failures, due to the fact that no biologic classification had been worked out, and consequently the serum was often of low titer for the particular strain causing the infection. With a biologic classification representative strains can be used and a more universally potent serum is produced.[5] The British Army, early in the war, had such an experience; the serum which was being used contained no antibodies against the particular strain which caused the epidemic. An investigation of the strains causing the epidemic and the inclusion of representatives in the production of the serum gave successful results. Besides saving a useful therapeutic agent from the scrap heap, the successful classification has been an aid in the search for carriers. The organism in the nasopharynx of the healthy carrier must correspond biologically with the organism causing the epidemic in order to prove the carrier to be a factor in the spread of the infection. A parameningococcus carrier can not be a source of an epidemic due to a "normal" meningococcus.

The epidemiology of streptococcus infections—pneumonia, sore throat, tonsillitis and bronchitis due to this group of organisms—is in much the same state as that of the pneumococcus previous to its classification into groups. It is known that many individuals carry these organisms in their throats and that chances for infection are constantly present. These organisms belong to several groups culturally, but there seems to be relatively little difference in the degree of infectivity between the various groups. Recently the hemolytic streptococci have been classified biologically[6,7] and it has been found that the cultural characteristics have no relation to the biologic grouping, the serologic types overlapping the cultural groups.[7] A further point which has been brought out in this study which, if corroborated, will prove to be an important epidemiologic factor, is that in a small series of fatal cases of streptococcus pneumonia studied the organisms isolated were all of one biologic type, indicating that this group is much more virulent than the others.

One more illustration will serve to show the practical importance of biologic groupings. Tetanus antitoxin was one of the first therapeutic serums to be used and has long been thought to be highly specific. Yet in a study of tetanus infections in the British Army several biologic groups of the bacillus were found.[8] The standard serum of the United States Public Health Service and of the British Government included only one of these groups, thus explaining the failure of antitoxin in a small number of cases due to the less common types. Tetanus antitoxin, by the inclusion of these other groups, can now be made more completely successful.

That a biologic classification of the colon-typhoid group may be of value to the epidemiologist seems probable. Satisfactory cultural standards for the differentiation of members of this important group are unsatisfactory, especially for differentiation of B. coli of fecal and nonfecal origin. Much clearer light could doubtless be thrown on this group of organisms by a classification according to their biologic characteristics.

One thousand deaths from diphtheria occur every year in New York City alone[9] in spite of the increasing use of antitoxin. An investigation of the serologic properties of the diphtheria bacillus might show biologic differences as in the case of the pneumococcus and the tetanus bacillus.

Only a few striking instances of the value of studying the biologic characteristies of bacteria have been cited. However, the importance of further investigation of the serologic properties of the different pathogenic groups has been shown by these actual cases and the fact that practical interest in these organisms lies largely in this field adds to the interest of such a classification. To the epidemiologist such work as has been done has proved of immense value and every new discovery that aids in the precise recognition of etiologic factors is of the utmost importance.

BIBLIOGRAPHY

[1]Dochez, A. R., and Gillespie, L. J.: Jour. Am. Med. Assn., 1913, lxi. 727.
[2]Birge, E.G., and Havens. L. C.: New York Med. Jour., March 29, 1919.
[3]Olmstead. M.: Proc. Soc. Biol. and Med., 1918, xv, 83-85.
[4]Public Health Reports: November 1, 1918.
[5]Amoss, H. L.: Jour. Am. Med. Assn., 1917, lxix, No. 14. p. 1137.
[6]Avery, O. T., and Dochez, A. R.: Jour. Exper. Med., 1919, xxx, 3.
[7]Havens. L. C.: Jour. Infect. Dis., 1919, xxv, No. 4, p. 315.
[8]Tulloch, W. J.: Jour. Hygiene, 1919, xviii, No. 2, p. 103.
[9]Public Health Reports, May 16, 1919.

LABORATORY METHODS

THE ICE-BOX FIXATION METHOD IN THE PERFORMANCE OF THE WASSERMANN REACTION*

By R. G. Owen, M.D., and F. A. Martin, M.D., Detroit, Mich.

HISTORICAL

WHILE certain radical changes in the technic of the Wassermann reaction have been advocated by Noguchi, Hecht-Weinberg, Stern, and others. the fundamental principles, the original method of Wassermann, Neisser and Bruck is still followed by the majority of serologists.

The most important changes in technic have been the adoption of smaller amounts of the various ingredients which enter into the test, the substitution of plain alcoholic or cholesterinized heart, human, beef and guinea pig, for the original watery liver extract of Wassermann and various refinements in the standardization of the hemolytic system, such as, using a fixed amount of amboceptor and titrating the complement for each set of tests; yet, to date, it has been impossible to get serologists to adopt any uniform method, each man being satisfied with his own peculiar technic and, perhaps, with justice.

Nevertheless, partly because of such varying technic, the Wassermann reaction has been unjustly criticized on account of discordant reports rendered on the same serum by different workers. The true worth of this reaction has been most aptly expressed by Vedder, who says: "One is impressed by the fact that the Wassermann reaction must be a test of most surprising merit to have survived all the clumsy technic that has been perpetrated in its name."

While the use of cholesterinized antigens gives a much higher percentage of positive results in cases of known syphilis, nevertheless the consensus of recent opinion is that such antigens undoubtedly give a not inconsiderable number of strongly positive reactions in cases where syphilis can be definitely excluded. The published figures of such false positive results run as high as 10 to 20 per cent, and the gain in detecting known cases of syphilis is certainly not compensated for by this considerable error. It is far better to get negative results in a few cases of syphilis than it is to attach the stigma of syphilis to an innocent person, for while we serologists insist that the Wassermann reaction should only be considered as one of the most constant symptoms of syphilis, nevertheless we know full well that in most cases the diagnosis is based entirely on results of the blood examination, even weak positive results being considered diagnostic of lues.

Any method, therefore, which will increase the percentage of true posi-

---

*From the Serological Department of the Detroit Clinical Laboratory, Detroit, Mich.

tive reactions without giving false results in nonsyphilitic conditions should have our most careful consideration.

Such a method, or rather, a variation of the older methods is now coming into use which fulfills these two requirements.

In the original Wassermann method the serum, antigen, and complement were left at 37.5° C. for one hour to permit the fixation of complement. Bordet, Gengou, and Wassermann tried various time limits and also the effect of various temperatures on complement fixation, and found that the process was a gradual one, occurring best at body temperature and they also determined that fixation of complement was practically complete in one hour, while longer periods at this temperature led to deterioration of the complement.

In 1910 Jacobstahl[1] advocated carrying out this first phase of the reaction in the ice box at about 4° C., where the tubes were left for one and one-half hours.

He found 2 per cent more positives, testing 200 bloods, when ice box fixation was used, but apparently missed the main reason for the superiority of such low temperature fixation, namely, that the reagents could be left in contact with each other for much longer periods without deterioration of complement. He did not try periods longer than one and one-half hours, and considered that the increased sensitiveness of his technic was due to better precipitation of the lipoidal extract with absorption of complement, such precipitation occurring better at 4° C. than at 37° C. He gives no details as regards the antigen used.

Guggenheimer[2] ran 623 sera with preliminary incubation at 0° C. and at 37.5° C., keeping both sets at the desired temperature for one and one-quarter hours.

Five hundred thirty four sera showed no difference in the two methods, being either negative or strongly positive; 89 cases showed a difference, but in 69 the difference was mainly a slight quantitative one which in no way affected the diagnosis; 20 cases, however, showed a radical difference in results, 12 being positive only at 0° C. and 8 only at 37° C., these 20 cases being clearly luetic. He used syphilitic fetal liver extract as antigen.

McNeil[3] was the first American observer to report cases tested in this way, and his method was adopted as the standard technic of the New York City Board of Health.

He used crude alcoholic tissue extracts, employing the Wassermann technic with inactivated serum, and found that a fixation period of four hours at 8° C. to 12° C. was best. Testing 466 cases he got 37.7 per cent of positive reactions with incubator fixation against 48 per cent of like results when fixation was carried out in the ice box. He failed, however, to give any histories of these cases, so we are left at a loss as just how to interpret his findings.

Altman[4] also claims to have obtained more satisfactory results when ice box fixation was used. Like Guggenheimer, he reports that certain bloods are positive at 37.5° C. which failed to react at the ice box temperature.

Favorable results with the ice box fixation have also been reported by Leredde and Rubinstein[5].

Coca and L'Esperence[6] report 828 sera run at 37.5° C. for one hour and in the ice box at 7° C. for eighteen to twenty-four hours. They use a special technic of their own devising, with an acetone-insoluble antigen. They report 584 bloods negative with both methods; 203 positive at 7° C. and 37.5° C., while 28 were positive only at the ice box temperature and 13 positive only at 37.5° C.

Smith and MacNeal[7] have reported similar favorable results with the ice box fixation method. They compared the results of cholesterinized antigen at 37.5° C. in incubator for one hour with plain alcoholic heart extract left a similar time at 37.5° C. and at ice box temperature, 8° C., some for four hours, others for sixteen to eighteen hours. They make no remarks concerning the best length of time for the ice box fixation. Testing 110 cases of known syphilis, they found 58 per cent of positives with cholesterinized antigen with incubator fixation against 77 per cent with plain antigen with ice box fixation, and only 32.2 per cent of positives when the plain antigen was used in the incubator method. With 43 patients, probably syphilitic, they got 65.9 per cent positive with cholesterinized antigen, and 75 and 36.3 per cent, respectively, with plain antigen in ice box and incubator. Fifty-nine patients, probably not syphilitic, yielded 40 per cent, 5 per cent, and 1.6 per cent, respectively, by the three methods. Two hundred sixty five nonsyphilitic patients were negative by all three methods.

They used human, beef, and guinea pig hearts as antigen, extracting 10 gm. of tissue with 100 c.c. of absolute ethyl alcohol and diluting this extract with from 10 to 31 volumes of salt solution. No details as to how the antigens were titrated are given.

The high percentage of positive results with cholesterinized antigen in the group "probably not syphilitic" is hard to reconcile with the lower figures given by this antigen in the "known syphilitic" and "probably syphilitic" groups, especially when it is considered that they report no positive reactions whatever with cholesterinized antigens among 265 nonluetic patients. We can not reconcile their 40 per cent of positive results with cholesterinized antigen among probable luetics with their negative results on 265 negative cases.

Their figures would indicate that cholesterinized antigens give no false positives with nonluetics, while yielding a very high percentage of positive results in doubtful cases and lower figures than plain antigen, ice box fixation, with known syphilitics.

It seems to us on theoretical grounds, and this belief is substantiated by our own figures, that cholesterinized antigens will uniformly give a higher percentage of positives in known syphilitics, doubtful, and nonsyphilitic cases.

In a personal communication, Dr. Smith informed us that cholesterinized antigens when used with ice box fixation gave a very high percentage of false positives, and our own investigations fully corroborated his results. These authors do not report any cases strongly positive with incubator method, with plain antigen, and negative with ice box fixation, but they did find 3 specimens giving ++ with plain antigen in ice box which gave +++ + reactions in the incubator test.

Ottenberg[8] considers ice box fixation with plain antigen as giving by far the most delicate and accurate results. He quotes Swift who, in conjunction with

Walker, first advocated cholesterin reinforced antigens in America, as saying that plain antigens with ice box fixation give results identical with cholesterinized antigens with incubator fixation.

With weakly positive sera Ottenberg[8] found that fixation was not as good at 0° C. to 2° C. in ice box as in the incubator but at 8° C. to 10° C. he found results just as good when left in ice box for one hour and even better when a period of four hours was used.

He states that fixation periods of twelve to eighteen hours are not as satisfactory as a four-hour time.

Like Smith and MacNeal and ourselves he finds that cholesterin antigens can not be used with ice box fixation.

Kaliski (quoted by Ottenberg[8]) combines incubator and ice box fixation, leaving the serum, complement, and antigen in the ice box for two hours, followed by one hour in the incubator.

TECHNIC

With our technic we use the following quantities:

1. Serum, 0.1 c.c. freshly inactivated at 56° C. for one-half hour.
2. Complement, (1 to 10 dilution) 2 units.
3. Sheep cells, 5 per cent suspension, 0.5 c.c.
4. Antigen—
   a. Cholesterinized, (1 to 10 dilution) 0.1 c.c. to 0.15 c.c.
   b. Plain alcoholic, (1 to 10 dilution) 0.3 c.c. to 0.7 c.c.
5. Amboceptor, 2 units.
6. Salt solution, q.s. to make vol. of 2.5 c.c.

The amboceptor unit is determined by using 0.5 c.c. of 1 to 10 dilution of complement with 0.5 c.c. of 5 per cent sheep cells and salt solution to make volume up to 2.5 c.c. This amboceptor unit is found after using several pooled complements. Using two units of amboceptor, a daily titration of complement is done and the unit determined. In the actual tests two units of complement and two units of amboceptor are employed.

We have found that such complement titration gives much more reliable results than when a fixed amount of complement is taken as two units and the amboceptor unit determined. If complement be not in excess, the presence of more than two amboceptor units, whether added or present in the serum makes little difference in the results. If, however, a fixed amount of complement be taken as two units and then two amboceptor units are used, the presence of natural hemolysins may cause false negative results, owing to the excess of complement often present in such arbitrarily chosen amounts.

In getting the daily complement dose we use three amounts of amboceptor with increasing amounts of 1 to 10 complement dilution. Thus if two amboceptor units be considered as 0.5 c.c. of a 1 to 1000 dilution, in the daily titration we would test 0.4 c.c., 0.5 c.c., and 0.6 c.c. against increasing doses of complement. The complement unit is then determined from that one of the three titrations which will make the daily dose (2 units) 0.5 c.c. or less; and is used with the corresponding amboceptor dose (2 units). This three-way standardization allows for any variation in the complement in use on that certain day and renders restandardization unnecessary.

We always inactivate the sera within an hour or two of testing them, as we have occasionally had a blood negative with cholesterinized antigen when tested immmediately after inactivation which would react positively if tested twelve to eighteen hours after inactivation.

The antigens are made up daily from the alcoholic extract, blowing the extract into the proper amount of salt solution, a 1 to 10 dilution in salt solution being used.

We determine the antigen value of each antigen by testing it against a series of pooled, strongly positive sera, and find that nearly all cholesterinized antigens, whether made from human, beef or guinea pig hearts, give complete fixation with our method (0.1 c.c. of serum) in amounts varying from 0.01 c.c. to 0.015 c.c. of 1 to 10 dilutions.

Even relatively poor alcoholic extracts were made good by adding cholesterin which seems to act as a sort of stabilizer. To the original alcoholic extracts was added 0.4 per cent of cholesterin.

With the plain alcoholic extracts, the fixation point varies from 0.03 c.c. to 0.07 c.c. Only those giving fixation with less than 0.07 c.c. were considered fit for use.

Having thus found the antigenic unit, we use 10 such units in our tests, provided this amount is not over one-half the beginning anticomplementary dose when tested against pooled sera. In the present work we used 0.1 c.c. of a 1 to 10 dilution of cholesterinized antigen and 0.5 c.c. of the plain.

Our standardization of antigens and our daily titrations are all carried out at 37.5° C., using one hour time periods for fixation and for the second phase of the reaction.

When ice box fixation was employed, the tubes were left at 7° C. to 10° C. for four hours. Amboceptor and sheep cells were then added, and the tubes put in a water-bath at 37.5° C. for twenty to thirty minutes, at which time the negative controls would be cleared. The sets run in the incubator were allowed one hour for fixation, and were read after about one hour, or when the negative controls showed complete hemolysis.

Each specimen was run with three plain alcoholic heart antigens in the ice box method, and in addition, plain and cholesterinized antigen sets were run at 37.5° C. The reactions were graded from 0 to ++++ according to the degree of fixation.

We found that every specimen positive in the incubator set with plain antigen, was equally as strong and often more strongly positive by the ice box fixation method.

We, therefore, do not see the necessity of running duplicate sets in incubator and ice box. We find that from four to six hours in the ice box is amply sufficient for complement binding, and that when bloods are left at this temperature for twelve to eighteen hours, occasional doubtful or weakly positive results are found with known negative bloods.

Intervals longer than four to six hours did not yield any higher percentage of positive results in known syphilis.

RESULTS

We examined sera from 1113 patients. Five hundred of these gave a definite history of lues or else showed symptoms of a syphilitic nature. Among these cases were many giving histories of very long standing, some also had gone years without symptoms, while others had been recently subjected to vigorous treatment. If we had included only the cases of active lues, we feel certain that our percentage of positive results would have been much higher.

Another 500 sera were from patients without any history or symptoms of lues, including cases of tuberculosis, cancer, nephritis, pernicious anemia and diabetes, with and without diacetic acid.

The remaining 113 cases were classed as doubtful, either because of an indefinite history or owing to the fact that the symptoms did not accord with the history or a clinical diagnosis of lues.

We have grouped together as positive reaction those sera giving +++ and ++++ results. The ++ and + reactions have been classed as doubtful.

The results obtained with the 500 cases of known syphilis are shown in Table I.

TABLE I

REACTIONS OBTAINED ON SERA OF 500 CASES OF KNOWN SYPHILIS

TEMP. OF FIRST STAGE	TIME	ANTIGEN	POSITIVE		DOUBTFUL		NEGATIVE	
			No.	%	No.	%	No.	%
37.5° C.	1 hr.	Cholesterinized	383	76.6	23	4.6	94	18.8
37.5° C.	1 hr.	Plain	258	51.6	35	7	207	41.4
7-10° C.	4 hrs.	Plain	353	70.6	16	3.2	131	26.2

It will be noted that while the plain antigen with ice box fixation gives but 6 per cent less of diagnostic reactions than does the cholesterin reinforced preparation, this same plain antigen when incubated at 37.5° C. for one hour, gives only 51.6 per cent of positive results, about 20 per cent less than the figures obtained by the ice box method.

Another point in favor of this technic is the sharpness of the reading found, doubtful reactions not being obtained nearly as often as is the case with the older method.

While the cholesterinized antigen shows 6 per cent more of strongly positive results among this group, we feel that an examination of the cases described below (Table II) will show that from the diagnostic standpoint, the ice box fixation method falls but little below the cholesterin antigen results.

It will be observed that most of the cases positive only with cholesterin were old latent cases absolutely free from clinical symptoms.

The advisability of subjecting these long-standing latent cases to treatment simply on the ground of such a result is, we think, open to grave doubt.

Cases 4, 7, 8, 12, 13, 15, 16, 19, 24, 26, 27, 28, 29, and 30 were all over ten years' standing, and had shown no symptoms since the disappearance of their secondaries. Some of them had taken rather irregular and intermittent treatment, but not enough, from our experience, to change their serologic reactions.

In fact, we do not think that any amount of treatment will ever get such cases negative if tested against cholesterinized antigens.

Cases, 1, 3, 5, 6, 17, 21, and 22 showed signs of an active syphilitic process at the time the serologic examination was made and represent among 500 known syphilitic cases, those where the diagnosis would have been seriously affected by dependence on plain antigen alone. This represents an advantage of 1.4 per cent in favor of cholesterinized antigen, but this slightly increased sensitiveness is more than offset by the high percentage of false positives which such antigens give.

The remaining cases, while free from symptoms, have all had more or less recent treatment, and are mostly cases of comparatively short standing, so that it is difficult to judge the relative value of the two antigens.

TABLE II

KNOWN SYPHILITIC CASES STRONGLY POSITIVE ONLY WITH CHOLESTERINIZED ANTIGEN

CASE NO.	ANTIGEN			HISTORY
	CHOLESTERINIZED 37.5° c.	PLAIN 37.5° c.	PLAIN 7-10° c.	
1	4*	0	0	Congenital—age 24 months. Treated since birth.
2	3	0	0	Infected 2 years ago. 3 doses of 606 and Hg at time. Treated up to 2 months ago. No symptoms at present.
3	4	0	0	Congenital lues, age 7 years. Never treated.
4	3	0	0	Infected 12 years ago. No symptoms in past 11 years. Treated off and on.
5	4	1	0	Infected 23 years ago. Treatment at time. Symptoms of beginning tabes.
6	3	0	0	Chancre 3 months ago. Malignant secondaries in mouth and throat and on body. Fever and marked debility.
7	4	0	0	Infected 17 years ago. Treated 2 years at time. Complains of pains in both knees.
8	4	0	0	Infected 12 years ago. ++++ W. R. with ice box method 3 months ago. Since then has had 4 doses of 606 and Hg to date. Latent.
9	3	0	0	Infected 9 years ago. Treated intermittently. Latent.
10	3	0	0	Infected 1 year ago. Hg and sod. cacodylate injections to date.
11	3	0	0	Date of infection not known. Tertiary ulcers 8 months ago. 4 doses 606 and Hg since.
12	3	0	0	Infected 23 years ago. Latent since. In past two years has taken 8 doses 606 and many injections of Hg without affecting Wass. reaction.
13	3	0	0	Infected 19 years ago. Treated at intervals since. No symptoms since secondaries.
14	3	0	0	Secondaries 1 year ago. Cleared up under 606 and Hg. Later developed iritis which cleared up under treatment. Husband is luetic. Latent.
15	4	0	0	Infected 18 years ago. Several secondaries. Treated at Hot Springs 3 months. No treatment since. Latent.

TABLE II (CONT'D)

CASE NO.	ANTIGEN			HISTORY
	CHOLESTER-INIZED 37.5° C.	PLAIN 37.5° C.	PLAIN 7-10° C.	
16	4	0	0	Infected 11 years ago. Treated 2 years. No symptoms since. Spinal fluid is negative.
17	3	0	0	Infected 4 years ago. Treated by mouth for 3 years. Now has ulcer of septum.
18	3	0	0	Infected 8 years ago. Treated off and on since. 12 doses 606 and Hg in past 5 years. Latent past 7 years. W. R. with cholesterinized antigen has been 4 or 3 always.
19	4	0	0	Infected 17 years ago. Tertiary ulcers on both shins 10 years ago. Nothing since. No treatment in 10 years.
20	4	0	0	Secondaries 6 months ago. 6 doses 606 and Hg to one month ago.
21	4	0	1	Infected 10 years ago. Multiple subcutaneous gummata.
22	4	0	0	Infected 6 years ago. Little treatment. Has double iritis now.
23	4	0	0	Infected 7 years ago. 5 years ago took 6 doses of 606 and Hg for 3 months. No symptoms since secondaries.
24	4	0	2	Infected 12 years ago. Treated 3 years. No symptoms since. Spinal fluid is negative.
25	3	1	1	Infected 3 years ago. Several doses 606 and Hg intermittently to 6 months ago. Latent.
26	4	0	0	Infected 19 years ago. No symptoms since. 4 doses of 606 in past three months.
27	4	0	0	Infected 35 years ago. Irregular treatment. No symptoms since.
28	4	0	0	Infected 27 years ago. No symptoms since secondaries. No treatment in 20 years.
29	4	0	0	Infected 11 years ago. Severe secondaries. No symptoms or treatment in 10 years.
30	4	1	1	Infected 30 years ago. Latent since. No treatment since secondaries disappeared.

Note: The name 606 in these tables has been applied to all the various forms of salvarsan and neosalvarsan.

*4 = +++, 3 = ++, 2 = ++, 1 = +, 0 = negative.

Taking up now the results obtained in the examination of 500 patients without history or symptoms of lues we obtained the figures shown in Table III.

Here is to be noted, not only the absence of false positive reactions with the ice box method, but also, as with the known cases of lues, the comparatively low percentage of doubtful reactions.

The one case in this group which gave a strong positive reaction with the ice box method was also positive with cholesterinized antigen and is No. 7 in Table IV, which gives in detail the histories of these cases showing false positive reactions.

This particular serum was from a man suffering from a rather severe anemia, apparently of a secondary type, who showed no improvement under mercury and

TABLE III
REACTIONS OBTAINED ON SERA OF 500 CLINICALLY NEGATIVE CASES

TEMPERATURE OF FIRST PHASE	TIME	ANTIGEN	POSITIVE		DOUBTFUL		NEGATIVE	
			No.	%	No.	%	No.	%
37.5° C.	1 hr.	Cholesterinized	19	3.8	33	6.6	448	89.6
37.5° C.	1 hr.	Plain	0	0	7	1.4	493	98.6
7-10° C.	4 hrs.	Plain	1	0.2	3	0.6	496	99.2

TABLE IV
NEGATIVE CASES GIVING POSITIVE REACTIONS WITH PLAIN AND CHOLESTERINIZED ANTIGENS

CASE NO.	ANTIGEN			HISTORY
	CHOLESTER-INIZED 37.5° C.	PLAIN 37.5° C.	PLAIN 7-10° C.	
1	4	0	0	History negative. Dementia precox.
2	4	0	0	History negative. No symptoms.
3	4	0	0	History and examination negative. Has healthy six-week-old baby which gives a negative Wassermann reaction.
4	4	0	0	History negative. Has a severe acne.
5	4	0	0	History negative. Has a severe nephritis with albumin and casts.
6	4	0	0	Tuberculous glands of neck.
7	4	0	3	Anemia not improved under Hg and KI. Improved under iron and arsenic.
8	4	0	0	Morphine fiend. Mental symptoms clearing under treatment, for drug addiction.
9	4	0	0	Nine-year-old child with spina bifida. Father and mother healthy.
10	4	0	0	History and examination negative.
11	4	0	0	History and examination negative. Has wrenched back.
12	4	0	0	Chancroid 6 weeks ago. W. R. negative. 2 months later no clinical or serologic evidence of lues.
13	4	0	2	No symptoms. Father paretic. Mother healthy and has negative Wassermann.
14	4	0	0	History and examination negative. Has psoriasis.
15	3	0	0	History and examination negative. Healthy adult.
16	3	0	1	History negative. Has severe weeping eczema.
17	3	0	0	History and examination negative. Healthy adult.
18	3	0	0	History negative. Has Lichen planus.
19	3	2	0	History negative. Persistent headaches. Spinal fluid is negative.

potassium iodide but who picked up wonderfully under the administration of iron and arsenic. A very careful investigation failed to show any symptoms suggestive of lues, and the history, which we considered dependable, was absolutely negative. We feel, therefore, that this should be classed perhaps as a false positive reaction.

Among the cases in this group, positive only with cholesterin antigen, we feel that syphilis can be excluded with reasonable certainty. When such a positive reaction with cholesterin antigen only was found, a thorough and careful reinvestigation of the patient's history and clinical condition was instituted to determine whether any evidence of lues could be found.

The 113 patients whose serologic examinations are tabulated in Table V were classed as doubtfully syphilitic, and either gave a history or showed sypmtoms leading to such diagnosis.

TABLE V

REACTION OBTAINED ON SERA OF 113 CASES CLASSED AS DOUBTFULLY SYPHILITIC

TEMPERATURE OF FIRST PHASE	TIME	ANTIGEN	POSITIVE		DOUBTFUL		NEGATIVE	
			No.	%	No.	%	No.	%
37.5° C.	1 hr.	Cholesterinized	45	39.8	13	11.5	55	48.7
37.5° C.	1 hr.	Plain	4	3.5	9	7.9	100	88.5
7-10° C.	4 hrs.	Plain	8	7.0	8	7.0	97	86.0

The figures found in the examination of this class of cases are of little value, of course, in establishing the relative worth of the different methods of performing the Wassermann reaction, but there should be noted the wide divergence of the results obtained with cholesterinized antigen.

Personally, we feel that most of the cases strongly positive with plain antigen in incubator or ice box, represent syphilitic cases, but this belief could not be reconciled with the history and clinical findings as noted by the attending physicians.

Deducting the 7 per cent of strongly positive with plain antigen in the ice box from the 39.8 per cent of such positives found with cholesterinized antigen leaves 32.8 per cent more strongly positive reactions in this group when tested with cholesterinized heart extract.

Just why the two antigens should differ so widely among the patients of this group, while showing a difference of 6 per cent and 3.6 per cent, respectively, among the known syphilitics and known negative cases we can not explain, but judging from the figures obtained with the two known groups we would certainly feel that much more evidence than a positive Wassermann reaction performed only with cholesterinized antigen should be adduced before making a definite diagnosis of lues in the presence of doubtful histories and physical findings.

We have appended below a brief history of the patients in this group who gave serologic reactions of diagnostic strength.

CONCLUSIONS

1. Simple alcoholic heart extracts give the most reliable Wassermann reactions, provided the first phase of the reaction is carried out at 7° C. to 10° C.

2. A period of four to six hours at this temperature gives the best results. Longer periods (twelve to eighteen hours) may give doubtful or weak positive reactions.

3. We have found human heart extracts more dependable than beef or guinea pig heart preparations.

TABLE VI
DOUBTFUL CASES GIVING POSITIVE REACTIONS

CASE NO.	ANTIGEN			HISTORY
	CHOLESTER-INIZED 37.5° C.	PLAIN 37.5° C.	PLAIN 7-10° C.	
1	4	0	0	Sore 3 months ago. Few spots on body later on. Slight general adenitis.
2	4	0	3	Suspected chancroid 10 years ago. No secondaries. Has itching, scaling palmar rash of both hands.
3	4	2	2	Husband luetic. Patient very nervous and irritable.
4	4	0	2	Scrofula when a child. Anemia and debility.
5	4	0	0	Father luetic. Has had 3 abortions. No clinical evidence of lues.
6	4	0	0	Indefinite. Has severe anemia with chronic nephritis.
7	4	0	0	Husband luetic. Has had chronic diarrhea which improved under antiluetic treatment.
8	4	0	0	Several sores at different times. History of doubtful rash which was probably acne.
9	2	0	4	No history. Prostitute, has general adenitis.
10	4	0	0	Sore 5 years ago. Low grade meningitis now. Spinal fluid not examined.
11	4	0	0	Prostitute. No history or symptoms.
12	4	0	0	No history. Psoriasis-like rash which has not improved under 606 and Hg.
13	4	0	2	Husband of Case 5. No history or symptoms except enlarged cervical glands.
14	4	0	0	Prostitute. No history or symptoms.
15	4	1	0	Prostitute. No history. Has eczema-like eruption on hands and feet.
16	4	3	2	No history. Underdeveloped boy of 16 years. Normal mentally. Parents apparently normal.
17	4	1	0	Sore 2 weeks ago. Appeared 3 weeks after exposure. General adenitis. Six weeks later sore healed. No clinical or serological change.
18	4	0	0	Sore 8 years ago. History of indefinite secondaries.
19	4	0	0	Gonorrhea 4 years ago. Now has persistent nocturnal headaches, not relieved by glasses. Spinal fluid negative.
20	4	0	0	Sore 1 year ago. Doubtful rash at time of sore. No symptoms now.
21	4	0	0	Prostitute. Denies primary. Had rash and sore throat six months ago. No clinical signs at present.
22	4	4	4	Prostitute. Denies primary or secondaries. Has ulcerated sore throat diagnosed as tbc, or lues.
23	1	1	4	Recent pregnancy. Baby healthy. History of recurrent abortions. Husband is luetic.

TABLE VI (CONT'D)

CASE NO.	ANTIGEN			HISTORY
	CHOLESTER-INIZED 37.5° C.	PLAIN 37.5° C.	PLAIN 7-10° C.	
24	4	0	0	Prostitute. Denies primary or secondaries. Shows general adenitis. Has a few scars on tibia.
25	4	0	0	Prostitute. Denies history. Has an anemia which has improved under Hg and KI.
26	4	0	0	History negative. Paralysis of hands, feet and vocal cords. Spinal fluid is negative.
27	4	0	0	History negative. Has scaling palmar rash.
28	4	0	0	Sore 10 years ago. No secondaries. Small ulcer on leg 4 years ago. Cured with S. S. S.
29	4	4	3	Sore 4 years ago. Later developed rash diagnosed as Lichen planus. No symptoms at present.
30	4	0	1	Denies primary. Severe rash over body, face, and scalp 6 years ago, which disappeared under local treatment. No symptoms now.
31	4	0	0	Prostitute. Sore but no secondaries 1 year ago. 2 doses 606 at time of sore. No symptoms now.
32	3	0	0	Sore 7 years ago. No secondaries. Hg. by mouth for 18 months.
33	4	0	4	Denies primary. History of blood poisoning 16 years ago. No symptoms, but general health improved under specific treatment.
34	4	0	0	No history of primary or secondaries. Has chronic ulceration of throat.
35	3	0	0	Possible secondaries 2 years ago.
36	4	4	4	Denies primary and secondaries. Has syphilitic child.
37	3	0	0	Prostitute. Sore on two occasions. Denies secondaries.
38	4	0	0	Denies history of lues. Has copper-colored spots on shins and periostitis of both tibia.
39	4	0	0	Doubtful history of possible infection 20 years ago.
40	4	2	1	Sore 18 years ago. Diagnosed as chancroid. Has arthritis which does not improve under specific medication.
41	4	1	4	History doubtful. 1 abortion. 1 child died at 6 weeks with suspected lues. Husband insane.
42	4	0	1	Sore 1 year ago. Treated 3 months. Now has atypical rash on face and hands.
43	4	1	0	Sore 6 years ago. No secondaries. Has inequality of pupils, sluggish reflexes, and is very nervous.
44	3	0	0	Sore 3 months ago. 3 doses 606 and Hg at time. No treatment in 6 weeks.
45	3	0	0	Prostitute. Denies lues. Has periostitis of frontal bone.

4. Cholesterinized antigens even when used in small quantities will give false positive reactions in a considerable number of cases.

Recent experiments, which we have carried out and which we hope to report later, tend to show us that a fifteen-hour fixation time gives a slightly higher percentage of positive results than is obtained with a four-hour fixation time. No better results have been obtained by extending the fixation time up to twenty-four hours.

NOTE: Since this article was written, Ruediger: Jour. Infect. Dis., 1918, xxiii, 173; and Wile: Jour. Am. Med. Assn., 1919, lxxiii, 1526, have reported uniformly better results obtained with ice box fixation than with the older method of preliminary incubation at 37.5° C. Berghausen: Jour. Am. Med. Assn., 1919, lxiii, 996, likewise advocates ice box fixation, but states that he finds cholesterinized antigen very satisfactory and a fixation period of eighteen to twenty hours at 0° C. the best.

BIBLIOGRAPHY

[1]Jacobstahl: München. med. Wchnschr., 1910, lvii, 689.
[2]Guggenheimer: München. med. Wchnschr., 1911, lviii, 1392.
[3]McNeil: Collected Studies of the Bureau of Laboratories, Department of Health, City of New York, 1912-13, vii, 325.
[4]Altman: Arch. f. Dermat. u. Syph., 1913, cxvi, 871.
[5]Leredde and Rubinstein: Bull. Soc. franc. de dermat. et de Syph., 1913, No. 2, p. 93.
[6]Coca and L'Esperence: Jour. Immunol., 1916, i, 129.
[7]Smith and MacNeal: Jour. Immunol., 1916, ii, 75.
[8]Ottenberg: Arch. Internal Med., 1917, xix, 457.

A COMPARATIVE STUDY OF THE WASSERMANN TEST AND THE HECHT-WEINBERG-GRADWOHL MODIFICATION*

BY A. J. BLAIVAS, BROOKLYN, N. Y.

DURING the past few years many papers have been published describing and discussing the various modifications of the Wassermann test. Kolmer[1], in one of his publications, states his conclusions that the Hecht-Weinberg-Gradwohl reaction is superior to that of the Wassermann test. He found that 92 per cent of sera are satisfactory for the modified test, and that only a small percentage contains sufficient natural complement and amboceptor to hemolyze more than 0.5 c.c. of a 5 per cent sheep cell suspension. In routine work of the Hecht-Weinberg-Gradwohl test, therefore, larger doses of sheep cells are not required to determine the hemolytic indices of the sera.

The following are the results obtained by Kolmer. "In 7 per cent of the sera the hemolytic activity was too weak for the conduct of the Hecht-Weinberg-Gradwohl tests. Eighty-five per cent of the sera agreed with the Wassermann reaction so far as positive and negative were concerned. In 12 per cent, the Hecht-Weinberg-Gradwohl were positive and the Wassermann reaction negative with all antigens."

*From the Serological Laboratory of the Brooklyn Diagnostic Institute, Brooklyn, New York.

Kolmer[2] also claims that in every instance of a positive Hecht-Weinberg-Gradwohl modification, notwithstanding the negativeness of the Wassermann test, either the history or the clinical diagnosis, or both justified a diagnosis of syphilis, thus proving the superior delicacy of the Hecht-Weinberg-Gradwohl modification. The majority of sera he used were from known syphilitic persons under active treatment. However, in one to two per cent of the total number of cases the Hecht-Weinberg-Gradwohl tests were found NEGATIVE while the Wassermanns were POSITIVE. The sera of two of these patients were tested again about a week later, when a positive reaction was obtained in both the Wassermann and the Hecht-Weinberg-Gradwohl tests.

In another series of cases Kolmer mentions similar discrepancies between the Wassermann and Hecht-Weinberg-Gradwohl tests. In explanation, Kolmer suggests that the positive Wassermann and the negative Hecht-Weinberg-Gradwohl tests of the sera may have been due to "technical errors." In a later article, however, he says as follows:

"These results are quite similar to those previously reported in which the Hecht-Weinberg-Gradwohl and Wassermann reactions yielded similar results with 82 per cent of 362 sera. In the former series, I found six sera, or about two per cent yielding positive Wassermann and negative Hecht-Weinberg-Gradwohl reactions and in the present series, a similar result was observed. While in the former series two sera yielded pseudopositive or proteotropic reactions, none occurred in the present series, a result which I ascribe to the use of acceptable extracts of acetone-insoluble lipoids as antigens after titration with human instead of guinea pig complement."

In our own experiments, we have never met with a simultaneous positive Wassermann and negative Hecht-Weinberg-Gradwohl reaction. Such a contradiction in our opinion, is in all probability due to technical errors.

Regarding the reliability of the Hecht-Weinberg-Gradwohl test, Gradwohl[3] offers the following evidences:

"We found that in no case where we obtained a positive Hecht-Weinberg-Gradwohl and a negative Wassermann was our work at fault or the serologic diagnosis a surprise to the clinician. We must confess that there are certain cases of syphilis in which both tests were negative which were really syphilitic, as proved by true clinical manifestations and later the appearance of positive reactions in one or both tests at a subsequent examination. These were invariably cases of latent syphilis in robust individuals. We wish to add too, that the use of cholesterinized antigens does not measure up in accuracy to the use of the Hecht-Weinberg-Gradwohl test for syphilis."

It is my experience in over 10,000 comparative tests that many final readings in the Hecht-Weinberg-Gradwohl modification show a faint inhibition of hemolysis in tubes No. 12 and No. 13 or No. 13 only, the latter containing the largest amount of antigen.

Such reactions make a positive diagnosis of syphilis doubtful, unless the patient gives also a positive clinical history, or one permitting the assumption of the existence of a latent state.

TABLE I

	NAME	SEX*	WASSERMANN	H. I.**	H. W. G.***	REMARKS
1	K. C.	F	—	5	—	
2	B. S.	M	—	2	—	
3	J. D.	M	—	4	—	
4	E. S.	F	—	4	—	
5	K. M.	F	—	5	±	Faint inhibition of hemolysis in tube No. 13
6	J.A.P.	M	—	6	—	
7	D. S.	M	—	5	—	
8	S. G.	M	—	6	—	
9	G. G.	M	—	3	—	
10	I. L.	F	—	no index	—	
11	O. B.	M	—	5	±	Faint inhibition of hemolysis in tube No. 13
12	J. P.	M	—	no index	—	
13	P. C.	M	++++	no index	—	
14	M.W.	M	++++	6	+	Strongly positive ++++
15	E. W.	F .	—	8	—	
16	S. H.	M	—	4	—	
17	A. B.	M	—	5	+	Positive in tubes 12 and 13
18	A. A.	M	—	2	—	
19	E. K.	M	—	3	±	Faint inhibition of hemolysis in tube No. 13
20	M.L.	M	—	1	±	Faint inhibition of hemolysis in tube No. 13
21	O. L.	M	—	3	—	
22	G. H.	M	—	2	—	
23	T. F.	M	— —	5	+	Early locomotor ataxia
24	J. F.	M	—	1	—	
25	M. G.	M	—	3	—	
26	G. K.	M	—	5	—	Nephritis
27	A. V.	F	±	8	+	
28	T. K.	F	—	5	—	
29	Dr. G	M	—	no index	—	Nephritis
30	M. H.	F	—	4	—	
31	R. C.	F	++	5	+	Known case of syphilis
32	J. R.	F	++++	5	+	Patient's husband has paresis
33	M. M.	M	—	no index	—	
34	J. M.	F	±	2	+	
35	A. V.	M	—	7	—	
36	C. V.	M	—	6	—	
37	T. F.	M	++	7	+	H. W. G. strongly positive ++++
38	G. O.	M	—	4	—	
39	D. J.	M	±	8	+	Treated case (1 injection)
40	D. J.	M	—	6	—	Treated case (1 injection)
41	G. T.	F	—	5	—	
42	P. H.	M	—	no index	—	
43	G.J.G.	M	—	9	—	
44	F. K.	M	—	7	—	
45	K. M.	F	—	no index	—	
46	J. P.	M	—	2	—	
47	R. L	F	—	5	—	
48	S. F.	M	—	2	—	Treated case
49	A. A.	M	—	4	—	Locomotor ataxia
50	J. C.	F	—	3	+	H. W. G. strongly positive ++++
51	R. M.	F	—	2	—	
52	J. S.	M	—	3	—	Treated case (2 injections)
53	S. S.	F	—	2	—	
54	D. K.	F	+++	5	+	Pregnant woman. Syphilis known
55	F. J.	M	—	4	—	
56	M. S.	M	—	8	—	
57	J. K.	M	—	7	—	
58	N. T.	M	—	6	—	Arthritis

*F. Female. M. Male. **H. I. Hemolytic Index. ***H. W. G. Hecht-Weinberg-Gradwohl.

TABLE I (CONT'D)

	NAME	SEX*	WASSERMANN	H. I.**	H. W. G.***	REMARKS
59	M. A.	F	—	4	+	Weakly positive (in tube 13)
60	C. M.	F	—	4	—	
61	R. M.	F	—	7	—	
62	C. W.	M	—	no index		
63	K. M.	F	—	3	+	Weakly positive (in tube 13), see Case 5
64	H. S.	F	—	5	—	
65	J. S.	M	—	4	—	Treated case (3 injections)
66	S. F.	M	++++	2	+	Known case of syphilis
67	M. D.	M	—	3	—	
68	M.W.	F	—	3	—	Pregnant
69	W. W.	F	—	no index		
70	N. N.	M	—	no index		See Case 5
71	K. M.	F	—	4	+	Inhibition in 12 and 13
72	O. M	M	—	4	+	Inhibition in 12 and 13
73	C. Z.	M	—	no index		
74	J. B.	M	—	1	—	
75	F. S.	M	—	no index		
76	S. S.	F	—	2	+	Inhibition in 12 and 13
77	J.E.B.	F	—	5	—	
78	F. D.	M	—	2	+	Inhibition in 13
79	J. A.	M	—	3	—	
80	T. F.	M	+	2	+	Early locomotor
81	M. R.	F	—	no index		
82	E. M.	M	—	2	—	
83	M. A.	F	—	3	+	Inhibition in 13
84	B. J.	F	—	2	+	Inhibition in 12 and 13. Pregnant woman
85	M. K.	F	—	no index		
86	M. P.	M	—	no index		
87	M. W.	F	—	3	—	
88	Dr. B.	M	—	3	—	
89	M. M.	F	—	4	—	
90	R. W.	F	—	5	—	
91	G. E.	M	—	3	—	
92	M. M.	F	—	4	—	
93	E. S.	F	—	2	—	
94	B. J.	F	—	1	—	2 days after delivery
95	L.A.T.	—	—	2	—	
96	S. N.	F	—	no index		
97	A. B.	F	—	3	—	Pregnant
98	F.A.B.	F	—	2	+	Very faint inhibition in No. 13
99	T. F.	M	—	2	—	Early locomotor
100	D. T.	—	—	no index		

*F. Female. M. Male. **H. I. Hemolytic Index. ***H. W. G. Hecht-Weinberg-Gradwohl.

Gradwohl claims that 98 per cent of the sera contain natural antisheep amboceptor. This may be true perhaps if the patient's blood is examined shortly after withdrawal or, at the latest, within a period of twenty-four hours. If correct, then it would necessitate working with the Wassermann test in the ordinary laboratory daily. My experience, however, does not seem to coincide with the statement presented by Gradwohl, as of the 100 cases shown in Table I, 17 per cent contained either no natural complement or antisheep amboceptor or neither of the two.

The average hemolytic index in our series was four, i. e., 0.1.c.c. of serum contained enough natural complement and amboceptor to hemolyze 0.4 c.c. of a 5 per cent suspension of sheep cells. The technic used in the Hecht-Weinberg-

Gradwohl test was exactly the same as done by Gradwohl in his laboratories which is as follows:

Place 0.1 c.c. of unheated serum into each of the fourteen test tubes which are placed in the special rack as shown in Fig. 1. Put 1 c.c. of normal salt in Tube 1, 0.9 c.c. in Tube 2, 0.8 c.c. in Tube 3, 0.7 c.c. in Tube 4, 0.6 c.c. in Tube 5, 0.5 c.c. in Tube 6, 0.4 c.c. in Tube 7, 0.3 c.c. in Tube 8, 0.2 c.c. in Tube 9, 0.1 c.c. in Tube 10, 0.2 c.c. in Tube 11, 0.15 c.c. in Tube 12, 0.1 c.c. in Tube 13, 0.3 c.c. in Tube 14. The first ten tubes are used to determine the hemolytic index of the blood under examination. In other words, the object is to find the amount of natural complement and amboceptor in the suspected serum. With Tubes 11, 12 and 13 the actual test is carried out. Tube 14 is the serum control tube. Now add 0.1 c.c. of a 5 per cent suspension of sheep cells to Tube 1, 0.2 c.c. to Tube 2, 0.3 c.c. to Tube 3, 0.4 c.c. to Tube 4, 0.5 c.c. to Tube 5, 0.6 c.c. to Tube 6,

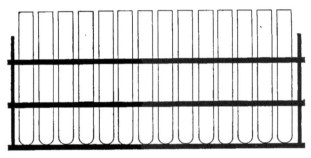

Fig. 1.

0.7 c.c. to Tube 7, 0.8 c.c. to Tube 8, 0.9 c.c. to Tube 9 and 1.0 c.c. to Tube 10. Place 0.1 c.c. of titrated ether-soluble, acetone-insoluble antigen into Tube 11, 0.15 c.c. of the antigen into Tube 12 and 0.2 c.c. of the antigen into Tube 13. These three tubes (11, 12, and 13) are the tubes in which the final readings are made and for that reason the antigen is added to them alone. Tube 14 being the serum control tube, received, of course, NO antigen. The tubes are now well shaken and placed into a water-bath for one-half hour at 37.5°C. At the end of this time the rack is removed from the water-bath and the last tube which shows complete hemolysis is the hemolytic index. For example, if Tube 5 is the last where complete hemolysis occurs, the hemolytic index is five. This means that 0.1 c.c. of the serum will hemolyze 0.5 c.c. of a 5 per cent suspension of sheep cells. In order to determine the amount of sheep cells to put into Tubes 11, 12, 13 and 14, Gradwohl has worked out the following table:

If the hemolytic index is from,

1 to 4 add 0.1 c.c. of sheep cells to the last four tubes.

5 to 7 add 0.15 c.c. of sheep cells to the last four tubes.

8 to 10 add 0.2 c.c. of sheep cells to the last four tubes.

After the addition of the sheep corpuscles to the last four tubes, the contents of the tubes are well shaken and again placed in the water-bath for one-half hour at 37.5° C. The rack is then removed and the results read just as in the Wassermann test.

Of the 19 cases which showed a positive or a borderline Hecht-Weinberg-Gradwohl test and a negative or a borderline Wassermann test, we have been able to obtain only 14 histories. In the other 5 cases data relating to luetic infection were unobtainable inasmuch as they were cases either referred special diagnosis or for special reasons were not questioned in that direction.

In most of the 14 cases in which a discrepancy between the Wassermann and its modification was found, there were direct evidences either of an early infection, or of a mild easily overlooked case of syphilis or of a syphilitic association or consanguinity. Perhaps a short resume of the histories of these cases, in which a negative or borderline Wassermann and a positive or suspicious Hecht-Weinberg-Gradwohl test were obtained might not be amiss.

CASE No. 5.—K. M., American, age 31, female. Negative personal history. The patient's husband contracted lues about fifteen years ago, with secondary but no tertiary manifestations later. Has two perfectly healthy children, but soon after last confinement, patient developed an eruption on the dorsal surfaces on the upper and lower extremities, copper-colored, circular, giving no subjective symptoms. The Wassermann negative, the Hecht-Weinberg-Gradwohl reaction positive in tubes 13 and 14. Six-tenths of a gram of salvarsan was given intravenously, after which the eruption disappeared completely, also. the headaches of which the patient complained previous to the injection.

CASE No. 21.—A. V., Russian, age 32, female. Negative family history. At the age of eight the patient had an unknown arthritic affection. Patient is married ten years and has had *four miscarriages*, and finally had one living child. Had nasal troubles for many years and was in a hospital eleven years ago for some abscess, the character of which is not related. Patient has had intensive treatment in a hospital and also privately with salvarsan, mercury, and iodides. This case seems to serve as a good illustration of the superiority of the Hecht-Weinberg-Gradwohl reaction over the Wassermann test, inasmuch as it represents a known and treated case of syphilis, giving a negative Wassermann but still showing a positive in the Hecht-Weinberg-Gradwohl test.

CASE No. 39.—D. J., Italian, age 32, laborer, male. The patient presents himself with a typical chancre of the right index finger. A dark-field microscopic examination proved the presence of Spirochete pallida. The patient, skeptical of the diagnosis first, refused the use of salvarsan, but returned several weeks later for a blood test. The Wassermann and the Hecht-Weinberg-Gradwohl tests disclosed. a four-plus positive reaction. After the injection of salvarsan, the Wassermann showed a borderline reaction and the Hecht-Weinberg-Gradwohl still remained strongly positive, illustrating again the higher qualifications of the Hecht-Weinberg-Gradwohl test over the Wassermann reaction. After further injections of salvarsan, both the Wassermann and the Hecht-Weinberg-Gradwohl tests cleared up.

CASE No. 59.—M. A., Italian, age 28, female. Patient was married nine years ago, but has never become pregnant. Had her left ovary removed four years ago. The patient had an iritis, also an enlarged right axillary gland. The Wassermann test in August, 1918, showed a two-plus positive, but the examination at the present time was negative. The gonorrheal complement-fixation test also showed a two-plus positive reaction. This case serves as another good example where the Wassermann becomes negative at an earlier date than the Hecht-Weinberg-Gradwohl test.

CASE No. 65.—J. S., Italian, age 28, longshoreman. male. The patient gave clinical evidences of syphilis and also a history of having a chancre and secondary signs. The Wassermann and the Hecht-Weinberg-Gradwohl tests were both four-plus positive. After injections of salvarsan, the Wassermann and Hecht-Weinberg-Gradwohl tests became negative. At a later date another blood test was made and a negative Wassermann and a strongly positive Hecht-Weinberg-Gradwohl reaction was obtained. The patient, however, felt perfectly well and refused further treatment. The fact, though, remained that the modified test reappeared earlier than the Wassermann did.

CASE No. 72.—O. M., American, age 33, salesman, male. Patient had a chancre thirteen years ago with following secondary eruptions. Had undergone intensive syphilitic treatment. The last injection of salvarsan was administered about a year and a half ago. He is married five years and has two healthy children. His wife (Case 5) was treated for secondary eruptions six months ago at which time she was nine months after her last pregnancy. This is a case of undoubted previous infection.

CASE No. 78.—F. D., Italian, age 36, laborer, male. Contracted syphilis nine years ago. Patient is married. His wife had been pregnant three times, but has no living child. His blood gave a four-plus Wassermann reaction four years ago. One year ago, it showed one plus. The patient has never had any salvarsan injections, but has received 100 intramuscular mercurial treatments. For one year treatment was stopped. The following year the patient received 24 intramuscular injections of mercury. the last one two weeks before the blood test was made. This is another undoubted case of syphilis, and illustrates again how the Hecht-Weinberg-Gradwohl modification is superior to the Wassermann test.

CASE No. 76.—S. S., Austrian, age 40, female. Married 23 years and has four children living and well. No miscarriages. Mother died of cancer. Patient was operated for uterine tumor four years ago. She complains of attacks of acute pains in the heart region, cyanosis, faint feeling, and palpitation. The attacks occur mostly at night. The patient is inclined to be obese and is mentally very apathetic. She shows a moderate exophthalmos and Mobius in the left eye. The pupils react sluggishly to light, and her reflexes are exaggerated. In this particular case, lues as the basis of the above symptoms can not be excluded, and it may therefore be counted as very suspicious. Perhaps the future will disclose further additional data to justify the diagnosis of latent lues, which makes it necessary to have further blood tests made.

CASE No. 83.—M. A., Irish, age 29, unmarried, female. Patient was admitted to the Prospect Heights Hospital, Maternity Ward, to be confined with a second child; both children are living and well. She denies syphilitic infection. Her mother died of asthma, her father is living, is a habitual drinker and has heart trouble. Her four brothers and three sisters are living and well. She complains of severe headaches and backaches. She also presents a positive Romberg, and clinically seems to be very suspicious of syphilis. She refused a recital of her previous history and also refused to submit to physical examination. Perhaps promiscuous intercourse may have caused mild infection of syphilitic nature and thus the cause of the positive Hecht-Weinberg-Gradwohl test.

CASE No. 84.—B. J., American, age 20, unmarried, female. This is the *girl's* first childbirth, both her parents are alive and well, also the rest of her family. Patient denies syphilitic infection or previous abortions. She has suffered fainting spells about once a week, from her seventeenth year. She also complains of severe headaches. Such a case deserves further watching, perhaps she may have had a syphilitic infection which she either denies or does not know of. She also refused a physical examination.

CASE No. 17.—A. B., Russian Hebrew, age 38, male. Married nine and a half years and has three healthy children. Suffers from pulmonary phthisis. Family history negative. He gives no history of venereal disease, and shows no clinical evidences of syphilis. This case may be classed as *very* doubtful.

CASE No. 11.—O. B., Russian, age 24, female. Venereal history negative. Married four years and has two children. No venereal history in husband who is, however, an excessive drinker. Shows no clinical manifestations, either objective or subjective of lues. Admits also of having had some throat troubles soon after marriage and never before. Patient now suffers from achylia gastrica without any pathologic basis as proved by a very careful clinical and laboratory analysis. This case permits suspicion of an early infection with secondary manifestations in the throat. Nevertheless the physician should not make a diagnosis of syphilis unless further proof is obtained.

CASE No. 50.—J. C., Italian, age 54, female. Married 34 years, pregnant fifteen times and seven were miscarriages. Patient has been ailing for the past seven years and has aches all over the left half of the body, with headaches either on the top or the left side. Also suffers from lack of weight. Shows gastrointestinal symptoms due to gall bladder disease. A physical examination disclosed a very sluggish left pupil, an appreciable enlargement of the left lobe of the liver and very highly increased reflexes. This case presents sufficient data permitting the assumption of a possible latent syphilis, in spite of the absence of definite data regarding such a state from the patient's history.

CASE No. 19.—E. K., Hungarian, age 40, baker, male. The patient had gonorrhea at 20, now complains of backaches, pain in pectoral region, numbness of extremities, pains in back of head, and noises in the right ear. Patient is also constipated and has an enlarged prostate. There seemed to be no history or physical signs of syphilis. A positive diagnosis of syphilis on the grounds that the blood of this patient showed a positive in the Hecht-Weinberg-Gradwohl modification is not therefore justifiable. This case, therefore, must also be classed as *very* doubtful.

In the aforegoing histories something suspicious was found in every case which gave either a positive or borderline reaction in the Hecht-Weinberg-Gradwohl test except two (see Cases 17 and 19). Nevertheless, in my opinion the Hecht-Weinberg-Gradwohl test should *never* be used alone, but only in conjunction with the Wassermann test, as at the present time there is not sufficient data available to justify its independent use and reliability. It is also unfortunate that some sera do not contain any natural complement. With such bloods the Hecht-Weinberg-Gradwohl test can not be used at all. In bloods that have no hemolytic index, we must depend upon the Wassermann test alone. The clinician must also exercise caution in diagnosing a case as syphilis when the Hecht-Weinberg-Gradwohl test *alone* is positive, while the Wassermann test is negative. When such results are obtained, a very careful clinical history must be taken and a very careful physical examination made before a diagnosis is pronounced.

SUMMARY

The following are the results with 100 comparative tests:

The above cases were not selected ones, but cases applying to the Brooklyn Diagnostic Institute for general diagnosis.

1. In 65 per cent of the sera the Wassermann and the Hecht-Weinberg-Gradwohl tests were either positives or negatives in both tests.

2. Nineteen per cent of the sera showed a positive or borderline in the Hecht-Weinberg-Gradwohl test and a one-plus or a borderline in the Wassermann reaction.

3. Seventeen per cent had no hemolytic index. (Of course in these cases the Hecht-Weinberg-Gradwohl test could not be employed.)

4. Five per cent showed a strong positive in the Hecht-Weinberg-Gradwohl test, and a negative in the Wassermann.

5. Five per cent showed a positive in Tubes 12 and 13 in the Hecht-Weinberg-Gradwohl test and negative in the Wassermann.

6. Four per cent showed a positive in Tube 13 in the Hecht-Weinberg-Gradwohl test and a negative in the Wassermann.

7. Two per cent showed very doubtful reactions. (See cases 17 and 19.)

8. Our average hemolytic index was four, not including those sera that had no index at all.

Gradwohl claims that only 2 per cent of the sera lack enough natural complement for the Hecht-Weinberg-Gradwohl test. This may be the case if the test is made on fresh sera. As already mentioned our tests were performed three times a week, so that some of the sera were about 48 hours old. Perhaps this may serve as an explanation of the 17 per cent that had no hemolytic index. We are now making the tests on the day the blood is withdrawn so as to determine what per cent of the sera lack enough natural complement to perform the Hecht-Weinberg-Gradwohl test under those circumstances.

Gradwohl claims that in the Hecht-Weinberg-Gradwohl test, a complete inhibition of hemolysis is obtained and states it thus:

"Furthermore, I wish to be understood as stating, that when I speak of negative Wassermann and positive Hecht-Weinberg-Gradwohls, we do not mean a faint inhibition of the latter and a complete hemolysis in the former. The results are astonishingly different and striking, on the one hand, a clean cut negative Wassermann, on the other a definite and distinct positive Hecht-Weinberg-Gradwohl."

My experiences with the Hecht-Weinberg-Gradwohl test, not only in this series herein reported, but also of former work, permit me to state that the Hecht-Weinberg-Gradwohl gives not only a faint inhibition of hemolysis, but sometimes a complete hemolysis in Tubes 11 and 12 and a complete or faint inhibition of hemolysis in Tube 13. It may also give a complete hemolysis in Tube 11 and a faint or complete inhibition in Tubes 12 and 13, and finally it may give a faint inhibition in Tubes 11, 12, and 13. Any of these reactions would be termed borderline reactions.

BIBLIOGRAPHY

[1]Kolmer, J. A.: The Hecht (Gradwohl Modification) Complement Fixation Reaction in Syphilis with Special Reference to Cholesterinized Antigens, Jour. Immunol., 1916, ii, 23-37.
[2]Kolmer, J. A.: Serum Diagnosis of Syphilis and Gonorrhea Employing Human Complement, Am. Jour. Syph., 1919, ii, No. 4, pp. 739-754.
[3]Gradwohl, R. B. H.: The Hecht-Weinberg-Gradwohl Test in the Diagnosis of Syphilis, Jour. Am. Med. Assn., 1917, lxviii, 514-520.
Butler, C. S., and Landon, W. E.: Technic for the Absorption Test for Syphilis Using Human Complement, U. S. Naval Bull., January, 1916, pp. 1-9.
Hecht, H.: Eine Vereinfachung der Komplement Bindungs Reaktion bei Syphilis, Wien. klin. Wchnschr., 1909, xxii, 338-340.
Health, O.: The Wassermann Test: A Method Not Necessitating the Use of Guinea Pigs as the Source of Complement, Brit. Med. Jour., June 19, 1915, i, 1041-1043.

A METHOD FOR PREPARING BACTERIOLOGIC MEDIA CONTAINING ASCITES FLUID*

By Linwood G. Grace, D.D.S., Cleveland, Ohio

THE use of broth to which certain amounts of ascites fluid are added has been advocated for some time for cultivating streptococci and other organisms. The usual directions given for its preparation are that the sterile fluid be added to the broth which has been previously made and sterilized. The method requires most careful attention to details and offers numerous sources for contamination. If the fluid has not been collected aseptically, it can, of course, be sterilized by passing through an unglazed porcelain filter. There still remains, however, the problem of getting it into tubes of broth in definite quantities without contamination. H. Bierry (Comptes Rendus des Seames de la Société de Biologie, 1916, No. 7, p. 270) called attention to the fact that ascites and other albuminous fluids may be autoclaved at 112° C. without coagulating, if previously rendered alkaline. It may then be neutralized and reautoclaved and still remain clear. Or it may be added to broth or agar, the reaction of which is adjusted as required, and autoclaved without causing coagulation or precipitation in the media.

It is quite obvious that such a process infinitely simplifies the preparation of such a media. The ascites can be added to the broth or agar in definite amounts before it is tubed. This is far more accurate than adding it to the media after it has been tubed and also less laborious.

In order to determine the minimum amount of alkali necessary to add to ascites fluid to prevent coagulation when autoclaved, we carried out the following experiment:

The sample of ascites on hand was nearly neutral. Phenolphthalein was used as the indicator. Twenty test tubes were selected and into each test tube were placed 10 c.c. of ascites fluid. Definite amounts of alkali were added to each tube and all autoclaved at 15 pounds pressure, 118° C., for 15 minutes. This is slightly higher than the temperature suggested by Bierry, but is the standard we have used for some time for autoclaving media. After autoclaving, all those which were still liquid were filtered. The results are noted in the accompanying table, together with the amounts of alkali added to each tube. A separate tube in which no alkali was added was run as a control. As a final test a few drops of a normal acid solution were added to each tube. A flocculent precipitate was thrown down in each case upon the addition of the first drop of acid.

From the table it would appear that six or seven drops of 40 per cent NaOH to each 10 c.c. of ascites, or about 2½ per cent alkali, gave the best results. However, before adding the alkali, the ascites should be titrated, as a more acid fluid would undoubtedly need a greater amount of alkali to produce the same results. It is better to add small quantities of a strong alkali than large quantities of a weak one on account of diluting the fluid.

*From the Laboratories of the Research Institute of the National Dental Association, Cleveland, Ohio.

253

When the ascites is received it is rendered alkaline by adding 2½ per cent of 40 per cent NaOH, autoclaved 15 pounds at 118° C. for 15 minutes and stored in the ice box until ready for use. When the media is made up this ascites is added in the required amounts, usually 5 per cent, the reaction of the entire batch adjusted, filtered, tubed, and autoclaved 15 pounds at 118° C. for 15 minutes. We have been using this method for over a year, and results have shown that all organisms tested grow equally as well as in media prepared by the old method.

TUBE NO.	AMOUNT OF ALKALI ADDED	APPEARANCE AFTER AUTOCLAVING	APPEARANCE AFTER FILTERING
1	0.1 c.c. N/1 NaOH	Entirely coagulated. Appear almost the same as tube without alkali	Not filtered
2	0.2 c.c. N/1 NaOH	Nearly all coagulated. Very little liquid left	Not filtered
3	0.3 c.c. N/1 NaOH	Same as 2	Not filtered
4	0.4 c.c. N/1 NaOH	Partly coagulated. Coagulum in suspension	Same as before filtering
5	0.5 c.c. N/1 NaOH	Same as 4	Same
6	0.6 c.c. N/1 NaOH	Same as 4	Same
7	0.7 c.c. N/1 NaOH	Same as 4	Same
8	0.8 c.c. N/1 NaOH	Same general appearance as 4. Slightly less coagulum	Same
9	0.9 c.c. N/1 NaOH	Same as 8	Same
10	1.0 c.c. N/1 NaOH	Same as 8	Same
11	1 drop 40% NaOH*	Nearly all coagulated	Not filtered
12	2 drops 40% NaOH	Partly coagulated. Coagulum in suspension	Same as before filtering
13	3 drops 40% NaOH	Same as 12	Same
14	4 drops 40% NaOH	Very little coagulation. Precipitate at bottom of tube	Cleared a little
15	5 drops 40% NaOH	Very little if any coagulation. Precipitate at bottom of tube	Fairly clear
16	6 drops 40% NaOH	Almost entirely clear. Precipitate at bottom of tube	Clear
17	7 drops 40% NaOH	Same as 16	Clear
18	8 drops 40% NaOH	Not as clear as 16	Not as clear as 16
19	9 drops 40% NaOH	Same as 18	Same
20	10 drops 40% NaOH	Same as 18	Same

*The pipette used to drop the 40% NaOH dropped about 0.04 c.c. to a drop, as nearly as could be measured.

THE EARLY DIAGNOSIS OF TYPHOID AND PARATYPHOID INFECTIONS*

By Henry J. Goeckel, Ph.D., Plainfield, N. J.

THE extensive employment of typhoid and paratyphoid vaccine for immunization is liable to render the Widal agglutination reaction on the blood serum as usually employed of doubtful value in many cases of suspected typhoid infection.

While blood cultures may prove a valuable aid in such cases and in others before a typical Widal reaction is obtainable, the method is time-consuming and it is neither convenient nor a desirable procedure in many cases.

I have recently had several cases of suspected typhoid infection referred to the laboratory, which either failed to give the agglutination reaction for typhoid and paratyphoid bacilli or gave only a partial agglutination of doubtful diagnostic value.†

In the first case which led to the investigation incorporated in this paper, the blood serum failed to show any agglutination. On the very day that the Widal reaction was made, the pathologic interne, while making the urine examinations, noted a moderate number of pus cells and numerous motile rod bacteria in the urine from this case. The specimen had been obtained at least four hours before the blood. As it was not secured aseptically, another one was obtained with a sterile catheter directly into a sterile container. This urine likewise showed pus and numerous motile rod bacteria.

Upon subjecting the lightly centrifuged bacterial suspension (without washing) to a series of agglutination tests, they proved to be paratyphoid bacilli, Type B.

The agglutinating sera employed had the following titer: typhoid, 1-4000; paratyphoid Types A and B, each 1-10,000; coli, 1-2000. They were employed in the following dilutions; Typhoid, 1-2000; paratyphoid A and B, each in 1-5000, and the coli serum in 1-1000 dilution. All gave an entirely negative test except the paratyphoid B serum.

The blood count showed 73% polymorphonuclear neutrophile leucocytes, 22.6% lymphocytes, and 4.4% mononuclear leucocytes.

The temperature was 104.2° F., the highest attained until discharged.

The urine showed a distinct trace of albumin, moderate indican test, moderate pus; few oxalate crystals and numerous motile rod bacteria.

The very next day a case was sent into the hospital for observation as a suspected case of appendicitis.

Child, 4 years, 11 months, 9/24/19. The day of admission the maximum temperature was 101.8° F. dropping to 99.9° F. The white cell count showed 17,000 cells per c.mm. of which 76% were polynuclear leucocytes and 24% mononuclear cells.

The Widal reaction on the blood showed partial agglutination for typhoid only in the 1-20 dilution. A catheterized urine as in the preceding case showed a moderate number of

*From the Clinical and Pathological Laboratory of Muhlenberg Hospital, Plainfield, N. J.
†Suspensions of live bacilli are employed by the hanging drop microscopic method. Agglutination and inhibition of motility are both noted in dilutions of 1-20 to 1-120.

255

isolated leucocytes and a moderate number of motile rod bacteria. These when tested with agglutinating sera of the same dilutions as in the preceding case, proved to be typhoid bacilli.

9/25/19.—Widal reaction on blood agglutinated to 1-60 dilution.

9/28/19.—Highest temperature was attained, 103.8° F.

10/1/19.—Widal reaction on blood agglutinated to 1-120 dilution.

10/3/19.—W. C. C. 18,000; polynuclear leucocytes 52%; mononuclear cells 45%; eosinophiles 3%.

10/5/19.—Routine urine examination was negative.

In the third case in the series the data given was that a month previous, the patient (a boy of 10 years) showed a temperature of 104° F. At the same time the lower right abdominal quadrant proved tense and tender. Upon consultation it was decided to remove the appendix which was found to be moderately inflamed. The case apparently made an uneventful recovery only to show the same temperature elevation four weeks later without any apparent physical distress, etc.

10/3/19.—Blood count showed 5,800 white cells of which 45.5% were polynuclears; 39% lymphocytes; and 15.5% were mononuclear leucocytes.

10/4/19.—Widal reaction positive for typhoid. On the same day the urine showed a moderate number of motile rod bacteria, no pus and no casts. The bacteria were concentrated by centrifuging at high speed. Most of the supernatant urine was decanted, and the residue was thoroughly agitated to break up any possible clumps resulting from the centrifuging. When subjected to a series of agglutination tests as were the preceding cases, they proved to be typhoid bacilli.

SUMMARY

In the first case while the Widal reaction and the blood count were in no way indicative of a typhoid or paratyphoid infection on the day of examination, the paratyphoid bacilli were identified in the urine.

In the second case the blood count was likewise of no value, in fact it was somewhat suggestive of a leucocytosis. The Widal reaction was doubtful, while the bacilli in the urine were identified as typhoid bacilli seven days before a typical Widal reaction was obtained and nine days before the blood count was typical.

In the third case the bacilli were identified at the same time that the blood count and Widal reaction showed typical for typhoid.

CONCLUSIONS

Although it is stated that the typhoid and paratyphoid bacilli appear in the urine some time after the second week of infection, the cases examined showed:

1. That it is possible to obtain and identify them in the urine by agglutinins before the blood shows a positive Widal reaction or a typical cell count.

2. By this means a prompter report was given than if blood culture had been resorted to.

3. It is a more definite method of identification of the infection than is identifying agglutinins in the patient's blood serum.

4. It is more positive and eliminates reliance on the Widal reaction on blood serum.

5. It should be resorted to whenever possible in patients who may have a natural or acquired agglutinating capacity due to previous infection or through the use of vaccines.

HEXAMETHYLENAMINE INTERFERES WITH THE TEST FOR INDOXYL IN URINE*

By Henry J. Goeckel, Ph.D., Plainfield, N. J.

KNOWING that formaldehyde when added to urine prevents the Obermeyer hydrochloric acid-ferric chloride reagent from reducing the indoxyl compounds to indican, I wish to call to the attention of those using this reagent that the administration of hexamethylenamine (i.e., urotropin, formin, etc.,) likewise prevents the reduction to indican.

This can be easily demonstrated by taking a urine high in indoxyl content, mixing with it some urine from a person taking hexamethylenamine, and applying the test.

The result will be a negative or very slight indican production while a control with an equal volume of the original urine will give a pronounced indican test.

DEVICE FOR WITHDRAWING BLOOD FROM VEINS

By Clyde L. Cummer, M.D., Cleveland, Ohio

A NUMBER of devices have been suggested for the withdrawal of blood from the veins for serologic, bacteriologic or chemical examination. The instrument long in vogue and still extensively utilized is the syringe. With a well made Luer syringe excellent service is obtained, since the use of washers or packing about the piston is obviated. The chief drawback is the expense, which is especially an item if much work is being done. Unfortunately, the vacuum in certain makes is often far from perfect. A needle is used by many for obtaining blood for the Wassermann reaction without the employment of negative pressure. This is reasonably satisfactory for serologic or chemical work, but is slow and can not be employed when cultures are to be made, on account of the likelihood of contamination. A larger needle is needed than is required when vacuum is utilized. While the Keidel tube is well adapted for serologic work and may be modified for bacteriologic work, it represents a definite expense, since it can not be resterilized and used again. In the writer's opinion the most practical instrument is the MacRae needle, which has been on the market for a number of years. It is, however, made of steel and corrodes readily. When it is frequently employed, the needle point is likely to lose its temper and the cannula portion so weakened by rust that it breaks off when this accident is least expected and least desired. Stitt has devised an extremely simple apparatus, employing a similar principle, made of glass, a piece of rubber tubing connecting the glass tubing which serves as an inlet to the needle. This is a disadvantage, since one hand

*From the Clinical and Pathological Laboratory of Muhlenberg Hospital, Plainfield, N. J.

must be used to introduce the needle and one to hold the apparatus. We have attempted to combine the good features of the MacRae and the Stitt outfits in an apparatus which is illustrated in the sketch.

A is a piece of glass tubing the distal tip (C) of which is ground to receive the Luer needle (D) by slip-joint connection. A collar or flange is blown into the tubing at the point (B) to prevent the tube from slipping down through the opening to the rubber stopper (E). A second piece of glass tubing (F) of approximately the same bore is bent slightly at an angle at one end, is introduced into a second hole in the rubber stopper (E). The lower end of the glass tube (A) should project about one-half inch or more below the bottom of the rubber stopper than does the lower end of glass tubing (F). To the upper end of glass tubing (F) is attached a piece of rubber tubing (H) about six inches long into

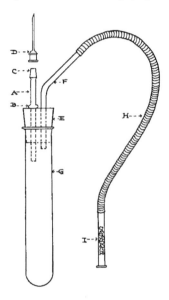

whose distal end is inserted a section of glass tubing (I) which is stuffed lightly with cotton and serves as a mouthpiece. The rubber stopper (E) should be such a size that it will fit snugly into the mouth of the test tube, flask or bottle which is to be employed for receiving the specimen.

With this apparatus a vacuum is secured by exhaustion of the air from the tube or flask by the operator, who sucks out the air through the rubber tubing. There is no danger of blood being drawn into the operator's mouth if the lower orifice of the tube (F) is kept above the lower orifice of the tube (A) when the apparatus is in use. Further security on this score is given by the cotton stopper in the mouthpiece. The entire apparatus may be handled with one hand, the tube serving as a handle, the rest of the outfit, except for the rubber tubing, forming a rigid unit. The other hand is left free for handling the tourniquet, steadying the patient's arm, etc. There are no parts to rust or corrode, except the needle. Any size Luer needle may be used, which is of distinct advantage. For bacteriologic or chemical work, the outfit may be sterilized by boiling, while if. it is desired to use the outfit for blood cultures, it may be wrapped in cloth and sterilized in the autoclave. The apparatus is convenient for bacteriologic work since the blood may be drawn directly from the vein without contact with outside atmosphere into a container charged with sodium citrate or with citrated physiologic salt solution, stoppered with a sterile stopper, and taken to the laboratory, where cultures may be made as desired. Cleaning is readily effected by inserting the stopper into the outlet of the cold water faucet and letting the water run through.

The apparatus has been made for me through the cooperation of the Will Corporation of Rochester, N. Y., from which it may be obtained.

TRAUMATIC HEMOLYSIS AND THE WASSERMANN REACTION

By George Manghill Olson, M.D., Minneapolis, Minn.

THE red blood cells of man and animals are rather fragile in structure, in comparison with the other body cells.

The destruction of red blood cells is evidenced by hemolysis, and is caused by thermal changes, by bacteria, by chemicals, by drying and trauma or rough handling.

The fragility of the red blood cells of various animals varies considerably, the red blood cells of the dog being most fragile and sheep's blood most resistant to mechanical or chemical injury.*

Rous and Turner quoted by Kolmer and Brown* found that human blood was more resistant than sheep's blood. I have found that over half of the specimens of human blood for the Wassermann reaction, when collected from a vein by the syringe method, show marked hemolysis when the serum has separated. The serum is often tinted to a degree resembling port wine. This traumatic hemolysis is due to the force required in discharging the blood from the syringe into the vial, and occurs even when the specimen is placed immediately in the ice box.

Marked traumatic hemolysis also often occurs when specimens of blood are obtained by puncture and squeezing from the finger.

In order to avoid this hemolysis which may yield false positives, specimens of blood for the Wassermann reaction should be obtained from a vein, the blood flowing through the needle into a vial.

Hemolysis of sheep's blood can easily be produced by even moderate trauma when washing with salt solution. Sheep's corpuscles, when placed in salt solution and centrifuged, tend to cling to the bottom of the tube. When the supernatant salt solution is removed and more salt solution added, it requires thorough shaking to remove the corpuscles from the bottom of the tube. This shaking often re-

*Kolmer, J. A., and Brown, C. P.; Am. Jour. Syph., April, 1919.

sults in slight hemolysis, even when perfectly fresh sheep's blood is used. Repeated washings serve only to increase the trauma, so that the fourth or fifth washing may show more hemolysis than the second.

The use of these red blood cells in the Wassermann reaction may result in complete hemolysis in the positive controls, or as a rule in slight hemolysis in the positive controls.

To avoid traumatic hemolysis, I use the following method in washing sheep's corpuscles:

Two or three c.c. of sheep's blood are poured into 50 c.c. centrifuge tubes filled with 0.9 per cent cold salt solution. The tubes are centrifuged at moderate speed. The supernatant salt solution is removed. The tubes are again filled with salt solution. A small bit of cotton is wound around the tip of a wooden applicator. With this cotton tipped applicator the corpuscles are carefully removed from the bottom of the tube and gently stirred. Two washings are sufficient.

SUMMARY

1. Specimens of blood for the Wassermann reaction should be collected from a vein, the blood flowing through the needle into the vial or tube.

2. The syringe method of collecting blood from the vein and the method of collecting blood from the finger should be abandoned.

3. In order to avoid hemolysis in washing sheep's corpuscles, thorough shaking of the centrifuge tubes should be avoided, a uniform suspension can be obtained by gentle stirring with a cotton tipped wooden applicator.

The Journal of Laboratory and Clinical Medicine

Vol. V.   JANUARY, 1920   No. 4

Editor-in-Chief: VICTOR C. VAUGHAN, M.D.
Ann Arbor, Mich.

ASSOCIATE EDITORS

DENNIS E. JACKSON, M.D.	CINCINNATI
HANS ZINSSER, M.D.	NEW YORK
PAUL G. WOOLLEY, M.D.	CINCINNATI
FREDERICK P. GAY, M.D.	BERKELEY, CAL.
J. J. R. MACLEOD, M.B.	TORONTO
ROY G. PEARCE, M.D.	CLEVELAND
W. C. MACCARTY, M.D.	ROCHESTER, MINN.
GERALD B. WEBB, M.D.	COLORADO SPRINGS
E. E. SOUTHARD, M.D.	BOSTON
WARREN T. VAUGHAN, M.D.	BOSTON

EDITORIALS

The Functional Pathology of Surgical Shock

BY CONCERTED investigation in experimental medicine in England and in this country, remarkable progress was made during the last two years of the war in the elucidation of the causes of the condition known as shock. There are several varieties of this condition, the two most characteristic of which are surgical shock met with in the operating room and after severe accidents in civic practice, and secondary trench shock met with at the battle front. In every essential particular these two conditions appear to be alike, and a condition apparently identical with them can be produced in laboratory animals by various experimental procedures. It is largely because of the availability of this experimental material that it has been possible to throw so much light on the problem. This but serves once again to illustrate the necessity of animal experimentation in the furtherance of medical and surgical knowledge. Had it not been for the work done on shock in the laboratory by Bayliss, Cannon, Dale, Erlanger, and others, the war might have ended without our being any further advanced in our knowledge of this mysterious and fatal condition. It may be of interest here to review very briefly some of this experimental work.

We shall consider first of all the investigations by Dale,[1] and Laidlaw and Richards[2] on the shock-like condition which is produced by injections of histamine (iminazylethylamine). This substance is derived by removal of the carboxyl group, as CO_2, from histidine, one of the most important of the building stones of the protein molecule. Injected quickly into etherized animals in very minute dosage (1 mg. per kg. body weight) histamine soon causes the arterial blood pressure to fall to the shock level of 30-40 mm. Hg. For a brief period preceding the fall there is a rise in pressure due to constriction of the arterioles, and this constriction persists while the pressure is falling. So far as the obvious vascular changes are concerned, therefore, the condition is strictly comparable with those found in shock—low blood pressure and constricted arterioles. By the time the pressure has fallen to near the shock level the cardiac pulsations disappear from the tracing. The respirations also cease, but if the animal be kept alive by artificial respiration and the thorax opened for inspection of the heart this organ will be observed to be beating quite vigorously, with, however, a pronounced deficiency of blood in the auricles and in the large veins both of the thorax and abdomen. This observation affords positive proof that in this form of shock at least the fundamental cause for the condition is inadequate blood flow to the heart. The question is, what becomes of the blood? Either it must pass out of the blood vessels into the tissues, or the capacity of the former must be increased. Loss of blood itself could scarcely occur short of hemorrhage—of which there is no evidence in histamine shock—but the water with some of the soluble constituents (plasma) might become extravasated, leaving in the vessels blood excessively rich in corpuscles. Such extravasation actually occurs in acute histamine shock, as revealed by measurement either of the concentration of hemoglobin or of the corpuscles, but this in itself can not explain all of the loss in circulating blood, for if the histamine be given slowly (over a period of 20-30 min.) it takes much longer for the shock to become established, and the blood does not show any increase in the percentage of hemoglobin or in the number of corpuscles. In these cases we are driven to conclude that much of the blood must be withdrawn from currency by stagnation in dilated vessels. Direct evidence for this important conclusion has been secured by determination of the volume of circulating blood, by means of the vital red method of Keith, Rowntree and Geraghty,[3] described elsewhere.

Although the oligemia is due in great part to dilatation of the capillaries and venules of the intestine, as can be shown by inspection, it is also partly dependent upon dilatation of vessels elsewhere, since histamine shock can be induced in animals from which all of the intestines have been removed. The vessels of the skeletal muscles are probably the chief extraabdominal vessels affected, for although no dilatation of these can ordinarily be seen in histamine shock, it becomes quite evident in animals which have been transfused before being shocked. The capillaries (and venules) in these areas evidently lose their tone so that they become too roomy for the available blood. As a matter of fact Dale and Richards[2] have shown that histamine abolishes the tone of capillaries at the same time that it increases the permeability of the walls and so permits the plasma to leak through. It is on account of this latter action that histamine when it is rubbed on the scarified skin soon causes the formation of a wheal like that following the lash of a whip.[4]

When histamine is given to unanesthetized animals about ten times as much can be withstood as in those that are anesthetized with ether.[5] At first sight this result might seem to discount the observations on etherized animals, but on the contrary they greatly enhance their importance. They indicate that whereas the normal animal is able to combat the toxic action of histamine, ether greatly depresses this power, an observation which agrees remarkably with the clinical experience that administration of ether is most dangerous in persons who are threatened with shock. The poisoning effect of ether persists for some time after the anesthetic is removed, and it is no doubt dependent upon a toxic action on the endothelium of the capillaries, for it is particularly in such animals that concentration of the blood is evident after histamine. It is of great significance that histamine did not readily produce shock in nitrous oxide anesthesia.

Hemorrhage also greatly predisposes to histamine shock, but in this case the blood is not nearly so concentrated as ordinarily because of the passage of plasma from the tissue spaces into the vessels, which, it will be remembered, is the natural reaction of an animal to hemorrhage alone. The cause of shock in such animals is mainly the opening up of the vessels.

Many bacterial toxins, both when applied to scarified skin and when injected intravenously, have effects very like those of histamine. It is also well known that shock is peculiarly common after injuries in which there has been extensive destruction of tissue. The facts warrant the suggestion that shock may be due to liberation from damaged tissues, particularly the muscles and the viscera of toxic substances acting like histamine. This conforms with the fact that shock is most common when there has been extensive destruction of muscle, or when the liver or intestines are roughly handled. It is possible also that the shock of intestinal obstruction is fundamentally due to absorption into the blood of similar substances from the closed loop of intestine. Whipple and Hooper's discoveries that absorption of a proteose is responsible for the shock-like symptoms of intestinal obstruction are very suggestive in this connection.[6]

But to return to surgical shock. Is it possible that the condition is dependent upon intoxication by histamine-like substances absorbed from greatly damaged tissues? To test this hypothesis Cannon[7] and others have investigated the effects of crushing the muscles of the hind limbs, without external hemorrhage, by blows from a heavy hammer. It was found that an immediate fall in blood pressure occurred, followed by a more gradual decline to the shock level, with a decrease in the CO_2-combining power and a marked concentration of the blood. This result was not due to irritation of afferent nerves, causing excessive stimulation of the vasomotor centers, since it persisted in animals in which all nerves of the limb had been cut; neither was it caused by any local loss of circulating fluid (by dilatation of vessels or extravasation). It was due to the discharge into the circulation of some toxic material, since no shock resulted when the vessels of the damaged limb were clamped. Removal of the clamp some time after the damage resulted in the immediate appearance of the symptoms which could again be caused to disappear somewhat by its reapplication. As to the nature of the toxic material, the first possibility to be considered is that it is unoxidized acid (lactic), which, it is well known accumulates quickly in muscular tissue whenever this is destroyed, or when the circulation through the tissues is greatly curtailed. As a matter of fact it was found that the CO_2-carrying power of the blood became greatly depressed whenever the toxic material was permitted to enter the circulation by removal of the clamp, and it is well known that there is also a decided depression in the blood carbonates in surgical shock. Acid intoxication can not, however, be the main factor, and for the following reasons: 1. Injections of lactic acid intravenously do not cause shock, neither do they predispose an animal to it. 2. Copious injections of bicarbonate solution do not prevent shock. 3. Extracts of damaged muscle made with isotonic saline do have a shock-like effect, but this is just as great when the lactic acid in the extracts is neutralized with bicarbonate, as when they are unneutralized. Moreover the fall in the blood carbonate does not coincide with, but rather precedes, the development of the shock symptoms. An excess of lactic acid in the blood has been noted in the later stages of many cases of shock (Wiggers and Macleod), but this is a secondary effect, and it is doubtful whether it is the only cause for the depressed CO_2-carrying power of the blood.

In one or two cases the muscles were crushed in unanesthetized cats, with the result that shock did not invariably follow, but this does not invalidate the observations on anesthetized animals; it only shows that, as in histamine poisoning, the anesthetic weakens the resistance. When the normal animals were bled before the crushing operation, shock supervened with certainty.

Taking the results as a whole and comparing them with clinical experience a very strong case is made for the hypothesis that surgical shock is essentially due to intoxication by materials derived from damaged tissue. Shock is particularly common after severe tissue damage; rough handling of the wound greatly aggravates it, whereas rigid care to render the wounded part immobile is a valuable safeguard; the administration of ordinary anesthesia, (ether) to a shock patient is notoriously dangerous, whereas rapid amputation under nitrous oxide often ushers in a steady recovery. All these clinical facts conform admirably with the experimental findings.

With regard to the diagnostic value of measurement of the blood volume, it has been shown by Erlanger, Gasser and Meek[8] that concentration of the blood becomes evident before the shock symptoms are pronounced. This concentration is no doubt a most important factor in causing curtailment of the volume of circulating fluid, not only because of loss of plasma, but also because it causes the corpuscles to become contiguous so that they have a tendency to jam in the capillaries and so lead to a progressively increasing under-nutrition of the tissues and the production of more toxic material.

It remains for us to show that the foregoing conclusions drawn from observations made on laboratory animals are applicable to the clinical condition known as surgical shock. It will then be advantageous to consider the principles which determine successful treatment. The unusual opportunity afforded at the front to study shock has led to a furtherance of our knowledge of its causes, which might have taken many years of investigation in time of peace, and by far the most important contributions have come from those who have been intimately familiar with the experimental as well as the clinical aspect of the problem. N. M. Keith[9] estimated the total volume of circulating blood by the vital red method and the relative amounts of plasma and corpuscles by measurement of hemoglobin or by means of the hematocrit, and as a result of his investigations has divided the cases of secondary shock into three groups which vary from one another with regard to: 1. The total volume of blood in circulation and (2) the relative amounts of plasma and corpuscles in the blood. The differentiation is not only of great prognostic value, but also invaluable as a guide to the proper plan of treatment. In group 1 are the *compensated cases*, in which the blood volume is reduced to not more than 80 per cent of the normal, but in which the plasma is relatively greater, being reduced only to 85 or 90 per cent of the normal. In other words these cases have reacted like cases of hemorrhage, i. e., there has been a migration of fluid from the tissues into the blood. If kept warm and given fluid per rectum, the patients recover. In the second group, called *partially compensated*, the blood volume is reduced to 65-75 per cent, with little, if any, evidence of dilution of plasma (i. e., the plasma is also reduced to 65-75 per cent). Treatment by transfusion either with blood (citrated blood by Robertson's method,[10] or with gum solutions (*vide infra*) is necessary and in most cases, if the proper technic is followed in the transfusion, recovery is likely. It is important, however, that the plasma volume be measured a few hours after the transfusion to see whether the desired reaction, namely, a migration of fluid into the plasma, has set in. If not so, a second transfusion is indicated. In favorable cases the plasma volume increases more rapidly than that of total blood, and *pari passu* the arterial blood pressure rises.

In the third or *uncompensated group*—the blood volume is below 65 per cent and the blood is more concentrated than normal, i. e., there is relatively a greater decrease of plasma. Treatment must be energetic in these cases, but the prognosis is unfavorable because the transfused fluid readily leaves the vessels, causing the lungs and tissues to become edematous.

With regard to the rationale of the transfusions, it is clear that the added fluid makes good the blood that is lost by stagnation, etc., and so tends to maintain in the circulation a normal pressure for a sufficient time to enable the organism to destroy the toxic bodies. If the shock condition has existed for some time, so that the nerve centers are paralyzed, the injections are of no avail. Since many cases of shock in man have also suffered considerably from loss of blood, it is often difficult to decide whether shock really exists apart from the effects of hemorrhage, the cardinal symptoms of the two conditions being very much alike. The test is afforded by examination of the total blood and plasma volume, and by the reaction to transfusion. After hemorrhage alone there is great migration of plasma into the blood, making this very dilute, and transfusion has immediately beneficial results. In shock there is no migration of fluid into the blood, indeed the reverse is usually the case, and transfusion does not always succeed in reestablishing normal conditions.

Finally, with regard to the composition of the transfusion fluid, should this be human blood, or can a reliable substitute be found in saline solutions containing gum? There is much diversity of opinion over this question. Keith sums up by stating that there does not appear to be any decided advantage in blood over gum solutions, although the immediate restoration of natural color to the patient, which occurs with blood but not with gum solutions, may make the former appear to be the more satisfactory treatment.

Much painstaking work has been done by Erlanger and Gasser[8] to determine the exact conditions for success in using gum solutions. As their criterion for successful treatment, they did not merely see whether the blood pressure was restored, but they allowed the animals to recover from the effects of the anesthetic and then watched them to see whether they became restored to normal. Many animals might appear to be recovering, but nevertheless succumb within 24 hours. These workers point out that strong gum solutions owe their efficacy to the fact that they slowly attract water into the blood from the tissues, and once attracted the water remains in the vessels. Hypertonic solutions of crystalloids on the other hand, quickly attract water, but this is not retained long. These workers, there-fore, devised the scheme of combining the two factors, and they found that suc-cess depended on how this was attempted. In the shock produced by partial clamping of the vena cava about one-half of the animals died within 48 hours. Neither weak gum (6 per cent) and weak alkali (2 per cent) given in large amount (12 c.c. per kg.) nor strong gum (25 per cent) in strong alkali (5 per cent) given in smaller dosage (5 c.c. per kg.) decreased the above mortality; but if strong gum (25 per cent) were given along with strong glucose solutions (18 per cent) at the rate of 5 c.c. per kg. an hour, many more animals survived. The alkali was chosen to furnish the crystalloid, in many of the experiments, so that it might incidentally combat any existing acidosis. We have already seen, how-ever, that there is no reason to believe that acidosis is an important factor in shock. Two precautions are necessary to success in using the gum solutions, first they must be properly prepared, and second they must not be injected so rapidly that their high viscidity would slow the circulation and so embarrass the heart's action.

BIBLIOGRAPHY

[1]Dale, H. H., Laidlaw, P. P., and Richards, A. N.: Med. Res. Com. Special Report, 1919, No. 26, p. 8.
[2]Dale, H. H., and Richards, A. N.: Jour. Physiol., 1908, lii, 110.
[3]Keith, Rowntree, and Geraghty: Arch. Int. Med., 1915, xvi, 547.
[4]Sollman and Pilcher: Jour. Pharmacol. and Exper. Therap., 1917, xix, 309.
[5]Dale, H.H.: Med. Res. Com. Special Report, 1919, No. 26, p. 15.
[6]Whipple and Hooper: Am. Jour. Physiol., xl, 332, 349; ibid., xliii, 257, 264.
[7]Cannon, W. B., and Bayliss, W. M.: Med. Res. Com. Special Report, 1919, No. 26, p. 19.
[8]Gasser, H. S.: Erlanger, J., and Meek, W. J.: Studies in Secondary Traumatic Shock iv, v, vi, and vii, Am. Jour. Physiol., 1919, 1, 31, 86, 119, 149.
[9]Keith, N. M.: Med. Res. Com. Special Report, 1919, No. 27.
[10]Robertson and Bock: Med. Res. Com., Reports of the Special Investigation Com. upon Surgical Shock & Allied Conditions, Aug. 8, 1918, No. 6.

—J. J. R. M.

The Cause of Yellow Fever

A REVIEW of the history of bacteriology, showing as it does, within the short interval of fifty years, the discovery of the causative agents of so many diseases can not but make one most optimistic regarding future developments in that field. We are today intimately acquainted with the organisms causing several diseases whose etiology ten years ago, was quite unknown. Later developments have been especially concerned with the so-called filter passers, or filterable viruses, such as the globoid bodies found in poliomyelitis and the organisms of the spirochetal class. Further developments in the study of these filter passers may be expected to enlighten us on many more of the common infectious diseases.

Yellow fever has been described until the present time as a disease due to an unknown ultramicroscopic virus, capable of passing through a porcelain filter. Noguchi announces the discovery of an organism in the blood and tissue of cases of yellow fever, allied morphologically and biologically to the parasites of the spirochete class, and which, when transferred experimentally into guinea pigs, produces a disease, similar both clinically and pathologically to yellow fever in man.

This organism he designates as leptospira icteroides, and describes as 'an extremely delicate filament measuring 4 to 9 microns in length and 0.2 of a micron in width, along the middle portion. It tapers gradually toward the extremities, which end in immeasurably thin sharp points. The entire filament is not smooth but is minutely wound at short and regular intervals, the length of each section measuring about 0.25 microns. The windings are so placed as to form a zigzag line by alternate change of direction of each consecutive portion at an angle of 90 degrees. The organism is unrecognizable by translucent light, but becomes quite visible under a properly adjusted dark-field illumination. It possesses active motility consisting in vibration, rotation, rapid bipolar progression and sometimes of twisting of parts of the filament. When it encounters a semisolid substance it penetrates the latter by a boring motion, and while passing through the body assumes a serpentine aspect with few undulations, the elementary windings undergoing no modification.

"The organism manifests remarkably flexibility to almost any angle while changing its course of progression in a semisolid medium. In a fluid medium it has fewer and quite characteristic movements. One end is usually bent in the form of a graceful hook, and, while rapidly rotating, the organism proceeds in the direction of the straight end, the hooked end apparently serving as a sort of rear propeller. When extricating itself from an entanglement, the same hooked end seems to act like the front propeller of an airplane. Many specimens are seen with both ends hooked, the organism then rotating in a stationary position unless one hook is larger and more powerful as a propeller than the other. The rapid rotation makes the organism appear like a chain of minute dots. From the dynamic point of view the portions which include the several windings from the extremities, represent the motor apparatus of the organism."

Staining of the organism is difficult, and best results are obtained by Giemsa's method after osmic acid fixation.

The parasite is not an anaerobe, and requires a certain amount of oxygen for growth. Blood serum is essential. The organism is highly sensitive to the reaction of the medium, and best growth occurs in a solution slightly alkaline to litmus. Bacterial contamination usually rapidly destroys the parasite.

Best results were obtained by cultivation in media consisting of one part blood serum and three parts Ringer's solution. The organism grows slowly and produces no macroscopic change in the culture media.

It is highly virulent, has been known to kill a guinea pig in a dose of .000001 c.c. and retains its virulence for at least thirty-seven days. After four months, the organism had lost some of its virulence, but this was brought back by animal passage.

It has occasionally been found in the blood and tissues of individuals and animals sick with the disease, usually being present in the blood two to three days after infection. In the moribund the organisms were decidedly less frequent both in the blood and the organs.

The description of this organism as being present in cases of clinically characteristic yellow fever, and as being the probable cause thereof must be accepted as the most satisfactory explanation of the etiology that has so far been produced. This germ, isolated in pure culture has been shown to produce a similar disease when reinoculated into laboratory animals, and from them it can be again obtained in pure culture.

Further proof will depend upon immunologic reactions. These have been developed in Noguchi's work, but have evidently not been completed. Guinea pigs inoculated with the blood of yellow fever patients, which survived, and were subsequently reinoculated with organ emulsions obtained from experimentally infected animals as a rule did not die from the second injection, whereas controls did die. We must notice here, that pure cultures were not used.

Intraperitoneal inoculation of convalescent patients' serum together with cultures of the organism was found to result in a positive Pfeiffer phenomenon in 83 per cent of cases. Moreover these pigs had fewer deaths after this inoculation than the controls. The latter showed no Pfeiffer phenomenon.

Noguchi was able to reproduce the experimental disease in guinea pigs from bites of Stegomyia mosquitos which had over 12 days previously fed on yellow fever patients, or over 8 days previously fed on animals sick with the experimental disease.

The close resemblance of the leptospira icteroides, in all respects, to the leptospira icterohemorrhagica of infectious jaundice, and the fact that this latter disease is found in the locality where the yellow fever studies were made, call for considerable discretion and convincing proof before their identity has been denied. The rather close clinical resemblance between the two diseases must also be remembered. This renders the work particularly difficult, with both diseases occurring in the same community.

Noguchi studied the leptospira found in several rats captured in the vicinity, and found them to be those of infectious jaundice. He further differentiated them from the icteroides by their immunologic reactions.

The sera of rabbits immunized against the leptospira found in rats at Guayaquil agglutinated the leptospira icterohemorrhagica and protected guinea pigs when inoculated with a mixture of this serum and the infectious jaundice organism, while they had little or no agglutinating action on the leptospira icteroides or protective action when inoculated together with it.

Guinea pigs inoculated with the killed rat organism proved resistant to infection with leptospira icterohemorrhagica. Noguchi does not state that pigs inoculated with the killed rat organism were not protected against the leptospira icteroides.

Finally, we must remember that this organism was demonstrated only in a small proportion of the cases studied.

Further studies and further refinements of methods will give us additional immunologic data from which to judge, and may enable the observers to find the parasite in a higher proportion of the cases. We shall also expect to see further reports on experiments with Stegomyia calopus mosquitos as the carrier of this organism or some phase of its life cycle.

BIBLIOGRAPHY

Noguchi, H.: Jour. Exper. Med., 1919, xxix, 547-564, 565-584, 585-596; ibid., xxx, 1-8, 9-12, 13-30, 87-94, 95-108. 401-410.

—*W. T. V.*

Agglutination of B. Anthracis*

NOBLE has investigated this matter. Previous experimenters have reached diverse and even contradictory conclusions. Sobernheim in a review of the subject states that the agglutinating action on anthrax bacilli may be demonstrated both microscopically and macroscopically, but on account of the immobility of the bacilli and their tendency to clump spontaneously, the test is unsatisfactory; that some serums give distinct reactions in high dilutions, while others from highly immunized animals fail wholly. Sacwtschenko states that horse serum, whether from normal or immunized animals always agglutinates the anthrax bacillus, while dog serum never does. Cavins claims to have obtained serum from vaccinated animals, which agglutinate in high dilutions, from 1-50000 and even as high as 1-500000.

After studying the literature Noble comes to the conclusion that the difference in results has been due to failure to secure homogeneous emulsions and this he claims to have done by the following method: The bacillus is transplanted daily for ten days on plain agar at 42.5 degrees until a sporeless and vigorous growth is obtained. It is then grown on the same medium and at the same temperature in quart whiskey flasks for 12 hours. These growths are washed off with physiologic salt solution to which 0.5 per cent formalin has been added (about 100 c.c. to a flask). These suspensions are shaken in a mechanical shaker for forty-eight hours and allowed to stand for several days, during which time they are tested for sterility. Then a shaking for twenty-four hours follows. After standing overnight, the supernatant part is filtered several times through four thicknesses of sterile cheesecloth. The suspensions are now diluted with physiologic salt solution containing 0.5 per cent formalin to a point corresponding to a suspension of B. typhosus containing 2000 million bacteria per c.c. Suspensions of b. anthracis thus prepared are perfectly

*Jour. of Immunology, iv, 105.

homogeneous and stand at 37 degrees for at least forty-eight hours without spontaneous clumping and are suitable for agglutination tests.

These suspensions were tested with the serums from thirteen horses which had been immunized first with vaccines and then with increasing doses of the virulent organism and contrasted with similar tests with the serums of seven untreated horses. The tubes with the serums of the normal animals ran from 1-80 to 1-200, while with the serums of the immunized horses it ran from 1-6400 to 1-20000.

In order to secure homogeneous suspensions the cultures must be sporeless and free from old organisms, not more than eighteen hours old. The suspensions must be well shaken, the clumps allowed to settle, and carefully strained.

—*V. C. V.*

Classification of Spiral Organisms (Spirochete, etc.).

IN CONJUNCTION with the study of an organism of the spirochete type as the probable cause of yellow fever, it is of interest to review briefly the later classifications of this family of parasites. The group has been known for so short a time, and new forms are being added so constantly, that numerous changes will undoubtedly be necessary before a standard classification will be attained.

The spirochete originally described was a large organism, more closely allied to the vegetable or protozoal form of life, nonparasitic, living in fresh water. We agree with Noguchi and others who prefer to keep that name for that particular type of organism. Two other organisms belonging to the family of spirals are included in the classification, but they are much more closely allied both in size and habitat to the original spirochete as described. Of these, the latter cristispira, is parasitic in the alimentary canals of fish, while the saprospira is purely saprophytic. All other genera have pathogenic forms. The three first genera have then been included, as a help in the comparative differentiation of the pathogenic members of the group.

Spironema is the word used to designate the organisms more familiarly known as spirilla, while treponema is used for the generic name of organisms similar to the Treponema pallidum. This name was preferred even by Schaudin himself, to the more usual designation of spirochete.

The accompanying table of classification following Noguchi, is the best classification of the spiral organisms, with which we are acquainted.

It has many drawbacks. Former standards required that organisms presenting transverse division be classed as bacteria, while those dividing longitudinally be called protozoa. Such a standard would require the designation of the original spirochete the saprospira and critispira as bacteria, which they obviously are not. Again the presence of an undulatory membrane, or crista, would place the cristispira also among the protozoa. Finally the possibility of longitudinal fission would throw the spironemata and treponemata also into this class.

CLASSIFICATION OF SPIRAL ORGANISMS

GENUS		SPIROCHAETA ("COIL-HAIR")	SAPROSPIRA ("PUTRID-COIL")	CRISTISPIRA ("CRESTED COIL")	SPIRONEMA ("COIL-THREAD")	TREPONEMA ("TO TURN, THREAD")	LEPTOSPIRA ("FINE-COIL")
Measurements	Length	Microns—100 to 150	100 to 120	45 to 90	8 to 16	6 to 14	7 to 9 or 14
	Diameter	—Microns 0.5 to 0.75		1.0 to 1.5	0.35 to 0.5	0.25 to 0.3 Cylindrical	0.25 to 0.3
	Width of spiral	2				1.0 Regular Rigid	0.45 0.5
	Length of spiral	1.5 Regular				0.8 to 1.0 Very constant	0.3 Regular
Ends	Shape	Blunt		Blunt	Pointed	Pointed	Pointed
Waves	In addition to finer spirals	Several large, inconstant, irregular	Large, inconstant, shallow, irregular. 3 to 5 in number	Two to five or more Large, regular, shallow	Large, wavy spirals. usually five	One or more slight undulating wave.	One or more gently throughout entire length. One or both ends circularly hooked when in liquid media. Serpentine in semisolid media. Extremely flexible.
Axial Filaments		Present (flexible elastic)	Absent	Absent	Present (?)	Doubtful	Absent
Chambered Structure		Absent	Present	Present	Absent	Absent	Absent
Membrane		Absent	Present (flexible elastic)	Present (flexible elastic)	Delicate flexible double contoured	Doubtful	Absent
Terminal	Finely spiral filament	Absent	Absent	Absent	Present	Present	Not recognized
Flagella		Absent	Absent	Absent	Absent	Absent	Absent
End	Highly motile end portion	Absent	Absent	Absent	Absent	Absent	Well developed in last 6-8 spirals
Crista	Undulating membrane	Absent	Absent	Present ridge-like membrane spirally about body.	Absent	Absent	Absent
Division	Character	Transverse	Tranverse	Transverse	Transverse possibly also longitudinal	Transverse possibly also longitudinal.	Transverse
Habitat		Fresh or Marine water	Foraminiferous sand	Parasitic in alimentary canals of fish	Numerous pathogenic and non-pathogenic varieties.	Two pathogenic and several harmless parasites.	Two pathogenic and one possibly nonpathogenic varieties.
Action of Chemicals	Trypsin Digestion	Axial filament resistant		Membrane resistant Crista and chambers disappear.		Resists for many days.	
	Bile Salts 10%	Becomes shadowy, pale but is not dissolved.		Crista destroyed. Body not attached.	Complete disintegration.	Disintegration complete	Easily dissolved
	Saponin 10%	Lives 30 minutes, later becomes shadowy, pale but not dissolved.		Crista becomes fibrillar and then indistinct. Body not affected	Immobilized in thirty minutes. Broken up in a few hours.	Broken up in time.	Completely resistant.

Just as there are dogs and horses and cattle, so in the microscopic forms of life, there are numerous varieties which can not be compressed by an artificial nomenclature into one species. Disease may be caused by bacteria, by protozoa, by organisms corresponding to the spiral species, which we prefer to consider apart from both of the preceding, by vegetable parasites, and by organisms of the globoid body type. And the list is probably not yet completed.

—*W. T. V*

The Teaching of Preventive Medicine in Medical Schools

THE national board of medical examiners which examines graduates of only our best medical schools after at least one year of hospital service finds practically all the candidates who come before the board lacking grossly in their knowledge of preventive medicine. This is because of the fact that they have had no adequate instruction along this line. The whole curriculum of our medical schools is devoted to curative medicine, and no adequate instruction is given in the prevention of disease. Early in the war the Surgeon General authorized one of his assistants to select and place in each camp and with each division a competent epidemiologist. A few medical men who had served as health officers of cities were found to be qualified for this position, but the rank and file of the medical profession did not know the A B C of preventive medicine. Very few knew how to compute an annual death rate, and the ignorance concerning the methods of tracing infection and preventing its spread was appalling. It was necessary to turn over the whole question of water supply and its purification to sanitary engineers, and, with a few exceptions mentioned above, members of the engineering profession supplied the best epidemiologists. We are not complaining; we are simply stating facts. It is probably right that the medical school should devote its chief attention to curative medicine. But we must face the facts and determine whether or not the practice of preventive medicine is to be assumed by some other profession. In most of our medical schools the chair of bacteriology is combined with that of pathology, and all attention is centered on the lesions produced by bacteria, and but little thought given to the control and limitation of infectious diseases. Preventive medicine is coming more and more rapidly to the front. The commissioner of health in the state of Ohio is seeking a competent health officer for each county in the state. Will he be able to find these men in the medical profession, and if found, will they demonstrate their fitness? We must recognize the fact that our medical schools do not fit their students for the practice of preventive medicine, and this must be made a specialty to be acquired by the pursuit of specially arranged courses extending for one or two years after graduation in medicine.

—V. C. V

Sir William Osler

THE cable brings us the sad news that Sir William Osler died at his home, Oxford, England, December 29. Last November Dr. Osler was stricken with pneumonia, but about the middle of that month it was reported that he was convalescing favorably. Then came more doubtful reports, but these left a ray of hope. On Christmas day he cabled his greetings to his old friends at the Johns Hopkins Hospital and announced that he was making a good fight after an operation for empyema. The cable, however, announces his death.

William Osler was the sixth son of an English clergyman and was born in Canada. He had his education at Trinity College, the University of Toronto and McGill University. After graduation he spent some time in Europe and became a member of the faculty of McGill University. Later he was called to the Professorship of Medicine in the University of Pennsylvania. When the medical school of John Hopkins University was organized about 1880 the board of trustees with great wisdom selected three eminent men to determine the destinies of that school. These three men were Osler, Welsh, and Halsted. This is not the place to dwell upon the great service that these men have rendered to American medicine. We must content ourselves with noting that each became the most potent factor in the scientific development of his specialty.

Dr. Osler represented a distinguished family; distinguished for strength of character, thoroughness in work, and the highest ideals. One of his brothers became a great financier and played an important part in the economic and financial development of Canada. This brother was knighted in 1912. Another brother became a member of the Supreme Court of Ontario and was noted for his wisdom and justice. A third brother for many years was one of the most distinguished members of the Canadian bar.

Every medical student in this country and Canada who has pursued his studies during the past forty years has had close association, intellectually if not personally, with Doctor Osler. His work on the practice of medicine in the various editions in which it has appeared, has had more influence upon the physicians of this country than any other book. In excellent and classical English he has initiated thousands of young men into the mysteries of disease and pathology. Doctor Osler was a close, keen, and accurate observer. He kept records of all his cases and was able to speak at all times and about all diseases with the certainty of one who had seen for himself. Doctor Osler is dead. This will be said thousands of times and always with the deepest regret. But his spirit and his work will long remain bright and shining lights to guide. not only those who are now living, but those who are to be born in the path of scientific medicine.

Doctor Osler's only son, an officer in the English artillery, was killed in France. The grief which this death caused bore heavily upon the distinguished father, but his home in Oxford was always open to medical men from this country. He assisted young and old medical officers from this side who went over early or late to give their service in the great emergency. His house was a Mecca to which all American medical officers traveled with deepest reverence and where they found a cheerful welcome and an ever ready helping hand.

The world has lost a great man. In Canada, England and the United States his death will be universally mourned. He was known not only to the medical profession, but to the educated world at large.

—*V. C V.*

Spirochetes

IT is only very recently that we have obtained anything like a satisfactory understanding and a classification of those interesting parasitic microorganisms generally classified under the name of Spirochetes. The very nature of spirochetes, whether animal or vegetable, has been the subject of continued discussion. Originally regarded as plant forms, they were subsequently considered in certain of their examples as animal parasites, but the consensus of opinion today would seem to place them as intermediate between the two, and more in the nature of plant than animal. (Chandler.[1])

The reasons for regarding spirochetes as more like bacteria than protozoa rests on the fact that they have no nucleus, that they divide by transverse division, and show no evidence of a sexual process. The less weighty arguments that have been offered for regarding them as protozoa are that some of their members have a crista-like membrane which suggests the undulating membrane of the trypanosomes, that they stain with difficulty, as do many of the protozoa, and that they frequently require insect intermediate hosts for their transmission.

[1]Chandler, Asa C.: Animal Parasites and Human Disease, 1918, John Wiley & Sons, New York.

Owing to the difficulty in cultivating spirochetes, of studying them in their living condition, and often of staining them in a satisfactory manner, much confusion has arisen as to the varieties that may be legitimately made in these interesting microorganisms. Noguchi[2] recently has suggested the first comprehensive and apparently thoroughly satisfactory classification of spirochetes. He divides them into six different genera—Spirochæta, Saprospira, Cristispira, Spironema, Treponema, and Leptospira. Of these groups the first three are of no particular pathogenic significance.

The first organism of the spirocheta group was the first spirochete to be described and was due to Ehrenberg in 1838. Several species of this genus have since been found in salt and fresh water and are characterizd by their considerable length (100 to 500 micra), by the fact that they have no membrane, that they contain plasmic spirals and volutin granules. Thesè characteristics, as indeed those of the subsequent genera to be mentioned, are far better visualized in Noguchi's admirable diagrammatic representations, than understood by mere descriptive terms.

Members of the saprospira group were described first by Gross in 1911. They are also long forms, though not so long as the spirocheta, and have a chambered structure. They occur in sand.

The cristispira group, also described by Gross (1910), is exemplified in the Cristispira balbiani, an inhabitant of the crystalline style of shell fish.

Numerous members of the next, or spironema genus are of pathogenic significance. They are small, (8 to 16 micra) twisted microorganisms with a permanent spiral filament and include many organisms that are the causative agents of the different forms of recurrent fever in man, formerly referred to as the Spirochetes of Obermeyer, etc. Among them may be mentioned *Spironema recurrentis, S. carteri, S. duttoni* and the like.

The spironema group may be easily separated from the treponema group in typical examples according to Noguchi. The treponemata as first described by Schaudinn (1905) in connection with the causative agent of syphilis are somewhat shorter (6 to 14 micra) than the spironema organisms, and are characterized by pointed ends, a spiral filament and regular and rigid spirals. The causative agent of syphilis (*Treponema pallidum*) and of yaws (*Tr. pertenue*) would be placed in this group, as well as certain nonpathogenic members of the group, like Tr. microdentium and Tr. macrodentium.

Last of all comes the genus newly differentiated by Noguchi (1917) of Leptospira. These organisms have pointed and hooked ends, a corkscrew-like appearance, and differ from other spirochetes in that they are very resistant to the action of saponin. Their locomotion, which is extremely active, differs somewhat in nature from the other varieties. The most important members of this genus that have hitherto been described are the leptospira of ichtero-hemorrhagic fever (L. icterohemorrhagiæ) and the recently described Leptospira icteroides which is regarded by Noguchi as a causative agent in yellow fever.

—*F. P. G.*

[2]Noguchi, H.: Morphological Characteristics and Nomenclature of *Leptospira (Spirochaeta) Ictero-haemorrhagiae* (Inada and Ido), Jour. Exper. Med., 1918, xxvii, 575.

The Journal of ·
Laboratory and Clinical
Medicine

| Vol. V. | St. Louis, February, 1920 | No. 5 |

ORIGINAL ARTICLES

BACTERIOLOGY AND PATHOLOGY IN SIX CASES OF ENCEPHALITIS LETHARGICA*

By P. F. Morse, M.D., and E. S. Crump, M.D., Detroit, Mich.

THIS report is based on material from six cases of 'Lethargic Encephalitis" coming to autopsy within seven days of one another. They represent the fatal portion of a larger series of cases which will be reported from the clinical standpoint by Freund, Lockwood, and Crump.

BACTERIOLOGIC PART

Isolation and Growth Characteristics of Organism.—Cultures were obtained at autopsy using the following technic. The brain was removed from the cranium and placed, vertex upward, on a dissecting board. The posterior horns of the lateral ventricles were opened under aseptic precautions by an incision through the after part of the cerebrum. Fluid was aspirated with a sterile pipette and planted on bouillon and several loops of material were taken with a platinum loop and planted on agar, blood serum, human blood agar, Kligler's medium and gelatin.

In 24 hours the bouillon was very cloudy, showing a diffuse growth and some precipitate, but no evidence of stalactite or pellicle formation. There was practically no odor to the culture. The colonies on the agar slants were small and discrete with well-defined borders slightly raised from the surface, glistening and yellowish white in color.

On Kligler's lead acetate modification of Russel's triple sugar medium the colonies were similar in morphology, faintly pink in color, with diffuse reddening of the medium. No gas and no browning of stab was noted.

---

*From the Buhl Memorial Laboratory, Harper Hospital, Detroit, Mich.

On blood serum the colonies were similar, but showed some digestion of the surrounding medium.

The glucose agar stab grew well throughout its length and was villous in character, without gas formation.

On human blood agar the growth is at first slight as noted by a few isolated colonies surrounded by a brown zone. Some of the primary cultures on human blood agar showed no growth at all, but subcultures grow well.

Gelatin stab cultures incubated at room temperature for 24 hours show finely villous growth throughout length of stab without liquefaction.

Transplants were made in xylose, saccharose, lactose, dextrose, salicin, mannite and plain bouillon with fermentation tubes and brom-cresol-purple as indicator. Fermentation took place in tubes containing lactose and dextrose with acid formation in twenty-four hours. There was slow and feeble fermentation with acid formation in saccharose. No gas formation took place in any of the tubes. The bouillon culture is not soluble in bile.

The growth, when removed from an agar slant, is mucoid in character, spreads freely on dry glass, has a tendency to agglutinate spontaneously when mixed with saline, and is then difficult to break up.

The organism is a nonmotile coccus, small in young cultures, as large as a staphylococcus in old cultures, with a tendency to grow in diplo and tetrad forms and to bunch in small clusters. It divides similarly to a staphylococcus in three planes, stains readily with the aniline dyes, and is Gram-positive.

Pure cultures were obtained from six consecutive autopsies, the organism found being identical in each case.

Agglutination.—Sera were obtained from two convalescent and three cases still at the height of the disease.

The two convalescent cases showed partial but incomplete agglutination in dilutions up to 1:40, but the agglutination was not complete in any dilution.

Of the three sick cases, one, who is still sick and will probably die, agglutinates the organism completely at 1:50 and partially at 1:100. The other two sick cases showed partial agglutination in dilutions of one to ten.

Control experiments with the serum of normal persons did not show agglutination.

ANIMAL EXPERIMENTS

EXPERIMENT I.—*To determine pathogenicity of the organism for rabbits.* A full grown rabbit was injected subdurally with 1 c.c. of a 24-hour bouillon culture under general anesthesia and aseptic precautions. Recovery from the operative procedure was prompt, and the animal was apparently well six hours later. The next morning the head was extended on the spine, the hind legs flaccid, and the forelegs showed continuous tremors. The respiration was slow but regular and rhythmical. It was very restless, shifting and throwing itself about the cage in an aimless manner. Active stimulation, such as a loud noise or jar, partially aroused the animal and caused it to make incoordinate movements with forelegs and head. These symptoms continued for two days, after which time it became quieter, and the respirations slower and more shallow. These symptoms progressed until its death, six days after injection. The autopsy showed no exudate on the meninges or base of the brain. The findings were similar to the findings observed in the human cases. The brain cortex was cherry red and there was passive congestion of the vessels of the pia and cerebrum. Cultures were taken of the posterior horns of the ventricles by searing the sur-

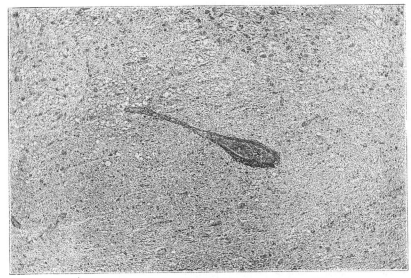

Fig. 1.—Perivascular infiltration. Blood vessel in the upper portion of the pons.

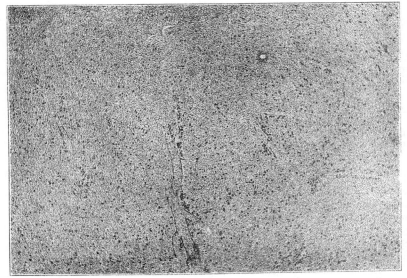

Fig. 2.—Small arterioles of the centrum semiovale showing perivascular collections of round cells.

face with a hot spatula and plunging a platinum loop into the brain. The organism was recovered in pure culture and found to be identical with the one injected.

EXPERIMENT II.—*To determine whether the organism was pathogenic by the intravenous route.* A full grown rabbit received 2 c.c. intravenously of the same culture as was used for Experiment I. No effects were noted, and at present, twelve days later, the animal is normal.

EXPERIMENT III.—*To determine the pathogenicity of the filtered culture.* The bouillon culture used for experiments one and two was allowed to grow five days. It was then filtered through a water-dammed Berkefeld "N" filter with a negative pressure of one-half atmosphere. One c.c. of this filtrate was used for subdural injection. The rest of the filtrate was incubated and also subcultures from it were incubated to determine its sterility. Both the original filtrate and the subcultures on all media· including bouillon are still sterile. One c.c. of the .five-day bouillon culture filtrate was injected subdurally in a full grown rabbit. There was immediate primary recovery from the operation, which was done about 6 P. M. The following morning the rabbit was in the typical lethargic state with symptoms exactly similar to those of the animal in Experiment I. This animal lived four days, and at autopsy showed intense injection of the meninges, brain edema, but no purulent exudate. Cultures were made by the same technic as in Experiment I and were all sterile. Intravenous injection of three c.c. of the bouillon culture filtrate in another animal produced no effect, and one c.c. intraperitoneally in a guinea pig was without result.

This result in Experiment III raised the question as to whether the pathologic effect was due to a toxin generated by the organism or to a filterable virus, as Loewe and Straus[3] believe, or to the bouillon itself. Certain manifestations of the disease clinically, as well as the fact that a purulent exudate was never found, either in the human autopsies or in the animal experiments, strongly suggested the toxin or filterable virus idea. It was evident that if a filterable virus was present it grew well in bouillon, therefore, the bouillon filtrate transplants in bouillon could be used to determine this point. The following experiments were therefore carried out.

EXPERIMENT IV.—*Bouillon control.* Two c.c. of sterile bouillon of the same batch as that so far used for cultures was injected subdurally. No effects were noted. The animal remained entirely normal.

EXPERIMENT V.—*Injection of the bouillon subcultures from Berkefeld filtrate.* Two c.c. of the bouillon subcultures from the primary toxic filtrate were injected subdurally as in the previous experiments. No effects resulted, and the rabbit remained well. As before noted, these cultures were morphologically sterile and the toxic effect of the primary culture was removed by .the dilution incident to subculturing.

Of course, another possibility remains that a filterable virus might still be present which would not grow except in symbiosis with the other organism and also that the organism itself might have a filterable stage in its development with unknown conditions for propagation. We leave this question as speculative and not subject to experimental elucidation.

Four attempts were made to grow the organism directly from the spinal fluid obtained at lumbar puncture without a success. One c.c. of spinal fluid from a sick case injected subdurally in a rabbit was without result. The search for the organism in smears of the sedimented spinal fluid has been negative. In smears from the ventricular fluid at autopsy there were found coccus-like bodies which could not be definitely diagnosed as the organism. In this connection it should

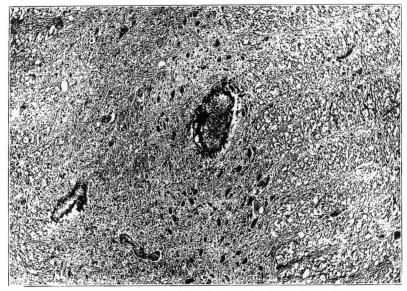

Fig. 3.—Vessel of the formatio reticularis in the region of the nucleus ambiguus.

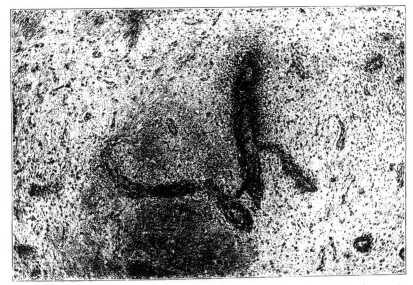

Fig. 4.—Thalamic region. Unusually intense lesion with multiple miliary hemorrhages and intense perivascular infiltration.

be remembered that the localization of the disease seems to be entirely cerebral and in the brain stem, and as the pathologic study shows, especially of the white matter of the basal ganglia and pons. To get the cultures from the posterior horns, several loopfuls were planted on each tube or several drops of spinal fluid from a sterile pipette dropped into bouillon. Even then in one of our cases only one colony was found on two tubes and none on the other tubes. The organism probably inhabits the perivascular spaces of the deeper portions of the brain, and the cultures and intravenous injections show that it probably does not grow well in body fluids.

SUMMARY OF BACTERIOLOGICAL FINDINGS

1. A staphylococcus-like organism has been isolated in primary pure cultures from six consecutive cases dying of encephalitis lethargica.

2. This organism when injected subdurally produces a fatal lethargic state in rabbits and the organism is recovered from the brain in pure culture.

3. The filtered culture contains a poison which produces a fatal lethargic state in rabbits.

4. Evidence is offered in favor of this effect being due to a poison (toxin?) generated by the growth of the organism rather than by a filterable virus.

5. Controls are reported to show that the lethargic state in animals was not due to the bouillon used for injection.

6. Agglutination experiments with patients' serum both in recovered and in sick cases are not productive of definite results, but are strongly suggestive.

In the August, 1919, number of this JOURNAL, C. M. Stafford[1] describes an organism obtained by spinal puncture of a lethargic patient which answers the same general description as the one we have isolated. Stafford's organism was nonpathogenic for rabbits intraspinously.

AUTOPSY FINDINGS

The autopsies were performed from one and one-half to three hours after death.

A summary of all the gross and microscopic findings will describe the pathologic picture better than to take up the individual protocols in detail. The intensity and distribution of the lesions varied somewhat and will be noted.

No abnormal external appearances of note are found. The scalp and tissues over the calvarium are normal. On removing the skull-cap there are no bone lesions. The dura is not adherent, and is white and glistening. The superior longitudinal sinus is empty. Upon removal of the dura we find the brain substance much redder than usual, due to the marked overfilling of the fine capillaries of the cortex. The pia is quite cloudy and looks thick and opalescent due to a marked edema of the leptomeninges. The superficial veins are distended. There are no gross hemorrhages, except very fine pin-point spots here and there on the cortical surface surrounding a tiny vessel.

The fluid in the cranial cavity is not usually increased, and the fluid in the ventricles is not much greater in amount than normal. The brain substance itself gives a definite impression of being moister than normal and has a dough-like character.

On section all the vessels of the brain substance are found to be engorged and bleed freely from the cut ends. The spinal cord presents the same picture of congestion and distended venules, and, when handled with forceps, is definitely dough-like and soft.

The other organs of the body presented no changes of importance. In one case there was a terminal lobular pneumonia in an early stage of development. This case also had areas of focal necrosis in the liver. These areas were invaded by wandering cells and resembled closely those found in typhoid fever. The other cases did not show these areas and they are possibly due to intensive treatment with arsphenamine that this man at first received under the impression that he was suffering from cerebrospinal syphilis. The gastrointestinal tract and urinary tracts are normal. The heart has been normal in each case, and the lungs have showed occasional healed tubercles but were otherwise normal except for the case of terminal lobular pneumonia. One case had a pregnancy of about three weeks in utero. The sinuses in each case were thoroughly explored with negative results in all.

THE BRAIN LESIONS

Material was removed from the frontal, paracentral, calcarine, and hippo-campal gyri, from the basal ganglia, thalamus, pons and medulla and cerebellum and fixed in formol, Zenker's, Cajal fluid and alcohol and stained by various methods.

The findings can best be classified according to location in meninges, cortex, basal ganglia, pons, medulla, and cord.

The meningeal findings are very characteristic and consist of marked edema of the pia and a moderate infiltration with wandering cells of different types. Neither the edema nor the infiltration is uniform in the leptomeninges, but is present in an irregular patchy manner. As in other meningeal inflammations, the findings are especially intense between the convolutions and the edema, and exudate dips down into the sulci.

The wandering cells consist of lymphocytes and plasma cells with large mononuclears scattered here and there. The infiltrating cells are usually scattered loosely through the edematous pia and do not tend to collect in dense foci except occasionally at the side of a vessel. The disease seems to stimulate a definite though feeble increase of the connective tissue, since young fibroblasts are present in the edematous infiltrated areas in increased numbers. The disease process in the affected areas of pia when dipping down into a sulcus are apparently definitely in relation to the perivascularly infiltrated vessels of the underlying cortical white matter.

The striking characteristic of the meningeal lesion is its apparent mildness.

The cortex: Some writers[2] have laid stress on the degenerative changes noted in the cortical pyramidal cells. Although Calhoun[3] lays more stress on the changes in the white matter at the base, Wegeforth and Ayer[4] found no changes of importance in the cortex. So far as our examinations go, we are impressed with exactly the opposite picture. Taking the gray matter of the cortex as a whole, only occasionally is a cell found definitely degenerated. We are making the study of the finer changes in cell structure by special methods, a matter of a separate report, but judged from the work so far done, we believe that the degenerative changes in the cortex pyramidal cells are slight and unimportant. The tigroid substance is well seen for the most part. Only very rarely is a definite "satellitosis" and "neurophagia" seen and the blood vessels of the cortex, except occasionally in the white matter beneath a sulcus, are free from the characteristic perivascular infiltration so characteristic of the white matter of the basal portions of the brain. In the face of the very definite, and even destructive lesions of the lower portions of the brain, it seems to us unreasonable to ascribe undue importance to slight changes in the cortical pyramidal cells when many fields must be searched to find a degenerating cell. The cells of the gray matter of the cortex do not seem to us to show greater changes than cases of uremia or diabetes dying in coma. The white matter of the cortex and of the centrum semiovale shows an occasional small vessel with perivascular infiltration.

The basal ganglia: The changes in the basal ganglia, the caudate and lenticulate nucleus and the thalamus, are marked and consist of intense perivascular infiltration and perivascular edema of the white matter. Here again the lesion is essentially interstitial. The vessels of the white matter are involved and the ganglionic areas lying contiguous to the involved areas are affected secondarily by edema and occasionally by the margin of a small hemorrhage. The changes are in most cases most intense in the thalamus.

Pons and medulla and cord: Throughout the extent of the pons and medulla, the characteristic lesion is the perivascular infiltration of the white matter accompanied by edema and an occasional miliary hemorrhage. As we pass down the cord, the changes become less intense and in the cervical cord only an occasional vessel of the posterior horn is found infiltrated.

The pathologic findings may be summed up as follows:

1. Low grade leptomeningitis with edema and moderate round-cell infiltration.

2. Perivascular infiltration of the vessels of the white matter, especially of the caudate and lenticulate nuclei, optic thalamus, pons, medulla, and posterior horns of the cord with resulting edema and miliary hemorrhages of surrounding parts.

CLINICAL SIGNIFICANCE OF THE LESIONS

It seems to us that an *a priori* opinion could be arrived at regarding the essential nature of the lesion from a consideration of the clinical symptoms. In the first place the fact that, in spite of a profound lethargic state lasting over weeks, the patient is often restored to normal speaks decidedly against any extensive parenchymatous brain lesion. Degenerated brain cells that could be diagnosed by "neurophagia" etc., probably do not recover even if the patient lives, and we can not explain the return to normal on the basis of a destructive, degenerative lesion of the gray matter. The few degenerations found are probably due to edema and to injury of the nerve fiber as it passed outward through one of the

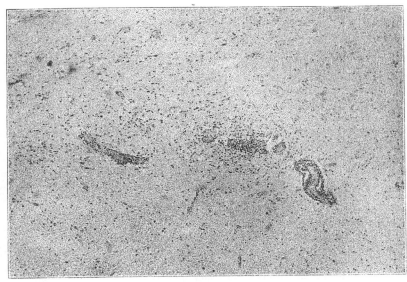

Fig. 5.—Infiltrated vessels on the posterior horn of the cervical cord.

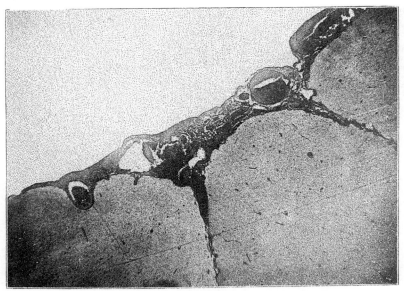

Fig. 6.—Low power of cortex showing engorgement and rupture of pial veins.

involved areas lower down. Much might be said for this point of view as to the relative unimportance of the degenerative lesions of the Betz cells by an analysis of the mental state of the patients, but this question is more properly discussed in a clinical paper.

The involvement of the cranial nerves, probably the most constant single clinical manifestation of the disease is evidently due to the close admixture of white and gray matter in the pons and medulla. This point is well illustrated by the photographs which show areas of severely involved white matter contiguous to cranial nerve nuclei. We have been interested in the fact that we never find involvement of the motor cells of the anterior horn, but frequently find the vessels supplying the posterior root in the cord markedly affected. This finding correlates well with the fact that although the reflexes are frequently lost at the height of the disease, paralysis is not present. This finding, both pathologically and clinically, sharply distinguishes this affection from Heine-Medin disease.

In short "encephalitis lethargica" is not a true encephalitis in the sense that we speak of general paresis or the cerebral form of poliomyelitis as examples of encephalitis, because ganglion cell and pyramidal cell destruction does not characterize lethargic cases. But we are dealing here with a typical example of low grade "meningomyelitis" the characteristic lesions being in the meninges and white matter of the basal ganglia, pons, and upper cord. It has come to our attention through Dr. Camp of the University of Michigan that Marie in 1890 described cases similar to "encephalitis lethargica" and called them "acute multiple sclerosis." From a pathologic, as well as clinical, point of view, this term has much to justify its use.

BIBLIOGRAPHY

[1]Stafford, C. M.: Jour. Lab. and Clin. Med., iv, No. 11.
[2]Bassoe and Hassin: Arch. Neurol. and Psychiat., ii, 24.
[3]Calhoun, Henrietta A.: Ibid., iii. p. 1.
[4]Wegeforth and Ayer: Jour. Am. Med. Assn., lxxiii., 5.
[5]Loewe and Strauss: Ibid., lxxiii, 1056.

PROTEIN FEVER
THE EFFECT OF EGG WHITE INJECTION ON THE DOG*

By Seymour J. Cohen, Chicago, Ill.

SPEAKING of his theory of fever, Victor C. Vaughan[1] and his coworkers reported some time ago that "It occurred to us, that if the above given ideas be correct, we should be able to induce in animals a continued fever by repeated subcutaneous injections of a soluble protein. We have done this with bacterial proteins, but since vitalistic dogmas cling so closely, we intend to present herewith an illustration of the result that we have obtained by repeated subcutaneous injections of egg white dilutions in rabbits * * * *

"We think that these investigations show that fever results when a foreign protein is introduced into the blood. This foreign protein is not necessarily of bacterial origin, though under natural conditions this is usually the case in continued fevers."

In other words, these investigators conclude that repeated subcutaneous injections of a protein into animals produce a fever which is similar to the temperature curve found in typhoid fever. Friedberger[2] in 1910 while working on the relation between anaphylaxis and injection, also came to the same conclusion, that repeated parenteral injections of a protein produce a continued fever. Both of these investigators were able at will to produce a continued, intermittent or remittent fever, by varying the frequency and size of the injections.

This idea of the production of fever by parenteral injection of protein is not a new one. Roques, Gamallia, Charrin and Ruffer, Buchner, Krehl and Matthews and a score of other investigators have shown that parenteral injections of a foreign protein, bacterial or nonbacterial, may produce fever.

So far as could be determined, most of these former investigators did their work on either rabbits or guinea pigs. This present investigation was undertaken to review some of the earlier work but chiefly to determine the effect of parenteral injections of protein on larger animals, namely, the dog.

I. THE EFFECT OF EGG WHITE INJECTIONS ON THE GUINEA PIG

The same method was used as was described by Vaughan. A series of guinea pigs was weighed. A normal temperature was recorded for 10 days, then 2 c.c. of diluted egg white (one part egg white to one part .5 per cent phenol) were injected subcutaneously every 2 hours, over a period of 10 hours for 6 days. During this period the guinea pigs received a total of 60 c.c. of diluted egg white, injected 5 times a day. By examining Tables I and II and Figs. 1 and 2, it will be noted that the normal temperature of guinea pig I during the 10 days, varied between 97.3° and 100.1° and guinea pig II, between 98° and 100.7°. After the injection of the protein, the temperature began to rise on the second day and reached its maximum of 104.5° and 104.3,° respectively, on the sixth day, when

*From the Laboratory of Pharmacology, University of Illinois, College of Medicine, Chicago, Ill.

the injections were stopped; after which the temperature gradually fell to normal. The animals themselves, showed all the signs of infection, during the high temperature. They were inactive and quiet; and remained in the corner of the cage huddled together. They did not eat much and consequently lost weight.

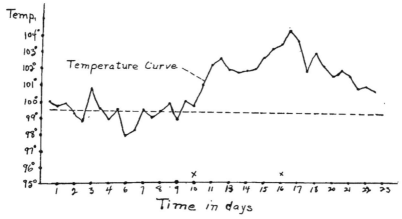

Fig. 1.—Showing the effect of subcutaneous injection of egg white on the temperature curve of Guinea Pig A.
X, injection begun; X, injections stopped.

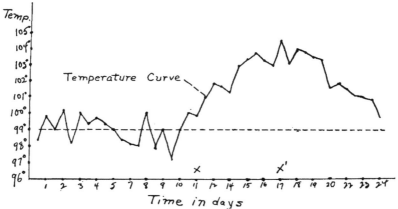

Fig. 2.—Showing the effect of subcutaneous injection of egg white on the temperature curve of Guinea Pig B.
X, injection begun; X', injections stopped.

These results agree quite uniformly with those of the previous investigators, that parenteral injection of protein in guinea pigs, at least, produces a continued fever.

II. THE EFFECT OF EGG WHITE INJECTIONS ON THE DOG

The injections of foreign protein into dogs were carried out along the same lines as those in the guinea pigs. A series of animals was prepared. Each animal was weighed and the urine examined before the experiment was begun. At

TABLE I

SUMMARY OF EXPERIMENT 1 SHOWING THE EFFECT OF SUBCUTANEOUS INJECTIONS OF EGG WHITE IN GUINEA PIG A

| DATE | TEMPERATURE AND INJECTIONS | | | | | WEIGHT |
	9:00	11:00	1:00	3:00	5:00	
5/14	100.0°				99.7°	370 gms.
5/15	99.8				99.4	
5/16	98.8				100.8	
5/17	99.6				99.8	
5/18						
5/19	99.6				98.	356 gms.
5/20	98.4				99.6	
5/21	99.2				99.5	
5/22	100.				99.0	
5/23	100.1				99.9	
	2 c.c.	2 c.c.	2 c.c.	2 c.c.	2 c.c.	
5/24	101.1				102.3	
	2 c.c.	2 c.c.	2 c.c.	2 c.c.	2 c.c.	
5/25						
5/26	102.7				102.	355 gms.
	2 c.c.	2 c.c.	2 c.c.	2 c.c.	2 c.c.	
5/27	102.8				102.0	
	2 c.c.	2 c.c.	2 c.c.	2 c.c.	2 c.c.	
5/28	102.4				102.8	
	2 c.c.	2 c.c.	2 c.c.	2 c.c.	2 c.c.	
5/29	103.4				103.6	
	2 c.c.	2 c.c.	2 c.c.	2 c.c.	2 c.c.	
5/30	104.0				103.4	
	2 c.c.	2 c.c.	2 c.c.	2 c.c.	2 c.c.	
5/31	102.0				102.1	
6/1						
6/2	102.3				101.7	352 gms.
6/3	102.1				101.8	
6/4	102.0				101.	
6/5	101.3				100.	

TABLE II

SUMMARY OF EXPERIMENT 2 SHOWING THE EFFECT OF SUBCUTANEOUS INJECTIONS OF EGG WHITE IN GUINEA PIG B

| DATE | TEMPERATURE AND INJECTIONS | | | | | WEIGHT |
	9:00	11.00	1:00	3:00	5:00	
3/14	99.0°				100.1°	335 gms.
5/15	98.2				100.4	
5/16	99.4				99.6	
5/17	99.4				99.2	
5/18						
5/19	98.4				98.1	325 gms.
5/20	98.				100.2	
5/21	97.8				99.	
5/22	97.2				99.	
5/23	100.0				99.8	
	2 c.c.	2 c.c.	2 c.c.	2 c.c.	2 c.c.	
5/24	101.				101.8	
	2 c.c.	2 c.c.	2 c.c.	2 c.c.	2 c.c.	
5/25						
5/26	101.6				101.3	305 gms.
	2 c.c.	2 c.c.	2 c.c.	2 c.c.	2 c.c.	
5/27	103.				103.4	
	2 c.c.	2 c.c.	2 c.c.	2 c.c.	2 c.c.	
5/28	103.7				103.3	
	2 c.c.	2 c.c.	2 c.c.	2 c.c.	2 c.c.	
5/29	103.1				104.5	
	2 c.c.	2 c.c.	2 c.c.	2 c.c.	2 c.c.	
5/30	103.1				104.0	
	2 c.c.	2 c.c.	2 c.c.	2 c.c.	2 c.c.	
5/31	103.8				103.5	
6/1						
6/2	103.4				101.6	302 gms.
6/3	101.9				101.5	
6/4	101.1				101.	
6/5	100.9				99.8	

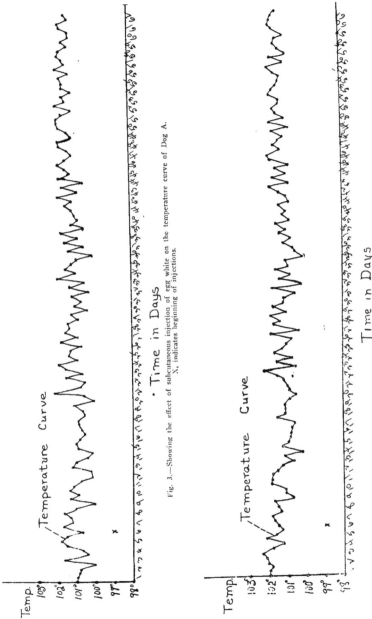

Fig. 3.—Showing the effect of subcutaneous injection of egg white on the temperature curve of Dog A.
X, indicates beginning of injections.

Fig. 4.—Showing the effect of subcutaneous injection of egg white on the temperature curve of Dog B.
X, indicates beginning of injections.

the end of each week the dog was weighed and the urine reexamined, making in all 10 determinations.

Results.—As practically all the animals reacted in the same way, only results on two dogs will be described.

Dog I.—*Black and white spotted female dog, weight 7 kilos. Urine negative, contains no sugar or albumin.* A normal temperature was taken for 5 days, averaging about 101°. Then 3 c.c. of diluted egg white were injected subcutaneously 3 times a day for 3 days. This was followed by injection of 5 c.c. 4 times a day for 12 days. Then 8 c.c. were injected 5 times a day for 6 days. This was finally followed by injections of 10 c.c. of diluted protein 5 times a day for 36 days. This made a total of over 2300 c.c. of diluted egg white injected 4 and 5 times a day for a period of 57 days. By examining Chart 3 and Figure 3, it will be noticed that the temperature did not vary any more during the injections than before the injections. The temperature during the injection varied between 100° and 102.4°. As the normal temperature for this animal was around 101°, this variation can not be called fever. In addition it will be observed that the urine was always free from albumin and sugar except at one time, when there was a trace of albumin present. This animal gained in weight from 7 kilos to 8.1 kilos.

Dog. II.—*Brown female dog, weight 5.1 kilos. Urine negative.* A normal temperature was taken for 5 days averaging about 101.5°. The diluted egg white was injected subcutaneously in the same way as in the first animal. This animal also received over 2300 c.c. of diluted egg white, injected 4 and 5 times a day for a period of 57 days.

By examining Chart 4 and Figure 4, it will be seen that the temperature is practically uniform and analogous to the temperature curve of the first animal. In this case the temperature varied from 100.3° to 102.4°. This also can not be considered fever, when the average temperature of the animal before the injections was about 101.5°. The urine of this animal was at all times free from albumin or sugar. This animal gained in weight from 5.1 kilos to 6.3 kilos. The animals were not injected nor the temperature recorded on Sunday. At no time during the injections did the animals appear to be sick. They were always active and barking. The stools were well formed. There was never any diarrhea or any vomiting. During all these injections only one abscess developed, which lasted only a few days. Dog A is still alive and in good health at the present time, one year after the last injection. Dog B was also in good health several months after the last injection, when he was used for some crucial experiment.

These results on the series of dogs are practically identical and uniform with each other, but are so strikingly opposite from those obtained on the guinea pigs, that they deserved some consideration and discussion. Injections of egg white solutions (foreign proteins) produce no effect on the temperature curve of the dog. This is a fact. The egg white is absorbed from the place of injections, because the lump disappears in a few minutes. If the egg white injections were not absorbed, but became encapsulated and underwent fibrous changes; then the back of the dog should be nodular due to so many hundred injections, but this was not the case. The back of the animal, a few hours after the last injection, was as smooth and level as before the injections were begun.

The idea that the egg white in the dog is excreted without being broken down can be disproved by the fact that the urine in all cases was free from albumin. If the egg white was excreted by the bowel, it seems that there might be some intestinal disturbance, either a diarrhea or a severe constipation, but neither of these factors were present. The injected egg white was absorbed and must have been broken down in the tissue without producing any effect on the general constitution of the animal, chiefly a rise in temperature.

TABLE III

SUMMARY OF EXPERIMENT 3 SHOWING THE EFFECT OF SUBCUTANEOUS INJECTIONS OF EGG WHITE IN DOG A

DATE	INJECTIONS AND TEMPERATURE					WEIGHT		URINE
	9:00	11:00	1:00	3:00	5:00			
2/8	101.0°				100.8°	7	K	no albumin no sugar
2/9	100.8				100.0			
2/10								
2/11	101.6				100.4	7.3	K	no albumin no sugar
2/12	100.6				101.5			
2/13	101.8				101.5			
2/14	100.6		100.8°		101.7			
	3 c.c.		3 c.c.		3 c.c.			
2/15	101.2		101.5		101.3			
	3 c.c.		3 c.c.		3 c.c.			
2/16	101.6		101.8		101.0			
	3 c.c.		3 c.c.		3 c.c.			
2/17								
2/18	100.0	100.1°	100.4	101.3°		7.6	K	no albumin no sugar
	5 c.c.	5 c.c.	5 c.c.	5 c.c.				
2/19	100.9	100.3	100.5	101.3				
	5 c.c.	5 c.c.	5 c.c.	5 c.c.				
2/20	101.1	101.3	100.9	100.6				
	5 c.c.	5 c.c.	5 c.c.	5 c.c.				
2/21	100.1	100.5	101.0	100.2				
	5 c.c.	5 c.c.	5 c.c.	5 c.c.				
2/22	101.2	100.9	100.7	101.0				
	5 c.c.	5 c.c.	5 c.c.	5 c.c.				
2/23	100.4	100.9	100.5	100.1				
	5 c.c.	5 c.c.	5 c.c.	5 c.c.				
2/24								no albumin no sugar
2/25	100.9	100.5	100.3	101.0		7.5	K	
	5 c.c.	5 c.c.	5 c.c.	5 c.c.				
2/26	100.8	101.0	100.9	100.5				
	5 c.c.	5 c.c.	5 c.c.	5 c.c.				
2/27	100.7	101.0	100.9	100.8				
	5 c.c.	5 c.c.	5 c.c.	5 c.c.				
2/28	100.9	101.0	101.2	100.5				
	5 c.c.	5 c.c.	5 c.c.	5 c.c.				
3/1	100.7	100.9	101.0	101.1				
	5 c.c.	5 c.c.	5 c.c.	5 c.c.				
3/2	100.0	100.6	100.7	100.5				
	5 c.c.	5 c.c.	5 c.c.	5 c.c.				
3/3								no albumin no sugar
3/4	102.1	101.9	101.8	101.6	100.7	7.8	K	
	8 c.c.	8 c.c.	8 c.c.	8 c.c.	8 c.c.			
3/5	100.5	100.7	101.0	101.6	101.5			
	8 c.c.	8 c.c.	8 c.c.	8 c.c.	8 c.c.			
3/6	100.6	101.8	101.0	101.6	101.5			
	8 c.c.	8 c.c.	8 c.c.	8 c.c.	8 c.c.			
3/7	101.9	101.7	101.8	101.6	100.9			
	8 c.c.	8 c.c.	8 c.c.	8 c.c.	8 c.c.			
3/8	101.4	100.9	101.5	100.8	101.3			
	8 c.c.	8 c.c.	8 c.c.	8 c.c.	8 c.c.			
3/9	100.6	101.	100.9	101.5	101.8			
	8 c.c.	8 c.c.	8 c.c.	8 c.c.	8 c.c.			
3/10								no albumin no sugar
3/11	100.8	101.2	100.9	101.	101.5	8	K	
	10 c.c.	10 c.c.	10 c.c.	10 c.c.	10 c.c.			
3/12	101.3	101.2	101.	100.9	101.4			
	10 c.c.	10 c.c.	10 c.c.	10 c.c.	10 c.c.			
3/13	100.8	101.2	101.0	101.1	101.2			
	10 c.c.	10 c.c.	10 c.c.	10 c.c.	10 c.c.			
3/14	100.4	100.9	101.5	100.6	101.			
	10 c.c.	10 c.c.	10 c.c.	10 c.c.	10 c.c.			
3/15	100.6	101.2	101.1	100.9	101.2			
	10 c.c.	10 c.c.	10 c.c.	10 c.c.	10 c.c.			
3/16	100.3	100.8	100.5	101.	101.3			
	10 c.c.	10 c.c.	10 c.c.	10 c.c.	10 c.c.			
3/17								trace of albumin no sugar
3/18	100.5	101.	101.5	101.7	101.9	8	K	
	10 c.c.	10 c.c.	10 c.c.	10 c.c.	10 c.c.			
3/19	101.	100.8	101.0	101.2	101.5			
	10 c.c.	10 c.c.	10 c.c.	10 c.c.	10 c.c.			
3/20	101.2	100.9	101.0	101.2	100.9			
	10 c.c.	10 c.c.	10 c.c.	10 c.c.	10 c.c.			
3/21	100.	100.3	100.7	101.	101.3			
	10 c.c.	10 c.c.	10 c.c.	10 c.c.	10 c.c.			
3/22	100.5	100.9	101.0	101.4	101.5			
	10 c.c.	10 c.c.	10 c.c.	10 c.c.	10 c.c.			
3/23	100.9	101.3	101.4	101.8	101.6			
	10 c.c.	10 c.c.	10 c.c.	10 c.c.	10 c.c.			
3/24								

TABLE III (CONT'D)

SUMMARY OF EXPERIMENT 3 SHOWING THE EFFECT OF SUBCUTANEOUS INJECTIONS OF EGG WHITE IN DOG A.

DATE	INJECTIONS AND TEMPERATURE					WEIGHT	URINE
	9:00	11:00	1:00	3:00	5:00		
3/25	100.5	100.6	101.	101.4	101.2		no albumin
	10 c.c.	10 c.c.	10 c.c.	10 c.c.	10 c.c.	7.8 K	no sugar
3/26	100.8	100.7	101.1	100.9	101.		
	10 c.c.	10 c.c.	10 c.c.	10 c.c.	10 c.c.		
3/27	101.1	101 5	101.3	101.2	101.5		
	10 c.c.	10 c.c.	10 c.c.	10 c.c	10 c.c.		
3/28	101.2	101.	101.2	101.7	101.9		
	10 c.c.	10 c.c.	10 c.c.	10 c.c.	10 c.c.		
3/29	100.8	101.4	101.6	101.9	101.6		
	10 c.c.	10 c.c.	10 c.c.	10 c.c.	10 c.c.		
3/30	100.5	100.8	101.4	101.1	101.8		
	10 c.c.	10 c.c.	10 c.c.	10 c.c.	10 c.c.		
3/31							no albumin
4/1	101.3	101.7	101.7	101.9	101.5		no sugar
	10 c.c.	10 c.c.	10 c.c.	10 c.c.	10 c.c.	8.1 K	
4/2	101.9	101.4	101.7	101.2	101.5		
	10 c.c.	10 c.c.	10 c.c.	10 c.c.	10 c.c.		
4/3	101.2	101.5	101.7	101.8	101.3		
	10 c.c.	10 c.c.	10 c.c.	10 c.c.	10 c.c.		
4/4	101.8	101.3	101.7	101.5	101.9		
	10 c.c.	10 c.c.	10 c.c.	10 c.c.	10 c.c.		
4/5	101.2	101.5	101.4	101.8	101.4		
	10 c.c.	10 c.c.	10 c.c	10 c.c.	10 c.c.		
4/6	101.8	101.5	101.0	101.6	101.9		
	10 c.c.	10 c.c.	10 c.c.	10 c.c.	10 c.c.		
4/7							no albumin
4/8	101.9	101.6	101.3	101.4	101.6		no sugar
	10 c.c.	10 c.c.	10 c.c.	10 c.c.	10 c.c.	8.2 K	
4/9	101.2	101.8	101.5	101.9	102.0		
	10 c.c.	10 c.c.	10 c.c.	10 c.c.	10 c.c.		
4/10	101.5	101.7	101.5	101.8	101.6		
4/11	101.2	101.1	101.4	101.4	101.6		
	10 c.c.	10 c.c.	10 c.c.	10 c.c.	10 c.c.		
4/12	101.4	101.0	101.4	101.2	101.7		
	10 c.c.	10 c.c.	10 c.c.	10 c.c.	10 c.c.		
4/13	101.3	101.5	101.9	101.6	102 0		
	10 c.c.	10 c.c.	10 c.c.	10 c.c.	10 c.c.		
4/14							no albumin
4/15	101.5	101.6	101.3	101.4	101.6		no sugar
	10 c.c.	10 c.c.	10 c.c.	10 c.c.	10 c.c.	8.3 K	
4/16	101.9	102.0	101.8	101.5	101.8		
	10 c.c.	10 c.c.	10 c.c.	10 c.c.	10 c.c.		
4/17	101.4	101.7	101.5	101.9	101.7		
	10 c.c.	10 c.c.	10 c.c.	10 c.c.	10 c.c.		
4/18	101.3	101.1	101.3	101.6	101.4		
	10 c.c.	10 c.c.	10 c.c.	10 c.c.	10 c.c.		
4/19	101.8	101.5	101.4	101.7	101.9		
	10 c.c.	10 c.c.	10 c.c.	10 c.c.	10 c.c.		
4/20	101.4	101.2	101.5	101.3	101.5		
	10 c.c.	10 c.c.	10 c.c.	10 c.c.	10 c.c.		

Another factor which must not be overlooked is that of dosage. A guinea pig weighing approximately 250 grams received 2 c.c. of egg white, while a dog of about 7000 grams received only 10 c.c. In other words if the weight of the animal is taken as a basis, then the dog should have received twenty times as much, instead of only five times as much as the guinea pig. Consequently if this held good, then the dog should have received 40 c.c. of egg white five times a day. In the first place this amount is not only a huge one but also an unnecessary one. In the second place "Friedberger has in a most exact way confirmed the statement that large doses of foreign protein do not, while small doses do, elevate the temperature."

Why there should be a difference between the reaction in a guinea pig and the reaction in a dog to parenteral injection of proteins is difficult to explain. But this factor is apparent. A dog's temperature is much more constant than a guinea pig's or a rabbit's temperature. It is possible to increase the temperature of a guinea pig or rabbit by rough handling or by fright or excitement. In the

TABLE IV

SUMMARY OF EXPERIMENT 4 SHOWING THE EFFECT OF SUBCUTANEOUS INJECTIONS OF EGG WHITE IN DOG B

DATE	INJECTIONS AND TEMPERATURE					WEIGHT	URINE
	9:00	11:00	1:00	3:00	5:00		
2/8	102.				101.9°	5.1 K	no albumin
2/9	102.1°				102.2		no sugar
2/10							
2/11	102.4				101.8	5.2 K	no albumin
							no sugar
2/12	101.3				102.2		
2/13	101.7				101.4		
2/14	101.5		101.7°		101.6		
	3 c.c.		3 c.c.		3 c.c.		
2/15	101.8		101.6		101.4		
	3 c.c.		3 c.c.		3 c.c.		
2/16	101.5		101.7		101.6		
	3 c.c	.	3 c.c.		3 c.c.		
2/17							
2/18	100.7	101. °	100.8	101.1°		5.4 K	no albumin
	5 c.c.	5 c.c.	5 c.c.	5 c.c.			no sugar
2/19	101.2	100.8	101.1	101.9			
	5 c.c.	5 c c.	5 c.c.	5 c.c.			
2/20	·101.8	101.5	101.6	101.8			
	5 c.c.	5 c.c.	5 c.c.	5 c.c.			
2/21	101.5	101.4	101.7	101.3			
	5 c.c.	5 c.c.	5 c c	5 c.c.			
2/22	100.7	101.2	100.9	101.1			
	5 c.c	5 c.c.	5 c.c.	5 c.c.			
2/23	100.2	100.6	100.7	101.2			
	5 c.c.	5 c.c.	5 c c.	5 c.c.			
2/24							
2/25	101.0	100.8	100.5	100.9		5.7 K	no albumin
	5 c.c.	5 c.c.	5 c.c.	5 c.c.			no sugar
2/26	100.8	100.7	101.1	100.8			
	5 c.c.	5 c.c.	5 c.c.	5 c.c.			
2/27	100.6	100.9	101.0	101.5			
	5 c.c.	5 c.c.	5 c.c.	5 c c			
2/28	101.2	100.9	101.8	101.1			
	5 c.c.	5 c.c.	5 c.c.	5 c.c.			
3/1	101.2	101.1	100.2	100.9			
	5 c.c.	5 c.c.	5 c.c.	5 c.c.			
3/2	100.5	100.8	101.	100.9			
	5 c.c.	5 c.c.	5 c.c.	5 c.c.			
3/3							no sugar
3/4	101.	101.3	101.7	101.3	101.2	5.9 K	no albumin
	8 c.c.	8 c.c.	8 c.c.	8 c.c.	8 c.c.		
3/5	100 7	101.	101.3	100.9	102.2		
	8 c.c.	8 c.c.	8 c.c.	8 c.c.	8 c.c.		
3/6	100.5	101.2	100.9	101.6	101.5		
	8 c.c.	8 c.c.	8 c.c.	8 c.c.	8 c.c.		
3/7	100.7	101.0	100.9	101.3	101.6		
	8 c.c.	8 c.c.	8 c.c.	8 c.c.	8 c.c.		
3/8	101.3	101.	100.9	101.8	101.		
3/9	8 c.c.	8 c.c	8 c.c.	8 c.c.	8 c.c.		
3/9	100 7	101.1	100.0	101.3	101.9		
	8 c c	8 c.c.	8 c.c.	8 c.c.	8 c.c.		
3/10							no albumin
3/11	100.4	100.7	101.	101.5	101.6	5.8 K	no sugar
	10 c.c.	10 c.c.	10 c.c.	10 c.c.	10 c.c.		
3/12	101.4	101.4	101.2	101.	101.7		
	10 c.c.	10 c.c.	10 c.c.	10 c.c.	10 c.c.		
3/13	101.	101.0	101.3	101.4	101.6		
	10 c c.	10 c.c.	10 c.c.	10 c.c.	10 c.c.		
3/14	101.2	101.9	101.8	101.3	101.1		
	10 c c.	10 c.c.	10 c.c.	10 c.c.	10 c.c.		
3/15	100.5	101.	101.2	101.2	101.7		
	10 c c.	10 c.c.	10 c c.	10 c.c.	10 c.c.		
3/16	100.2	101.	100.9	101.1	101.4		
	10 c.c.	10 c.c.	10 c.c.	10 c.c.	10 c.c.		
3/17							no albumin
3/18	100.7	101.2	101.3	101.6	101.5	5.9 K	no sugar
	10 c c.	10 c.c.	10 c.c.	10 c.c.	10 c.c.		
3/19	100.9	100.6	100.9	100.7	101.0		
	10 c c.	10 c.c.	10 c.c.	10 c.c.	10 c.c.		
3/20	100.1	100.5	100.7	101.0	100.5		
	10 c c.	10 c.c.	10 c.c.	10 c c	10 c.c.		
3/21	100.6	101.	101.2	101.5	101.1		
	10 c c.	10 c.c.	10 c.c.	10 c.c.	10 c.c.		
3/22	100.7	101.	101.0	101.1	101.3		
3/23	10 c.c.	10 c.c.	10 c.c.	10 c.c.	10 c c.		
3/23	101.	101.7	101.2	101.1	101.5		
	10 c c.	10 c.c.	10 c.c.	10 c.c.	10 c.c.		
3/24							
3/25	100.8	100.4	100 7	100.9	101.1	6.1 K	no albumin
	10 c c.	10 c c.	10 c c	10 c.c.	10 c c		

TABLE IV (Cont'd)

Summary of Experiment 4 Showing the Effect of Subcutaneous Injections of Egg White in Dog B

DATE	INJECTIONS AND TEMPERATURE					WEIGHT	URINE
	9:00	11:00	1:00	3:00	5:00		
3/26	101.	100.9	101.3	101.1	101.3		
	10 c.c.	10 c.c.	10 c.c.	10 c.c.	10 c.c.		
3/27	100.8	101.0	100.8	101.1	101.0		
	10 c.c.	10 c.c.	10 c.c.	10 c.c.	10 c.c.		
3/28	101.4	101.5	101.3	101.6	101.9		
	10 c.c.	10 c.c.	10 c.c.	10 c.c.	10 c.c.		
3/29	100.8	101.0	101.2	101.4	101.7		
	10 c.c.	10 c.c.	10 c.c.	10 c.c.	10 c.c.		
3/30	101.	101.2	101.3	100.9	101.5		
	10 c.c.	10 c.c.	10 c.c.	10 c.c.	10 c.c.		
3/31							
4/1	100.8	101.0	101.3	101.6	101.8	5.9 K	no albumin
	10 c.c.	10 c.c.	10 c.c.	10 c.c.	10 c.c.		no sugar
4/2	102.	102.1	101.7	101.8	101.3		
	10 c.c.	10 c.c.	10 c.c.	10 c.c.	10 c.c.		
4/3	101.6	101.8	101.9	102.0	101.4		
	10 c.c.	10 c.c.	10 c.c.	10 c.c.	10 c.c.		
4/4	101.3	101.8	101.9	101.4	101.7		
	10 c.c.	10 c.c.	10 c.c.	10 c.c.	10 c.c.		
4/5	100.9	101.3	101.4	101.7	101.9		
	10 c.c.	10 c.c.	10 c.c.	10 c.c.	10 c.c.		
4/6	101.1	101.7	101.8	101.8	101.5		
	10 c.c.	10 c.c.	10 c.c.	10 c.c.	10 c.c.		
4/7							
4/8	101.7	101.4	101.6	101.5	101.4	6.2 K	no albumin
	10 c.c.	10 c.c.	10 c.c.	10 c.c.	10 c.c.		no sugar
4/9	101.4	101.9	101.3	101.7	101.9		
	10 c.c.	10 c.c.	10 c.c.	10 c.c.	10 c.c.		
4/10	101.7	102.	102.1	101.9	101.5		
	10 c.c.	10 c.c.	10 c.c.	10 c.c.	10 c.c.		
4/11	101.4	100.9	101.1	101.1	101.3		
	10 c.c.	10 c.c.	10 c.c.	10 c.c.	10 c.c.		
4/12	101.6	101.3	101.5	101.8	102.0		
	10 c.c.	10 c.c.	10 c.c.	10 c.c.	10 c.c.		
4/13	101.1	101.7	101.9	102.	101.8		
	10 c.c.	10 c.c.	10 c.c.	10 c.c.	10 c.c.		
4/14							
4/15	101.	101.4	101.3	101.6	101.4	6.2 K	no albumin
	10 c.c.	10 c.c.	10 c.c.	10 c.c.	10 c.c.		no sugar
4/16	101.6	101.8	101.7	101.3	101.5		
4/17	10 c.c.	10 c.c.	10 c.c.	10 c.c.	10 c.c.		
4/18	101.2	101.0	101.3	101.8	101.7		
	10 c.c.	10 c.c.	10 c.c.	10 c.c.	10 c.c.		
4/19	101.9	101.2	101.4	101.7	101.8		
	10 c.c.	10 c.c.	10 c.c.	10 c.c.	10 c.c.		
4/20	101.7	101.5	101.6	101.8	101.5		
	10 c.c.	10 c.c.	10 c.c.	10 c.c.	10 c.c.		

dog the temperature center or heat center seems to be more constant and less affected by external stimuli. But even this does not explain the wide difference in the reactions of these animals. However, it remains a fact that repeated subcutaneous injections of egg white will not elevate the temperature of a dog.

SUMMARY

1. Repeated subcutaneous injections of egg white in guinea pigs produce a constant fever, associated with most of the signs of infection. (Confirmatory of Vaughan.)

2. Repeated subcutaneous injections of egg white in dogs do not affect the temperature curve and do not produce fever.

3. The author is unable to explain the difference of reactions.

ADDENDUM

The author of the above paper has asked the editor of the journal to make comment upon his article. The result obtained by Dr. Cohen is interesting. He should now find out what becomes of egg white when injected subcutaneously in dogs. Is it changed in the blood or tissues, or is it eliminated through the liver into the intestines, there digested and absorbed? These matters can be decided by sensitizing guinea pigs with the blood and bile of dogs which have recently received subcutaneous injections of egg white.—Editor-in-chief.

BIBLIOGRAPHY

[1]Vaughan, Victor C.: Jour. Am. Med. Assn., 1909, liii, 629. Jour. Am. Med. Assn., 1911, lvii, 398. Jour. Lab. and Clin. Med., 1916, ii, 15. Protein Split Products, Phila., 1913, Lea and Febiger. Poisonous Protein, St. Louis, 1917, C. V. Mosby Co., p. 75.
[2]Friedberger: Berl. klin. Wchnschr, Oct. 1910, xlvii.
[3]Vaughan, Victor C.: Poisonous Protein, St. Louis, 1917, C. V. Mosby Co, p. 80.

LEUCOCYTES IN ANAPHYLAXIS OF SERUM SICKNESS

By Joseph H. Barach, M.D., Pittsburgh, Pa.

A RECENT contribution to the blood changes following intravenous injection of foreign protein, prompts me to record some observations made in a case of serum sickness with delayed anaphylactic reaction. The observations were made in 1912 and remained unpublished. But the findings of Cowie and Calhoun are so much in accord with mine that it seems worth while reporting them. .Particularly so since Cowie and Calhoun consider the blood pictures which they found due directly to the intravenous injection, while my findings, similar to theirs, occurred in a case of subcutaneous injection. Also in their conclusions Cowie and Calhoun state the "temperature reaction and clinical findings are not in the nature of an anaphylactic response, as is shown by the absence of an eosinophilia" while the case reported here is a genuine anaphylactic response and eosinophilia was not present.

I point out these facts not in any way to contradict the conclusions, derived from their admirable work, but rather to offer one more ray of light on a complicated and interesting problem.

Patient, Miss E. K., taken ill October 29, 1912, with sore throat, muscle pains, and general symptoms of fever. Examination of throat revealed a diphtheritic infection and antitoxin was administered as the accompanying table and chart show:

TIME	AMOUNT OF SERUM	DIPH. UNITS	LOCAL REACTION
1st day of illness	1.5 c.c.	3,000	Slight
2nd day of illness	2.5 c.c.	5,000	Marked in 3 hrs.
4th day of illness	1.5 c.c.	3,000	Moderate

The tonsillar patches disappeared within 48 hours after first injection and recovery seemed to be progressing uneventfully.

On the morning of the 9th day after the first injection, patient complained of itching, and there was an urticaria over the site of the injection, which subsided after an alcohol rub. Fifteen hours later—on the tenth day of her illness—at 12:30 a.m., patient awakened out of her sleep with an itching over the entire body. The nurse proceeded to give her an alcohol rub, during which patient complained of being cold and chilly. Her skin was cold and clammy, her entire body became pallid, respirations shallow and accelerated, pulse small, rapid and for a short time could not be counted at the wrist. Temperature dropped to 97½°. External heat was applied, an injection of strychnine and one of pituitrin was given by the resident physician. In about half an hour patient reacted from this state of shock, and a diffuse urticaria appeared. First at the site of injection, then on the back, arms, lower extremities, face, palms of hands, soles of feet and abdomen. In some places the lesion consisted of small papules, in others, large blotches. The urticaria lasted for about twenty-four hours. Typical urticarial lesions limited to portions of the body, recurred during the two following days. They were evanescent, lasting a few minutes to an hour. Twelve hours after onset of the general urticaria, the pharynx and larynx became edematous; this was evidently due to the same process. The swelling in the throat continued for twenty-four hours.

At the time of this urticaria, patient also complained of pains in the elbow joints, and there was glandular swelling and pain in the neck and axilla.

By the twelfth day all symptoms had subsided and patient felt perfectly well.

It is important to note that the patient never had diphtheria or antitoxin prior to this, and that several years previous, a sister of hers had diphtheria, was given antitoxin and also experienced an attack of serum sickness.

We have here, then, a typical case of serum sickness with a delayed reaction, accompanied by anaphylactic shock and collapse which seemed to threaten the patient's life.

The blood findings are shown in the following table:

TABLE OF WHITE CELL COUNTS.   (EHRLICH'S CLASSIFICATION)

TIME OF EXAM. 17 hours after	DAY OF DISEASE	LEUCOCYTES	POLY	LYMPHO.	LARGE MONO.	TRANS.	EOS.	MAST	MYELO-CYTES
Anaphylactic Shock	10th	20,000 pr cum.	81.25	16.25	1.5	0.5	0.5	0.0	0.0
2 days later	12th	3,200 pr cum.	56.0	27.50	5.5	0.0	0.0	0.5	10.5
4 days later	16th	3,400 pr cum.	54.0	37.0	3.5	1.5	3.0	1.0	0.5
8 days later	20th	13,800 pr cum.	68.0	24.5	4.5	1.0	1.5	0.5	0.5

THE BLOOD FINDINGS

Considering that the temperature, pulse rate, and general condition of the patient seemed normal in every way preceding the anaphylactic attack, even though we have no record on this point, it seems fair to presume that the leucocyte count was about normal, or perhaps it is best to say that the blood picture was unknown.

Seventeen hours after the onset of the attack we find a polynuclear leucocytosis. This is followed by a leucopenia. Accompanying this leucopenia, or more likely at the end of the leucocytosis, we find the increased presence of large mononuclears, Ehrlich's myelocytes in rather large numbers, and the smear showed a marked increase in the blood platelets. Ehrlich's myelocytes are known to occur in the blood when there has been a call upon the reserve forces of the blood-making organs. The second count, two days later, still showed a leucopenia, but the myelocytes have disappeared, showing that their presence is not part of the leucopenia; more likely a precursor of it. The last count, eight days after the attack, was made when the patient had fully recovered. The count then showed a leucocytosis with the various cells in about normal proportions.

One phase of the admirable work of Vaughan[2] on cancer proteid—in which extensive observations including more than 20,000 differential counts were carried out—is confirmatory of the findings in this case.

By sensitizing rabbits to the cancer cell—and upon reinjection. producing anaphylaxis and in some instances shock—Vaughan found a transitory increase in the large mononuclears after each injection. This occurred 490 times in 500 animal experiments.

A noteworthy feature of the counts in this case, and in the anaphylactic reactions in Vaughan's work, is the absence of eosinophilia, which has been found present in a number of conditions said to be due to anaphylaxis.[3]

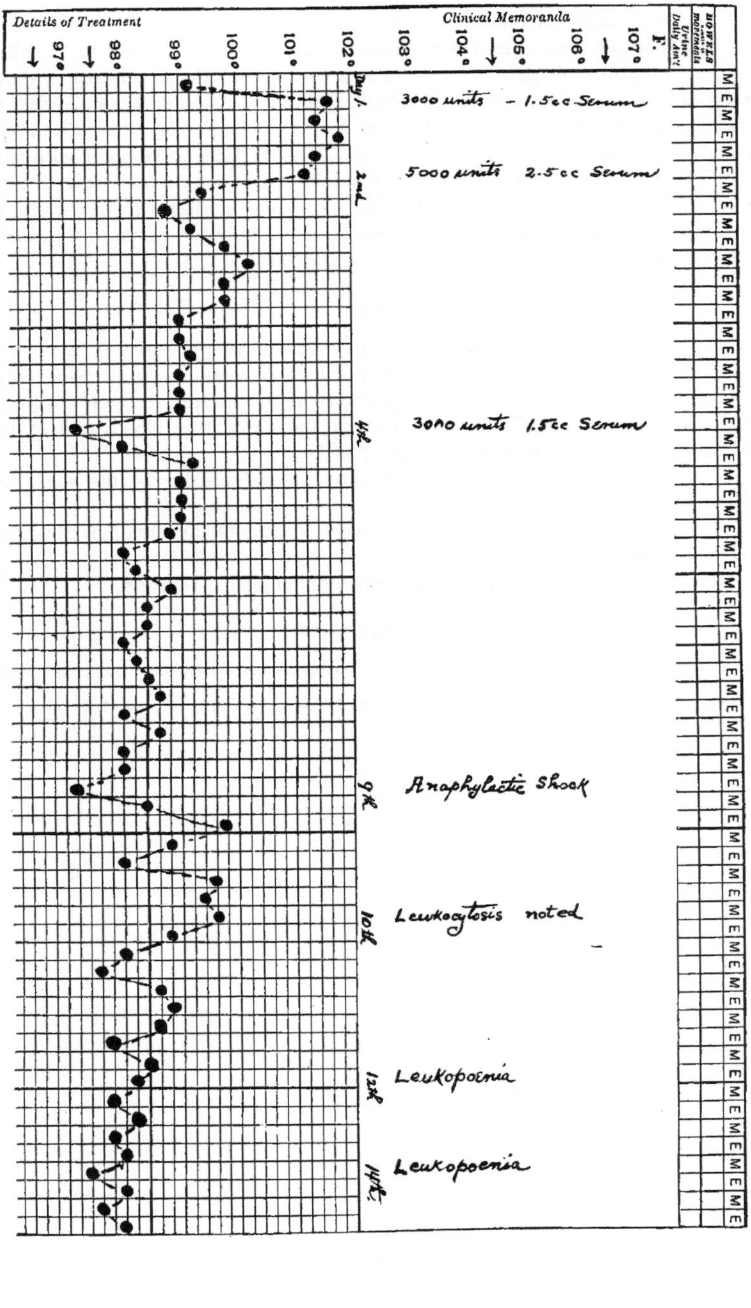

Details of Treatment
Clinical Memoranda
97°
98°
99°
100°
101°
102°
103°
104°
105°
106°
107°
F.
Urine Daily Am't
BOWELS movements
Day 1.
3000 units - 1.5cc Serum
2nd
5000 units 2.5cc Serum
4th
3000 units 1.5cc Serum
9th
Anaphylactic Shock
10th
Leukocytosis noted
12th
Leukopoenia
14th
Leukopoenia

It is also worthy of note that in this case when the leucocytes had reached only 20,000 per cu. mm., the reserve forces of the blood supply had to be called upon; while in other diseases we may have a leucocytosis thrice this size without the appearance of myelocytes in the circulation. The probable reason seems to be that in anaphylaxis the demand is very sudden, whereas in other conditions, particularly in inflammations, the organism has more time to respond with matured white blood cells. The blood picture in this case of anaphylaxis at its critical period, in some respects resembles that of the crisis in cases of pneumonia, in which we have a preceding polynuclear leucocytosis, and at the time of the crisis, myelocytes and increased numbers of blood platelets.

SUMMARY

1. A case of serum sickness with a delayed anaphylactic reaction.

2. Blood shows at the time of the anaphylactic reaction, a primary polynuclear leucocytosis followed by the appearance of myelocytes after the organism had appropriated the available leucocytes of the circulating blood, and at the same time an increased number of blood platelets.

3. A leucopenia followed; at which time the polynuclear counts were low and the mononuclears relatively high.

4. The eosinophilia, which has been said to accompany anaphylactic reactions in general, was absent throughout.

5. Eosinophilia is not the criterion of an anaphylactic reaction.

BIBLIOGRAPHY

[1]Cowie and Calhoun: Non-Specific Therapy in Arthritis and Infections, Arch. Int. Med., Jan., 1919, p. 69.
[2]Vaughan, J. W.: Cancer Proteid, Jour. Am. Med. Assn., Nov. 16, 1912, p. 1764.
[3]Moschowitz: Eosinophilia and Anaphylaxis, New York Med. Jour., Jan. 7, 1911, p. 15.

STUDIES IN THE METABOLIC CHANGES IN EXPERIMENTAL TETANY*

By Dr. Tokuji Togawa, Tokyo, Japan

O UR present view as to the cause of tetany is contradictory. It is even un-decided that the tetanic symptoms may be induced by a certain intoxication. Many facts in experimental tetany were studied and many theories in tetany were proposed by authors especially in America.

MacCallum and Voegtlin,[1] Medwedew,[2] Jacobson,[3] Underhill and Saiki,[4] Cooke,[5] Beebe and Berkeley,[6] Falta and Kahn,[7] Greenwald,[8] MacCallum and his coworkers,[9, 10] Wilson, Stearns, Janney and Thurlow,[11, 12] Burns and Sharpe,[20] Paton and Findlay,[13] Watanabe.[14,15]

The studies by Wilson, Stearns, Janney and Thurlow[11,12] showed that there is a condition of alkalosis after parathyroidectomy in dogs. This was proved by the studies on the dissociation of oxyhemoglobin, on the hydrogen-ion concentration of the blood, and on the carbon dioxide pressure of the alveolar air. They described further, that this alkalosis is neutralized by certain acids, probably by lactic acid formed during the tetanic period and in the next period an acidosis can be induced by overneutralization. Thus the periodic variations in the acid-base equilibrium cause the periodic attacks of tetany.

Studying on two dogs, parathyroidectomized, and on five dogs, subjected to gastric operation, W. S. McCann[16] found a marked increase in the carbon-dioxide-combining power of the blood plasma, coincident with the development of tetany.

In the recent studies by Watanabe,[15,16] it was demonstrated, that a marked acidosis appears in the condition of tetany caused by guanidine injection. He observed the same phenomenon in the parathyroid tetany and in idiopathic tetany.

The view seems therefore to be contradictory as regards the reaction of blood serum in experimental tetany.

So I have studied in the experimental puppies' tetany the carbon-dioxide-combining power of the blood plasma, the antitryptic power and the nonprotein nitrogen content of the serum.

The puppies were observed for three days at least and their normal condition assured. As method of operation the thyro-parathyroidectomy was chosen, because of its great simplicity and surety for removing all the parathyroid glands. Special attention was paid to leave a certain portion of the thyroid glands. All operative procedures were carried out without any narcotics.

1. DETERMINATION OF THE CARBON-DIOXIDE-COMBINING POWER OF THE BLOOD PLASMA

The apparatus of Van Slyke and Cullen[17] was used because of its great simplicity and accuracy. The blood sample was drawn usually from an ear vein directly into a paraffined centrifuge tube containing potassium oxalate. The

*From the Serochemical Laboratory, Medical College, Tokyo Imperial University.

299

plasma separated by centrifuging was saturated with alveolar air. The only variation from the original technic was the substitution of amyl alcohol for the caprylic alcohol. In the preliminary period the normal blood samples were obtained in three successive days. The average of the CO_2-combining power of these samples was taken as the normal value before operation.

2. DETERMINATION OF THE ANTITRYPTIC POWER OF THE SERUM

Bergmann and Meyer's method,[18] a little modified, was used, Gruebler's Trypsin sicc. being employed.

A. Titration of 0.1 per cent trypsin solution preceded the test proper. Into each of several test tubes were placed decreasing amounts of the trypsin solution as stated in Table I, A and II, A. To each tube 2.0 c.c. of 0.2 per cent casein solution were then added. After incubating for half an hour at 37° C., 1.0 c.c. of the acetic acid solution was added to each tube and the appearance of cloudiness was observed.

B. Determination of the antitryptic power of the serum. The fresh serum was diluted 20 times with salt solution. The mixtures of trypsin, casein, physiologic salt solution and serum were made as stated in Table I, B, I, C, and Table II, B. After incubating at 37° C. for half an hour 1.0 c.c. of acetic acid solution was added to each tube.

3. DETERMINATION OF THE NONPROTEIN NITROGEN CONTENT OF THE SERUM

Folin and Denis' method[19] was used. Five c.c. of the fresh serum were mixed with 50 c.c. of methyl alcohol. Twenty c.c. of the last filtrate were employed for nitrogen determination by Kjeldahl's method (duplicate determination).

PROTOCOLS

$C =$ Vol. percentage of combined CO_2, calculated to 0°C., 760 mm.
anti-T $=$ Antitryptic power of 1 c.c. serum.
$N =$ Amount of nonprotein nitrogen in 100 c.c. of serum.

Dog 1, Bodyweight 1120 gm.
    (i) Before operation.
    XI, 16. $C = 45.62\%$; anti-T $= 20$ (Table I, A and I, B)
        $N = 68.3$ mg.
    XI, 18. 10:30 A.M. operation.
    (ii) After operation.
    XI, 19. 4 P.M. slight stiffness of legs, walked not easy, no tremors.
    XI, 20. Marked stiffness, mild tremor, depression, no walking.
        11 A.M. blood drawn from carotid artery.
        Animal sacrificed.
        $C = 37.51\%$ (-8.11%); anti-T $= 40$ (Table I, A and I, C);
        $N = 94.5$ mg. (+26.2 mg.)

Dog 2, Bodyweight 520 gm.
    (i) Before operation.
    XI, 19. $C = 45.35\%$; anti-T $= 40$; $N = 65.7$ mg.
    XI, 22. 1 P.M. operation.
    (ii) After operation.
    XI, 24. Afternoon, stiffness of legs.

XI, 25. 10 A.M. marked stiffness, especially of forelegs, hyperpnea, marked cramps time to time.

Immediately blood was drawn from carotid artery.

Animal dead.

$C = 35.05\%$ (-10.3%); anti-T = 60 (Table II, A and II, B);

$N = 96.3$ mg. ($+30.6$ mg.)

Dog 3, Bodyweight 720 gm.

(i) Before operation.

XI, 26. $C = 49.0\%$; anti-T = 20; $N = 70.1$ mg.

XI, 27. 3 P.M. operation.

(ii) After operation.

XI, 28. Morning, stiffness.

XI, 29. Morning, shivering and contraction of the forelegs, exaggerated by stimulation, salivation. At 10:30 A.M. blood was drawn from femoral artery.

$C = 36.4\%$ (-12.6%); anti-T = 60; $N = 94.6$ mg. ($+24.5$ mg.)

Dog 4, Bodyweight 720 gm.

(i) Before operation.

XI, 28. $C = 54.04\%$; anti-T = 40; $N = 65.7$ mg.

XI, 29. 4 P.M. operation.

(ii) After operation.

XII, 1. Stiffness of legs.

XII, 2. Morning. Violent tetany, twitching and jerking, hyperpnea, profuse salivation, all legs stiffly extended, moribund. Blood drawn, animal sacrificed. Autopsy: only congestion of viscera.

$C = 39.89\%$ (-12.15%); anti-T = 60; $N = 109.0$ mg. ($+43.3$ mg.)

Dog 5, Bodyweight 560 gm.

(i) Before operation.

XI, 30. $C = 51.4\%$; anti-T = 20; $N = 100.7$ mg.

XII, 2. 3 P.M. operation.

(ii) After operation.

XII, 4. Morning. Stiffness, slight tremor. Exertion caused contractions. At 10 A.M. blood was drawn.

$C = 37.09\%$ (-14.31%); anti-T = 40 ($+20$); $N = 84.1$ mg.

Dog 6, Bodyweight 720 gm.

(i) Before operation.

XII, 3. $C = 47.37\%$; anti-T = 20; $N = 68.3$ mg.

XII, 4. 3 P.M. operation.

(ii) After operation.

XII, 5. Appeared bright, no sign of tetanic symptoms.

$C = 47.38\%$.

XII, 6. Stiffness and tremors of legs, hyperpnea, salivation. Lying on its side with legs extended. Blood was drawn. Dog sacrificed.

$C = 26.49\%$ (-20.88%); anti-T = 60; $N = 101.6$ mg. ($+33.3$ mg.)

Dog 7, Bodyweight 1700 gm.

(i) Before operation.

XII, 18. $C = 45.72\%$; anti-T = 40; $N = 112.1$ mg.

2 P.M. operation.

(ii) After operation.

XII, 20. Walking somewhat uneasy.

XII, 21. Morning. Violent tetany. Animal killed.

$C = 37.48\%$ (-8.24%); anti-T = 60; $N = 91.1$ mg.

TABLE I

THE ANTITRYPTIC POWER OF THE BLOOD SERUM BEFORE AND AFTER PARATHYROIDECTOMY (DOG 1)

A. TRYPSIN TITRATION

	1	2	3	4	5
Trypsin	1.0	0.8	0.6	0.4	0.2
NaCl	0	0.2	0.4	0.6	0.8
Casein	2.0	2.0	2.0	2.0	2.0
Acetic Acid	1.0	1.0	1.0	1.0	1.0
	+	+	+	+	-

B. ANTITRYPTIC POWER BEFORE OPERATION

	1	2	3	4	5
Trypsin	1.0	0.8	0.6	0.4	0.2
NaCl	0	0.2	0.4	0.6	0.8
Casein	2.0	2.0	2.0	2.0	2.0
Serum	0.2	0.2	0.2	0.2	0.2
Acetic Acid	1.0	1.0	1.0	1.0	1.0
	+	+	-	-	-

anti-T = 20

C. ANTITRYPTIC POWER AFTER OPERATION

	1	2	3	4	5
Trypsin	1.0	0.8	0.6	0.4	0.2
NaCl	0	0.2	0.4	0.6	0.8
Casein	2.0	2.0	2.0	2.0	2.0
Serum	0.2	0.2	0.2	0.2	0.2
Acetic Acid	1.0	1.0	1.0	1.0	1.0
	+	-	-	-	-

anti-T = 40

(+) = Clearness
(-) = Cloudiness

TABLE II

THE ANTITRYPTIC POWER OF THE BLOOD SERUM AFTER PARATHYROIDECTOMY (DOG 2)

A. TRYPSIN TITRATION

	1	2	3	4	5
Trypsin	1.0	0.8	0.6	0.4	0.2
NaCl	0	0.2	0.4	0.6	0.8
Casein	2.0	2.0	2.0	2.0	2.0
Acetic Acid	1.0	1.0	1.0	1.0	1.0
	+	+	+	-	-

B. ANTITRYPTIC POWER AFTER PARATHYROIDECTOMY

	1	2	3	4	5
Trypsin	1.0	0.8	0.6	0.4	0.2
NaCl	0	0.2	0.4	0.6	0.8
Casein	2.0	2.0	2.0	2.0	2.0
Serum	0.2	0.2	0.2	0.2	0.2
Acetic Acid	1.0	1.0	1.0	1.0	1.0
	-	-	-	-	-

anti-T = 60

Dog 8, Bodyweight 610 gm.
    (i) Before operation.
    XII, 19. C = 46.77%; anti-T = 40. N = 112.1 mg.
        2 P.M. operation.
    (ii) After operation.
    XII, 23. Morning. Tremor of all legs, would not eat, restless panting. At 11 A.M.
        Blood was drawn. Animal killed.
        C = 34.81% (-11.96%); anti-T = 60; N = 161.2 mg. (-49.1 mg.)

Dog 9, Bodyweight 1100 gm.
    (i) Before operation.
    XII, 20. C = 44.77%; anti-T = 40; N = 66.6 mg.
    XII, 21. 2 P.M. operation.
    (ii) After operation.
    XII, 23. Typical tetanic symptoms. Animal killed.
        C = 51.99% (+7.22%); anti-T = 60; N = 84.6 mg. (+18.0 mg.)

Dog 10, Bodyweight 1220 gm.
    (i) Before operation.
    XII, 24. C = 44.45%; anti-T = 60; N = 69.0 mg.
        2 P.M. operation.
    (ii) After operation.
    XII, 26. Walked about easily, appeared bright, slight stiffness of forelegs in excite-
        ment. Blood was drawn from ear vein.
        C = 38.58% (-5.87%).
    XII, 27. Morning. Violent cramps, restless groaning, moribund.
        C = 35.55% (-8.9%); anti-T = 60; N = 94.6 mg. (+25.6 mg.)

Dog 11, Bodyweight 1460 gm.
    (i) Before operation.
    1,18. (1919) C = 45.35%; anti-T = 60; N = 49.0 mg.
        4 P.M. operation.
    1,20. (ii) After operation.
        Slight stiffness of legs. C = 36.61% (-8.74%).
    1,22. Stiffness scarcely noticed, walked easily.
        C = 29.09% (-16.26%).
    1,23. Bodyweight 1120 gm., marked stiffness N = 110.9 mg.
    1,24. Stiffness and tremors, especially in excitement.
        C = 28.26% (-17.09%).
    1,25. C = 30.45% (-14.90%).
    1,27. Bodyweight 1000 gm., weakness increased, legs quite relaxed, no appetite since
        yesterday, moribund. Blood was drawn from femoral artery. Animal dead.
        C = 27.53% (-17.82%); anti-T = 60; N = 161.1 mg. (+112.1 mg.)

CONTROL TEST

    Four dogs were thyroidectomized, special attention was paid to leave the parathyroid glands as intact as possible. In no cases tetanic symptoms were observed.

Dog 12, Bodyweight 1200 gm.
    (i) Before thyroidectomy.
    1,10. C = 37.04%; anti-T = 40; N = 56.0 mg.
        1 P.M. thyroidectomized.
    (ii) After thyroidectomy.
    1,13. No sign of tetanic symptoms.
        C = 36.96%; N = 54.0 mg. (-2 mg.)
    1,14. C = 44.64% (+7.60%); anti-T = 40; N = 50.2 mg. (-5.8 mg.)

1,15. almost normal. C = 37.60% (+ 0.56%).

1,16. Bodyweight 1040 gm; C = 44.98% (+ 7.94%) ; anti-T = 40; N = 56.0 mg.

1,17. Weakness and emaciation gradually increased, walked easily.
C = 44.76% (+7.72%).

1,18. C = 44.63% (+ 7.59%) ; anti-T =60; N = 63.0 mg. (+ 7.0 mg.)

1,20. Since yesterday no appetite, Dog moribund. Blood was drawn from femoral
artery. Animal killed.
Autopsy: Bronchopneumonia.
C =38.49% (+1.45%) ; anti-T = 60; N = 105.1 mg. (+ 49.1 mg.)

Dog 13, Bodyweight 2320 gm.
  (i) Before thyroidectomy.
  1,13. C = 42.19%; anti-T = 40; N = 84.1 mg.
      4 :30 P.M. thyroidectomized.
  (ii) After thyroidectomy.
  1,17 Almost normal.
      C = 46.0% (+3.81%) ; anti-T = 40; N = 49.0 mg. (- 35.1 mg.)
  1,18. No tetanic symptoms. C = 45.35%.
  1,21. C = 48.32% (+ 6.13%) ; N = 49.0 mg. (- 35.1 mg.).
  1,22. C = 43.09% (+ 0.9%).
  1,23. Bodyweight 2020 gm.; C = 48.98% (+ 6.79%) ; N = 52.9 mg. (- 31.2 mg.)
  1,24. C = 46.64%.
  1,25. C = 47.23%.
  1,27. Bodyweight 2000 gm.; C = 46.15%.
  1,28. Bodyweight 1920 gm.; C = 41.64%. anti-T = 60.
  1,31. Morning. Dog found dead. Autopsy: Bronchopneumonia.

Dog 14, Bodyweight 1420 gm.
  (i) Before thyroidectomy.
  1,21. C = 36.08%; anti-T = 60; N = 56.0 mg.
      3 P.M. thyroidectomized.
  (i) After thyroidectomy.
  1,22. C = 44.22% (+ 8.14%).
  1,23. Bodyweight 1320 gm.; C = 40.40% (+ 4.32%).
  1,24. C = 33.95% (- 2.13%) ; anti-T = 60.
  1,25. C = 37.70% (+ 1.62%).
  1,27. C = 39.14% (+ 3.06%).
  1,28. Morning. Found dead.

Dog 15, Bodyweight 1440 gm.
  (i) Before thyroidectomy.
  1,22. C = 38.9%; anti-T = 60; N = 56.0 mg.
      3 :30 P.M. thyroidectomized.
  (ii) After thyroidectomy.
  1,23. C = 43.54%.
  1,24. C = 39.72% ; anti-T = 60; N = 59.5 mg.
  1,25. C = 36.44%.
  1,27. C = 38.17%.
  1,28. C = 36.0%.
  1,31. C = 38.64%. N = 91.1 mg.

From the preceding protocols or in the Table III it will be seen that the
parathyroidectomized dogs, showing the tetanic symptoms, had not any sign of
alkalosis. An acidosis, on the contrary, was observed almost constantly. The
only exception was Dog 9, in which a slight alkalosis appeared after the parathyroidectomy.

TABLE III

THE CO_2 COMBINING POWER OF THE BLOOD PLASMA, THE ANTITRYPTIC POWER AND THE NONPROTEIN NITROGEN CONTENT OF THE BLOOD SERUM IN PARATHYROIDECTOMIZED DOGS

DOG	C		ANTI-T		N	
	BEFORE OP.	AFTER OP.	BEFORE OP.	AFTER OP.	BEFORE OP.	AFTER OP.
1	45.62	37.51	20	40	68.3	94.5
2	45.35	35.05	40	(60)	65.7	96.3
3	49.0	36.4	20	(60)	70.1	94.6
4	54.04	39.89	40	(60)	65.7	109.0
5	51.40	37.09	20	40	100.7	84.1
6	47.37	26.49	20	(60)	68.3	101.6
7	45.72	37.48	40	(60)	112.1	91.1
8	46.77	34.81	40	(60)	112.1	161.2
9	44.77	51.99	40	(60)	66.6	84.6
10	44.45	{ 38.58 } { 35.55 }	(60)	(60)	69.0	94.6
11	45.35	32.39	(60)	(60)	49.0	{ 110.9 { 161.1

TABLE IV

THE CO_2 COMBINING POWER OF THE BLOOD PLASMA, THE ANTITRYPTIC POWER AND THE NONPROTEIN NITROGEN CONTENT OF THE BLOOD SERUM IN THYROIDECTOMIZED DOGS

DOG	C		ANTI-T		N	
	BEFORE OP.	AFTER OP.	BEFORE OP.	AFTER OP.	BEFORE OP.	AFTER OP.
12	37.04	38.92	40	40	56.0	{ 55.8 { 105.1
13	42.19	45.93	40	{ 40 { (60)	84.1	50.3
14	36.08	40.48	(60)	(60)	56.0	
15	38.90	38.75	(60)	(60)	56.0	{ 59.5 { 91.1

In the tetanic animals the antitryptic power of the serum was always increased. In Dogs 10 and 11, the antitryptic power of the serum was unusually strong, both before and after the operation.

As the time was not observed, any change of the antitryptic power due to the tetany can not be stated.

The amount of nonprotein nitrogen of the serum was usually increased by parathyroidectomy. Dogs 5 and 7, which had a rather high value of the nonprotein nitrogen content of the serum before the operation, did not show any increase.

In control animals, thyroidectomized but with a certain number of the intact parathyroid glands, acidosis could not be observed, but on the contrary a slight alkalosis condition was usually induced (Dogs 12, 13, 14). The antitryptic power and the non-protein nitrogen content of the serum did not show any marked variation. An increase observed directly before the death can not be considered to be related to the condition of athyreosis (Table IV).

SUMMARY

1. In parathyroidectomized dogs, showing typical tetanic symptoms, an acidosis condition is always observed.

2. The antitryptic power and the nonprotein nitrogen content of the blood serum are usually increased.

3. In thyroidectomized dogs, showing no tetanic symptoms, an acidosis condition is never observed. A slight alkalosis condition, on the contrary, is sometimes induced.

4. The antitryptic power and the nonprotein nitrogen content of the blood serum remain almost unchanged.

I desire to express my hearty thanks to Prof. S. Mita, to whom I am greatly indebted for his suggestions and help.

BIBLIOGRAPHY

[1]MacCallum, W. G., and Voegtlin, C.: Jour. Exper. Med., 1909, xi, 118.
[2]Medwedew, A.: Ztschr. f. physiol. Chem., 1911, lxxii, 410.
[3]Jacobson, C.: Am. Jour. Physiol., 1910, xxvi, 407.
[4]Underhill, F. P., and Saiki, T.: Jour. Biol. Chem., 1908-09, v, 225.
[5]Cooke, J. V.: Jour. Exper. Med., 1911, xiii, 439.
[6]Berkeley, W. N., and Beebe, S. P.: Jour. Med. Research, 1909, xx, 149.
[7]Falta, W., and Kahn, F.: Ztschr. f. klin. Med., 1911, lxxiv, 108.
[8]Greenwald, I.: Jour. Biol. Chem., 1913, xiv, 363 and 369.
[9]MacCallum, W. G., and Vogel, K. M.: Jour. Exper. Med., 1913, xviii, 618.
[10]MacCullum, W. G., Lambert, R. A., and Vogel, K. M.: Jour. Exper. Med., 1914, xx, 149.
[11]Wilson, D. W., Stearns, T., and Janney, J. H.: Jour. Biol. Chem., 1915, xxi, 169.
[12]Wilson, D. W., Stearns, T., and Thurlow, M. DeG.: Jour. Biol. Chem., 1915, xxiii, 89.
[13]Paton, D. N., and Findlay, L.: Quart Jour. Exper. Physiol, 1916, x, 203 and 315.
[14]Watanabe, C. K.: Jour. Biol. Chem., 1918, xxxiii, 253.
[15]Watanabe, C. K.: Journ. Biol. Chem., 1918, xxxiv, 65, 73 and 51.
[16]McCann, W. S.: Jour. Biol. Chem., 1918, xxxv, 553.
[17]Van Slyke, D. D., and Cullen G. E.: Jour. Biol. Chem., 1917, xxx, 317.
[18]Bergmann and Meyer, K.: Berl. klin. Wchnschr., 1908, xlv, 1673.
[19]Folin, O., and Denis, W.: Jour. Biol. Chem., 1912, xi, 527, ibid., 1913, xiv, 29.
[20]Burns, D., and Sharpe, J. S.: Quart. Jour. Exper. Physiol., 1916, x, 345.

BACILLUS BRONCHISEPTICUS AS THE CAUSE OF AN INFECTIOUS RESPIRATORY DISEASE OF THE WHITE RAT*

By H. Preston Hoskins, V.M.D., and Alice L. Stout, A. B., Detroit, Mich.

THE importance of Bacillus bronchisepticus as a pathogenic microorganism has been firmly established by the investigations of numerous workers, both in this country and abroad. A search of the literature dealing with the bacteriology of various diseases of the smaller animals, for the past thirty years, leaves no doubt that B. bronchisepticus was frequently encountered by the investigators who studied these diseases. In the majority of the reports the completeness of the data does not permit a positive statement, now, to the effect that this or that organism was the same as the one we now call B. bronchisepticus, but the fragmentary evidence dealing with the morphology and cultural characteristics, together with certain statements as to the symptoms shown by the infected animals, really leaves little room for doubt as to the identity of some of these organisms with B. bronchisepticus, especially in the light of our present knowledge regarding it and its pathogenic powers.

BRONCHISEPTICUS INFECTIONS OF OTHER ANIMALS

It remained for Ferry[1] to publish the first complete description of the organism, to which he first gave the name B. bronchicanis, having isolated it from dogs suffering with distemper. In pursuing his investigations further, Ferry found that the organism did not confine its pathogenic activities to the dog, but that it was associated with distemper-like diseases of other small animals. This caused Ferry[2] to rename the organism B. bronchisepticus. This work was confirmed by the publications of M'Gowan[3] and Torrey and Rahe,[4] which followed shortly after Ferry published his findings. Up to this time B. bronchisepticus has been reported as having been isolated from dogs, cats, rabbits, guinea pigs, ferrets, monkeys and man, but not from rats. M'Gowan[3] made bacteriologic examinations of rats in his laboratory, while studying infections among his laboratory animals, but did not find B. bronchisepticus in cultures made from the lungs, trachea, back of the nose and heart blood.

It is the purpose of this report to record the finding of B. bronchisepticus in pure culture as the apparent cause of a serious distemper-like disease among white rats. The white rat (Mus Norwegicus albinus) is now being extensively used in certain laboratory investigations, especially in work with glandular substances, vitamines and other accessory food substances, in the study of dietary deficiency diseases. In many laboratories the rats are kept in the same buildings with other small animals, such as guinea pigs and rabbits, or even in close proximity to dog kennels, thereby affording favorable conditions for the spread of such an infection as B. bronchisepticus, probably the most common pathogenic organism found among laboratory animals.

*From the Research Laboratories, Parke, Davis & Co., Detroit, Michigan.

NATURE OF THE DISEASE

The symptoms shown by affected rats are rather constant. These include loss of appetite, dullness, loss in weight, and respiratory disturbances. The latter are quite characteristic and sometimes are present without the other symptoms mentioned. There is a nasal discharge, which varies in consistency, color and amount, in different cases. Accompanying this are frequent paroxysms of sneezing and a peculiar "rattling" breathing sound. For this symptom the name "snuffles" has been casually applied by laboratory attendants, probably on account of the similarity of the rat disease with the well-known "snuffles" of rabbits. Diarrhea was not noted in any of the cases observed.

The disease may run a protracted course or end suddenly. Few recoveries have been noted. Usually a pneumonia has been found in those cases terminating fatally. No attempt has been made to treat cases of the disease for obvious reasons. It has been on the part of economy to destroy all rats showing symptoms and start over again with new stock, placed in thoroughly cleaned and disinfected quarters. There have been times when it was very difficult to obtain healthy stock from commercial rat-breeding establishments. Shipments have been made of apparently healthy stock, only to have them arrive with some of the rats showing symptoms.

BACTERIOLOGIC EXAMINATIONS

Material for study consisted of sick rats in various stages of the disease and rats dead of the infection. Cultures were made by plating material from the upper respiratory tract, trachea, lungs, and heart blood. Table I shows that B. bronchisepticus was isolated from two rats dead of the infection, and from eleven others killed for autopsy and cultural purposes. The organism was isolated from the nostrils, nasal sinus, trachea, lungs, and heart blood. Usually the cultures from the trachea were pure, as well as those from the lungs and heart blood in the two cases where the organism was recovered from these sources. Cultures made from the upper respiratory tract, nostrils and nasal sinuses, frequently

TABLE I

Data on Rats from Which B. Bronchisepticus Was Isolated

RAT NO.	KILLED OR DIED	SYMPTOMS	ORGANISM
2	K	Sick; "rattling" breathing	Sinus
3	K	Sick; "rattling" breathing	Sinus
4	K	Sick; "rattling" breathing	Sinus
7	K	Sneezing, "rattling" breathing	Trachea
14	K	Sneezing	Nostril
19	D	Not observed	Heart Blood*
21	K	Sneezing	Trachea*
24	K	Sneezing	Trachea*
25	K	Sneezing	Trachea*
26	K	Sneezing	Trachea*
28	K	Sneezing	Sinus
29	K	Sneezing	Sinus
31	D	Not observed	Lung*

*B. bronchisepticus in pure culture.

yielded B. bronchisepticus, as well as other organisms, such as staphylococci and pyocyaneus. Gas producers were not found.

At the same time that rats Nos. 20-29 were killed, samples of blood were taken, the serum removed and subsequently used for a series of agglutination tests, against B. bronchisepticus isolated from rats in the present outbreak, as well as cultures of the organism obtained from dogs. (See Table II.)

In the isolation and identification of B. bronchisepticus, suspected colonies

TABLE II

AGGLUTINATION TESTS

(1) B. bronchisepticus (rat) suspensions against homologous rat sera.
(2) B. bronchisepticus (rat)* suspensions against rat sera.
(3) B. bronchisepticus (dog) suspensions against rat sera.
                    *(Strain obtained from Rat 31)

(1) Suspension of B. bronchisepticus against the serum of the rat from which the strain was isolated.

DILUTIONS	RAT 21	RAT 25	RAT 28
1-8	++	+++	+++
1-16	+	++	+++
1-32		++	+++
1-64		++	++
1-128		++	+
1-256		+	
1-512			
1-1024			
Controls			

(2) Suspension of B. bronchisepticus (Rat 31) against sera of rats sick with disease.

DILUTIONS	RAT 21	RAT 22	RAT 23	RAT 24	RAT 25	RAT 26	RAT 27	RAT 28	RAT 29
1-8	+++	+++	+++	+++	+++	+++	+++	+++	+++
1-16	+++	+++	+++	+++	+++	+++	+++	+++	+++
1-32	++	+++	+++	+++	+++	+++	+++	+++	+++
1-64	++	++	++	++	++	++	++	++	++
1-128	++	++	++	++	++	++	++	+	++
1-256	+	++	++	+	+	+	+	+	+
1-512	−	+	+	−	−	−	−	−	+
1-1024	−	−	−	−	−	−	−	−	−
Controls	−	−	−	−	−	−	−	−	−

(3) Suspension of B. bronchisepticus (Canine Strain) against sera of rats sick with disease.

DILUTIONS	RAT 20	RAT 21	RAT 22	RAT 23	RAT 24	RAT 25	RAT 26	RAT 27	RAT 28	RAT 29
1-8	+++	+++	+++	+++	+++	+++	+++	+++	+++	+++
1-16	+++	+++	+++	+++	+++	+++	+++	+++	+++	+++
1-32	+++	+++	++	+++	+++	++	++	+++	+++	+++
1-64	++	++	++	+++	++	++	++	++	++	+++
1-128	++	++	++	++	++	+	++	++	++	++
1-256	++	+	+	++	+	+	+	++	+	++
1-512	++	+	+	−	+	+	−	++	−	+
1-1024	++	−	−	−	−	−	−	−	−	−
Controls	−	−	−	−	−	−	−	−	−	−

were picked from the agar plates and transferred to various media. All organisms which were ultimately designated B. bronchisepticus failed to produce gas or acid in fermentation tubes containing dextrose, lactose, and saccharose bouillon. The closed arm remained clear with turbidity in the open arm. Litmus milk was permanently alkalined in 48 to 72 hours, and the growth on potato was yellowish brown (tan). All organisms were actively and progressively motile, Gram-negative, nonspore forming, and failed to produce indol.

DISCUSSION

It will be noted that with two exceptions the agglutination titers were fairly uniform. One exception, where the serum of Rat 21 was run against the homologous strain of B. bronchisepticus, the suspension did not show any agglutination above a dilution of 1 to 16. The same serum agglutinated a strain of the organism from another rat at a dilution of 1 to 256. The organism from Rat 21 was typical of B. bronchisepticus in all respects. The other exception was in the case of the serum from Rat 20, which strongly agglutinated a canine strain of the organism at a dilution of 1 to 1024. At autopsy this rat showed pneumonic areas in the lungs. We were unable to determine the agglutination titer of the serum of normal rats. All rats on hand had been exposed to the disease and efforts to locate healthy stock were unsuccessful. Serum from normal rabbits does not usually agglutinate B. bronchisepticus above a dilution of 1 to 10.

SUMMARY

1. Bacillus bronchisepticus has been isolated from nostrils, nasal sinuses, trachea, lungs and heart blood of white rats affected with a serious disease of a distemper-like character.

2. The organism was recovered in pure culture in about one-half of the cases. Other organisms were found with B. bronchisepticus, in the nostrils and nasal sinuses, and once in the trachea.

3. Agglutination tests pointed to the identity of the rat organism and B. bronchisepticus from a canine source.

4. The serum of rats affected with the disease agglutinated both homologous as well as heterologous strains of B. bronchisepticus in comparatively high dilutions. One rat serum showed strong agglutination at a dilution of 1 to 1024.

BIBLIOGRAPHY

[1]Ferry, N. S.: A Preliminary Report of the Bacterial Findings in Canine Distemper, Am. Vet. Rev., 1910, xxxvii, No. 4, pp. 499-504.
[2]Ferry, N. S.: Further Studies on the Bacillus Bronchicanis, the Cause of Canine Distemper, Am. Vet. Rev., 1912, xli, No. 1, pp. 77-79.
[3]M'Gowan, J. P.: Some Observations on a Laboratory Epidemic, Principally Among Dogs and Cats, in Which the Animals Affected Presented the Symptoms of the Disease Called "Distemper," Jour. Path. and Bact., 1911, xv, No. 5, pp. 372-426.
[4]Torrey, J. C., and Rahe, A. H.: Studies in Canine Distemper, Jour. Med. Res., 1913, xxvii, No. 3, pp. 291-364.

BACTERIOLOGY AND CONTROL OF CONTAGIOUS NASAL CATARRH (SNUFFLES) OF RABBITS*

By N. S. Ferry, Ph.B., M.D., and H. Preston Hoskins, V.M.D., Detroit, Michigan

THE condition among rabbits commonly referred to as 'snuffles" has been, more or less, a disturbing element to laboratory workers ever since the animal in question was first used so generally for experimental purposes. It has also of late bid fair to become of considerable economic importance, as the practice of breeding and raising rabbits by many individuals in this country as a means of augmenting the family exchequer has recently developed into an industry of extensive proportions.

On account of the general distribution of this industry and the prevailing custom of exhibiting pure bred rabbits at the meetings of the various state and local rabbit associations, together with the opportunity offered for the spread of the infection in pet shops and bird stores, the disease has necessarily become rapidly and widely disseminated. This has resulted in an increasing demand for a more comprehensive bacteriologic study of the infectious process, as it now exists, and the development, if possible, of a means of protection against it.

PREVIOUS BACTERIOLOGIC FINDINGS

One of the earliest descriptions of an epizootic, of bacterial origin, of the respiratory tract of rabbits was given by Beck[1] in 1893. He described an infectious rabbit disease accompanied by a catarrhal pneumonia and often a fibrinous pleuritis caused by a small bacillus which was aerobic, nonmotile, negative to Gram and which could not be grown on potato, although it thrived on other alkaline media. This bacillus was found to kill rabbits within five days after intrapulmonary inoculations. It took eight or ten days, however, to kill after inoculations directly into the blood or on the uninjured nasal mucous membranes. The organism proved pathogenic for mice and guinea pigs.

In 1897 Kraus[2] described an epizootic in rabbits which resulted in pneumonia with purulent pleuritis and pericarditis, accompanied by a purulent nasal catarrh and an inflammation of the antrum of Highmore. The infection was produced by a small, Gram-negative, aerobic, motile bacillus which developed a yellowish-brown growth on potato.

Volk[3] in 1902 described a contagious disease of rabbits which always appeared to attack the pleura, pericardium and endocardium. As the cause of the infection Volk reported a small, aerobic, nonmotile bacillus, negative to Gram, which was able to grow luxuriantly on potato. This organism appeared to be extremely virulent, killing rabbits within 36-48 hours with a dose of 0.000001 c.c. of a 24-hour bouillon culture after an intraperitoneal or intrapleural inocula-

*From the Research Department, Parke, Davis & Co., Detroit, Mich.
Presented at the meeting of the Society of American Bacteriologists, Boston, Mass., Dec. 29-31, 1919.

tion. This amount inoculated into the uninjured nasal membranes took three days to kill, while 0.005 c.c. injected into the trachea resulted in death within ten days.

Südmersen in 1905[4] described an infectious rabbit pneumonia in which a fibrinous pleuritis and catarrhal lung inflammation appeared. The cause of the disease was a short, thin, occasionally double, actively motile bacillus which was Gram-negative and easily stainable with the ordinary aqueous aniline dyes. On potato it formed a yellowish-brown, wax-like growth and produced gas and indol.

In 1910 and 1911 one of us (N. S. F.)[5, 6] described an organism as causing distemper in dogs and later, 1912[7, 8] and 1914,[9] as producing snuffles in rabbits and a disease similar to distemper in other small animals. This organism, which the above author ultimately named Bacillus bronchisepticus, is recognized by the following characteristics: It is a short, slender bacillus, usually found single, but often in pairs. In liquid media it may be seen in long chains or filaments and, when cultivated directly from the animal body, may be larger and more oval in form. It does not stain by Gram but stains with most aniline dyes and with Löffler's methylene blue often gives a typical bipolar appearance. The organism is actively and progressively motile. It gives a filiform translucent growth on solid media. On potato and Koch's serum it produces a tan colored moist growth. It does not liquefy gelatin, and does not produce acid or gas in sugar. It gives an alkaline reaction to litmus milk. In broth it produces a persistent clouding with a rather viscid sediment. Indol is negative.

The disease as it was found in rabbits was briefly described by Ferry[9] as follows: "Loss of appetite and flesh with decreased activity are usually the initial symptoms. Diarrhea is an invariable symptom, while a discharge from the nose and eyes (purulent very early) is recognized in most cases; wherein it differs from the guinea pig. Death in the majority of cases is found in from two to ten days, although the disease is not as fatal as with the guinea pig. Incubation period from five to seven days. In the early stages B. bronchisepticus is usually found in the respiratory tract in pure culture. It may also be found in the blood and abdominal organs. In later stages of the disease this microorganism is associated with pyogenic organisms of secondary infections."

Ferry also mentioned an uncommonly acute infection which was present among his rabbits, at the same time, due to a bacillus of the hemorrhagic septicemia type. This disease was of extremely short duration and invariably fatal. "Often a slight discharge was observed at the nostrils but this was not so profuse nor so purulent as in snuffles due to B. bronchisepticus. At autopsy a general invasion of the body with the specific microorganism was the rule." An observation was made at that time which appears to have been substantiated by later facts that "slight discharge (of the nostrils) seems to be a common symptom of most infections in the rabbit."

In 1911 M'Gowan[10] described an organism found in an epidemic among laboratory animals, including the rabbit, (presenting the symptoms of the disease called distemper) which proved identical to the organism just preceding (B. bronchisepticus). The condition among M'Gowan's rabbits was, no doubt, typical snuffles.

In 1913 and 1917 Davis[11, 12] described a Gram-negative, nonmotile, polar staining minute bacillus which was found in subcutaneous abscesses and in snuffles in rabbits.

PRESENT INVESTIGATIONS

Culture material was obtained from rabbits of various ages and during all stages of the disease, particular attention being paid, wherever possible, to rabbits showing early symptoms of the disease. All cultures were obtained by streaking the material on plates or planting in broth. Previous work, as well as preliminary experiments during the present investigations, showed that the predominating and most consistent colonies were small, round, grayish, translucent and small, round, white, opaque. These two types alone were employed for isolation work. Smears from other colonies were studied, however, but the findings proved conclusively that they had nothing in common with the primary infectious process.

During the life of the rabbits, cultures were obtained from the nares by passing sterile swabs as far into the nasal cavity as possible. At autopsy cultures were obtained from the nasal sinuses, trachea, heart's blood and various organs of the body.

Access was afforded the investigators for a thorough study of this disease as it presented itself in rabbitries in various parts of the country and under conditions ideal for such a line of work, so that the conclusions are in no way influenced by conditions prevailing in any one locality. Entire rabbitries were placed at the disposal of the investigators for bacteriologic observations as well as for further experimental work, and as a result, a large number of animals were studied either experimentally or clinically. With these rabbits, also, were included many which were under observation for the effect of specific bacterial vaccine treatment, both prophylactic and therapeutic.   ·

RABBITS STUDIED BACTERIOLOGICALLY

1. Private stock (6 mos. old doe, Flemish Giant). June 16, 1919. Symptoms 7 months. Thick discharge from nose; sneezing. Cultures from nares. Numerous colonies of a small bacillus (B. bronchisepticus) and a few colonies of Staph. albus.

2. Private stock (young buck, Flemish Giant). June 16, 1919. Sick four weeks. Thick discharge from nose; sneezing. Cultures from nares. Numerous colonies of a small bacillus; B. bronchisepticus in large numbers; few Bact. lepisepticum and few Staph. albus.

3. Private stock (young doe, Flemish Giant). June 16, 1919. Just showing signs of illness; slight watery discharge from nose. Cultures from nares. Small bacillus in large numbers; plate contaminated; B. coli only organism isolated.

4. Private stock (young doe, Flemish Giant). June 16, 1919. Sneezing 3 to 4 days. Cultures from nares; small bacillus in large numbers which proved to be B. bronchisepticus; Staph. albus also isolated.

5. Private stock (buck, Flemish Giant). June 19, 1919. Sick six months; thick discharge. Cultures from nares. Several organisms present; gas producing organisms of the colon type isolated.

6. Private stock (young doe, Flemish Giant). June 19,1919. Sick six weeks. Thick, white discharge. Cultures from nares. Numerous colonies of small bacillus; B. bronchisepticus in pure culture.

7. Private stock (young suckling, Flemish Giant). June 19, 1919. Nursing sick mother; sneezing. Killed and posted. Cultures from nares, blood, trachea and nasal sinuses. Numerous colonies in large numbers; B. bronchisepticus in nares and trachea in pure culture; Bact. lepisepticum in sinus.

10. Laboratory rabbit. June 18, 1919. Length of illness not known; thick purulent discharge. Killed and posted. Cultures from nares, trachea and blood. Several unidentified organisms in nares only.

11. Laboratory rabbit. June 18, 1919. History not known; thick purulent discharge. Killed and posted. Cultures from nares, trachea and blood. Bact. lepisepticum in blood; unidentified organisms from nares.

12. Laboratory rabbit. June 18, 1919. History not known; thick discharge. Killed and posted. Cultures from nares, trachea and blood. Bact. lepisepticum in blood; unidentified organisms from nares.

13. Laboratory rabbit. June 18, 1919. History unknown; watery discharge. Killed and posted. Cultures from nares, trachea and blood. Unidentified organisms from nares only.

14. Laboratory rabbit. June 18, 1919. History unknown; thick purulent discharge. Killed and posted. Cultures from nares, trachea and blood. Unidentified organisms from nares only.

15. Laboratory rabbit. June 18, 1919. History unknown; thin watery discharge. Killed and posted. Cultures from nares, trachea and blood. Unidentified organisms from nares; Bact. lepisepticum from blood.

17. Laboratory rabbit. June 19, 1919. History unknown; watery discharge. Killed and posted. Cultures from nares, trachea, sinus and blood. Bact. lepisepticum and B. coli from nares; B. bronchisepticus and B. coli from trachea.

18. Laboratory rabbit. June 19, 1919. History unknown; slight discharge. Killed and posted. Cultures from nares, trachea, sinus and blood. Unidentified organisms from nares; Bact. lepisepticum from sinus.

19. Laboratory rabbit. June 20, 1919. History unknown; watery discharge. Killed and posted. Cultures from nares, trachea, sinus and blood. Bact. lepisepticum from sinus.

20. Laboratory rabbit. June 20, 1919. History unknown; slight discharge. Killed and posted. Cultures from nares, trachea, sinus and blood. Unidentified organisms from nares; Bact. lepisepticum from trachea and sinus.

21. Laboratory rabbit. June 18, 1919. History unknown; thick purulent discharge. Cultures from nares. Organisms unidentified.

22. Laboratory rabbit. June 18, 1919. History unknown; thin watery discharge. Cultures taken from nares. Organism unidentified.

23. Laboratory rabbit. June 30, 1919. History unknown; slight watery discharge. Killed and posted. Cultures from nares, trachea, sinus, blood, spleen and kidney. B. bronchisepticus in large numbers in nares and also in pure culture in the trachea and sinus.

24. Laboratory rabbit. June 30, 1919. History unknown; slight discharge. Killed and posted. Cultures from nares, trachea, sinus, blood, spleen, liver and kidney. B. bronchisepticus from trachea and sinus in pure cultures.

25. Laboratory rabbit. June 30, 1919. History unknown; sneezing; no discharge. Killed and posted. Cultures from nares, trachea, sinus and blood. Unidentified organism from nares.

31. Private stock (2 months old doe, Flemish Giant). Aug. 11, 1919. Ill four days; dead six hours; slight watery discharge. Posted. Cultures from nares and sinus. B. bronchisepticus in pure culture from sinus; B. bronchisepticus with other organism from nares.

32. Private stock (young doe, Flemish Giant). Aug. 11, 1919. Sick few days; slight watery discharge and sneezing. Killed and posted. Cultures from nares and sinus. B. bronchisepticus in pure culture from both situations.

33. Private stock (young doe, Flemish Giant). Aug. 11, 1919. Sick five days; slight watery discharge. Killed and posted. Cultures from nares and sinus. B. bronchisepticus in pure culture from sinus.

34. Private stock (buck, fourteen months old, Flemish Giant). Aug. 12, 1919. Sick six months; thick white discharge. Cultures from nares. Staph. albus; B. coli and other gas producers.

35. Private stock (young doe, common rabbit, wet nurse). Aug. 12, 1919. Sick few days; slight watery discharge. Killed and posted. Cultures taken from sinus. B. bronchisepticus in pure culture.

36. Private stock (young wet nurse, common rabbit). Aug. 12, 1919. Sick one week. thick discharge. Killed and posted. Cultures from nares and sinus. B. bronchisepticus from sinus in pure culture; B. bronchisepticus associated with other organisms from nares.

37. Private stock (11 months old doe, Rufus Red). Aug. 12, 1919. Sick three weeks; thick white discharge. Killed and posted. Cultures from nares and sinus. B. bronchisepticus in pure culture from both places.

43. Private stock (young doe, New Zealand Red). Aug. 13, 1919. Symptoms one week; slight watery discharge. Killed and posted. Cultures from sinus. B. bronchisepticus in pure culture.

44. Private stock (young doe, New Zealand Red). Aug. 13, 1919. Sick few days; slight discharge. Killed and posted. Cultures from sinus. B. bronchisepticus.

46. Private stock (doe, with young, New Zealand Red). Aug. 13, 1919. Sick few days. Young rabbits perfectly healthy. Cultures from nares. Staph. albus.

50. Private stock (young rabbit, Flemish Giant). Well when brought in Aug. 13, 1919; rubbing nose, Aug. 16, 1919; dead Aug 18, 1919. Cultures from sinus. Unidentified organism.

51. Private stock (young rabbit, Flemish Giant). Sick when brought in Aug. 13, 1919; discharge from nose, Aug. 15, 1919; sneezing and very sick, Aug. 16, 1919. Killed and posted, Aug. 18, 1919. Cultures from sinus and blood. Bact. lepisepticum in sinus.

52. Private stock (young rabbit, Flemish Giant). Slight symptoms when brought in Aug. 13, 1919; considerable discharge, Aug. 15, 1919; very sick, Aug. 16, 1919. Killed and posted, Aug. 18, 1919. Cultures from sinus and blood. Bact. lepisepticum in sinus.

53. Private stock (young rabbit, Flemish Giant). Well when first seen, Aug. 13, 1919; no symptoms, Aug. 16, 1919; killed and posted, Aug. 18, 1919. Cultures from sinus and blood. Bact. lepisepticum in sinus.

54. Private stock (young rabbit, Flemish Giant). Slight symptoms, Aug. 13, 1919; rubbing nose, Aug. 16, 1919. Killed and posted, Aug. 18, 1919. Cultures from sinus. Staph. albus.

55. Private stock (young rabbit, Flemish Giant). Well when first seen, Aug. 13, 1919; slight symptoms Aug. 15, 1919; nose moist, Aug. 16, 1919. Killed and posted, Aug. 18, 1919. Cultures from sinus and blood. Unidentified.

60. Private stock. (Flemish Giant.) Chronic case; thick discharge. Cultures from nares. Gas producer and Staph. aureus.

61. Private stock (Flemish Giant). Chronic case; thick purulent discharge. Cultures from nares. Gas producer and B. bronchisepticus.

Total rabbits examined—40.

CONTROL OF THE DISEASE

If the control of snuffles is to be attempted it must be handled as any contagious disease of bacterial origin; namely, by the observance of the ordinary sanitary precautions and hygienic measures and the use of specific therapy wherever applicable.

In 1914 one of us (N. S. F.)[8] reported the control of a severe local outbreak of an infection with B. bronchisepticus in rabbits by means of prophylactic inoculations with a specific vaccine containing 100 million bacteria per cubic centimeter. Each animal received the vaccine every third day, starting with one cubic centimeter and doubling the dose at each subsequent injection until three injections had been given. At the same time the author reported the unsuccessful attempt to control an infection due to a bacillus of the hemorrhagic septicemia type; later experiments, however, have taught us that the dose was probably much too small. The most recent work of the authors has shown that a larger dose of both organisms may be given with more satisfactory results; in fact, they recommend the use of a vaccine containing 400 million each of B. bronchisepticus and Bact. lepisepticum and 200 Staph. albus as the initial dose.

According to reports from various localities relative to the use of this vaccine it would appear that about 90 per cent of the rabbits were protected after prophylactic inoculation, and of those cases where treatment was instituted after the disease was well established, about 50 per cent were relieved of symptoms.

DISCUSSION

From the results of the present as well as former investigations, it is very evident that snuffles in rabbits is not a single entity, due to any one microorganism, but is more or less of a symptom following an infection of the upper respiratory tract with any one or more of several organisms. To further substantiate this statement, in addition to the findings of the authors already quoted, Ward[13] experimentally produced snuffles in rabbits by the intravenous injections of B. ozenæ, B. proteus and B. bronchisepticus.

It seems to be evident that the ordinary form of snuffles as encountered in the various rabbitries in this country, characterized by a variable nasal discharge accompanied by sneezing and rubbing the nose, with more or less loss of appetite and weight and a rather subacute or chronic course (which constitutes the large majority of cases), is caused by B. bronchisepticus; while the more acute form and the most fatal, in the majority of instances is due to Bact. lepisepticum. This statement is not based on absolute findings, as both organisms have been encountered in various types of cases, but is the opinion of the authors, judging from the well recognized pathogenic powers of the two organisms and a general picture of all the cases they have observed taken as a whole.

It seems to be a fact, also, from a careful perusal of the literature relating to infections of the respiratory tract of rabbits, that these conditions are becoming less severe and are changing from acute general infections, with the most prominent symptoms associated with the lungs and surrounding tissues to a more subacute and chronic condition, with symptoms referring to the upper respiratory tract only. Formerly all the epizootics seemed to be sporadic in nature and extremely severe, while at the present time the infection appears to be constantly with us, spreading over the entire country, now and then increasing in severity in certain localities.

In this connection it might be stated that the opinion is rather general among those who have examined available literature on the subject of snuffles, that it is a form of hemorrhagic septicemia. This no doubt is explained for the reason that veterinary textbooks give a prominent place to the rabbit septicemia organism in diseases of rabbits. This is probably due to the tendency of previous workers to investigate acute diseases of these animals, and give less attention to a chronic nonfatal disease as is characteristic of snuffles at the present time.

The fact should be kept in mind that certain members of the hemorrhagic septicemia group of organisms have been isolated from the respiratory tract of apparently healthy animals, and for this reason these organisms are classed with others such as the pneumococcus, for example, which is believed to become pathogenic under conditions which tend to lower the resistance of the host. The work of Davis, previously referred to, has shown that the "carrier" state in rabbits, as concerns the hemorrhagic septicemia organisms, is a condition to be reckoned with. One of the present writers (H. P. H.)[14] has called attention to the liability to obtain misleading results from rabbit inoculations, on account of the fact that the rabbits may actually be harboring the organisms at the time they are inoculated with suspected material for diagnostic purposes. In the event of the death of the rabbit, and obtaining a pure culture at autopsy, there is no way of determining definitely the actual source of the organism. The conditions under which hemorrhagic septicemia organisms are transformed from saprophytes to pathogens are probably quite varied, and in the disease being discussed in some cases, at least, we may have a double infection to deal with, probably a bronchisepticus infection supervening upon a previous hemorrhagic septicemia invasion, or vice versa.

The organism found most frequently as a secondary invader, and which probably is responsible for the purulent condition of the nasal discharge and perhaps for the chronicity of many of the cases, was Staph. albus. This organism was observed in almost every case.

Oddly enough the streptococcus, which is usually considered a common secondary invader in all infectious processes, especially of the respiratory tract, was not present in one of our cases. We must conclude, therefore, that the streptococcus is infrequently harbored by the rabbit and is not a factor to be reckoned with when undertaking to control diseases of this animal.

CONCLUSIONS

1. Contagious nasal catarrh of rabbits, commonly called "snuffles," may be caused by any one of several microorganisms.

2. B. bronchisepticus is responsible for the majority of cases of the ordinary snuffles encountered in this country at the present time.

3. Bact. lepisepticum is an important etiologic factor, as it was found in a large number of cases, and is probably responsible for many of the acute types of the disease which result fatally.

4. Staph. albus, probably present in the nature of a secondary invader, was found in practically all cases with purulent nasal discharges.

5. Many other organisms, especially gas producers of the B. coli type, were isolated but in such small numbers as to preclude their relationship to snuffles from an etiologic standpoint.

6. The streptococcus is probably not a factor to be considered in infections of the respiratory tract of the rabbit, as it was not found in a single case.

7. The disease can, in a large measure, be controlled with a vaccine composed of the three most prominent microorganisms mentioned above, especially if the conditions surrounding the animals are at all sanitary.

BIBLIOGRAPHY

[1]Beck: Ztschr. f. Hyg., 1893, xv, 363.
[2]Kraus: Ztschr. f. Hyg., 1897, xxiv, 396.
[3]Volk: Centralbl. f. Bakteriol., 1902, xxxi, 177.
[4]Südmersen: Centralbl. f. Bakteriol., 1905, xxxviii, 343.
[5]Ferry: Am. Vet. Rev., 1910, xxxvii, 499.
[6]Ferry: Jour. Infect. Dis., 1911, viii, 399.
[7]Ferry: Am. Vet. Rev., 1912, xli, 77.
[8]Ferry: The Vet. Jour., 1912, lxviii, 376.
[9]Ferry: Jour. Path. and Bacteriol., 1914, xviii, 445.
[10]M'Gowan: Jour. Path. and Bacteriol., 1911, xv, 372.
[11]Davis: Jour. Infect. Dis., 1913, xii, 42.
[12]Davis: Jour. Infect. Dis., 1917, xxi, 314.
[13]Ward: Jour. Infect. Dis., 1916, xix, 153.
[14]Hoskins: 22nd. Ann. Rpt. U. S. Live Stock Sanitary Assn., 1918, p. 123.

THE QUESTION OF THE TOXICITY OF LUNG EXTRACTS

By Plinn Morse, M.D., Detroit, Mich.

MOST laboratory workers, sooner or later in their experimental work, encounter the fact that lung extracts are highly poisonous when given rapidly by the intravenous route. This result without proper controls has undoubtedly led many into errors in interpreting their results. Some years ago, in trying to prove a tissue specificity of lung tissue for the tubercle bacillus, V. C. Vaughan, Jr., and the writer encountered this phenomenon, and for a while gave it some attention under the impression that it constituted an original observation. In association with Miss Stott the subject was pursued further, and lung tissue was found more toxic than that of other organs, but the extract of scrapings from the intima of the aorta was far more potent than any organ extract examined. The poison did not pass a Berkefeld filter and did not dialyse, and the conclusion was reached that it was apparently related to the phospholipin content of the tissue. Heating to 70 degrees destroyed its toxic properties, but heating to 56 degrees had no effect. We always found the poison confined with the nucleoprotein fraction of the protein precipitate, but thymus nucleic acid made by ourselves, and yeast nucleic acid purchased from Merck did not contain the poison. The mode of death was suggestive of anaphylaxis, but postmortem quickly showed that death was due to massive coagulation of the venous blood in the large veins and right heart. The conclusion was arrived at that the extract of endothelial cells contained a powerful activator of coagulation which was probably identical with that present in leucocytes and might be classed with those substances loosely called thrombokinase. We found by referring to the literature that all these facts were well known and that a considerable bibliography already existed covering all the points we had determined and many others in addition.

The effect of tissue extract as a coagulin led Loeb to give the name "Tissue Coagulins" to these substances and the literature of the subject is closely bound up with that of coagulation of the blood. It is the writer's impression, from inquiring among laboratory workers, that the lethal action of lung extract due to the "Tissue Coagulin" content is quite well known to those who have worked along the lines of experimental pathology. Nevertheless, in the last fifteen years very little has been written about this particular phenomenon and textbooks have no occasion to call it to the attention of students.

Several articles have appeared recently which have revived the interest in lethal organ extracts. Wherry and Ervin have called attention to the toxicity of lung extracts and publish their findings as original observations without a bibliography. From the context of the article one gathers the impression that they believed they were dealing with a hitherto unobserved phenomenon. They did not determine that death was due to intravascular clotting, but did find that the blood found in the vessels at autopsy had a delayed clotting time, a fact that is clearly stated in the older literature.

319

Wherry and Ervin noted that though in many ways the manner of death resembled that due to anaphylaxis, there were important differences in that the lungs collapsed on opening the thorax of lung-extract killed animals and that atropin does not protect. They also found, again confirming earlier work, that a sublethal dose of organ extract protected against a lethal dose of lung extract given an hour later. This "negative phase" of coagulability is a well-known phenomenon following organ extract injections.

Later Kowsaku Kakinuma studied the toxicity of lung extracts. Kakinuma was apparently well aware that the subject was not new and appends a partial bibliography of the previous work on this subject. He showed that glucose and adrenalin had each a certain power to protect against the lethal action of the lung extract and that the blood sugar of an animal was raised after a sublethal dose.

Kakinuma gives Dold (1911) the credit for observing that intravenous administration of extract of normal lung killed animals, but this phenomenon was observed before this and is referred to by Loeb.

The most exhaustive articles on the subject that have come to the writer's attention are those of Loeb (1904) (1907) the latter with a very complete bibliography. Still more recently C. A. Mills, believing that Wherry and Ervin had been the first to observe this phenomenon studied the question further and determined that lung tissue was more toxic than that of other organs, although Loeb had already shown that an extract of the scrapings of the aortic intima was the most toxic of all. Mills rediscovered the fact that death was due to intravascular clotting.

The articles of Wherry and Ervin and of Mills have been of service in that they have called attention in the recent literature to a fact that seems to have disappeared from current printed pages in the last few years.

A partial bibliography, including the more important of the older articles, is appended. Very complete bibliographies are given by Loeb and Morawitz, and Kakinuma mentions several important articles.

BIBLIOGRAPHY

Aronson: Berl. klin. Wchnschr., 1913, No. 6.
Dold: Ztschr. f. Immunitatsf., x (see also bibliography bv Kakinuma).
Doyon · Arch. Path. and Physiol., 1912, xiv, 229.
Gutman, L. H.: Ueber die Blutveranderungen bei der Vergiftung mit Organextrakten, Ztschr. f. Immunitatsf., 1913, No. 4, pp. 362, 372.
Howell: Am. Jour. Physiol., 1911, xxix, 187.
Izar Palane: Ztschr. f. Immunitatsf., xiv.
Kakinuma, Kowsaku: Am. Jour. Physiol., l, 9.
Kuster, Hermann: Ergebn. d. im Med. u. Kinderheilk., 1913, xii, 666, 732.
Loeb, Leo.: Biochem. Centralbl., 1907, iv, 829; also Bull. Univ. of Penn. Med., 1904, xvi, 382.
Mills, C. A.: Jour. Biol. Chem., vl, 425.
Morawitz: Ergebn. d. Physiol., abt. 1, 1904, iv, 307; also Handbuch d. Biochem., 1908, ii, 40.
Muraschew: Deutsch. Arch. klin. Med., 1904, lxxx. 187.
Wherry and Ervin: Jour. Infect. Dis., xxiii, 240.
Wohlgemuth: Biochem. Ztschr. xxv.

A SIMPLIFIED METHOD FOR THE DETECTION AND ESTIMATION OF THE DISTRIBUTION OF MORPHINE*

By Sergius Morgulis and Victor E. Levine, Omaha, Nebr.

THE observations here recorded arose out of an attempt to simplify the procedure of testing for the presence of morphine, which we applied to a sample of poisoned meat sent to our laboratory for investigation. As a result of our effort a method has been worked out which can be easily employed in a clinical laboratory for the detection of morphine in food, body tissue or fluids.

The specimen under examination is finely minced and heated on the water-bath for 30 minutes with 100 c.c. of a 2 per cent aqueous tartaric acid solution for every 20 gm. of substance. The morphine, when present, is converted to soluble morphine tartrate. The material is cooled, preferably in the ice chest to facilitate the solidification of all the fatty matter. The material is then strained through cheesecloth which retains most of the solid particles, and washed until the washings are no longer acid. The liquid portion upon refiltering through paper gives a clear, usually somewhat opalescent fluid. The filtrate is evaporated to a thick consistency and sodium bicarbonate is added in small amounts until effervescence ceases; after which a small excess is added. The morphine tartrate is thus decomposed and the alkaloid set free. The pasty mass is now evaporated to dryness, ground to a fine powder i an mortar and extracted with chloroform.

In order to establish the sensitiveness of the reaction, an aqueous solution of morphine sulphate was prepared, 1 c.c. of which corresponded to 0.01 mg. morphine. Definite volumes of this solution were evaporated on the water bath in a porcelain crucible and after cooling, five to ten drops of a freshly prepared selenious-sulphuric acid reagent (0.5 gm. selenium dioxide in 100 c.c. concentrated sulphuric acid) were added to the residue. We found that 0.01 mg. morphine equivalent to 0.025 mg. morphine sulphate yielded a positive reaction, while 0.005 mg. morphine corresponding to 0.0125 mg. morphine sulphate gave a faint but recognizable positive test. Selenium dissolves in concentrated sulphuric acid and forms selenosulphur trioxide, which gives a green solution. It is probable that reduction of selenious acid to free selenium through the reducing action of morphine occurs, leading to the production of a green color, owing to the interaction of the selenium and the sulphuric acid. In the presence of moisture the selenosulphur trioxide is decomposed, giving brick-red selenium which may remain in colloidal form or which may precipitate out. The color developed in the test with morphine disappears on standing, heating, or on adding water; it is replaced by a reddish brown color.

To determine how much morphine can be recovered when mixed with biologic material two experiments were performed with meat and one with liver. Twelve portions of 20 gm. each of the finely minced material, containing respectively (1) 0.00 mg.; (2) 0.005 mg.; (3) 0.01 mg.; (4) 0.05 mg.; (5) 0.1 mg.; (6) 0.2 mg.; (7) 0.3 mg.; (8) 0.4 mg.; (9) 0.5 mg.; (10) 0.6 mg.; (11) 0.7 mg.; (12) 1 mg. were heated on the water-bath with 100 c.c. 2 per cent

*From the Biochemical Laboratory, Creighton University, College of Medicine, Omaha, Nebr.

tartaric acid for one-half hour and examined for morphine, in the manner already described using 50 c.c. chloroform for extraction. No less than 0.2 mg. morphine equivalent to 0.5 mg. morphine sulphate could be detected.

The first one to report a selenium compound as an alkaloidal reagent was Brandt, who, in 1875, made use of concentrated sulphuric acid containing selenic acid for the detection of morphine and narcotine. Morphine gave at first a bluish green, then grass-green, which quickly changed into reddish yellow and reddish brown. Narcotine first produced a blue color, which became green and, finally, also changed to reddish yellow or reddish brown. The limit of reaction for morphine he gave as 1/5 to 1/6 mg. and for narcotine as 1/10 mg. In 1885 Lafon used ammonium selenite in concentrated sulphuric acid. He obtained green colorations with codeine or morphine. The limit of sensitiveness for codeine was reported as 0.1 mg. In 1891 Ferreia da Silva obtained the characteristic reaction with morphine, codeine, narceine, and narcotine. In 1899 Mecke described experiments with an alkaloidal reagent consisting of 0.5 gm. selenious acid in concentrated sulphuric acid. He highly recommended its use in deteeting the opium alkaloids. Morphine gave an evanescent blue, then intense blue, then green to persistent olive green; codeine, blue quickly changing to emerald green, and later to persistent olive; narceine, faint greenish yellow, then violet; narcotine, greenish steel blue, later cherry red; papaverine, greenish, dark steel blue, then deep violet resembling methyl violet; thebaine, deep orange, gradually paling; apomorphine dark blue, violet. Mecke made a number of comparative tests with the selenium reagent, and with several others. He found the selenium test more sensitive than the Pellagri test, nitric acid test, and Froehde's test. The characteristic color developed with the selenium appears in the cold. In practical work which involves the testing of alkaloids in tissues, the heat necessary for the extraction process gives rise to brown impurities, which often hide the color produced by alkaloidal reagents. The characteristic selenium reaction is apparent even under such conditions, provided no water is present.

The selenium reagent, sometimes called Lafon's reagent, or Mecke's reagent, gives a characteristic bluish or olive green coloration with the opium alkaloids mentioned, except thebaine, which gives a deep orange gradually paling. We have also found heroine and dionine to give the bluish olive green reaction and Lafon observed that oxydimorphine gives a brownish violet color changing to violet. On account of its sensitiveness and specificity for the opium alkaloids the reagent should be a very useful indication for them.

Several animal experiments were performed with the idea of determining the distribution of morphine as identified by the selenious-sulphuric acid reagent, which has been but recently introduced into toxicology. Our experiments represent acute morphine intoxication so that our findings would be of value from a forensic point of view as the deaths usually reported from morphine poisoning are those of the acute type. The only record we have been able to find on the use of the selenious-sulphuric acid reagent in the literature, was in the case of a Portuguese physician (1891-3) who was accused of having poisoned three of his wife's nephews, and of having brought about the death of one of them by poison given in enemata.   The symptoms were those caused by opium in part only. Morphine, narcotine and delphinin were found in the urine and in the viscera. The presence of morphine was revealed by the iodic test, Froehde's and the selenious-sulphuric acid reagents.

To determine the distribution of morphine in the animal organism, we adopted the following procedure.   The organs were weighed and treated according to the method already outlined and of the final chloroform extract the smallest quantity was found, which, when evaporated, gave a positive reaction with the selenious-sulphuric acid reagent.   The amount of morphine in the total extract was obtained in the following calculation:

$$\frac{V \times 0.01}{v} = \text{Mg. Morphine in sample.}$$

V = the volume of the total extract; v = volume of extract giving a positive reaction.   The smallest amount of morphine that can be detected with certainty is 0.01 mg.

EXPERIMENT No. 1, MAY 27, 1919.*

May 10. Male rabbit, 1.5 kg. subcutaneous injection of 450 mg. morphine sulphate.
May 27. injected 800 mg. of morphine; found dead next morning.

	ORGAN	WEIGHT OF ORGAN IN GRAMS	RELATIVE MORPHINE CONTENT
1	Liver	66	100
2	Bladder and urine	3.5	91
3	Lungs	16.8	57
4	Kidneys	18.9	19
5	Brain	8.0	14
6	Heart	7.7	4
7	Spleen	1.0	3
8	Stomach* and contents	121.5	0.5
9	Pancreas	7.0	trace
10	Small int. and contents	72.0	—
11	Large int. and contents	44.0	—
12	Cecum and contents	120.2	—

*The chloroform extracts of stomach, small and large intestines and cecum were greenish owing to the chlorophyl of the ingested food.   On evaporation a greenish residue was left.   Since it was impossible to apply the selenium reagent to the colored residues, these were extracted with ether, in which morphine is insoluble.   The ether extracts were filtered through paper, and again dissolved in chloroform.   On evaporating this second chloroform extract, negative reactions were obtained with small and large intestines and cecum, while the stomach yielded a slight positive test.

The trend of opinion is that morphine is eliminated principally by the alimentary canal.   Alt first demonstrated its elimination by the stomach and Vogt first detected morphine in the stools of a morphinist.   The latter found on washing the stomach after hypodermic injection of morphine about one-half the amount recoverable in that organ, and that the elimination began in from one to three minutes and ceased completely in from fifty to sixty minutes.   Hamburger reported both morphine and meconic acid in the stomach washings in the case of opium poisoning *per os.*   Binz in experiments on men found morphine in the stomach contents two and a half minutes after the hypodermic injection of 0.03 gm. morphine.   Tauber, with dogs, recovered after hypodermic injection 41.3 per cent in the feces; and Faust in similar experiments recovered 70.9 per cent while 62.2 per cent morphine has also been detected in the feces after hypodermic administration.   In experiments with rabbits Neuman and Tetze failed to obtain

EXPERIMENT No. 2, JUNE 23, 1919

Rabbit, 2.1 Kg. given by mouth one gram morphine sulphate.

	ORGAN	WEIGHT OF ORGAN IN GRMS	RELATIVE MORPHINE CONTENT
1	Stomach and contents	94.	100
2	Urine	(28 cc)	64
3	Small int. and contents	74.5	12
4	Cecum and Contents	109.0	8
5	Large int. and contents	48.5	4
6	Lungs '	19.0	2
7	Liver	53.0	1.5
8	Brain	8.5	1.0
9	Kidneys	15.2	0.9
10	Blood	9.5	0.6
11	Heart	7.5	0.3
12	Pancreas	3.5	0.23
13	Urinary bladder	1.5	0.19
14	Spleen	1.5	0.17
15	Gall bladder	0.5	0.03
16	Muscle	52.0	

so large a proportion in the feces as those found by Tauber and Faust with dogs, probably because of the greater reabsorption in the large intestines of rabbits.

It is evident from laboratory findings that morphine, however administered, will most probably be detected in the alimentary canal in the material removed from the stomach by vomiting or by lavage. Analyses performed for medico-legal purposes have very frequently failed to demonstrate the presence of morphine in well marked and known cases of opiate poisoning even when made soon after the ingestion and under conditions apparently favorable. Witthaus cites very many cases where morphine could not at all be detected in the stomach. It does not seem that the pathway of elimination or that the distribution follows any regular scheme.

In a number of undoubted opiate poisonings as well as in cases of morphinists taking large quantities, analyses of the urine have failed to show the presence of morphine. In others, however, morphine has been demonstrated repeatedly in the urine. Bischoff in some of his postmortems found nothing in the stomach and but traces in the urine. Lesser reported morphine in the urine, but nowhere else in the cadaver. It is believed that renal elimination plays a secondary part to that of the alimentary canal and with small doses may be inoperative. Our experiments indicate that renal elimination of morphine is probably of no less importance than elimination through the alimentary canal. especially in acute poisoning, and that from a toxicologic standpoint the examination of urine is essential.

Marcelet in his study of the localization of morphine in different portions of the organism of an addict records the following relative distribution:

Liver + + + +
Stomach + + +
Kidney + + +
Heart +
Brain +
Lungs +

These results compare well with our experiment on the rabbit which received morphine by subcutaneous injection. Marcelet's addict was doubtless also taking morphine hypodermically. In both instances the liver is found to contain the largest amount of the alkaloid, while the kidneys (and urine) contain only somewhat less than the liver. These independent analyses suggest the probability that in morphine poisoning the liver assumes an important part if the morphine is given as a subcutaneous injection. From a forensic point of view these experimental findings are significant in that they emphasize the necessity of determining the relative amounts of morphine in alimentary canal, liver, kidney and urine.

The fact that morphine is not always detected in the urine has led to the supposition that the alkaloid is modified and rendered undetectable in the system. Rubsamen has shown that certain proportions of injected morphine disappear in the bodies of rats and that these proportions become larger by habituation. The disappearance is ascribed to oxidation or conjugation. Marme reported in urine a substance which differed from morphine in giving a nontypical test with the Husemann and Froehde reagents. He believed this substance to be identical with the oxydimorphine obtained by oxidation *in vitro* but Donath and Stolnikow and also Marquis failed to confirm the finding. Marquis claimed morphine to be eliminated in part at least in the form of a conjugated compound. Although morphine through its phenolic hydroxyl has the power of forming ester sulphates similar to those normally present in the urine, monomorphyl sulphate is not found in the urine after administration of morphine. The proportion of ethereal sulphate in the urine, however, is nevertheless increased. The occurrence in urine after the administration of morphine of a reducing substance argued for a glycuronic pairing, but recently the experiments of Spitta have demonstrated that the carbohydrate component is not glycuronic acid but an unknown acid related to laiose. In our experiments the fact that large quantities of morphine were recovered in the urine probably indicates that the selenious-sulphuric acid can detect morphine even in a modified or paired condition.

Our experimental findings point to the precaution that in the chemical examination of a cadaver for morphine no portion of the body should be overlooked. Even the salivary secretion is of importance in this respect, for Rosenthal, in a patient receiving hypodermically therapeutic doses of morphine, found considerable quantities of the alkaloid in the saliva.

SUMMARY

Morphine can conveniently be determined in food, or in tissues and body fluids by heating with 2 per cent tartaric acid (if solid, the material should first be ground or finely minced) to convert all morphine into the soluble tartrate. The mixture is rapidly cooled, preferably on ice, to solidify the fatty material. The solid residue is removed by straining through cheese cloth, and washed until the washings are no longer acid to litmus. The liquid, after being filtered through paper, is evaporated to a pasty consistency. The tartrate is then decomposed by the addition of an excess of solid sodium bicarbonate which sets the alkaloid free. The evaporation is then continued to complete dryness, the mass powdered and extracted with chloroform to remove the free morphine. The volume of the chloroform extract is noted, and the smallest quantity of the extract is found which on evaporation (in a porcelain crucible over the water-bath) leaves a residue which yields a definite morphine test. In this way the relative amount of morphine in several extracts can be determined; besides, knowing the limit of sensitivity of the reaction an approximate estimate of the amount of morphine in the original sample is possible.

The various alkaloidal tests can be applied to the residues after the evaporation of portions of the chloroform extract. The reagent we employed, selenium dioxide dissolved in concentrated sulphuric acid, is very sensitive towards the opium alkaloids. While the limit of sensitivity for morphine may be regarded as 0.005 mg. yet for practical purposes the smallest amount that can be unmistakably identified as morphine with this reagent is 0.01 mg.

We conclude from our experiments with rabbits that morphine whether given subcutaneously or by mouth is widely distributed throughout the animal body, finding its way into almost every tissue. The morphine is invariably found in appreciable quantities in the urine and kidney. Also large quantities may be present in the alimentary tract, liver, lungs and brain. According to our results especially large amounts of morphine were present in the alimentary tract and excretory organs after administering the poison by mouth, while after injecting under the skin it was recovered principally from the liver, excretory organs, and also from the lungs and brain.

We conclude furthermore, that it is not advisable to limit the toxicologic examination for morphine to the alimentary tract alone, an examination of at least the kidney and urine, and liver being indispensable.

BIBLIOGRAPHY

Autenrieth, W.: Detection of Poisons, translated by W. H. Warren, ed. 4. p. 108.
Brandt, C.: Ueber eine neue Alkaloidreaction mit Selen-und Tellursäure, Dissertation, Rostock, 1875; Jahresb. ü. d. Pharm., 1875, p. 341.
Ferreira da Silva, A. J.: Sur l'emploi du sulfo-sélénide d'ammoniaque poui characteriser les alcaloides, Jour. de pharm. et de chim., 1891, xxiv, 102.
Lafon, P. L.: Action des séléniates et des sélénites sur les alkaloides, Compt. rend. Acad. sc., 1885, c, 1543.
Mecke: Ein neues Reagens auf Alkaloide, Nachweis von Opium, Ztschr. f. öffentliche Chemie, 1899, v, 351.
Marcelet, H.: Localization of Morphine in the Human Body, Bull. sc. pharm., 1918, xxv, 292.
Witthaus, R. A.: Medical Jurisprudence, Forensic Medicine and Toxicology, New York, W. Wood & Co., iv.

LABORATORY METHODS

WASSERMANN RESULTS WITH ANTICOMPLEMENTARY SERA

By Miles J. Breuer, M.A., M.D., Lincoln, Nebr.

WHEN a serum turns out to be anticomplementary, as a rule no other thought occurs to the serologist than to discard it and request another specimen. I had never given the matter any other thought until the following case was met with, in doing serologic work at a Base Hospital Center in France:

A specimen was sent into the laboratory by the medical officer in charge of the genitourinary ward, and was found to be anticomplementary. The serum was perfectly clear, about 24 hours old when the test was made, and had been kept cold. Another specimen was requested, in the routine manner, and was again found to be anticomplementary. This time I saw the ward surgeon personally, and requested that all possible precautions be taken in obtaining the third specimen. This was taken at once into the laboratory, and the serum separated immediately after clotting had taken place; and the test run on the same day. The serum was again anticomplementary. For some reason this patient's serum possessed the property of absorbing complement; specimens taken a month and two months later were identical in the possession of this property.

As it was very desirable to get a Wassermann result on this man, the complement-fixing power of the serum was titrated as follows: A series of ten tubes was set up, containing 1 c.c. of normal salt solution, 0.1 c.c. of the patient's serum, and quantities of complement from 0.1 c.c. to 1.0 c.c. in steps of 0.1 c.c. This was incubated for an hour, and then amboceptor and cells added, and the incubation continued for 30 minutes. The first tube showing complete hemolysis was the seventh. The dose of complement being 0.4 c.c. the anticomplementary power of the serum was represented by 0.3 c.c. of the complement. The 0.7 c.c. represented the dose of complement required in the reaction, including the excess over the normal dose represented by the serum's anticomplementary power. With this amount of complement a satisfactory double-plus Wassermann result was obtained, differing in no way from the results with the rest of the sera. Consistent results were obtained upon repeating the test a month and two months later. No Wassermann result could have been obtained on this patient without this procedure.

Upon resuming serologic work in civil practice, this method suggested itself when anticomplementary results were obtained on sera sent into the laboratory by physicians in general practice. In military work, or in a large hospital, when a serum is found anticomplementary, it is a small matter to get another specimen. In private practice there is a good deal of hesitation in asking patients to allow themselves to be punctured a second time; the procedure is none too popular. In case of sera shipped from a distance, the matter of delay also enters. As a rule, the delay makes little difference in the actual course of the disease, but makes a great deal of difference in the mental attitude of the patient. There are very few people who will not become difficult to handle as private patients, if they have to wait a week for a report, and then instead of getting one, find they have to have the needle in their arm a second time.

The titration of the anticomplementary power of serum was therefore tried out in seven cases of sera which were found to be anticomplementary. The results are here shown:

SERUM	ANTICOMPLEMENTARY POWER	DOSE OF COMPLEMENT	SPECIMEN HEMOLYZED	APPROXIMATE AGE OF SPECIMEN	RESULT
1	0.7 c.c.	0.5 c.c.	yes	4 days	+ +
2	0.4 c.c.	0.6 c.c.	yes	4 days	+ +
3	0.4 c.c.	0.5 c.c.	yes	6 days	+
4	0.2 c.c.	0.4 c.c.	no	24 hours	neg
5	1.0 c.c.	0.6 c.c.	yes	7 days	+ +
6	0.3 c.c.	0.5 c.c.	yes	3 days	+
7	0.4 c.c.	0.5 c.c.	yes	4 days	neg

In all of these cases, the results were clear cut, with the exception of the fifth. In this one, the control tube was not clearly hemolyzed, and it was considered advisable to report that another trial should be made. In all of these cases, the anticomplementary action was clearly due to deterioration or poor preservation, with the possible exception of No. 4. While the number of observations in this preliminary report is too small to warrant any definite conclusions, the following points are suggested: That a high anticomplementary power does not interfere with a clear-cut positive reaction, and therefore probably the syphilitic amboceptor is not concerned in the absorption of the complement occurring in anticomplementary action; that the anticomplementary action depends on hemolysis in most cases, and increases with the age of the specimen.

The question of whether or not it is practical to undertake this titration and repetition of the test after the main portion of the specimen has been run, in preference to getting another specimen, must be left with the individual worker.

BARRON'S POLYCHROME TOLUIDIN BLUE AS A SUBSTITUTE FOR METHYLENE BLUE IN THE EOSIN-METHYLENE BLUE METHOD OF MALLORY*

By R. C. WHITMAN, M.D., BOULDER, COLO.

SHORTLY after Barron published in this journal, (1918, iii, 432) his method for polychroming toluidin blue I began using his solution for staining sections cut frozen for rapid diagnosis. The results were so satisfactory that I soon found myself using the same solution as a routine substitute for alkaline methylene blue, and I have now been employing it for more than a year in this way, particularly in the eosin-methylene blue method of Mallory. I have been so pleased with the results obtained that I give the method herewith.

The toluidin blue solution is prepared by Barron's method as follows: Dissolve toluidin blue, 1, and potassium carbonate, 1, in distilled water, 400. Boil in a glass beaker to 300. Cool and add toluidin blue 2, sodium chloride 3, glacial acetic acid 12, and alcohol 15. It is ready for use at once, and in my experience seems to improve with age.

The staining method is:

1. Fixation in Zenker's, Orth's or Helly's fluid. Formalin is quite unsuitable.

2. Celloidin or paraffin embedding.

3. Fairly strong yellowish water soluble eosin. (I use 5 per cent), five or ten minutes.

4. Water

5. The above toluidin blue solution, diluted 5, 10, or 20 times with water, for five or ten minutes, or until the nuclei are stained about as deeply, or only slightly more deeply than it is desired they should appear in the finished preparation. The dilute solution keeps indefinitely.

6. Water.

7. 95 per cent alcohol to differentiate.

8a. Paraffin sections, absolute alcohol, xylol, balsam.

8b. Celloidin sections, clearing oil (I use Dunham's mixture), slide, balsam.

The following points of difference with Mallory's method may be noted:

a. Equally satisfactory results are obtained after any of the fixing fluids mentioned above, except formalin.

b. Differentiation is vastly less tricky. With paraffin sections overdifferentiation is almost impossible. Indeed, overstaining with the blue should be avoided. Celloidin sections seem to decolorize more readily, and therefore need to be watched more carefully.

c. The blue is not affected by clearing oil, (Dunham's), making the method more easily applicable to celloidin sections.

d. The toluidin blue is decidedly more opaque than methylene blue, and hence gives greater contrast in photographic plates.

The stain differentiates with extraordinary sharpness and brilliancy, and gives truly exquisite color gradations.

*From the Henry S. Denison Memorial Research Laboratories.

329

The Journal of Laboratory and Clinical Medicine .

VOL. V.   FEBRUARY, 1920   No. 5

Editor-in-Chief: VICTOR C. VAUGHAN, M.D.
Ann Arbor, Mich.

ASSOCIATE EDITORS

DENNIS E. JACKSON, M.D. - -	CINCINNATI
HANS ZINSSER, M.D. - - -	NEW YORK
PAUL G. WOOLLEY, M.D. - -	CINCINNATI
FREDERICK P. GAY, M.D. - -	BERKELEY, CAL.
J. J. R. MACLEOD, M.B. - - -	TORONTO
ROY G. PEARCE, M.D. - - -	CLEVELAND
W. C. MACCARTY, M.D. -	ROCHESTER, MINN.
GERALD B. WEBB, M.D. -	COLORADO SPRINGS
E. E. SOUTHARD, M.D. - - - -	BOSTON
WARREN T. VAUGHAN, M.D. - .	BOSTON

EDITORIALS

The Transmissions of Respiratory Infection

IN A STUDY of those infectious diseases in which the portal of entry appears to be the respiratory tract, we may divide the infection cycle for convenience into a number of subdivisions or phases. By infection cycle we would designate all the phenomena that occur from the time a virus leaves the body of one individual until it leaves that of a second, after having been transmitted in some manner to the second, having been deposited on the skin or mucous membranes, having actually invaded the tissues, and finally having been liberated from the surface to begin again its infection cycle. In its broader sense these phenomena will include, not only the life history and peregrinations of the organism, but will include all of the reactions of the infected host. It is fortunate that much of the work undertaken as a result of the influenza epidemic will be of great value in the study of the pathogenesis of other so-called respiratory infections and, conversely, that even though we may now have little or no influenza, increased knowledge of the pathogenesis of these other conditions will facilitate the ultimate description of the infection cycle in this greatest of pandemic diseases.

330

The three phases in the consideration of the pathogenesis of respiratory infections as described by Bloomfield[1] are: first, the means whereby the virus is conveyed to the individual; second, the fate of the organism from the time it reaches the mouth or nose until it is eliminated or until invasion takes place; and third, the actual invasion of the virus into the body. It might even be well to subdivide the first phase into first, manner of leaving the originally infected individual, and second, history up until its deposition on the mucous membrane or other locality of the exposed individual. We possess much valuable information concerning each of the phases, but many links in the chain are missing in all.

Means Whereby the Virus is Conveyed to the Individual.—Three factors in the transfer of virus from the infected to the healthy are receiving chief emphasis at the present time. First among these is "droplet infection," then contamination of hands, clothing, etc., and finally, contamination of eating utensils. Droplet infection, a mode of spread which has been recognized for many years, has, following particularly the work of Weaver,[2] received great emphasis. It has resulted, especially in the army, in the adoption of masks and the cubicle system. Weaver was able on diphtheria wards to reduce the incidence of diphtheria carriers among the nursing attendants from 23.25 per cent to 5.2 per cent by the use of face masks. Before the use of masks 8.0 per cent had developed scarlet fever whereas in the three years of their use no scarlet fever had occurred among the nurses.

Doust and Lyon,[3] and Haller and Colwell[4] published simultaneously reports on the relative efficiency of masks made of various cloths and of various sized weaves. This was followed by further work on this same subject by Weaver and Murchie.[5] They showed that sneezing and blowing through the nearly closed mouth produced the heaviest droplet contamination, while coughing with the mouth wide open or talking or whistling resulted in much less droplet contamination. In coughing with the lips only slightly parted there was also heavy contamination. The average range of spread of contagious droplets has been estimated at from eighteen inches by Lynch and Cumming[6] to ten feet by Doust and Lyon, while Weaver and Murchie assume about three feet to be the droplet radius of contagious importance.

From their work it would appear that coughing with the mouth wide open presents less danger so far as droplets are concerned than does the spray-producing explosion resulting from an attempt to smother with closed lips the inevitable cough. In either event we have been taught that we must cover the mouth with the hand when coughing. This brings us to the second means of transmission—the infected hand.

This mode of spread has been emphasized during the influenza epidemic by Lynch and Cumming who ascribed to it even greater importance than droplet infection. Brown, Petroff and Pasquera[7] produced tuberculosis in guinea pigs with the washings from the hands of heavily infected tuberculous patients who had previously coughed onto their hands. They were not able to infect guinea pigs with washings from sterile door knobs which tuberculous patients with demonstrated contaminated hands had handled, or with washings from the hands of individuals who had shaken hands with these patients. On the other hand, Weaver and Murchie showed that at one time or another 35.6 per cent of forty-five pupil nurses on a diphtheria ward showed hemolyzing streptococci either on the palmar surface of the fingers or under the nails, or in both places. Three per cent of these nurses carried in the same manner diphtheria bacilli. These cultures were made after routine washing of the hands. The same authors cultivated hemolyzing streptococci in 5.8 per cent and diphtheria bacilli in 4.4 per cent of 137 cultures from door knobs in the wards.

Contaminated eating utensils, especially if not properly sterilized, are a potent source of infection. Lynch and Cumming showed that the mess kit rinse water as usually used in the army messes was an excellent spreader of organisms from the utensils of one individual to those of another. Brown, Petroff and Pasquera in a study of the transmission of tubercle bacilli were able to infect guinea pigs with the washings from spoons, forks, glasses, and cups immediately after use by patients with numerous tubercle bacilli in the sputum. Washings from knives and plates did not produce the disease in guinea pigs.

The three modes of conveyance above described have received chief attention but they by no means exhaust the possibilities. Kissing as a means of infection has been studied by the last named authors. They produced tuberculosis in guinea pigs with washings from sterile petri dishes which tuberculous patients had kissed, both immediately and ten minutes after coughing. Dust, particularly the dust of rooms, has been shown to harbor tubercle bacilli, fixed type pneumococci and other organisms, but it has not been conclusively shown that the role played by contaminated dust is of great importance in the spread of infection. This subject requires further investigation. Spread through flies and contaminated food is possible. Calmette[8] states that all cases of tuberculosis which expectorate have tubercle bacilli in the dejecta. The occurrence of organisms causing other respiratory infections in feces has not so far as we know been seriously studied. Maxcy[9] introduced B. prodigiosus into the conjunctival sac and recovered the organism from the stools after twenty-four hours. It may not be venturing too far into the realm of the impossible to suggest that further studies in this field might resurrect the old subject of water-borne infection as in typhoid fever, as one of the means of spread in influenza.

The importance of the eye as a possible portal of entry is emphasized by Maxcy and by Vincent and Lochon.[10] The former introduced B. prodigiosus into the conjunctival sac and recovered it within five minutes from the nose and within fifteen minutes from the throat. The face mask as usually employed, for the prevention of droplet infection does not protect against infection of the throat through the eyes. Maxcy points out that respiratory infections such as acute coryza, measles and influenza begin with conjunctivitis, and that although this symptom in certain cases is simply a suffusion and a part of a general mucous membrane reaction, yet in others the priority and prominence of this symptom indicate rather a primary relationship with the disease. He further states that in the great epidemics of plague that have from time to time swept over the Old World, masking of the entire face, eyes included, has been wonderfully effective.

Most of the experimental work on the use of face masks has been in their ability to prevent the discharge of organisms in droplets from infected individuals, while the application of the principle has been for the protection of those exposed, which is in reality quite another problem. Maxcy has shown that infection with B. prodigiosus can take place through the conjunctival and lacrymal duct even though the mouth and nose be masked. He suggests the use of goggles. Vincent and Lochou recommend the use of a mask which will surround the entire head and which prevents the gauze from touching the face. They found that a thickness of five layers of the gauze used was necessary.

Fate of Organism from the Time It Reaches the Exposed Individual Until Eliminated or Until Invasion Takes Place.—Maxcy reports that the lacrymal secretion is not bactericidal. The sterility of the conjunctival sac is probably maintained by mechanical irrigation through the lacrymal duct. Maxcy recovered in man B. prodigiosus from the nose within five minutes after it had been introduced into the conjunctival sac. Stort[11] found that colon bacilli instilled onto a rabbit's conjunctiva had disappeared within an hour, but that after ligation of the lacrymal duct, the organisms remained present over a much longer period.

Bloomfield, in a study of the mechanism present in the upper air passages for disposing of bacteria, inoculated individuals with pure cultures of sarcina lutea. These organisms applied in large amounts to the tongue, the nasal mucosa or crypts of the tonsils disappeared within a short time, usually within an hour. In one case they were recovered from the nose after twenty-four hours. He enumerates the factors of this protective mechanism in the upper air passages as: (1) mechanical, (flushing action of secretions, with swallowing and ejection of nasal and mouth secretions, and the action of ciliated epithelium; (2) chemical, (including the reaction of mouth and nose secretions with other possible bacterial inhibitory factors); and (3) biologic (including such processes as phagocytosis and the effect of bacteria already present on the invader).

He was unable by cleansing the mouth with one liter of saline to reduce the bacterial content of the mouth secretion below 50 per cent. Fluids with hydrogen ion concentration similar to those of several specimens of saliva had no inhibitory action on the growth of sarcina lutea. This organism did not die out when kept in saline solution or in a mixed growth of normal mouth flora, but did die out, usually within one hour, when it was introduced in varying concentration into saliva. Bloomfield concludes that the rapid disappearance of sarcina lutea from the nose and mouth was due chiefly to the bactericidal effect of the saliva and mouth secretions.

Why is it that with this bactericidal substance in the oral and possibly also the nasal secretions some pathogenic organisms, as for instance the meningococcus, do grow apparently quite freely on the mucous membranes? This subject requires further investigation. Stillman[12] has been able to obtain the influenza bacillus in carriers from the postpharyngeal wall and Sailer[13] and his associates discovered fixed type pneumococcus carriers through the use of nasopharyngeal cultures. Kligler[14] reports that small amounts of nasal secretions added to culture media at times favored the growth of meningococcus organisms. This does not appear to be true for all bacteria.

Interest in streptococcus and diphtheria bacillus carriers has centered chiefly on the bacteriology of the contents of the tonsillar crypts and follicles. Numerous observers have shown that these organisms localize in the tonsillar tissue, and Moss[15] has concluded from experimental evidence that intermittent diphtheria carriers may show positive cultures at those times when the colonies in the follicles or caseous plugs break forth at the tonsillar surfaces, and become negative when they are entirely within the tonsillar tissue. That this is but one phase of the story is evidenced by failures to cure diphtheria carriers through tonsillectomy.

That the nasal accessory sinuses may serve as reservoirs is shown by the work of various observers. Crowe and Thacker-Neville,[16] found B. influenzæ in 26 per cent of infected maxillary antra during the period of the influenza epidemic and in 21 per cent in a series observed during six years when there was no epidemic.

The Mode of Invasion of the Virus into the Body.—A discussion of this phase in the pathogenesis of respiratory infections will be reserved for a later review.

BIBLIOGRAPHY

[1]Bloomfield, Arthur L.: Bull. Johns Hopkins Hosp., 1919, xxx, 317.
[2]Weaver, George H.: Jour. Infect. Dis., 1919, xxiv, 218.
[3]Doust and Lyon: Jour. Am. Med. Assn., 1918, lxxi, 1216.
[4]Haller, D. A., and Colwell, R. C.: Jour. Am. Med. Assn., 1916, lxxi.
[5]Weaver, G. H., and Murchie, J. T.: Jour. Am. Med. Assn., 1919, lxxiii, 1924.
[6]Lynch, C., and Cumming, J. G.: Mil. Surg., 1918, xliii, 597.
[7]Brown, L., Petroff, S. A., and Pasquera, G.: Jour. Am. Med. Assn., 1919, lxxiii, 1576.
[8]Calmette, A.: Ann. de l'Inst. Pasteur, 1919, xiii, 60.
[9]Maxcy, Kenneth F.: Jour. Am. Med. Assn., 1919, lxxii, 636.
[10]Vincent and Lochon: Bull. l'Acad. Med., 1918, lxxx, 348.
[11]Stort, A. G.: Arch. f. Hyg., 1891, xiii, 395.
[12]Stillman, E. G.: Jour. Exper. Med., 1919, xxxiii.
[13]Sailer et al.: Arch. Int. Med., 1919, xxiv, 600.
[14]Kligler, I. J.: Jour. Exper. Med., 1919, xxx, 3.
[15]Moss, W. L.: Personal communication.
[16]Crowe, S. J., and Thacker-Neville, W. S.: Bull. Johns Hopkins Hosp., 1919, xxx, 322.

—*W. T. V.*

Immunization Against Diphtheria by the Employment of a Toxin-antitoxin Mixture. A Caution

ONE of the most brilliant and most useful discoveries of modern medicine is that which has given us diphtheria antitoxin. This wonderful agent has robbed this distressing disease of much of its horror. I well remember, and indeed shall never forget, the scene in one of the lecture rooms of the University of Budapest in 1894 when Roux read his paper on the employment of this agent. Before that time Von Behring had announced the discovery and published some confirmatory results. Even the Germans present at that meeting were hesitating about accepting Von Behring's claims, but in that mingled audience there was no one who was at all in doubt concerning either the honesty or the skill of Roux. Some years before Roux and Yersin had discovered diphtheria toxin and all assembled that day were ready to accept any statement that Roux might make. He read his paper giving in detail the preparation of the antitoxin and the results which he had obtained in using it in the treatment of diphtheria in children. When he concluded, hats were thrown to the ceiling, grave scientific men arose to their feet and shouted their applause in all the languages of·the civilized world. I had never seen and have never since seen·such an ovation displayed by an audience of scientific men. Each of the delegates of that section of the International Congress of Hygiene left Budapest with a bottle of antitoxin in his grip and thus its use was begun in the most distant parts of the earth. Twenty-five years have elapsed since that eventful day at Budapest and it is now conceded that everything claimed for this discovery at that time has been more than justified. Many of us remember when the death rate from diphtheria in many epidemics ran to 70 per cent and even higher. Now we know that when used on the first appearance of the membrane in the throat there are practically no deaths. The neutralization of the toxin by the antitoxin is as sure as that of the neutralization of an alkali by an acid. Hilbert has shown that when the antitoxin is administered late in the first day, the death rate is 2.2. This increases as follows:

On the second day   7.6
On the third day   17.1
On the fourth day   23.8
On the fifth day   33.9
On the sixth day   34.1
After the sixth day 38.2

The value of this agent, however, is even greater than is indicated by the lowering in the death rate. For every sick child saved five are saved from being sick. While the curative value of diphtheria antitoxin is great, its preventive value is greater still. The physician called to a family in which one child has diphtheria gives a curative dose to the sick one and immunizing doses to all others. Even when the sick one has been neglected so long that the curative value of the agent is lost its preventive value is still potent. Diphtheria antitoxin has lowered not only the mortality rate but still more the morbidity rate. Unfortunately however, the immunity produced by diphtheria antitoxin is only temporary, lasting only from three to four weeks. This discovery, as valuable as it is. has not exterminated diphtheria.

Recently a toxin-antitoxin mixture nicely adjusted, so that there is no excess of toxin, has been used for purposes of immunization. The claim is made that permanent immunity against diphtheria is secured by this preparation. It is the purpose of this writing to call attention to the fact that there is danger in the use of this mixture. If it should happen that the toxin is in slight excess lives may be lost. Moreover, the claim that this mixture confers lasting immunity to diphtheria is without scientific justification. No manufacturer possesses the scientific data necessary to justify him in making any such claim for his product. In addition to this there is great responsibility resting upon the manufacturers of this preparation. Should the mixture be improperly balanced and contain an excess of toxin some day some health officer in trying to eradicate diphtheria ·from his community may find that his zeal has lead him into .a most embarrassing situation.

—V. C. V.

Full Time Medical Professors

MUCH has been said in the last few years concerning full time clinical professors in our medical schools. This is a question of considerable importance to the future of medical education in this country. The board of regents and the faculty of the University of Michigan Medical School will make an attempt to demonstrate the value of full time chairs. The regents have decided that hereafter all appointments in this school shall be for full time. There will be no divided allegiance. From the head of the department down to the humblest assistant all shall give full time to university work. The clinical professors will be paid two salaries, one as a teaching professor and the other as a clinician. The first salary will be equal to the salaries paid men of equal rank in the other departments of the University and the second salary will be paid from the hospital funds. This school now has a hospital of over 400 beds, but these fail to accommodate all the patients who come to Ann Arbor. The legislature has authorized the board of regents to build and equip a new hospital which will furnish 800 additional beds. This should give ample accommodation for a time at least. The hospital is a part of the University and a state institution. The state makes special appropriations for the hospital and it seems willing to pay the men who serve in this institution in taking care of the sick and injured people in the state. The hospital salary will be determined by the skill and ability of the individual filling the position. In other departments of the University the teacher has but one market value and that is as a teacher. On the other hand the clinician has two market values, one as a teacher and one as a clinician. This fact seems to justify the action taken by the board of regents. It must be quite evident that the full time plan will not work when it is not applicable to all members of the teaching and clinical staffs. In the new University of Michigan hospital, as in the old one, there will be neither free beds nor beds set aside for the financial support of members of the staff. Every patient is used or may be used for teaching purposes. It has been demonstrated that this may be done when good judgment is exercised not only without injury to the patient but actually to his benefit. Of course it will be understood that the University can not pay to any of its professors the great sums now being earned by many men in private practice. But the University intends to pay a liberal salary to its clinical men and it is believed that good men will be found on these terms. They will not have extravagant incomes but they will have enough to live upon decently, support their families in comfort, attend medical societies, go abroad and keep up with the profession. In addition they will have opportunity to do consecutive scientific work, to contribute to the advancement of their specialties and to make for themselves reputations both as teachers and as contributors to scientific knowledge. While there may be still some doubt as to the success of this plan there can be no question that part time clinical instructors do not give satisfactory results. The man whose time is divided between earning a living and seeking the comforts and even the extravagances of his family, and his duty as a teacher is almost certain to be influenced most largely by the former. There has been a marked evolution of the medical school in this country. Less than a century ago a group of ambitious medical men in any city could charter a medical school, bring in students and lecture or hold clinics whenever they were not engaged in private practice. This resulted in a large number of medical schools giving poor instruction and failing to adequately instruct students. The members of such faculties as a rule did not expect to make money directly out of their schools but they did seek to enhance their reputations and expected their graduates would call upon them when in need of consultation. Later it became the custom to pay the men in the medical schools who were engaged in laboratory and more strictly scientific work. This has resulted in great advance in teaching the fundamental sciences in our medical schools. So great has been this advance that it is probably no exaggeration to say that our best medical schools today are giving the scientific fundamentals as well as they are taught in any part of the world. To do the same for the clinical branches it will be necessary to secure the full time of those who instruct in these subjects. The outcome of this move in the department of medicine and surgery of the University of Michigan will be watched by the profession with interest.

—V. C. V.

Medical Veterans of the World War

UNDER the above name there was organized at the last meeting of the American Medical Association, June, 1919, a society for which a constitution and by-laws were adopted and officers for the year elected. Those eligible to membership include the following groups:

1. All medical officers, contract surgeons of the United States Army and Act. assistant surgeons of the United States Public Health Service who have served in the medical corps of the United States Army, United States Navy and the United States Public Health Service.

2. All medical members and medical examiners of local medical advisory and district boards, officially appointed by the President of the United States, the Provost Marshall General of the United States Army and the Governors of the various states.

3. Members of the medical profession of allied nations who have been in the service of their governments during the world war shall be eligible to associate membership.

The officers are a president, vice-president at large, one vice-president for each state and territory and a secretary-treasurer. The vice-president for each state with two other members from such state shall constitute a state council.

Each member shall pay one dollar to the treasurer as annual dues. The treasurer is Colonel F. F. Russell, M.C., U.S.A., Army Medical School, Washington, D. C., to whom application for membership should be made.

It is hoped that a chapter will be formed in each state. The next meeting will be held in New Orleans. La., at the time of the annual meeting of the American Medical Association. The present membership of this society is about 2200. It is estimated that there are about 50,000 men eligible to membership.

The objects of the association must be self-evident. In the first place it is desirable to have at least annual meetings when the good comradeship begun in camp or field may be renewed. In the second place it is desirable to perpetuate the memory of the hundreds of the profession who gave their lives in the great conflict. And finally those who fought to make the world safe for democracy should have some interest in determining what kind of democracy we are to enjoy. It is not the intention of the founders of this society that it should become a political organization but it is expected that this association will interest itself intelligently and unitedly in every policy which promises good to the nation as a whole and will oppose every move to the contrary. If the world is to advance in the right direction the medical profession must aid in such advancement. Individually the medical man has but little influence but collectively he can speak with a voice which will be heard even to the most remote parts of the country. Nearly one half or more of the legally qualified physicians of this country of military age responded to their country's call in time of need. No other profession or group of men made such a record. In the hospitals in this country and in France the sick and wounded American soldier was ministered to by men for the most part unaccustomed to war and only recently removed from civil practice. To this duty the American physician gave the best that was in him. Whether we remain in peace or be again involved in war the medical profession must prove a mighty factor in the evolution of the race. It is to be hoped that the muster roll of the Medical Veterans of the World War will become longer and longer until it includes every eligible name.

—V. C. V.

The Required Year of Hospital Work

SOME years ago certain medical schools, with best intentions, decided to require a hospital year of all their students before graduation. This example has been followed by other schools and an attempt has been made to have all Class A medical schools adopt this requirement. Is this wise? No medical school in this country is today prepared to guarantee to all its students who finish their fourth year satisfactory hospital appointments. At best the medical school controls only a limited number of appointments as interns in its own hospital or in hospitals dominated by members of the faculty. It follows from this that the faculty can not supervise, properly direct or in any thorough way control the hospital instruction which its students receive. It must therefore give credit for work over which it has had no direction. Is this wise? It should furthermore be borne in mind that all those who go to medical schools are not to become practitioners of medicine. Some, and it is to be hoped that among these will be found the brightest students in the class, have no intention of practicing medicine; they are going into medicine in order to do scientific work. I am aware of the fact that it has been proposed that these students should be provided for by allowing a year of laboratory work to count for an equal time in the hospital. But it has happened in at least one state that when the legislature was asked to pass a law requiring a year of hospital work before graduation in medicine, the law makers failed to make any provision for the substitution of laboratory for hospital work. You can hardly expect a young man who intends to go into pathology or physiology to delay his work along these lines by taking a hospital year; probably in some hospital where he serves only as an orderly and the highest type of scientific work that he is called upon to do is to test samples of urine for albumin or sugar or occasionally to examine microscopically a bit of tissue or more rarely to make an autopsy. The result of requiring a hospital year of medical students before graduation is going to be most disastrous to the fundamental scientific branches of medicine. It will be found more and more difficult to fill the laboratory positions with competent medical men. From this one of two things must follow. First, the scientific work in our medical schools will be done more and more by nonmedical men. Students who intend to work in physiology and pathology will not graduate in medicine because to do so would compel them to spend a year in hospital work, most likely under conditions which would be unpleasant and by no means helpful. The second alternative is that the scientific work will be done by medical graduates who have been compelled to take the hospital year and in doing so have acquired a dislike for medical practice. This is a serious matter and already the heads of laboratory departments are complaining because the brightest students are lured into clinical medicine or surgery. There is still a bigger problem, one which possibly may influence greatly the future of the profession. The demand for full time health officers is growing day by day and it is not beyond the range of possibility that within twenty-five or fifty years every city of twenty-five thousand or more inhabitants and every densely populated county will demand full time health officers. There is nothing in the ordinary routine of a hospital year which in any way fits a man for the duties of a health officer. He gets in the hospital no instruction in epidemiology and but little in the control of infectious diseases. He learns only the rudiments of the influence of diet on health and the effects of various foods upon disease remain unknown to him. In view of all these things I suggest that the medical schools that have not already required a hospital year before graduation of their students should stop and think.

The question of a hospital year before admission to the practice of medicine is another question. There is no doubt about the wisdom of this requirement. Therefore the only conclusion is that the requirement of a hospital year in medicine should lie with state boards of medical examiners and not with medical faculties. —*V. C. V.*

A New Book on Pellagra*

NO one, in this country at least, is more competent to write upon this subject than the author of the volume which now lies before us, Dr. H. F. Harris, of Atlanta, Ga. Dr. Harris has made a most important contribution to the literature of this interesting disease. He has given us a most faithful and accurate résumé of the work done on this subject, especially that of Italian physicians. As is well known the author is a firm believer in the theory that this disease is caused by maize or Indian corn. However, he modifies the maize theory inasmuch as he believes that Indian corn must be eaten through two or more generations before it develops the disease. His conclusions are so well stated by himself that we herewith reproduce them as follows:

*Pellagra, by H. F. Harris, M.D., The Macmillan Co., 1919.

"Pellagra is an extremely chronic affection of temperate and subtropical countries, i. e., where Indian corn is grown and much eaten. While the malady has been generally thought in the past to be the consequence of inanition, the result of an adequate diet, it has been more recently regarded as the effect of the habitual consumption of Indian corn, and possibly in rare instances of eating other starchy foods that have been acted upon by low vegetable forms. If this theory should be found to be correct the disease is probably more directly the result of the action of certain phenol poisons, produced by moulds while growing in these cereals, and possibly of albuminous and ferment toxins contained in sound maize, all of which together, acting from one generation to another, and not unlikely intensified by bad hygienic conditions and insufficient and imperfect food, ultimately culminate in a frank outbreak of the classical symptoms of this disease. Finally, it can not be too strongly urged that the malady is probably always hereditary, no person ever in his lifetime eating enough maize to produce the disease."

The author rejects all theories founded upon the belief that the disease is of bacterial origin or is contagious. In this he is undoubtedly right. The transmission of pellagra to the lower animals, to apes, and to man, has been tried in every conceivable manner and has always ended in failure. Certainly we are justified in concluding that pellagra is not an infectious disease.

The half baked and visionary theory of Sambon that pellagra is transmitted by the bite of a gnat receives the ridicule which it deserves. Sambon seems to have been a Dr. Cook who hurried to Italy to announce a discovery which the best Italian physicians had been seeking for centuries. The distinguished Roumanian bacteriologist, Babes, expresses himself concerning Sambon and his announced discovery as follows: "An English Commission, which had probably never seen pellagra, on arriving in a region where the disease was common, and after seeing the pellagrins, and observing that there was a small gnat which produced a redness on the skin immediately after biting, promptly telegraphed to the world that the insect was the cause of pellagra."

We must admit that however much we have enjoyed and profited by Dr. Harris' new book, we fail to see where he has done justice to Goldberger and his associates. The author scarcely mentions the work of Goldberger. Having seen the results that have followed the change in diet as recommended by Goldberger, especially as demonstrated in the large asylum at Milledgeville, Ga., we think that Goldberger's conclusions deserve more consideration than is shown them by Dr. Harris. However, no one interested in this disease should fail to read the book by Doctor Harris.

—*V. C. V.*

The Pathogenesis of Pulmonary Tuberculosis

OUR ability to distinguish human and bovine strains of the tubercle bacillus has been of assistance in studies of the mode of invasion of those organisms into the body. It is now quite generally accepted that about 10 per cent of cases of tuberculosis in humans is due to the bovine tubercle bacillus, and that in all probability this type of infection, coming from cows' milk, passes through the tissues of the alimentary tract as a portal of entry. Infection of this type usually occurs in infancy or childhood, adults being relatively immune to the bovine organism.

Concerning the primary site of the thoracic lesion in pulmonary phthisis, there is still difference of opinion. One theory is that the lesion is usually primary in the lymph glands, particularly the glands around the hilus of the lungs, and that involvement of the lung parenchyma follows spread from these primary foci usually along the bronchi or the peribronchial tissues. The opposite tenet is held by some,—that the glandular involvement is usually or always secondary to invasion of the lung parenchyma. Ghon believes that the focus is primary in the lung and that at necropsy it is found to be small, varying in size from pinhead dimensions to that of a cherry, being most often about the size of a pea. It is often smaller than the "secondary," focus in the glands, the glandular material being particularly prone to hyperplastic changes, but Ghon explains that the apparent age of a lung focus is always as great or greater than that of the glandular process. It is chiefly on this pathologic distinction that he bases his theory of parenchymatous priority.

Ghon states that the mediastinal glands which one finds to be tuberculous are those that would become so from a primary focus in the lungs, and that on following out the drainage area from the involved glands into the lung tissue, a tuberculous lesion is almost always found in the latter area. The changes in the glandular structure never appear to be older than do those in the parenchyma.

The primary lung focus is described as usually single (72 per cent), rarely occurring as more than two or three lesions, usually situated immediately beneath the pleura which frequently becomes involved, and rarely located at the apices. It may occur in any lobe, being present in 31 per cent in the right upper lobe, in 23 per cent in the left upper lobe, in 22.5 per cent in the right lower and least frequently in the right middle lobe. The commonest site is in the anterior surface of the upper lobes, midway between apex and interlobar fissure. In the lower lobes the most frequent site is near the lower edge posteriorly.

Lymphatic drainage from these areas passes through the bronchopulmonary glands to the tracheobronchial group. The inferior tracheobronchial, those beneath the angle made by the right and left bronchi, receive the greater portion of the drainage from the lower portions of the lungs, while the right and left superior tracheobronchial systems, located in the angles between the bronchi and the trachea, receive from the upper portions. Ghon shows that the diseased glands lie in the drainage system collecting from the regions of the primary lung foci. Numerous anastomoses connecting the various sets of glands explain, according to him, apparent deviations from this rule.

Canti reaches conclusions similar to those described by Ghon. In sixteen cases studied, single lung foci were discovered in eight, and multiple in two. Among the remaining six no "lung foci" as described were found, but abdominal tuberculosis was present in all. Tuberculosis of the mediastinal glands, other than in acute miliary tuberculosis, was found in twelve of the sixteen cases. In ten the glands were located in anatomic relationship with a "lung focus" and in two no focus could be found. In these latter there was extensive accompanying abdominal tuberculosis.

The lung focus was usually caseous or fibrocaseous and averaged the size of a pea. One was calcareous, one was liquefying and one showed cavitation. The most severely infected mediastinal glands were recorded as being in caseous or fibrocaseous state.

Canti, in claiming that the lung focus when present is the original tuberculous lesion in the body, emphasizes the facts that the focus is usually single, that when it is present there is in the majority of cases no other lesion in other organs indicating another portal of entry, that when the portal of entry appears to be elsewhere, as in the intestines, there is usually no lung focus, and that there is a quite constant relationship between the occurrence of lung foci and tuberculous mediastinal glands.

The work of Ghon and Canti does not prove conclusively the priority of lung infection, but it does serve to remind us that the mode and site of invasion of the tubercle bacillus in pulmonary tuberculosis is still a debated question. It remains to be proved that in two such different tissue structures as lung parenchyma and glandular tissue a caseous or fibrocaseous process in the latter is necessarily of more recent duration than a calcified or cavitated lesion in the former. Ghon found only one case with lung focus which showed no involvement of the mediastinal glands, while there were seven showing diseased mediastinal glands without lung foci and with no evidence of a source of infection outside the lung. This appears somewhat contradictory to the theory.

BIBLIOGRAPHY

Ghon, A.: The Primary Lung Focus of Tuberculosis in Children, trans. by D. Barty King, Lond., 1918.
Canti, R. G.: Primary Pulmonary Tuberculosis in Children, Quart. Jour. Med., 1919, xiii, 71.

—*W. T. V.*

Dr. Elmer Ernest Southard

It is with the deepest sorrow that we record the death of one of the most brilliant members of our editorial staff. Dr. E. E. Southard was born in Boston, July 28, 1876. He took his A.B., A.M., and M.D. degrees from Harvard University, taking the last mentioned in 1902. Following his graduation in medicine he studied in Germany. In 1906 he married Dr. Mabel Fletcher Austin, of Boston.

He became successively Assistant, Instructor and Professor of Neuropathology in his Alma Mater. From 1906 to 1909 he was pathologist to the Danvers State Hospital. From 1912 to his death he was Director of the Boston Psychopathic Hospital. He was a member of the American Academy of Arts and Sciences, the Association of American Physicians, the American Medical Association, and the American Association of Psychologists.

Dr. Southard was a writer of forcible English and was thoroughly sound in all his conclusions. A few weeks before his death he completed a compendious work on Shell Shock. With Dr. Gay he contributed very largely to our knowledge of anaphylaxis. Readers of this journal have profited by some of his best writings. He died in New York City February 8, from influenza-pneumonia within forty-eight hours after he was taken ill. He was one of the most brilliant contributors in this country in his specialty.

We extend to his wife and children our deepest sympathy. The medical profession of this country has lost in early life one of its most brilliant and productive workers.   —*V. C. V.*

The Journal of
Laboratory and Clinical
Medicine

| VOL. V. | ST. LOUIS, MARCH, 1920 | No. 6 |

ORIGINAL ARTICLES

CHEMICAL CHANGES IN THE BLOOD IN DISEASE*

By VICTOR C. MYERS, PH.D., NEW YORK CITY

INTRODUCTION

ACCURATE data on the chemical composition of the blood, especially of the nonprotein fraction, are of comparatively recent origin, and are primarily the result of American observations with American methods. We owe largely to Folin, Benedict, and Van Slyke the development of the methods which have made this work possible. The practical information which these methods have made available has been especially helpful, since they have given us very valuable data on just those conditions on which the older methods of blood examination, cytology, bacteriology, serology, gave little information—reference is made principally to such constitutional conditions as nephritis, diabetes, and gout.

Although it is the primary object of the present paper to consider those observations which have served as a guide to the diagnosis and treatment of disease, it may be well at the outset to indicate the rather broad scope which chemical methods have recently taken in the study of the blood. They have included methods for the blood volume, the blood proteins, serum albumin and globulin, improved methods of hemoglobin estimation; methods for the determination of the nonprotein nitrogen and its individual components, urea, creatinine, uric acid, amino acids, creatine and ammonia; methods for sugar, and for the lipoid constituents, fat, lecithin and cholesterol; methods for the mineral constituents, chlorides, phosphates, calcium, magnesium, potassium, sodium and iron; methods for the blood gases, carbon dioxide, carbon monoxide and oxygen, and methods for the hydrogen ion, the acetone bodies, phenol, and such enzymes as diastase, catylase, etc.

*From the Laboratory of Pathological Chemistry, New York Post-Graduate Medical School and Hospital.
This is the introductory part of a paper read in Symposiums on the Clinical Examination of the Blood before the New York Academy of Medicine on April 17, 1919, and the Cleveland Academy of Medicine on October 17, 1919. The present paper is the first of a series of papers to appear on this topic.

TABLE I

SIGNIFICANT CHEMICAL CHANGES IN THE BLOOD IN DISEASE*

CONDITION	UREA N	SUGAR	CO_2-COMBINING POWER	CREATININE	URIC ACID	NON-PROTEIN N	CHOLESTEROL	CHLORIDES AS NaCl	DIASTATIC ACTIVITY
	mg. to 100 12-15	per cent 0.09-0.12	c.c. to 100 50-75	mg. to 100 1-2	mg. to 100 2-3	mg. to 100 25-30	per cent 0.14-0.17	per cent 0.57-0.62	15-20
1. Normal	12-15	0.09-0.12	50-75	1-2	2-3	25-30	0.14-0.17	0.57-0.62	15-20
2. Beginning pathologic	20	0.15	-45	3.5	4	35	0.19	{ -0.55 +0.65	25
3. Renal diabetes		0.08-0.12							
4. Mild diabetes		0.15-0.30							25-40
5. Severe diabetes	20	0.30-1.20	50-10	2-4	4-10		0.2-0.8	0.5	35-75
6. Gout					4-10				
7. Early interstitial nephritis	15-25	0.12-0.15		2-3.5	5-12				
8. Acute nephritis	40-100	0.12-0.18	45-20	2-6	5-15				
9. Parenchymatous nephritis	20-50	0.12-0.20		2-4	2-5		high	to 0.75	20-50
10. Terminal interstitial nephritis	60-300	0.12-0.24	40-12	5-28	5-27	100-350	to 0.30	to 0.46	
11. Bichloride poisoning, to	300	0.12-0.20		33	15	370	0.35	0.5-06	
12. Double polycystic kidney, to	75	0.20		8	5				
13. Prostatic obstruction	12-40	0.11 0.16		1.5-3.5	3-9				
14. Acute intestinal obstruction	45-120					75-170			
15. Eclampsia	10-25		58-43			25-45	0.13-0.30		
16. Cholelithiasis							to 0.06		
17. Pernicious anemia									

*The data recorded in Table I are from our own observations except the figures under numbers 14, 15 and 16. The data on intestinal obstruction were taken from Tileston and Comfort,[1] on eclampsia from Losser and Van Slyke[2] and on cholelithiasis from Rothschild and Rosenthal.[3] The figures under 11 and 12 (to) simply indicate the maximal values we have observed in these conditions.

As already pointed out, these methods have yielded especially helpful information in diabetes, nephritis, and gout, while the data obtained in renal diabetes, infantile conditions such as tetany and the diarrheal acidoses, in eclampsia, malignancy, cholelithiasis, pernicious anemia, disorders of the ductless glands and various urologic conditions, have given us a new point of view regarding many of these disorders.

Before proceeding to a discussion of the pathologic variations in the composition of the blood, it may be well to indicate in tabular form the range of changes usually encountered in several common metabolic disorders. From an inspection of Table I it will be apparent that the tests furnish information of great value in diagnosis, prognosis, and treatment. Data are given on nine different blood constituents, the first five of which are regarded of special significance, and are arranged in order of their supposed clinical importance; viz., urea, sugar, CO_2-combining power, creatinine and uric acid.

A discussion of the various conditions will be taken up in the order in which they are presented in Table I. It is difficult to draw an arbitrary line indicating where normal findings end and pathologic begin, but it is believed safe, when the blood is taken after a 14-hour fast (in the morning before breakfast), to regard a urea nitrogen above 20 mg. and a sugar above 0.15 per cent as quite definitely pathologic, etc.

RENAL DIABETES

It will at once be noted in the case of renal diabetes that the blood sugar is perfectly normal, and it is only when a knowledge of this fact is at hand that a definite diagnosis of this rather uncommon condition can be made. Here the threshold point of sugar excretion is below the level of the normal blood sugar. Broadly considered, renal diabetes may be regarded as a condition of glycosuria (glycuresis[4]) not dependent upon a temporary increase of blood sugar in an individual free from symptoms of diabetes mellitus. It should perhaps be noted that mild glycosuria occasionally appears to be associated with parenchymatous nephritis[5] in which case a slight hyperglycemia may be present, but quite without influence on the glycosuria.

DIABETES MELLITUS

In diabetes the examination is primarily directed to the determination of the sugar, although in advanced cases the acidosis, as indicated by the CO_2, may assume greater significance. Here the condition of lipemia may develop, and of this the cholesterol is a particularly good index.

It should be remembered that the excretion of sugar by the kidney is simply one of the body's many factors of safety, in fact it may be compared with the safety valve of a steam boiler. The real condition to which attention should be directed is the hyperglycemia, and as the disease advances the glycosuria becomes less and less a safe criterion of this, since the permeability of the kidneys for sugar appears to be gradually lowered. Normally the blood sugar varies from 0.09 to 0.12 per cent and in early cases of diabetes one may note an excretion of sugar when the sugar of the blood rises above 0.16 or 0.17 per cent, but in advanced cases showing nephritic symptoms, blood sugar figures of 0.2 to 0.3 per cent, and even more, may be noted without the appearance of any sugar in the urine. We have observed that the diastatic activity[6] of the blood is proportional to the blood sugar in untreated cases and appears to be the blood sugar determinant. In those cases which develop a severe acidosis, the CO_2 determination of Van Slyke is a much more reliable and valuable index of the acidosis than any urinary determination. Any extended medical treatment or surgical interference should not be attempted on a severe diabetic without a knowledge of the blood sugar and the alkali reserve of the body as indicated by the CO_2 of the blood.

GOUT

The blood in gout is characterized by its rather high content of uric acid, figures of 4 to 10 mg. It should be borne in mind, however, that early cases of interstitial nephritis disclose similar figures, although here there is generally a tendency for uréa retention as well. Since a purine-free diet lowers the blood uric acid, treated gout cases may occasionally be encountered where the uric acid is only slightly elevated. The estimation of the blood uric acid is a valuable aid to the diagnosis of gout, but only when considered in connection with the clinical symptoms and other laboratory findings.

NEPHRITIS

There would appear to be little doubt that early cases of chronic nephritis are accompanied by an appreciable rise in the blood uric acid, although a rise in the blood urea can probably be taken as a safer sign of impaired kidney function. It is certainly true that the urea nitrogen falls within very narrow limits for perfectly normal individuals. As soon as one passes to hospital patients, however, figures above 15 mg. of urea nitrogen are found. Figures over 20 on the usual restricted diet of the hospital would suggest impaired kidney function. Creatinine appears to be more readily eliminated than either uric acid or urea, and it is not, as a rule, until the blood urea has doubled, or more than doubled the normal, that there is a very appreciable increase in this purely endogenous waste product derived apparently from muscle metabolism. The normal for the creatinine of the blood is approximately 1 to 2 mg. per 100 c.c. and figures over 3.5 mg. can be viewed with grave concern, while figures over 5 mg. are almost invariably indicative of an early fatal termination.[8] The only possible exceptions are cases where the retention is due to some acute renal condition, such as acute nephritis and mild bichloride poisoning. How these changes gradually come about is well brought out in the accompanying staircase table (Table II).

The inability to properly excrete the waste products of nitrogenous metabolism is only one of the difficulties which arise as the result of renal disease. As is well known, in parenchymatous nephritis, or nephrosis, the edema is probably dependent, in part at least, on the lowered permeability of the kidney for chlorides with their consequent retention. It is natural, therefore, to expect that the excretion of other salts should be deficient, although we have only recently come to appreciate the effect of the retention of phosphates. Normally, acid phosphate provides one of the most important mechanisms of eliminating acid. When the phosphate excretion is impaired, bringing about an increase in the (acid) phosphate of the blood[9] (and tissues), an acidosis results, which may be quite as

TABLE II

STAIRCASE RETENTION OF URIC ACID, UREA AND CREATININE IN NEPHRITIS*

DATE 1915-16	CASE	AGE	SEX	DIAGNOSIS	CONDITION	MG. PER 100 C.C. OF BLOOD			PHTHAL-EIN 2 HRS. PER CENT.	SYSTOLIC BLOOD PRES-SURE	URINE	
						URIC ACID	UREA N	CREAT-ININE			ALBU-MIN	CASTS
I												
9/17	H. L.	23	♂	Pulmonary tuberculosis	Unchanged	6.5	16	2.7	58	130	++	+
8/10	E. H.	41	♂	Pericarditis	Unchanged	5.6	13	2.1	45	150	-	-
10/12	F. D.	45	♂	Initial nephritis	Unchanged	5.5	12	2.5	37	185	-	+
3/6	B. D.	35	♀	Diffuse nephritis	Unchanged	9.6	19	2.4	45	175	+	+
II												
8/11	J. J.	65	♂	Early interstitial nephritis	Unchanged	9.5	25	2.5	13	185	+	+
7/21	D. S.	56	♂	Early interstitial nephritis	Unchanged	6.6	22	3.3	26	185	-	+
9/21	D. D.	52	♂	Early interstitial nephritis	Unchanged	8.7	20	3.6	20	100	+	+
8/3	C. M.	54	♂	Early interstitial nephritis	Unchanged	6.3	31	2.0	23	150	-	-
III												
1/6 }, 3/1 }	L. P.	57	♂	Moderately severe chronic interstitial nephritis	Improved	8.0 / 4.9	80 / 17	4.8 / 2.9	0 / 10	240 / 170	++	++
4/23 }, 5/21 }	J. P.	34	♂	Moderately severe chronic diffuse nephritis	Improved	8.3 / 5.3	72 / 21	3.2 / 1.9	25 / 43	238 / 145	+++	++
1/15 }, 1/28 }	W. C.	49	♂	Moderately severe chronic diffuse nephritis	Improved	9.5 / 2.5	44 / 19	3.5 / 1.9	38 / 52	210 / 120	++	++
IV												
4/11	E. C.	50	♀	Typical fatal case of chronic interstitial nephritis	Died	22.4	236	16.7	0	210	++	Pus
3/23	T. D.	34	♂	Typical fatal case of chronic interstitial nephritis	Died	15.0	240	20.5	2 - 3	225	++	+
1/25	S. H.	37	♂	Typical fatal case of chronic interstitial nephritis	Died	14.3	263	22.2	0	220	++	+
4/15	J. W.	34	♂	Typical fatal case of chronic interstitial nephritis	Died	8.7	144	11.0	Trace	225	+	+

*From Chace and Myers,[7] 1916.

severe as that resulting from diabetic ketosis, judging from the CO_2-combining power of the blood. All cases of advanced interstitial nephritis suffer from acidosis,[10] and in some cases this is apparently the actual cause of death. It may also be noted that cases of acute nephritis occasionally show marked acidosis. When this is relieved by the administration of alkali or otherwise, a simultaneous clinical improvement takes place.

In parenchymatous nephritis, if we may be allowed to use this term, the findings are quite different. Here the nitrogen retention is comparatively small, although, as noted above, the examination of the blood may disclose a retention of chlorides. The figures for urea nitrogen seldom exceed 30 mg. except in terminal stages of the disease, and generally fall between that figure and 15.

It is of interest in this connection to note that many advanced cases of malignancy,[11] possibly as a result of the toxemia, give the chemical blood picture of moderately severe nephritis, also that many cases of pneumonia show definite evidence of nitrogen retention, while in the terminal stages of the disease a severe acidosis quite generally develops.

It is apparent from the observations of Losee and Van Slyke[2] that eclampsia is accompanied neither by nitrogen retention nor severe acidosis. Although these observations are essentially negative, they are very helpful in that they show that this toxemia is not a 'uremia."

These facts regarding the nitrogen retention and acidosis of nephritis are worthy of consideration from a surgical as well as from a medical point of view, especially when one considers that a very appreciable fall in the CO_2-combining power of the blood may result from the use of a general anesthetic such as ether. When the acidosis is already pronounced, it is easy to imagine what may happen from the additional fall of 10 to 15 volumes per cent, such a fall being not uncommon in individuals without acidosis as the result of ether anesthesia.

PROSTATIC OBSTRUCTION

The blood urea has been found to be a very valuable preoperative prognostic test in cases of prostatic obstruction.[12] Cases showing urea nitrogen figures under 20 mg. per 100 c.c. of blood may be regarded as good operative risks so far as the kidneys are concerned. When the urea nitrogen figures are found between 25 and 30, the patient should be operated on with considerable caution and best after a period of preliminary treatment directed to relieve the nitrogen retention. Urea nitrogen figures over 30 mg. are very good evidence of renal involvement, and therefore afford a rather poor operative prognosis.

CHOLELITHIASIS

Since gallstones are largely composed of cholesterol, it is reasonable to suppose that their appearance might be associated with an increase in the cholesterol content of the blood. Although it seems quite probable that a hypercholesterolemia is present during the early period of the formation of the calculi, analytical data show wide variations in the blood cholesterol,[3, 13] the findings ranging from low normals to figures that are definitely increased. This being the case, it is not possible to employ the cholesterol estimation in the blood as a satisfactory means of diagnosing cholelithiasis.

PERNICIOUS ANEMIA

It is of interest that in pernicious anemia the cholesterol content of the blood plasma is markedly decreased.[13] When the antihemolytic action of cholesterol is recalled, it will be seen that this observation may possess some practical significance. The therapeutic administration of cholesterol in this condition has received attention from Italian investigators and has apparently been followed by beneficial results.

MISCELLANEOUS CONDITIONS

Sufficient has been said to indicate the practical value of the chemical analysis of blood in pathologic conditions, especially those of a constitutional nature, although many others might be mentioned. In the diarrheal acidosis of infancy the CO_2-combining power has been very helpful in pointing the way to an accurate diagnosis and therapy. Disturbances of an endocrine origin have long been recognized to be associated with a change in carbohydrate tolerance. The estimation of the blood sugar after the administration of a suitable amount of carbohydrate has afforded a much more reliable method of bringing out deviations in tolerance than the older technic of examining the urine. In leucemia it is of interest that we frequently find a very marked increase in the uric acid content of the blood.

DIFFERENTIAL DIAGNOSIS

The physician encounters many conditions where a knowledge of the chemical blood findings is of great assistance in differential diagnosis. One of these has already been mentioned, viz., renal diabetes. Without a knowledge of the blood sugar content it is scarcely possible to suitably differentiate this condition from diabetes. The estimation of the blood uric acid is often of considerable assistance in the differential diagnosis of gout and arthritis, the uric acid being essentially normal in the latter condition. Cases are sometimes encountered which clinically might be diagnosed as cases of essential hypertonia without a knowledge of the chemical blood findings, but these disclose a high uric acid, definite urea retention and figures for creatinine somewhat higher than one would ordinarily expect from the urea, a picture which appears fairly characteristic of nephritis of the arteriosclerotic type. In essential hypertonia one may find a fairly marked increase in the uric acid, but obviously no urea or creatinine retention. Cases of apoplexy present some of the clinical symptoms of uremia, but negative data on the urea and creatinine of the blood definitely exclude "uremia" as the cause of these symptoms. Such cases should not be passed over, however, without a knowledge of the CO_2-combining power, as cases of acute nephritis are sometimes encountered without nitrogen retention but with pronounced acidosis.[10]

COLORIMETRIC METHODS

It is perhaps appropriate that some remarks be made regarding the very sensitive quantitative methods which have been developed for the chemical analysis of blood. The determination of the nine constitutents for which data are given in Table I may all be made colorimetrically except for the CO_2-combining power and chlorides. Such extensive use of colorimetric methods is a development of the past fifteen years. In 1904 Folin introduced his accurate and surprisingly simple colorimetric method for the estimation of creatinine in the urine, and this gave a great impetus to the development of colorimetric methods. For this work Folin employed the Duboscq colorimeter and at the present time there are very few laboratories of physiologic chemistry that do not boast one or more of these instruments.

COLORIMETERS

Since the accuracy of colorimetric methods depends in considerable part on a satisfactory colorimeter, it may be of value to consider the mechanical principles upon which the several different instruments in common use are constructed. The instruments may be simply designated as the (1) plunger, (2) wedge or (3) dilution type. With the plunger type the intensity of the color of either the standard or unknown is varied by changing the depth of solution through which the light passes with the aid of a plunger. The Duboscq, Krüse, Kober and Bock-Benedict are of this type. With an instrument of the wedge type such as the Hellige, the standard is placed in a wedge and the unknown in a small cup with sides parallel to the wedge. The wedge is moved up and down until the intensity of the color is the same as the unknown. With the dilution type of instrument such as the Sahli hemoglobinometer and the inexpensive test tube instrument described by the writer, the unknown is diluted with water or some diluting fluid until it has identically the same color as the standard.

The instruments of the plunger type have been most extensively employed where accuracy and rapidity were required. Of the individual instruments on the market the Duboscq is the oldest and best known. Disadvantages of this instrument are the high cost and the fact that the cups and plungers are mounted in balsam and require frequent remounting. The original French instrument is very substantially constructed, however, and the glass parts are of excellent quality. This latter fact is very important, since good prisms are probably the most essential part of the instrument, otherwise it is not possible to make the two halves of the field appear the same. The Krüse model of the Duboscq, available before the war, contained some advantages over the French instrument, notably in the mounting of the cups and plungers, and was more reasonable in price, although in general it was hardly the equal of the Duboscq. The American-made Kober has many mechanical superiorities over the Duboscq and is less expensive. It has a much better arrangement for adjusting the stages than the old style rack and pinion, the vernier scale may be readily set at zero, the reflecting mirrors are divided, while the cups and plungers are of black glass with fused-on clear glass bottoms, thus making the field considerably sharper. With these cups, chloroform may be used with impunity. It should be noted, however, that the cups are much more fragile than in the Duboscq, and it is doubtful whether the prisms are as evenly matched as in the French instrument. A very simple and relatively inexpensive colorimeter has recently been introduced by Bock and Benedict.[14] In this instrument small reflecting mirrors have been substituted for the expensive prisms. The standard is put in a cell of known breadth through which the rays of light pass longitudinally, thus removing the necessity for more than one moving part. Colorimeter estimations may be made very rapidly with the instrument, and it is possible, when the instrument is precisely constructed to make exceedingly accurate colorimetric comparisons, owing probably to the fact that the glass prisms have been eliminated. Considerable personal experience with all four instruments mentioned has led the writer to choose this instrument for routine work.

The Hellige instrument has the advantage that permanent standards may be kept in individual wedges, but the disadvantages that few of these standards are really permanent and that the wedges need to be empirically standardized. When a wedge is carefully calibrated for a given purpose by the individual using the instrument, very satisfactory results may be obtained. However, just the individuals to whom this instrument especially appeals are the ones who will not insure the accurate calibration of the standard wedges.

With the dilution type of instrument such as the Sahli hemoglobinometer and the inexpensive test tube instrument described by the writer,[15] the unknown is diluted with water

*An improved model of this instrument is now sold by the C. M. Sorensen Co., Inc., New York City, who also distribute the Bock-Benedict and Kober colorimeters.

or some diluting fluid until it has identically the same color as the standard. Theoretically, the principle of diluting the unknown to the same intensity of color as the standard is excellent, but practically, it requires considerable care in execution and fairly large volumes of fluid in order to secure accuracy, since the diluting fluid must be added a drop or a few drops at a time. Where the volume of fluid is large enough that one or two drops of fluid more or less do not impair the accuracy of the test, as in the test tube instrument mentioned above, the method is perfectly satisfactory, especially for an occasional estimation, but in such very small instruments as the Sahli and Kuttner a large error is necessarily introduced.

REFERENCES

[1]Tileston and Comfort: Arch. Int. Med., 1914, xiv, 620.
[2]Losee and Van Slyke: Am. Jour. Med. Sc., 1917, cliii, 94.
[3]Rothschild and Rosenthal: Am. Jour. Med. Sc., 1916, clii, 394.
[4]Benedict and Osterberg: Jour. Biol. Chem., 1918, xxxiv, 258.
[5]Myers and Kast: Jour. Biol. Chem., 1920, xli (proceedings).
[6]Myers and Killian: Jour. Biol. Chem., 1917, xxix, 179.
[7]Chace and Myers: Jour. Am. Med. Assn., 1916, lxvii, 929.
[8]Myers and Killian: Am. Jour. Med. Sc., 1919, clvii, 674.
[9]Marriott and Howland: Arch. Int. Med., 1916, xviii, 708.
[10]Chace and Myers: Jour. Am. Med. Assn., 1920, lxxiv, 641.
[11]Kast and Killian: Proc. Soc. Exper. Biol. and Med., 1919, xvi, 141.
[12]Squier and Myers: Jour. Urol., 1918, ii, 1.
[13]Gorham and Myers: Arch. Int. Med., 1917, xx, 599.
[14]Bock and Benedict: Jour. Biol. Chem., 1918, xxxv, 227.
[15]Myers: Jour. Lab. and Clin. Med., 1916, i, 178.

A THIRD MODEL ILLUSTRATING SOME PHASES OF KIDNEY SECRETION*

By Martin H. Fischer, M.D., and George D. McLaughlin, Cincinnati, Ohio

I. INTRODUCTION

IT has been emphasized upon previous occasions[1] that it is necessary in discussing secretion to differentiate between (1) secretion of water and (2) secretion of the substances "dissolved" in the water. Secretions, in other words, are not formed "as such," but represent the result of those interacting circumstances which make primarily for the secretion of water and secondarily for what has been called a leaching out of available substances to be dissolved in the water. While secretions are usually thought of as materials strangely different from gland substance or from blood, this difference is more apparent than real. Secretions do not in general differ from their sources except in *quantitative* composition. A secreting cell may, of course, elaborate a new chemical entity, and in this way contribute to a secretion something not found in the blood, but, except for such, it is only a matter of the same or more or less of urea or salt or acid in the urine than in the kidney, or, to trace it all back to the first source, in the blood itself. Why such quantitative differences come to pass requires no recourse to vague "vitalistic" or "physiologic" concepts—mere differences in the distribution of dissolved substances (as determined by differences in solubility, in adsorption or in chemical composition) between three phases of different chemical or physical make-up (in other words, the secretion, the secreting parenchyma, and the blood) are sufficient to explain even the most marked of the existent quantitative differences.[2]

We purpose returning in these paragraphs to that half of the secretory process which has to do with the mechanism by which a glandular parenchyma separates *water* from the blood and thus fathers a secretion.

If we ignore the entirely purposeless efforts to explain such separation on a "physiologic" basis—which amount in essence to nothing more than the statement that a cell secretes because it secretes and that it fails to secrete because it can not—then the attempts to account for what is observed may be divided into two classes. The first of these is the filtration theory originally put forth by Bowman (as mere speculation based upon histologic studies) and later by Carl Ludwig and his followers upon an experimental basis. The second is properly not a theory at all, but really only a critique of the Bowman-Ludwig concept by R. Heidenhain and his successors, who, on the basis of various physiologic observations (in which the questions of the secretion of water and the secretion of various dissolved substances are hopelessly confused) negate the adequacy of the filtration hypothesis. A good illustration of the modern situation is furnished by the work of T. G. Brodie and his coworkers[3] who, from their experiments on urinary secretion, came to the conclusion that the secretion of water by such an organ as the kidney is paralleled by a consumption of oxygen. At times there was also an in-

*From the Eichberg Laboratory of Physiology in the University of Cincinnati, Cincinnati, Ohio.

creased carbon dioxide production. In plainer terms, such a parallelism means that in secreting water the kidney does work, that this work calls for a consumption of energy, and that the greater the amount of work thus done, the greater the consumption of energy. We have ourselves supported such a view.[4] The work of other authors is, however, opposed to such a conclusion, notably that of J. Barcroft and H. Straub[5] who noted an even twenty-fold increase in water output by the kidney, under the influence of injections of various salt solutions, with *no* appreciable increase in oxygen consumption. As must be apparent, the two observations are mutually exclusive for were they both correct, it would compel the conclusion that to secrete water the kidney must sometimes do work and sometimes not. Is there a less inconsistent way out?

In our opinion there is; provided we will stop confusing the two elements of the secretion of water and the secretion of dissolved substances, and bear in mind the conditions experimentally found necessary for every increase or decrease in the secretion of these two materials and the significance of such conditions in the body of the living animal from a colloid-chemical point of view.

Our previous studies have shown that the conditions making for the *absorption* of water by the colloid-chemical mass which we term a living animal, are the opposite of those which make for the secretion of this same substance. Thus water is absorbed only as the capacity of the body colloids for holding water is increased by any of various circumstances, while a separation or secretion of water follows as these conditions are reversed. Water is therefore best absorbed in those portions of the alimentary tract (the large intestine) which are bathed by the most venous blood (that richest in carbonic or other acids) while no such absorption occurs in the stomach during the "periods of digestion" when this viscus is supplied with highly arterialized blood. A *secretion* of water, after its absorption into the venous blood, becomes possible as soon as the acid content of this venous blood (carbonic acid under normal circumstances or other acids in states of disease) is diminished on passing through the lungs. At this point water becomes "free" and may be lost through any secretory organ. A first place of loss is in the lung itself, while the other places of loss of general importance are represented by the kidney and the sweat glands of the skin. To make possible a secretion of water, the following conditions must, therefore, be satisfied: (1) "free" water must be brought to the secreting parenchyma, (2) the blood carrying such free water must contain a sufficiently low concentration of various acids (and a sufficiently high concentration of oxygen) and (3) if the secretion of water is to cost the kidney or other secreting gland no work the secreting parenchyma must be "permeable" to the free water and not to the combined.

Upon previous occasions we have shown how the experimental data of other authors, as well as our own all support the first two of these conclusions. A water-starved animal is incapable of any secretion; and the injection of any amount of water in combined form (as whole blood, blood plasma or any proper hydrophilic colloid)* will not increase any secretion by a drop. Secretion in-

*This constitutes the scientific basis for the injection of proper colloid solutions to raise and maintain blood Pressure in shock. It seems to be largely forgotten by modern writers on this subject that the principles underlying the use of such solutions and the relative merits of blood, blood serum, gelatin and acacia mixtures were worked out in this laboratory over a decade ago. See Fischer, Martin H.: Oedema, New York, 1910, p. 186; Kolloidchem. Beihefte, 1911, ii, 324; Hogan, J. J., and Fischer, Martin H.: Kolloidchem. Beihefte, 1912, iii, 411; Fischer, Martin H.: Oedema and Nephritis. New York, 1915, ed. 2, p. 345; Hogan, J. J.: Jour. Am Med. Assn. 1915, lxiv, 721.

creases and is proportional to the amount of "free" water furnished the secreting organ (in other words, the amount available above that necessary for saturation of the colloids). When secretion-promoting substances like saline diuretics or materials of the type of caffeine and digitalis are used, the mechanism still remains in essence the same. In the first instance, the administered salts dehydrate the body colloids generally, and thus make available free water for secretion. while, in the second instance, they increase cardiac and respiratory efficiency, and by thus increasing the circulation through the tissues, decrease their content of carbonic and other acids, thus again making for the appearance of the free water necessary for secretion.

These ideas may be applied to such experiments as those of Brodie and his followers, and Barcroft and Straub. While insisting upon the general parallelism between amount of oxygen consumed and water secreted a study of the individual protocols and foot-notes of the first named of these authors indicates that he himself failed to discover such parallelism whenever a diuretic salt was administered; and this is the rule in all of Barcroft and Straub's findings. We would, in our own terms say that these facts compel the conclusion that the secretion of "free" water does *not* cost a kidney or other secreting organ any work. This conclusion is the logical one demanded by the colloid-chemical theories of absorption and secretion for which we have so long stood, but because such apparently finite experiments and deductions as those of Brodie stood against us we, too, insisted that water secretion represented an "active" process,[6] and thus failed to find in filtration and the "microcapillary" structure of the colloids (as illustrated in our first urinary secretion model[7]) an explanation of *all* the phenomena observed in a living animal. Therefore, if the secretion of water is essentially a filtration process, simple hydrated colloids of proper composition ought to behave like kidney parenchyma. The experiments described in this paper show that they do.

Since the colloid-chemical behavior of various hydrated soaps seems to be identical in every way thus far studied with the behavior of that hydrated protein mass which we call protoplasm (more specifically, for our purposes, with the parenchyma or hydrated colloid membrane which lies between any secretion like urine and its source, the blood) we decided to study the filtration properties of such hydrated soap systems in order to discover whether they showed any analogy to what is observed in biologic secretion.

II. EXPERIMENTS

We chose for particular study the system, hydrated sodium stearate. For filtration purposes this was cast into cylindrical cups measuring in the moist condition 7.2 cm. transversely by 5.2 cm. high with walls 1 cm. thick. The cups were made by supporting one calibrated beaker (of 120 c.c. capacity) within a second (of 350 c.c. capacity) and filling the intervening space with a hot sodium stearate solution. After the material had "set" by being cooled to room temperature, the soap model was removed from the mold and set up for experimental purposes as indicated in Fig. 1 except that the whole was covered so as to prevent undue evaporation. In the experiments to be described, the filtration properties of the cups were then tested by filling them with 80 c.c. of the solution to be filtered. The filtration pressure (the hydrostatic pressure) represented by this volume of fluid is 5 cm.

Water filters through such a soap cup in a fashion remarkably analogous to that observed in the various secreting organs of the body.

1. We tested out first the effects of the concentration of the hydrated sodium stearate system upon the filtration of water through it.   The amounts of water which will pass through a sodium stearate cup of different concentrations under the circumstances described for these experiments are indicated in Table I.

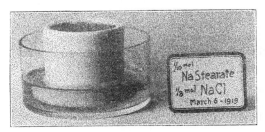

Fig. 1.

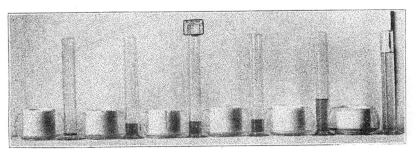

Fig. 2.

TABLE I

AMOUNT OF WATER WHICH FILTERS THROUGH SODIUM STEARATE CUPS OF DIFFERENT CONCENTRATIONS

HOURS ALLOWED FOR FILTRATION	CONCENTRATION OF SODIUM STEARATE CUP					
	1/2 m	2/5 m	3/10 m	2/10 m	1/10 m	1/20 m
2:45	0	0	0	0	3 c.c.	27 c.c.
4	1 c.c.	2 c.c.	1 c.c.	1 c.c.	6 "	34 "
5	1 "	3 "	3 "	2 "	8 "	42 "
6	2 "	3 "	4 "	2 "	10 "	46 "*
8	3 "	5 "	5 "	4 "	14 "	62 "
24:15	3 "	10 "	11 "	12 "	36 "	96 "
NEUTRALIZATION VALUE IN C.C. n/10 H₂SO₄ OF WHOLE FILTRATE	.1 "	.5 "	.6 "	6 "	1.2 "	1.4 "
NEUTRALIZATION VALUE PER C.C. OF FILTRATE	.033	.050	.054	.050	.033	.014

*25 c.c. more H₂O added to this cup.

These experiments show that the ease with which water filters through a hydrated sodium stearate decreases with every increase in the concentration of the colloid membrane. The filtration capacities of the different soap cups are so strikingly different that they are readily apparent to the naked eye as shown in Fig. 2, which is a photograph of this experiment at its end.

2. It was our next purpose to demonstrate the gross differences existent between the rate at which "free" water will filter through such a colloid cup and combined water as represented by a liquid colloid which in its physical constitution may be compared with blood. To this end we compared the filtration of water with that of a molar "solution" of sodium oleate. Since in the previous series of experiments 1/10 m sodium stearate cups had yielded a good average filtration rate we chose these for this experiment and the subsequent ones.

TABLE II

AMOUNT OF WATER WHICH FILTERS THROUGH 1/10 MOLAR SODIUM STEARATE CUPS WHEN
"FREE" OR "COMBINED" WITH A HYDRATABLE COLLOID

HOURS ALLOWED FOR FILTRATION	COMPOSITION OF LIQUID BEING FILTERED	
	H_2O	1/m sodium oleate
:30	2 c.c.	0 c.c.
1 :15	6 "	0 "
2 :15	9 "	0 "
3 :15	15 '	0 '
4 :15	19 '	0 '
5 :15	23 '	0 '
20	30 "	0 "

This experiment shows that water when combined with a hydrophilic colloid fails to come through a hydrated soap just as urine fails to come from blood when this contains no "free" water. That it is nothing specific about the sodium oleate which makes the filtration of water impossible but merely the fact that the water is bound to the sodium oleate is proved by the fact that mere dilution of the sodium oleate, sufficient to guarantee the presence of free water, at once allows some liquid to filter through. Its amount in no instance, however, equals that when pure water is used.

3. These colloid soap cups may be used to illustrate even the biological action of the various salines in increasing secretion. The saline diuretics owe their effects[8] to a dehydrating action upon the hydrophilic (protein) colloids of the body in general and upon those of the kidney in particular. By dehydrating the proteins of the body in general, they furnish "free" water for the kidney to secrete, while through such action upon the kidney specifically, they not only exhibit this function, but through it, obviously, the diameter of the capillaries must be increased which must be existent in the glandular parenchyma if mere filtration is presumed to be the mechanism by which free water is squeezed off from the blood.

The effects of the salines are different both as to their concentration and to their kind. Table III illustrates upon colloid soap how the "diuretic" effect of any salt is increased with every increase in its concentration.

The results of this experiment at the end of 7 hours are shown in Fig. 3.

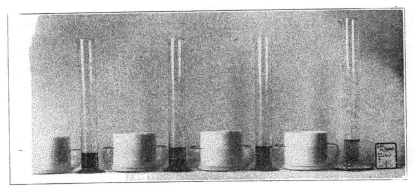

Fig. 3.

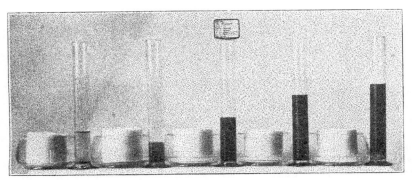

Fig. 4

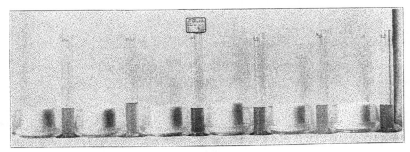

Fig. 5.

4. Table IV illustrates the difference in effects when equally concentrated (equimolar) solutions of salts possessed of a common acid but different basic radicals are filtered through a series of cups.

TABLE III

AMOUNT OF WATER WHICH FILTERS THROUGH 1/10 M SODIUM STEARATE CUPS FROM PURE WATER AND SOLUTIONS OF SODIUM CHLORIDE OF DIFFERENT CONCENTRATIONS

HOURS ALLOWED FOR FILTRATION	COMPOSITION OF LIQUID BEING FILTERED			
	H_2O	1/8 m NaCl	1/4 m NaCl	1/1 m NaCl
4	10 c.c.	13 c.c.	15 c.c.	20 c.c.
7	16 "	19 "	22 "	27 "

TABLE IV

AMOUNT OF WATER WHICH FILTERS THROUGH 1/10 M SODIUM STEARATE CUPS FROM EQUIMOLAR SOLUTIONS OF DIFFERENT SALTS

HOURS ALLOWED FOR FILTRATION	COMPOSITION OF LIQUID BEING FILTERED				
	H_2O	1/8 m NH_4Cl	1/8 m NaCl	1/8 m $MgCl_2$	1/8 m $CaCl_2$
:30	1 c.c.	3 c.c.	3 c.c.	3 c.c.	4 c.c.
1:15	2 "	6 "	8 "	10 "	10 "
2:15	6 "	9 "	14 "	20 "	23 "
3:15	9 "	12 "	20 "	29 "	35 "
4:30	15 "	14 "	27 "	40 "	50 "
5:30	19 "	16 "	33 "	52 "	64 "
6:30	23 "	17 "	38 "	58 "	70 "
7:50	30 "	18 "	42 "	62 "	72 "

The results of this experiment at its end are shown in the photograph of Fig. 4.

It is to be noted that the ammonium chloride leads to a *decrease* in secretion as compared with the effects of pure water. On the other hand, magnesium and calcium chloride are more powerful "diuretics" than sodium chloride. We return to a discussion of these findings later.

We tried next the effects upon filtration of equally concentrated (*either equinormal or equimola*r) solutions of salts containing a common basic radical with different acid radicals. Table V gives the results when equimolar solutions are used, while Table VI and Fig. 5 give the findings when equinormal solutions are employed. It will be observed that within the limits of experimental error there is *no change* in either case in amount of water secreted as compared with

TABLE V

AMOUNT OF WATER WHICH FILTERS THROUGH 1/10 M SODIUM STEARATE CUPS FROM EQUIMOLAR SOLUTIONS OF DIFFERENT SALTS

HOURS ALLOWED FOR FILTRATION	COMPOSITION OF LIQUID BEING FILTERED					
	H_2O	1/8 m NaCl	1/8 m Na_2SO_4	1/8 m Na acetate	1/8 m Na_2HPO_4	1/8 Na citrate
1	1 c.c.	1 c.c.	2 c.c.	1 c.c.	1 c.c.	1 c.c.
2:30	3 "	5 "	4 "	2 "	3 "	3 "
3:30	5 "	7 "	6 "	4 "	4 "	5 "
5:30	8 "	12 "	10 "	7 "	7 "	10 "
6:30	11 "	14 "	12 "	9 "	8 "	14 "
7:30	12 (?)	16 "	13 "	11 "	9 "	17 "
24:10	37 (?)	37 "	35 "	31 "	30 "	cup broken
NEUTRALIZATION VALUE IN C.C. n/10 H_2SO_4 FOR WHOLE FILTRATE	1.4 c.c.	.7 c.c.	.7 c.c.	.6 c.c.	.8 c.c.	

TABLE VI

AMOUNT OF WATER WHICH FILTERS THROUGH 1/10 M SODIUM STEARATE CUPS FROM EQUI-
NORMAL SOLUTION OF DIFFERENT SALTS

HOURS ALLOWED FOR FILTRATION	COMPOSITION OF LIQUID BEING FILTERED					
	H₂O	1/8 m NaCl	1/16 m Na₂SO₄	1/8 m Na acetate	1/24 m Na₂HPO₄	1/24 m Na citrate
1	1 c.c.	2 c.c.	2 c.c.	1 c.c.	1 c.c.	1 c.c.
2	2 "	4 "	3 "	1 "	2 "	2 "
3	4 "	6 "	4 "	2 "	2 "	2 "
4	5 "	7 "	6 "	4 "	4 "	4 "
5	6 "	9 "	7 "	5 "	5 "	5 "
6	8 "	11 "	8 "	7 "	7 "	7 "
7	9 "	13 "	9 "	8 "	7 "	8 "
22	30 "	32 "	27 "	28 "	24 "	28 "
NEUTRALIZATION VALUE IN C.C. n/10 H₂SO₄ FOR WHOLE FILTRATE	1.3 c.c.	.7 c.c.	.8 c.c	.7 c.c.	.8 c.c.	.5 c.c.

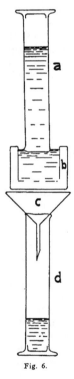

Fig. 6.

the effects of sodium chloride. In other words, the greater diuretic action of the acetates, citrates, phosphates and sulphates observed in living animals as compared with the diuretic action of
equally concentrated chlorides, bromides, or iodides does *not* appear in these filtration experiments with soaps. To the discussion
of this finding we also return below.

6. There exists a variable in all the described experiments
which may be made a constant when it is so desired. In the simple arrangement described above, the filtration pressure falls as
the amount of liquid which passes through the cup increases.
Since, besides, the filtrate is not removed as formed, more and
more accumulates about the cup and thus reduces the surface
available for filtration. Both objections may be overcome by
utilizing the filtration arrangement with constant level shown in
Fig. 6.

In Fig. 6 *b* represents in section a sodium stearate cup supported upon a coarse galvanized iron screen held in a ring stand.
In proper position above the cup is supported the inverted 100 c.c.
graduate *a*. At the beginning of the experiment the cup *b* and the
graduate *a* are filled with the liquid to be filtered, the filled graduate being inverted and placed in position as indicated in the figure. The filtration pressure is obviously determined by the height
of the liquid standing in *b*. As liquid filters through the cup
and its level falls in *b*, air enters the graduate, allowing the
liquid column in *a* to fall sufficiently to restore the old level in *b*.
In this way the filtration pressure available in *b* is kept constant.
Any liquid which filters through *b* is caught by the funnel *c* and
collected in the graduate *d* from which direct readings as to
quantity of filtrate may be made.

III. DISCUSSION

1. The model described above may be used also to demonstrate various facts
regarding *the secretion of dissolved substances*. A first point covers the matter

of how a secretion more alkaline may be derived from a less alkaline or even neutral source (parenchyma or blood). If phenolphthalein is added to the solution being filtered, is applied to the soap of the cup, and is added to the secretion escaping from the soap cup, in such an experimental series as indicated in Table III (where water and sodium chloride solutions of different concentrations are being filtered) the following facts may be observed. The original salt solutions leave phenolphthalein uncolored; so also do the sodium stearate cups; in the case of the filtrates, however, that from pure water turns the phenolphthalein brilliantly red. The same is true, though in decreasing intensity, as we examine the "secretions" from the cups containing increasingly strong sodium chloride solutions. The filtrate from the sodium chloride of highest concentration may leave the phenolphthalein practically uncolored.

Expressed in ordinary terms, alkaline secretions are here being derived from parenchymas or blood which are by themselves neutral or even acid. There is, however, nothing mysterious in the observed facts if a previous study on the composition of the lyophilic colloids and of the behavior of the colloid soaps toward indicators is kept in mind.[9] Distilled water and aqueous solutions of neutral salts are of course not expected to color phenolphthalein. The solid soap cups are essentially solutions of *water in sodium stearate* and such hydrated soap colloids also leave phenolphthalein uncolored. But upon diluting such a colloid, the soap dissolves in the water and such solutions of *soap in water do* color phenolphthalein. Hence the secretion which has passed *through* the solid sodium stearate is "alkaline" in reaction. This solubility of the soap in water decreases, however, as neutral salt is added to the water, hence less soap dissolves and hence less reaction to the phenolphthalein.

The biological significance of these findings (aside from the light which they throw upon the mechanism by which secretions more or less acid or alkaline may be obtained from allegedly more neutral sources) is of course great. In the terms of the pure physical chemists, the dilute soap solutions, as represented by the filtrates, are alkaline because, after hydrolysis of the dissolved soap, there is present an excess of hydroxyl ions. By the same reasoning the soap cups show no reaction to phenolphthalein because these are too "concentrated soap solutions." Even if we allow the correctness of such deductions—we are ourselves of the opinion that indicator methods are largely inapplicable here*—the necessary additional conclusions are still of small comfort to orthodox physiology. From a colloid point of view protoplasm behaves like the soap cup and blood and lymph like a concentrated liquid colloid of the type of sodium oleate. By the indicator methods these show no ions. Are the physical chemists who believe in the applicability of the laws of dilute solutions to living cells going to admit that solid protoplasm and blood and lymph under normal circumstances contain practically no ions, and that they have in consequence ascribed to the theories of dilute solutions, electrolytic dissociation, etc., an importance which they in no sense can exercise in normal living tissues? We believe, as a matter of fact, that normal *uninjured* protoplasm is, from a physical point of view, electrically neutral and that there are in it under normal circumstances as few or less electrically charged

* Because to our minds the system *soap dissolved in water* is something totally different from the system *water dissolved in soap.*

atoms and groups of atoms as in pure water or alcohol or ether or a dry crystal holding water of crystallization. Protoplasm is, in other words, a "solution" of water in hydrophilic colloid and this is a system to which the physico-chemical laws covering the dilute solutions may not be applied without the greatest reserve. Such laws may only be applied to the solutions of protoplasm in water, as to the more watery secretions from the body like urine, saliva or sweat.

2. If, instead of testing the "secretions" in the above experiments for alkalinity, we analyze them for content of fatty acid (in other words, for amount of soap dissolved in the secretion), it is found that most soap is dissolved when plain water is filtered through the cup and less and less as salt solutions of increasing concentration are employed. This too has its biological parallel. Distilled water can not, for example, be furnished secreting cells without damaging them, for the cells tend to dissolve in such distilled water. Thus the excessive consumption of distilled water makes for the appearance of albumin in the urine. To keep a colloid parenchyma (be it soap or protoplasm) from thus going into solution, salt must be added to the distilled water. This is one of the reasons why all cells are less damaged by a so-called physiologic salt solution than by plain water. In fact in the case of a kidney previously damaged by distilled water (or worse still by some powerful "solution"-producing agent like an acid) the progressive solution of the kidney in the urine (the albuminuria) may be cut down by perfusion of the organ with a proper salt solution.

3. We wish finally to return to the fact that if the rate at which distilled water filters through a soap cup is taken as the standard, the rate of such secretion from an ammonium chloride solution is less, while that from other salt solutions like sodium, magnesium or calcium chloride at an equivalent concentration is greater and in the order named. This, too, has its analogue in what may be observed in animals, and the explanation of what occurs in animals may be deduced, we think, from the action of these salts upon soap. Generally speaking all salts tend to dehydrate soaps and this in increasing amounts with increasing concentration. When sodium chloride is used there is therefore a progressive increase in dehydration of the hydrated sodium stearate constituting the soap cup and with the secondary enlargement of the capillary pores consequent upon this, filtration is made proportionately easier. When, however, a salt capable of entering into double decomposition with the sodium stearate is used, there is added to this first effect a secondary one incident to the production of a new soap. The hydration capacities of soaps of the commoner fatty acids with different bases runs in about the following order:

$$NH_4, K, Na, Mg, Ca.$$

(The solubility of these soaps in water also runs in this order). It will now become clear, when equally concentrated solutions of these different salts are filtered through sodium stearate, why ammonium and potassium salts lead to a lesser secretion of water than sodium, while magnesium and calcium salts lead to a greater one, and in the order named. After double decomposition and at least partial formation of the corresponding soaps, the original capillarity of the hydrated sodium stearate will be changed, being decreased in the first named, left largely unchanged in the middle member, and increased in the last named.

It was emphasized above that while the 'diuretic" action of equally concentrated but different salts differs when their basic radicals are different, such distinctions are largely missing when salts with a common base but different acid radicals are employed. In other words, these soap models do not show the greater diuretic action of the citrates, tartrates, phosphates and sulphates over chlorides, for example, which do animal kidneys or living cells in general. We expected this result as the necessary corollary of certain chemical differences between fatty acids and amino acids and the possibilities possessed by the latter of forming longer series of different salts.

The action of different bases upon a fatty acid may be compared with the action of the same bases upon the polymerized amino acid which we call protein. "Soaps" are formed in both instances with their varying hydration capacities. It is our belief, in other words, that if we write the formula for any fatty acid as:

$$x - COOH$$

that the colloid-chemical properties of the different soaps are dependent upon the substitution for the H in the above formula of the various metal radicals. If now we write the formula for an amino acid as:

$$x - COOH$$
$$|$$
$$NH_2$$

the effects of the metal radicals are again the same, and the colloid-chemical behavior of the pure proteins which are thus formed is again of the same kind as in the case of the soaps. Instead of soaps of fatty acids we get "soaps" of proteinic acid, the solvation and solution characteristics of both of which are largely the same. The fatty acids do not, however, possess the power of uniting with acid as do the amino acids. In the latter instance acids may unite with the NH_2 groups. In this fashion there can then be produced the chlorides, bromides, sulphates, phosphates, etc., of the polymerized amino acids each again possessed of its own solubility in water and solvent power for water. Since the cells of the living body are the hydrated salts of polymerized amino acids, the various salts may affect them "diuretically" not only through their basic, but also through their acid radicals.

IV. SUMMARY

The question is raised of the mechanism by which *water* is secreted by such a secreting parenchyma as a kidney. The experimental evidence is reviewed which indicates that only "free" water can be separated from the blood and that the separation of such water costs the kidney no work. This supports the conclusion that such separation is a mere filtration process, and since the secreting parenchyma of such an organ as the kidney is a hydrated colloid which has properties closely akin to a solid hydrated soap, the filtration properties of such a soap (sodium stearate) are studied to see whether any analogy exists between its behavior and what may be observed biologically.

1. Hydrated sodium stearate allows water to pass through it under slight hydrostatic pressure, the ease of such passage being increased as the concentration of the hydrated colloid is lowered.

2. While "free" water passes readily through such a hydrated colloid, water tied to a hydratable colloid (liquid sodium oleate) can not.

3. Salt solutions lead to a greater filtration of water than plain water and this (a) according to their concentration and (b) their kind, generally speaking. The higher the concentration of any salt, the greater the filtration of water. On the other hand, at given concentration, salts of ammonium or potassium produce less filtration than salts of sodium, and these less than those of magnesium or calcium. The findings on soaps are here identical with the behavior of these same salts upon the living organism. When, however, the effects of equally concentrated salts with the same basic radical but different acid radicals are compared, *no* such diuretic differences appear as occur in living animals.

4. The theory of the action of these effects is discussed, it being pointed out that because of the existent differences in chemical composition of fatty acids and of the polymerized amino acids known as protein it is possible in the former to produce only one series of salts as different bases are introduced into the fatty acid. In the case of the proteins a similar series may be produced, but because of the existence in the latter of NH_2 groups, a second series may be produced through the linking of acid with these groups. Colloid-chemical and physiologic behavior are then an expression of the solvation and solubility properties of the different compounds thus formed.

5. The dangers of applying without due reserve indicator methods and the laws of dilute solutions of electrolytic dissociation, etc., to the normal cells and fluids of the body but not to their secretions is reemphasized.

REFERENCES

[1]Fischer, Martin H.: Oedema, 1910, New York, pp. 180, 200; Oedema and Nephritis, 1915, New York, pp. 286, 324.
[2]Fischer, Martin H.: Nephritis, 1912, New York, p. 113; Oedema and Nephritis, 1915, New York. ed. 2. p. 510; Jour. Lab. and Clin. Med., 1920, v. p. 207.
[3]Barcroft, J., and Brodie, T. G.: Jour. Physiol., 1904, xxxii, 18; ibid., 1905, xxxiii, 52.
Brodie, T. G., and Cullis, W. C.: Ibid., 1906, xxxiv, 224.
Brodie, T. G.: Harvey Lectures, Philadelphia, 1909.
Cushny, A. R.: Secretion of Urine, 1917, London, pp. 34, 35.
[4]Fischer, Martin H.: Oedema and Nephritis, 1915, New York, ed. 2, p. 507.
[5]Barcroft, J., and Straub, H.: Jour. Physiol., 1911, xli, 145.
[6]Fischer, Martin H.: Oedema and Nephritis, 1915, New York, ed. 2, p. 314.
[7]Fischer, Martin H.: Ibid., p. 283.
[8]Fischer, Martin H.: Oedema, 1910, New York. p. 134; Oedema and Nephritis, 1915, New York, ed. 2, p. 295.
[9]Fischer, Martin H.: Science. 1918, xlviii. 143; ibid., 1919, xlix, 515; Chemical Engineer. 1919, xxvii, 184; ibid., 1919, xxvii, 271.

THE EPIDEMIOLOGY OF INFLUENZA-PNEUMONIA*

By Colonel Charles Lynch, Medical Corps, U. S. A., and Lieut.-Colonel James G. Cumming, Medical Corps, U. S. A. Port of Embarkation, Newport News, Va.

IT is noteworthy that as a result of the influenza epidemic the pneumonia death rate in civil life was 4.7 per 1000 population, while in the army this rate was 14.4 per 1000—a ratio of 1-3 comparing the two groups; in other words, per 1000 population, there were three times as many deaths in the army as in civil life.

What is the reason for this difference in the mortalities of the two groups? Is it age group susceptibility, air space, adequacy of clothing, fatigue, habits, crowding, food, or insanitary messing and other indirect contact incident to army life?

It has been argued because of the extreme prevalence of influenza in the military service and supposedly among civilians in the same age group that this age group is particularly susceptible, in short, that this is the susceptible age group. In order to get some definite data on this question certain information concerning children in public institutions, was secured.[1] As a result of this investigation it was found that among these children, 49,140, the influenza rate was 412 per 1000. Among 703,006 adults in similar institutions the rate was 203 per 1000. It should be added that these 49,140 children constituted the population of 131 institutions. These figures include children in a large number of institutions scattered throughout the United States. Since we found the rate highest among children it is obvious that in the young, we have the susceptible age group. This might be expected for in children we have a larger percentage of nonimmunes, while the adult population as a whole is partially immune as a result of previous attacks.

It is a fact that during the early part of the epidemic the disease prevailed most extensively among male adults, but was not this due to exposure to infection incident to their mode of life? In the days of typhoid prevalence it was recognized that young male adults, owing to their greater exposure—they eating in public places and obtaining their water from many sources—developed this disease more frequently than any other group. We have an analogy to this in influenza. The young adult is more subject to exposure owing to his mode of life. Fundamentally, infection results only from the introduction of the specific organism. Exposure is the primary factor; the secondary being the susceptibility of the individual, and this depends largely on the immunity conferred by a previous attack.

On this hypothesis we would expect the highest influenza rate in children, and the lowest among the aged. An investigation of the rates in public institutions confirms this theory.

*Read before the Medical Section of the American Life Convention, Chattanooga, Tenn., March 26, 1919. Authority to publish granted by Surgeon General's Office, Washington, D. C.

364

As a matter of fact all nonimmune individuals are susceptible whatever their age group, and will develop the disease upon the introduction of the infective agent, so that fundamentally the object to be sought is prevention of infection.

Epidemiologic studies show very definitely that air space, within moderate limits, adequacy of clothing, fatigue, habits, the kind and adequacy of food and water, play little or no part in the spread of the so-called respiratory diseases.

ARMY INFLUENZA

This leaves only insanitary messing and other indirect contact, and our recent laboratory studies and field investigations of troops show that in them the respiratory diseases are spread by indirect rather than by direct contact. Droplet infection in camps, in civil life, and in hospitals is believed to play but a minor role in the spread of sputum-borne diseases.

Indirect transmission of infection takes place by two routes of travel. But a distinction must be made between transmission in civil and that in army life. In the army the insanitary methods of washing mess gear were chiefly responsible for the high rates of sputum-borne infections. Unclean hands were then an important factor in the army.[2]

Each soldier washed his own mess gear in the same water, used by other soldiers in the same company. The companies were large—250 men. The water was inadequate in amount and with the washing of each successive mess gear it became more highly contaminated with mouth organisms from the whole company. These organisms were introduced from the mouth to the mess-kit wash water by two routes, the mess gear and the hands. The wash water was warm, sometimes hot, but the infective agents transferred to it were not killed, as it was not hot enough to do this. There was a cumulative action; the pollution of the water increased with the successive washing of mess gears, pollution by mouth and hand organisms. The washed mess gear and hands were thus contaminated by organisms from the mouths of many men. The organisms, newly acquired by the water, travel from the wash water to the mouth through two routes, through the eating utensils and the hands. From the frequency with which the hand visits the mouth it is more than probable that this is the major route.

The mess kit wash water is the focus; its use gives a common contact among troops, and this mess kit wash water is the most intimate and frequent point of indirect contact transmission for a group of mouths. Close observation of the messing of troops leads one to the above hypothesis. But have we any proof that this is actually so, and if so will it be possible to institute preventive measures? As troops were messed by two different methods it was possible to collect evidence which proved this hypothesis satisfactorily. For aside from troops, which eat from mess-kits, which they themselves wash, many organizations eat from tableware which is washed by the kitchen force. Under the latter conditions the contamination of the hands of each soldier by the common wash water, is eliminated. His hands are not exposed to the pollution by organisms common to dish water. He should then be more likely to escape infection. An investigation of the incidence of influenza among 66,000 troops, 31,000 of whom ate from tableware, and 35,000 from mess kits, proves that those who ate from tableware, which is washed by a limited force, were far less liable to infection.[3] The rate of infection in this group was 51 per 1000, while in that group which ate from mess kits, washed by the men themselves, the rate was 252 per 1000. The ratio in the two groups is 1 to 5, or per 1000 troops in the two groups, 84 per cent of the cases occurred among those whose hands were contaminated by the washing of their own eating utensils. It would seem that this is ample proof of our original hypothesis that the infection occurred by indirect contact through the use of tepid eating utensil wash water.

In order to institute corrective measures, which will prevent to a large extent the high mortality among troops, of foremost importance is the providing of boiling water for washing eating utensils. There is then no cumulative contamination of the water, infective organisms are killed, the eating utensils are more thoroughly cleansed, they are disinfected, and of far greater importance is the fact that hand contamination is prevented because of the use of boiling water.

CIVIL AND INSTITUTIONAL INFLUENZA AS AFFECTED BY THE METHOD OF WASHING DISHES

What then we consider proved up to the present stage in our paper is that the excess of influenza in troops, and excess mortality, were due to their promiscuity in messing, or in other words, to increased indirect contact from this cause.

Interesting and important as this is so far as the army is concerned, does it not possess a wider significance? The results of further study demonstrate that this is actually the case.

In order to extend the study of the theory of indirect contact transmission of influenza to the civil population and to apply it directly to the question of feeding, investigations were made in Chicago and Washington.

Machine Washed

	Persons	Cases	
Chicago Employees 12 Hotels & Restaurants	1350	13	
Chicago Employees 4 Department Stores	13500	181	
Washington Employees 2 Department Stores	2386	155	
	17236	349	20 per 1000.

Hand Washed

	Persons	Cases	
Chicago Employees 3 Restaurants	25	7	
Chicago Employees 1 Department Store	3100	259	
Washington Employees 2 Department Stores	1050	163	
	4175	429	103 per 1000.
Total	21411		

These 21,411 business men and women were employed in fifteen hotels and restaurants, and in nine department stores, where all or a part of the meals were provided.

These employees were divided according to whether they ate from machine-washed or hand-washed dishes. Among 17,236 who ate from machine-washed dishes there occurred 349 cases of influenza, while among 4175 who ate from hand-washed dishes were 429 cases. There was a rate of only 20 per 1000 in the former while in that group in which the dishes were not treated with boiling water, the rate was 103 per 1000. It appears that the chances of infection between the two groups are as one is to five, or exposure to infection among those eating from hand-washed dishes is five times greater than in that group which ate from the disinfected dishes.

Is not this a suggestion for sanitary dish washing by immersion in boiling water in the home, as well as in public eating places, and does it not give us a new conception of what we mean by crowd disease?

It was maintained that on the Panama Canal pneumonia was brought under control by segregating in huts the workmen with their families. The crowding in barracks was thereby eliminated, but it is to be pointed out that at the same time the common mess as well was abolished. In the light of our recent epidemiologic knowledge it is believed that the beneficial results were mainly from the abolition of the *common mess* rather than from the change in lodging arrangements.

The results in the two civilian groups studied dictated an extended survey of civilian fixed groups. Inasmuch as state and federal institutions have such fixed groups and would be able to furnish accurate data as to the recent influenza epidemic, questionnaires covering the information desired, were sent to such institutions; 593 replies were received.

Many of these replies had to be discarded because they were incomplete or because no cases of influenza occurred in the institutions. Accurate data covering 252,186 individuals was secured, however.

In the group eating from machine-washed dishes the rate was 108 per 1000, while in the group eating from hand-washed dishes the rate was 324 per 1000. This gives a ratio of 1 to 3 between the two groups, or 75 per cent of the cases occurring in that group which ate from dishes not disinfected with boiling water, in other words, hand-washed dishes.

Here we have fixed groups living under the same institutional conditions. Can there be any other explanation for this striking difference in the influenza rates, except the notable difference in methods of dish washing, disinfection in the one case and increased contamination in the other?

DURATION AND DAILY RATE OF INFECTION

It is interesting to note that in institutions where machine-washed dishes were used the average duration of the epidemic was 5.1 weeks, whereas in institutions where hand-washed dishes were used this period was 4.5 weeks. The daily rate of infection then was three times greater in the hand-washed group.

In the machine-washed group the major route of transmission through eating utensils was eliminated, resulting in reducing the number of infections, but in prolonging the epidemic. In the other group, where both major and minor routes of transmission, eating utensils and inanimate objects, freely took part as transmitting agents, the duration of the epidemic was shortened and the daily rate of infection was three times as great.

These findings are wholly in keeping with our theory as to the relative importance of eating utensils and inanimate objects as conveyors of infection.

COMPARATIVE MORTALITIES IN THE TWO GROUPS

In the two groups we find that among those using machine-washed dishes the mortality from pneumonia per 1000 population was less than one-half the mortality among those using hand-washed dishes. The difference in mortality is, in the ultimate analysis of any investigation, of prime importance. This especially holds true in our consideration of the influenza epidemic because influenza of itself but rarely kills. The recent pandemic might have come and gone without special comment and the fatalities would not have been more than a couple of thousand instead of 500,000 had the primary infection, influenza, been uncomplicated. Influenza, like measles and scarlet fever, is but rarely if ever the immediate cause of death, and reports of high death rates from influenza are to be accepted with caution.

The group of virus infections, influenza, measles, scarlet fever, are nonfatal primary infections. These prepare the soil for the highly fatal secondary invaders, the pneumococci and streptococci. It was then the pandemic of resultant pneumonia rather than that of the primary infection, influenza, which caused the heavy toll in deaths.

In normal times the body resistance is for the most part sufficiently high to ward off invasion by these secondary invaders which prevail in the throats of apparently normal individuals, producing a carrier state, a condition of potential danger to the carriers, as well as to others, because of the possibility of transmission.

These pneumonia-producing organisms lie in wait for the production by virus infections of favorable conditions for their invasion of lung tissue. The pneumonias are for the most part due to temporarily lowered resistance. a potential danger lingers in the throat of every carrier who harbors pneumococci or streptococci.

Was the high pneumonia death rate due wholly to the *absence* of a recent pandemic of influenza. or due entirely to what we may term recent increased promiscuity, increased communal intercourse, particularly community feeding? Of these two factors it is believed that community messing played the major role in this increased pneumonia mortality.

In former times community messing had its limitations. The working man carried his dinner bucket, now he goes to the restaurant. The clerk and the office man formerly returned home for lunch, now they patronize the cafeteria. Formerly when the farmer made a trip to town he took his lunch with him, but now he patronizes the restaurant. In the days of economy it was an event for even the first families of the community to gather at the hotel for a luxurious meal, and now that a premium is put on brawn even the laboring man considers a hotel party uneventful. But why should this increased patronage of common eating places influence the mortality from pneumonia?

Let us inquire further whether or not any advance has been made in our knowledge of the epidemiology of pneumonia as well as of the sputum-borne diseases? And let us not forget that upon this alone depends successful preventive measures. During the influenza epidemic the face mask was advocated and in many cities it was tried without beneficial results. Communities were quarantined against inter-city communication to no avail. All administrative effort on the part of the city, state, and federal health authorities was without result in limiting the spread of the contagion.

The quarantine of a city is impracticable. It can not be maintained over a sufficient length of time to be of value. There is only one example where quarantine has proved of practical value, and that is in state institutions where an absolute quarantine can be held in force for an indefinite time without jeopardizing commercial interests. There are a number of such institutions which escaped entirely by prolonged quarantine, and there are others in which a temporary quarantine resulted in the postponed admission of a convalescent or unrecognized case and spread of the contagion to practically all nonimmune inmates.

Influenza is highly contagious, but nonfatal, while pneumonia is moderately contagious, and, when the body resistance is temporarily lowered by a virus infection, highly fatal. In other words, the pandemic of influenza would be of no moment if unaccompanied by the fatal pneumonias.

Which of these infections is the more easily controlled, or are both controlled by the same preventive measures? Influenza virus is introduced and burns out quickly, while pneumonia organisms are continuously and insidiously spreading from carriers to nonimmunes where they prevail as a potential danger. The carrier state in question is not, as in the case of typhoid and immune diphtheria carriers, a danger only to others, but is a menace to the carrier as well. This distinction in types of carriers demands recognition by those interested in preventive medicine. In this connection let us study the comparative mortality per 1000 in New York City for 1890, 1891 and 1918.[4]

In comparing the pneumonia fatalities of New York during the influenza epidemies of 1890, 1891, with that of 1918, it is found that the mortality per 1000 population for the 1918 epidemic is twice as great as that of the former epidemics. Furthermore, the recent epidemic was of shorter duration, it was more explosive in character, indicating that our present day environment transmits with greater facility the infecting agent. With increased travel, increased eating in common eating places, increased congestion of urban districts, it may be concluded that the virus of influenza was transmitted with greater facility than ever before. With a large residual population of influenza nonimmunes, owing to the absence of a recent pandemic of the infection, and because of the increased facility with which the infective agent was transmitted, it may be further concluded that the recent pandemic has run its course, and that there will not be a second year recrudescence as in 1890 and 1891.

If one compares the mortality rates of cities in the registration area to the mortality rate for the entire population of the United States, it is found that the epidemic has spent itself, and assuming that the high mortality rates for the several years following 1890 and 1891 epidemics were due to an increased sporadicity of influenza-pneumonia, it may be concluded that the annual death rates following the recent epidemic will not be appreciably increased.

If the influenza virus is today transmitted with greater facility than in former times it is reasonable to assume that the organisms of secondary invasion are likewise more widespread than formerly; hence, we have this corresponding greater mortality from pneumococci and streptococci, secondary invasion resulting from a temporarily lowered resistance.

We have previously presented evidence showing that approximately 80 per cent of the influenza morbidity in the military service was due to insanitary messing facilities. Corrective measures for these defects can be instituted and effectively carried out. Furthermore, in two large civilian groups it was shown that in civil life about 80 per cent of the cases of influenza occurred among those using hand-washed eating utensils. In addition we have shown that 75 per cent of the morbidity in institutional population occurred among those eating from hand-washed dishes.

It appears that in camps as well as in civil and institutional life the use of only warm water for washing eating utensils is the chief sanitary defect. In the camps the contaminated hand and its auxiliary, the eating utensil, are probably equally responsible for the dissemination of the contagion, whereas in civil and institutional population, the auxiliaries of the hand, eating utensils, are primarily responsible, while the contaminated hand aside from its auxiliary eating utensil, plays a less important role.

It would appear from epidemiologic data secured in our recent investigations that influenza, as well as scarlet fever, and the bacterial infections may occasionally be food borne.

Our investigations would indicate that transmission by droplet infection through the air route by direct contact is at the most only of minor importance as compared to transmission by indirect contact through the hand to mouth, or hand auxiliary to mouth route of travel. The fallacy of wearing the mask in civil communities and cubicling patients on a hospital ward, without disinfecting the hands might well be compared to a surgeon who would wear a mask and fail to wash his hands. Transmission of the sputum-borne diseases is indirect through the hand to mouth route of travel and in order to obtain favorable results in the control of any infection the major avenues of travel must first be blocked, and as the air route of transmission is of such minor importance, the value of the face mask fades into insignificance.

CORROBORATIVE LABORATORY RESEARCH

If the foregoing deductions, which are based almost wholly on field and hospital observations, are correct, it should be possible to verify them by laboratory research. In regard to our laboratory investigations covering both direct and indirect contact transmission of infective organisms, the following salient facts may be presented.

In a former report it was demonstrated that the epidemic of streptococcus pneumonia, which swept through the camps last winter, and which for the most part followed measles, was not a hospital infection, but that at least 94 per cent of the pneumonia cases following measles were streptococcus carriers upon entering the hospital.[5] From this finding it is a question whether the cubicle system, as carried out on the so-called respiratory disease wards, was of any value. It was reported by some investigators that throat swabs of measles cases on successive days showed from day to day an increase in the number of streptococcus hemolyticus cases, and on this was based the conclusion that the infection was spread in the hospital, hence the cubicle system of segregation.

Our former reports did not support these contentions, and our recent laboratory researches show the fallacy of those reports on which the hospital infection theory was based. Serial throat swabs from average throats of troops show that the percentage of positive streptococcus carriers, while only 32 per cent on the first swabbing, may be as high as 82 per cent on the fourth swabbing, and this accounts for the apparent increase in positive cases on the hospital wards.

In all walks in civil life is there any more intimate and almost direct contact than at the public and private mess through the common spoon? The hand, contaminated by handling inanimate objects, and its auxiliary, the eating utensil, make up the busy avenues through which are spread the infective organisms of the sputum-borne diseases.

In infectious disease wards pathogenic organisms are invariably found in floor dust, while the examination of over 9000 cubic feet of air in these wards fails to reveal the presence of more than three hemolytic streptococci. By the spray and plate method it is found that even the finest spray has a rapid rate of fall. In three minutes 85 per cent of the organisms fall through a distance of two feet and in ten minutes the air is entirely free.

It then appears that the falling of even the finest spray expelled by an act of coughing may well be compared to an aeral barrage. Furthermore, we find that comparatively few organisms are expelled by coughing. By the sterile glove and cultural method it is found that this number rarely exceeds 1500 organisms.

From these findings it may be concluded that transmission by direct contact through the air route but rarely if ever takes place.

In contrast to this our recent research shows with what great facility organisms may be spread by indirect contact through inanimate objects by the hand to mouth route of travel. The number of organisms in the mouth runs into the billions; the number on the hand runs into the millions, and owing to the frequency of contact between the mouth and hands many hand organisms are of mouth origin. While only about 1500 organisms are expelled onto the floor by an act of coughing, a sterile glove wiped across the lips picks up about 2,000,000 organisms. Such organisms are readily transferred to inanimate objects which are handled by many people.

Hemolytic streptococci and pneumococci are isolated with great regularity from the hands of carriers or patients, from tableware, inanimate objects touched by these patients, and from floor dust, and diphtheria and tubercle bacilli have been isolated from the hands and eating utensils of patients.[6] These pathogenic organisms prevail so universally and in such number on the hands, on inanimate objects, especially on eating utensils, that the chances of transmission by indirect contact through the hand or hand auxiliary to the mouth, must outnumber the chance of spread through the air route by many hundred times. Furthermore, our epidemiologic data support this contention. We have secured most interesting and striking data in regard to the sanitation of washing dishes in both the home and public eating place. The average count of a large number of restaurant dishwater specimens is 4,000,000 bacteria per c.c. The temperature of this water is warm to the dish washers' hands, its average being 43° C. In restaurants where the hand method of washing is practiced the dishes are never scalded. The water is often so highly polluted that the dishes are more highly contaminated after they are washed than before the washing process. In the cycle which dishes make from table to kitchen and back again, the spoon or fork is often freer from organisms just after being used by the restaurant patron than when taken from the restaurant's polluted dish water. In the average restaurant where dishes are hand washed only about 50 per cent of the organisms are removed by the washing process.

In children there is less than 1 per cent hemolytic streptococcus carriers. In those of the adolescent age, the percentage is slightly higher—1.2 per cent. In the civilian adults we find another increase to 5 per cent, while in the military forces there is that enormous percentage, by a single swab, of 42. In the Southern Department during the winter of 1917-1918, this organism was the most common of all secondary invaders, and in the winter months it caused a case mortality equal to that of former plagues. In our recently acquired knowledge of the facility with which transmission took place at the soldiers' mess, we have the explanation of epidemic pneumonia among troops.

To the cost of lives on the battle field there must be added those fatalities in the civil population which result from the inevitable post-bellum epidemic. After the Spanish American War there was an increased typhoid mortality; after this World War there will be an increased pneumonia death rate.

If pneumonia mortality has not heretofore been decreased in civil life by preventive measures, and if our report showing the increased influenza rate incident to the use of hand-washed dishes is of value as an index for the facility with which contagion may be spread at public eating places, it may be predicted that with the demobilization of approximately two million hemolytic streptococcus carriers, there will result in civil communities an equal number of new foci for the further spread of this potential danger. In addition to hemolytic streptococcus carriers, concerning which we have accurate data, it may be assumed that there is also a relatively high percentage of carriers of the other pneumonia-producing streptococci and pneumococci. This demobilization will of itself immediately and automatically increase the carrier state of hemolytic streptococci alone in the civil population to approximately 8 per cent. With these new foci, in conjunction with the increasing patronage of public eating places, we may predict an increasing number of carriers with the increasing mortality incident thereto in the civil population from year to year.

Preventive measures alone can stem this rising tide of increasing mortality. Among these the most important are the hygiene of the hand and the disinfection of dishes, but there are multitudes of other details.

In a large number of tests we have been able to isolate pathogenic organisms almost without exception from eating utensils used by carriers and patients. These results show the facility with which infective agents may be spread at the common mess and suggests the necessity of the disinfection by boiling water of all eating utensils. In public eating places this is best accomplished by the mechanical dish washer in which it is essential to use scalding water in order to get the cleansing effect. Our investigation of the dishes washed in this manner shows a minimum degree of contamination.

Much has been gained by the prohibition of the roller towel and the common drinking cup, but our work shows the necessity of extending this same idea to include common eating utensils. In fact we believe that today the greatest ad-

vance in preventive medicine can be accomplished by requiring in public eating
places the disinfection of eating utensils. On the other hand, personal hygiene
of the hand is a measure which the individual must regulate himself. Instruction in this, however, might well be undertaken in the habit-forming or school
age.

There is nothing new in the theory of indirect contact, but the point is that as
a transmitting avenue it has been almost wholly neglected, perhaps because of its
simplicity. On the other hand the air-borne or droplet infection theory presented
a complex problem capable of endless mysticism.

CONCLUSIONS

It is believed that the results of our epidemiologic studies and laboratory
research show that indirect spread through the hand or hand auxiliary to the
mouth is by far the most important and major route of contagion dissemination. Granting that this is true, preventive measures will not consist of periodic masking of the populace, but simply an intensification of the rules of
personal hygiene, hand hygiene and especially the sanitation of eating utensils,
and the protection of food. The most ordinary social requirements demand clean
hands, clean eating utensils, and the protection of food supplies. But we must
extend this to include the actual sterilization of eating utensils both in the army
and in civilian life. In both, boiling water is essential for sanitary dish water.
In civil life this should be provided in restaurants and the like by washing
machines. In the army, if mess kits are utilized, the washing water must be
boiling for two reasons; viz., to sterilize the mess gear and to prevent soldiers
from putting their hands into it and so contaminating it or their hands as the
case may be.

REFERENCES

[1]A detailed report to appear later.
[2]Lynch and Cumming: The Role of the Hand in the Distribution of Influenza Virus and
the Secondary Invaders, Mil. Surgeon, December, 1918.
[3]Lynch and Cumming: The Distribution of Influenza Virus by Indirect Contact, Hands
and Eating Utensils, Am. Jour. Pub. Health, January, 1919.
[4]Monthly Bull. Dept. of Health, New York, December, 1918.
[5]Cumming, Spruit and Aten: Streptococcus Pneumonia. Jour. Am. Med. Assn., Mar. 8,
1919.
[6]A detailed report of this research to appear later.

STUDIES ON PATHOGENIC ANAEROBES*

I. Biology of Bacillus Welchii

By Benjamin Jablons, Major, M.C., Army Medical School, Washington, D. C.

E NOUGH evidence has now been accumulated to prove that the B. welchii represents a large group of bacilli which are anaerobic and have a large number of group characteristics in common, but which differ from one another in what might be considered to be minor characteristics. Thus Simonds[1] has been able to differentiate them into four groups on the basis of their sugar fermentations and serologically there are at least two varieties which fail to agglutinate by means of specific sera. This organism has been incriminated in so many disease processes during the past two decades that it might be valuable to review their best known characteristics, and to describe in detail the pathologic lesions that this organism is capable of initiating, as a result of its toxic and other secretions.

This bacillus is identical with the following bacteria:
B. of Achalme (1891).[2]
B. aerogenes capsulatus, Welch and Nuttall (1892).[3]
B. phlegmonis emphysematosæ, Eug. Fiænkel (1893).[4]
B. perfringens, described by Veillon and Zuber (1898).[5]
B. of Welch, Migula (1900)[6] (1).

It is customary to call this organism in France the 'B. perfringens because it was the first binominal designation given to this microorganism, the name suggested by Welch being a trinominal one. In justice to Welch, we feel, however, that the name suggested by Migula in 1900 should be retained.

The causal role of the Bacillus welchii in gas infections had been demonstrated by Eugene Fiænkel in 1893.[7] by Guillemot in 1898,[8] by Hitschmann and Lindenthal in 1899,[9] by Welch in 1900,[10] by Albrecht in 1902,[11] by Kamen in 1904,[12] etc. P. Simonds, in his monograph on the B. welchii published in 1915, collected 175 cases of gaseous gangrene or of gaseous phlegmon due to this microorganism, occurring before the war, with a mortality of about 45 per cent. This high figure indicates the importance of this organism in gaseous infections.

All authors agree that the bacillus of Welch plays an important role in the pathogeny of gas infections. Weinberg found this organism present more frequently than any other anaerobe in the series of gaseous infections which he studied. We have isolated this organism a great many times from cases of gaseous gangrene and infected wounds and have found that it has a definite number of characteristics by which it may be recognized.

A. Morphology

It appears as a thick rod, the ends of which are blunt and slightly rounded. It is nonmotile and capsulated, and forms spores only under certain conditions of culture. It retains the Gram stain.

*Published by permission of the Surgeon General. U. S. Army.

Form and Dimensions.—In pathologic exudates or in very young cultures in broth, this bacillus is usually characterized by its short, thick forms. The ends of the bacillus are almost always slightly rounded, the angles being slightly bulging. Frequently the bacilli are grouped in pairs, the two elements forming a prolongation of one another or forming an angle of 45°. In older cultures long or curved forms are sometimes observed. We have encountered on several occasions, strains which developed curved bacilli even in young cultures in glucose broth and in liver peptone water medium. Some strains even form fairly long filaments, which are thicker and not as long as those seen with other anaerobic germs. Many variations in the thickness of the bacillus occur. While the majority of the bacilli studied had a breadth of 1.2 to 0.8 microns, it is not un-

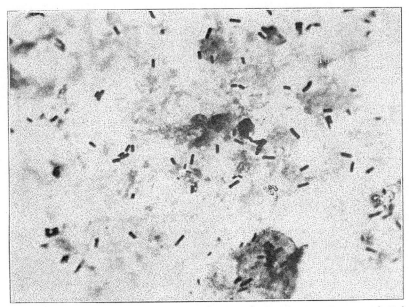

Fig. 1.—Bacillus welchii in muscle exudate. One sporulating bacillus close to center. (Army Medical Museum.)

common to see bacilli which are smaller and whose average breadth does not exceed 0.8 to 0.6 microns. These short forms usually showed extremities which were much more definitely rounded. The variations in form make the recognition of Bacillus welchii in stained smears difficult.

Motility Flagella, Capsule.—The Bacillus welchii is definitely nonmotile. The capsule can be stained, using fuchsin ink as a mordant and staining with steaming carbol fuchsin, and is best demonstrated in young cultures grown on slant agar. Rarely bacilli from cultures in gelatin show capsules when stained with carbol gentian violet and exudates from animals dying of B. welchii infections show capsules fairly frequently.

Spores.—The question of sporulation of B. welchii has been studied extensively, but still remains a subject of considerable controversy. Spores never occur in media in which the bacteria produce acidity. It seems pretty definitely established that this germ can only sporulate in neutral or alkaline media. In serous exudates spores are usually not present. Cultures grown for more than a year in sugar-free broth containing white of egg fail to show spores. Some strains occasionally sporulate more or less rapidly in this medium; whereas certain other strains sporulate abundantly only on coagulated horse serum. Direct examination is often insufficient to demonstrate the presence of spores; they are very rarely seen in smears stained with Gram. They are stained with difficulty by the Ziehl method, and in many cases can only be demonstrated by the heating method.[13] They are seen rarely in the serous exudate of necrotic muscle, more especially with toxic strains of the Bacillus welchii. Fig. 1 shows one such spore amidst numerous vegetating bacilli. Spores are oval, occasionally attaining large dimensions, and they are almost always free. Where they are enclosed in the body of the bacillus, they are median or subterminal, and extend beyond the body of the bacillus. The spores of the B. welchii, as a rule, show little resistance to heat. It is known that they are usually killed by boiling. Serous exudates heated for one to three minutes at 100° after inoculation in broth tubes usually fail to grow B. welchii. At times it is possible to obtain cultures of this bacillus in broths inoculated with pathologic fluids that have been boiled for three to five and even eleven minutes, provided media have been heavily inoculated (Weinberg).

B. CULTURAL CHARACTERISTICS

The bacillus of Welch can be grown fairly easily in anaerobic media. For a long time it was thought necessary to have strictly anaerobic conditions, and many anaerobic apparatuses were suggested for the cultivation of this microorganism:

It was first shown by Tarozzi[14] that this organism could be cultivated in broth tubes containing sterile pieces of liver tissue, and later by Ori and Wrzosek[15] that the addition of sterile raw or autoclaved pieces of potato or other vegetable matter would also permit of anaerobic cultivation in what was formerly considered aerobic media. Douglas, Fleming and Colebrook[16] and later Wright and Fleming[17] showed that the Bacillus welchii could be cultivated in tubes of glucose broth containing a small quantity of asbestos wool, or even ordinary absorbent cotton, wool, platinum black, a rusty nail, and even a fine capillary tube containing diluted Welch bacillus culture. Besides these substances, cultures have been obtained by the addition of pieces of vegetable, such as potato, carrots, white beans, bread, cabbage, as well as cheese, sterile earth, dried and powdered albumin. All of these substances apparently create a nidus which protects inoculated bacilli against the effect of dissolved oxygen of the medium and give the organism its initial growth. As it grows it creates further anaerobic conditions. It is the most easily grown anaerobic organism of those met with in gaseous infections.

It does not grow as well in ordinary agar as in agar to which protein and carbohydrate have been added. The addition of blood or serum to ordinary agar appreciably increases the vitality of the culture. Veillon's agar is a particularly good culture medium.

Veal Infusion Broth with 0.2 Per Cent Glucose.—Abundant growth with production of a large amount of gas. Clouds medium uniformly within the first 24 hours, and the culture settles slowly but progressively in several days at the bottom of the tube. The sediment packs down, and occasionally black pigment granules are present in the sediment. The culture has a butyric acid odor and the reaction is acid to litmus.

In *sugar-free broth*, to which a cube of coagulated egg white has been added, the same cultural characteristics are manifest. Egg albumin is slightly attacked at its margins or remains unaltered. After several months' incubation, it may become completely transparent, and is accompanied by a strong, disagreeable, nonputrid odor.

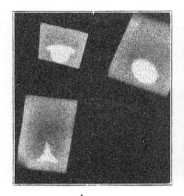 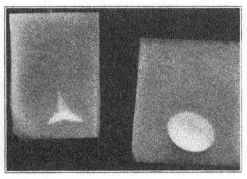

A.   B.

Fig. 2.—Various types of colonies of B. welchii. A. Low magnification. B. High mignification. (Army Medical Museum.)

Liver Cube Plus Peptone Water.—Same cultural characteristics as above except that gas bubbles arise from liver and medium clouds within six to twelve hours. The liver cube turns brick red.

In *blood broth*, hemolysis occurs, the medium taking on a brownish tinge. There is a pronounced butyric acid odor.

Trypsinized Serum of Wright.—The bacillus grows well if sterile trypsin is added in 1/25 of its volume to normal serum.

Veillon Agar.—Development with marked production of gas and fragmentation of the agar. The colonies occasionally grow up to the water of condensation on the surface. Colonies have well-defined margins and are lenticular in shape. Certain variations in the forms of the colonies are often seen. Often they begin as "yellowish heart-shaped" forms and later develop into small "brioche-like" shapes, as the results of growths of small protuberances from the notches of the previously described heart-shaped forms. Fig. 2 shows the various shapes of the colonies of B. welchii. On the surface of agar, colonies appear round in shape, with well-defined margins, grey in the center, and more transparent at the margins. Occasionally the lenticular colony develops a circular margin which has streaks radiating out toward the periphery, giving the colony an iris-like appearance. In glucose gelatin, colonies are of the same appearance as those seen in deep agar. Liquefaction of gelatin is slow and incomplete. It sometimes requires incubation over a period of months before the gelatin is liquefied to at least ⅓ or ¼ of its depth. Some strains liquefy gelatin completely after several months' growth.

On *blood agar* the colonies grow as well-defined, circular, slightly raised colonies with an opaque center which is granular and a periphery which is more translucent. The colony usually appears after 24 hours' incubation as small, opaque points and, after several days' growth, assumes typical colony shape. It is usually surrounded by a clear zone due to the hemolysis of the blood in the medium.

Deep Trypsin Agar.—B. welchii grows readily in this medium, producing a large amount of gas which fragments the medium, and forms lenticular colonies which grow up to within the water of condensation.

Andrade Veillon Agar.—The addition of 1 per cent solution of neutralized acid fuchsin to veillon agar inhibits somewhat the development of this bacillus. The colonies are less numerous and smaller, assume a light brick red color after several days' incubation, and the surrounding medium becomes tinged a light salmon color.

Litmus Milk.—Sometimes the litmus is reddened and sometimes it is completely decolorized. Coagulation occurs quickly en masse, owing to the large amount of acid produced. The clot then contracts, is riddled with gas bubbles, which gives it a sponge-like appearance, and floats on the clear whey. This reaction in milk is very characteristic and is spoken of as stormy fermentation. The milk has a butyric acid odor. This takes place within from 8 to 24 hours, provided fresh milk, which has been boiled and cooled previous to seeding, is used. Otherwise reaction is delayed for as long as 48 hours.

Coagulated Serum.—Very slightly attacked by some strains; usually is not changed at all, even after several days' incubation. Sporulation is at times very abundant in this medium. Swollen forms appear occasionally with free spores. Some bacilli staining with Gram often contain spores.

Meat Broth.—Culture is less abundant, media has a weak butyric acid odor, sporulation occurs at times, and meat assumes a brick red color.

Resistance.—Extremely feeble acidity corresponding to an H-ion concentration equal to that of a 1:30,000 N/HCl is sufficient to inhibit bacterial activity. (Wolf and Harris.)

Heat.—Heating above 90° is sufficient to stop the growth of the majority of strains.

C. BIOCHEMICAL PROPERTIES

1. *Saccharolytic Properties.*—The B. welchii contains a very powerful saccharolytic ferment and attacks carbohydrates, resulting in the production of gas, accompanied by a marked acidity. P. Simonds, who has studied twenty strains

derived from different sources, from this point of view, divides the B. welchii into four groups:

Group 1 ferments inulin and glycerin, resulting in the production of gas and acid, and no spores form in either of these media.

Group 2 ferments glycerin, with the production of gas and acid, but does not ferment inulin, and forms spores only in media containing inulin.

Group 3 ferments inulin, but not glycerin, and forms spores in media containing glycerin.

Group 4 ferments neither inulin nor glycerin and sporulates in both media.

This classification has been confirmed by H. Henry,[19] who has studied numerous strains of B. welchii isolated from war wounds. According to this author, B. welchii ferments constantly glucose, levulose, galactose, saccharose, maltose, raffinose, mannose, starch, dextrin and glycogen. Wolf and Harris have found that the B. welchii produces gas in media containing 3 to 4 per cent of lactose. The gas produced is 3.8 times the volume of the original medium. Gas is occasionally formed from certain amino acids which are glycogenetic. The gas is composed of hydrogen and carbon dioxide in the proportion of 2:1. Nitrogen has never been demonstrated in the gas that is formed. There is a latent period in gas production which lasts from four to eight hours when properly prepared medium is seeded with an active strain. Following this period there is a sudden drop in the production of gas, which seems due to a partial inhibition of the growth of the organisms by the products which are formed. There is then a secondary rise which reaches its maximum in about 24 hours.

During the latent period there is a slight rise in the H-ion concentration of the medium, and a maximum rise which corresponds with the production of acid during the sixth to the eighth hour.

The maximum gas production is attained when the H-ion concentration is that which corresponds to Ph = 4.52 to Ph = 4.56. When the acidity is increased, there is an inhibition of the metabolic activity of the microorganism.

The acids produced are 60 per cent volatile. These volatile acids consist chiefly of normal butyric acid varying from 5.4 grams to 8.3 grams per liter.

2. Proteolytic Properties.—The proteolytic properties of the B. welchii are still the subject of much discussion. It will liquefy gelatin slowly, will attack very feebly and slowly egg albumin, and does not seem to influence casein. Certain strains attack very slowly coagulated serum albumin. Tissier and Martelly consider the B. welchii an energetic proteolytic agent, particularly in sugar-containing media. In protein-containing media, the Bacillus welchii first forms amino acids before it begins to ferment carbohydrate substances. (Wolf and Harris.)

Peptolytic Power.—P. Simonds finds that it produces very little ammonia, even when inoculated into sugar broth, indicating that its power of breaking down noncoagulable nitrogen is negligible. Search for indol has given very contradictory results. The ability to produce indol seems to vary a great deal, depending upon the strains that are studied. In peptone water which contains 30 per cent of its nitrogen as amino acids, the Bacillus welchii forms, in addition, often as much as 20 milligrams of nitrogen contained in amino acid form. According to Wolf and Harris, the B. welchii is therefore peptolytic and, in media which contain only amino acids, it is also aminolytic. In media prepared from meat which is digested by trypsin and erepsin to the point where no biuret reacting substances are present, Bacillus welchii is still capable of metabolic activity, as shown by the increase in the amount of ammonia nitrogen and the reduction in the amount of amino acid nitrogen. According to Tissier and Martelly, the B. welchii secretes, in addition to a trypsin and an amylose, a fat-splitting ferment which saponifies fats.

D. SEROLOGIC CHARACTERISTICS

1. *Hemolysins.*—It secretes hemolysins for the blood corpuscles of man, rabbits, dogs, pigeons, white mice, hogs, cattle, sheep, horse, guinea pig, white rat, and hen. It dissolves hemoglobin out of the red cells of the guinea pig, rabbit, hen and pigeon. It destroys the red cells of the other animals. Young rabbits, dogs, and white mice show hemoglobinuria following injection of these substances. This hemolytic substance is destroyed by heating to 60° for one-half hour, prolonged incubation and exposure to light. It passes only partly through a Berkefeld filter.[22] It can be conserved in the ice chest. Cultures which have no hemolytic substances often contain hemagglutinins. Young cultures 15 to 16 hours in glucose broth contain an appreciable amount of hemolytic substances. One-tenth of a c.c. of total culture will hemolyze a dilution of red cells corresponding to 1/40 to 1/20 of a c.c. of packed red cells, 1.0 c.c. having therefore sufficient hemolysin to dissolve $\frac{1}{4}$ to $\frac{1}{2}$ of a c.c. of packed red cells. Forty-eight hour cultures rapidly lose their hemolytic substances. It is neutralized by the serum of a large number of animals. Horses have normally an appreciable amount of antihemolysin. White mice are very susceptible to the Welch hemolysin.

2. *Agglutinins.*—It has been possible to produce agglutinating substances by the injection of massive amounts of culture into rabbits and horses. The best agglutinating serum agglutinates its homologous strain in 1/500 and 1/2000 dilution, whereas a serum furnished us by Dr. Weinberg agglutinated a strain isolated from an infected war wound in a dilution of 1-800. A good agglutinating serum may be prepared by the injection either of washed bacilli or bacillary emulsions detoxicated by the addition of $\frac{1}{3}$ of its volume of Lugol's solution.

3. *Precipitins.*—McCampbell[23] produced precipitins in the serum of rabbits, and Korentchewsky[24] claims to have produced precipitins in the serum of animals injected per rectum and fed with filtrates from cultures of B. welchii.

4. *Bacteriolysins.*—McCampbell claimed to have produced bacteriolysins against the B. welchii. In 1915, we succeeded in producing bacteriolysins in a horse injected with small quantities of killed and living cultures of the B. welchii which had a bacteriolytic titer of 1:100 and $\frac{1}{2}$ c.c. of which protected against a lethal quantity of a 24 hour culture.

5. *Complement-Fixing Bodies.*—McCampbell found complement-fixing bodies in the serum of animals injected with B. welchii. Korentchewsky claimed similarly to have found complement-fixing bodies in the serum of dogs fed with culture filtrates. Rocchi[25] did not obtain uniform results.

6. *Toxins* have been isolated from cultures and are best separated from 18 to 24 hour cultures of the bacillus in glucose broth. Bull[26] has suggested the use of broth to which fresh pieces of rabbit muscle are added, whereas De Kruif[27] has suggested the addition of $\frac{1}{5}$ volume of horse serum. Antitoxins have also been prepared, but their method of preparation and titration will be more fully discussed in a subsequent paper.

<h3 style="text-align:center">D. PATHOGENIC POWER</h3>

The pathogenicity of the B. welchii is extremely variable, as is that of all the anaerobic bacteria encountered in gaseous gangrene. Strains isolated from fatal cases of gaseous gangrene are usually very pathogenic for the guinea pig, and are able to retain their virulence over a period of months. The pathogenic power is titrated by injecting 24 hour cultures of the bacillus in 0.2 per cent glucose broth into the muscles of the thigh of a guinea pig.

One-fourth to $\frac{1}{8}$ of a c.c. of 24-hour culture in glucose broth of the most pathogenic strains kills a guinea pig in 24 to 48 hours. The best strain studied at the Central Medical Department Laboratory of the A. E. F., killed a 350 gram guinea pig in less than 20 hours following injection of $\frac{1}{10}$ of a c.c. of a 20-hour culture in broth.

By separating the toxin from young cultures either by centrifugation or filtration through Berkefeld or Mandler filters, it is possible to obtain a toxin which will kill a guinea pig following intravenous injection of $\frac{1}{2}$ to 1.0 c.c. within five minutes.

The study of experimental infection with B. welchii has thrown a great deal of light on the pathogeny of gas gangrene. For a long time there was a great deal of discussion regarding this point. It was thought by many that B. welchii was always capable of producing so-called gas bacillus infection. Then Marbais[28] and others found that injection of large quantities of washed bacilli failed to produce any lesions whatsoever in both guinea pigs and monkeys. Other investigators then proved that lesions could be produced if lactic acid or powdered glass was injected with the bacilli, or if a slight injury to muscles preceded the injection.[29]

De Kruif[30] showed that the toxin of the bacillus exercised a very definite aggressive action on the bacilli. Washed bacilli in relatively enormous quantities produced no or very slight injury, whereas the addition of minimal quantities of toxin would produce rapidly a very fatal result.

The symptoms following injection of bacilli plus toxin or after injury to muscles are invariably the same. If culture is virulent, it is not uncommon to see swelling and induration of the region injected within four to six hours after inoculation. The swelling increases and in about six to eight hours crackling is perceptible. The swelling increases, and extends up to the abdomen. The animal holds its limb in a flexed position to relieve the tension of the tissues. Swelling is due chiefly to edema, and to gas infiltration. As the bacteria multiply, the symptoms of intoxication become manifest and are the same as those observed when sublethal doses of toxin are injected into the circulation of susceptible animals. They act on the nervous system, producing tremor, slight convulsion, hiccup, bristling of the hair, constipation by paralysis of the bowel. They affect the circulatory system as evidenced by the extreme rapidity of the pulse.

Before death, paralysis of the hind legs occurs and the animal refuses food. It remains hunched up and motionless, and its respirations are markedly increased. Death intervenes by respiratory failure rather than by cardiac paralysis.

· The lesions are those referable to the muscles, the blood vessels and the fat of the subcutaneous connective tissue. The muscles are first rendered necrotic by contact with the toxin which is a protoplasmic poison, and this has been shown experimentally *in vitro* by K. Taylor[31]. The carbohydrates of the necrotic muscle are then attacked in turn by the saccharolytic ferments of the bacilli which produce gas and acid. The gas infiltration results from this change. The edema which occurs has been ascribed by some authors to the acid produced,[19] whereas others maintain that it is due to the pressure of the infiltrating gas.

The toxin seems to exert a specific effect on the muscle fibers of the media coat of the blood vessels, with a tendency to rupture of the blood vessels and consequent hemorrhage. The exuded blood is hemolyzed by the hemolytic substances secreted by the B. welchii. This diffusion of laked blood is particularly noticeable with toxic strains.

REFERENCES

[1]Simonds: Studies in Bacillus Welchii with Special Reference to Classification and Its Relation to Diarrhea. Monograph No. 5, Rockefeller Institute for Medical Research, Sept., 1915.
[2]Achalme: Compt. rend. Soc. de Biol., July 25, 1891, pp. 651-656.
[3]Welch and Nuttall: Bull. Johns Hopkins Hosp., 1892, iii, 81-91.
[4]Fraenkel: Centralbl. f. Bakteriol., 1893, xiii, 13-16.
[5]Veillon and Zuber: Arch. d. Med. exper., 1897, x. 517-545.
[6]Migula: System of Bakterien, 1900, Jena, Fischer.
[7]Fraenkel: Ueber Gasphlegmone, 1893, Hamburg and Leipzig.
[8]Guillemot: Compt. rend. de la Soc. de Biol., Nov. 5, 1898, pp. 1017-1019.
[9]Hitschmann and Lindenthal: Sitzungsberichte der Kaiserlich Akademie der Wissentchafter in Wien, 1899, cviii, III Abt., pp. 67-239.
[10]Welch: Bull. Johns Hopkins Hosp., 1900, ii, 185-204.
[11]Albrecht: Arch. f. klin. Chir., 1902, lxvii, No. 3.
[12]Kamen: Centralbl. f. Bakt., I Abt. Orig., 1904, xxxv. 554-563, 686-712.
[13]Weinberg and Seguin: La Gangrene Gazeuse, Paris, 1918.
[14]Tarrozzi: Centralbl. f. Bakteriol., Abt. I, Orig., 1905, xxxviii, 619.
[15]Wrzosek: Centralbl. f. Bakteriol., Abt. I, Orig., 1907, xliii, 17.
[16]Douglas, Fleming, and Colebrook: Studies in Wound Infections, Growth of Anaerobic Bacilli in Fluid Media, Lancet, London, 1917, ii, 530-532.
[17]Wright, Fleming, and Colebrook: Sterilization of Wounds by Physical Agencies, Lancet, London, June 15, 1918.
[18]Wright and Fleming: Acidemia in Gas Gangrene, Lancet, London, Feb. 9, 1918.
[19]Henry, H.: Investigation of Cultural Reactions of Certain Anaerobes Found in Wounds, Jour. Path. and Bacteriol., xxi, 376.
[20]Wolf and Harris: Biochemistry of Pathogenic Anaerobes, ibid., xxi, 386.
[21]Tissier and Martelly: Recherches sur la Putrefaction de la Viande de Boucherie, Ann. de l'Inst. Pasteur, 1902, xvii, 540.
[22]Ouranoff, A.: Sur l'hemotoxine du B. Welchii (B. perfringens), Compt. rend. Soc. de Biol., 1903, 1917, lxxx, 706-708.
[23]McCampbell, E. F.: Toxic and Antigenic Properties of B. Welchii, Jour. Infect. Dis., 1909, vi, 537.
[24]Korentchewsky: Etude biologique du B. perfringens et du B. putritiens, Ann. de l'Inst. Pasteur, 1909, xxiii, 91-95.

[25]Rocchi: Centralbl. f. Bakteriol., I Abt. Orig., 1911, lx, 579-581.
[26]Bull and Pritchett: Jour. Exper. Med., July, 1917, pp. 119-138.
[27]De Kruif: Verbal communication.
[28]Marbais, C. R.: Soc. de Biol., 1914.
[29]Jablons: Pathology of War Surgery, Jour. Am. Med., Assn., July, 1915.
[30]De Kruif and Bollman: Mechanism of Infection with B. Welchii, Jour. Infect. Dis., 1917, xxi, No. 6, pp. 588-599.
[31]Taylor, K.: Factors Responsible for Gaseous Gangrene, Lancet, London, January 15, 1916, pp. 123-125.

LABORATORY METHODS

A METHOD FOR THE COLLECTION OF URINE FROM EACH KIDNEY SEPARATELY IN THE DOG*

By F. S. Hopkins, M.D., and W. C. Quinby, M.D., Boston, Mass.

IN the conduction of certain types of experimental investigation it is important to be able to obtain the product of each kidney separately, and especially is this importance noted in work dealing with experimental nephritis. Of course, in those cases where the experiment can be performed as an acute one, lasting at the most only a few days, it is quite feasible to collect the urine from each ureter, which has been provisionally delivered from the abdomen onto the surface of the skin in the loin. For prolonged observation, however, this method is not feasible on account of the unavoidable advent of infection which soon manifests itself and leads to definite pyelonephritis and death.

In the female dog it is possible to collect urine separately from the bladder by means of the cystoscope, but this method also has very definite limitations. In the first place one must be very adept at cystoscopic technic, because the use of this instrument in the dog's bladder is made more difficult than it is found to be in the human bladder on account of the fact that in the dog this viscus is practically an intraperitoneal organ, and therefore very movable. Furthermore, the dog's ureter, on leaving the bladder, takes a downward and sometimes a downward and forward course for approximately 1 cm., thus making the introduction of a ureteral catheter very difficult, but, as mentioned above, ureteral catheterization is possible in the dog, although it can not be performed widely and also can not be performed frequently because of the extreme sensitiveness of the bladder mucosa in this animal. This latter fact leads to hyperemia and edema about the ureteric orifice which has been catheterized, thus making the identification of the orifice at a second period quite difficult.

A further method of segregation of the dog's urine, and one which we believe to be superior to any other, is made possible by the use of the uterus as a receptacle of the products of one kidney while the normal relations between the bladder and other kidney are maintained. As will be seen from the diagram this is not an especially difficult procedure. Its description is as follows: By laparotomy the ureter on one side is delivered from behind the peritoneum and cut across at a convenient point above the bladder; the stump remaining attached to the bladder is tied off. The corresponding horn of the uterus is then incised by a small longitudinal cut, and an anastomosis is made between the ureter and uterus. This

*From the Laboratory of Surgical Research, Harvard Medical School, Boston.
Reported at the tenth annual meeting of the American Society for Clinical Investigation, Atlantic City, June, 1918.

union is made much easier by using as a splint a small No. 5 ureteral catheter. This is first passed up the ureter toward the kidney for a sufficient distance and then its lower end passed in through the incision in the uterus until it appears at the vulva. The ureter is then stitched to the uterus with a few interrupted stitches of blood-vessel silk. The cornu of the uterus above the point of anastomosis is then ligated in order to prevent the extension of urine in an upward direction, and similarly the opposite cornu is then closed and the catheter appearing through the

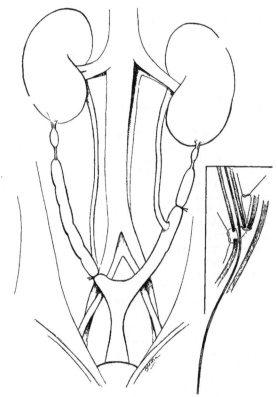

Fig. 1.—Semidiagrammatic sketch of anastomosis between ureter and left uterine cornu. Insert shows detail of anastomosis using ureteral catheter as splint.

vulva is cut off so as to be inaccessible to the dog. If it be intended to prolong the observations over a considerable period of time, it is easy to avoid the complications which might be caused by the advent of catamenia by the removal of the ovaries at the time the anastomosis is made.

We thus have established a condition in which the urine drains through the catheter into the vagina for a period of approximately 48 hours, after which the catheter can be safely withdrawn by forceps introduced into the vulva. At the end of one week it is possible to collect the products of each kidney in the follow-ing fashion: A glass tube is adjusted so as to fill the vulva and with this in place collection can be made over the required time period. The urine from the bladder is subsequently withdrawn by catheterization through the urethra. Analysis of the urine collected by this uterovaginal route shows it to be normal and similar to that from the other side, with the exception that it is apt to contain an excess of mucus.

SOME LIMITATIONS OF THE FLOTATION METHOD OF FECAL EXAMINATION*

By J. Daley McDonald, M.S., Berkeley, Cal.

THE brine flotation-loop method of fecal examination for intestinal worms was first employed by Kofoid and Barber[1] in the examination of troops of the United States Army.

This method is based on the fact that the specific gravity of the ova of the worms is considerably less than that of a saturated solution of sodium chloride. Barring interfering factors, this will result in the rise of the ova to the surface of the brine mixture of feces, while the heavy and the penetrable material will settle, thus producing a marked segregation. The authors give the following ac-count of the manner of procedure.

"The method finally perfected by us may be designated as the brine flotation-loop method. It consists in mixing a large fecal sample thoroughly in concen-trated brine, in a paraffined paper can of from two to three ounces capacity, fore-ing the coarse float below the surface by means of a disk of No. 0 steel wool, and then allowing the can to stand one hour for the ova to ascend. The surface film is then looped off with wire loops, one-half inch in diameter, and examined on a slide without a cover glass." [Page 1558.]

This method was adopted for making routine fecal examinations by the Division of Parasitology of the California State Board of Health in January, 1919. Its advantages over other methods in matters of rapidity, simplicity, and adaptability have already been demonstrated beyond doubt. During the first half of the year several hundred Orientals (residents of California) were examined both for intestinal worms and for intestinal protozoa. A small portion of each fecal specimen was set aside for the protozoan determination and the remainder examined by the flotation method as just described. Early in this work the ova of *Clonorchis sinensis* were found in the smears being examined for protozoa, while in the portion of the identical specimen, on which the flotation method had been previously employed, not a single ovum had been found. In the next 500 specimens examined, ten cases of *clonorchiasis* were diagnosed by means of the method used for protozoa. An equal number must have passed undetected, for the method of examination for protozoa necessitates the use of an extremely small sample of feces and permits little or no concentration. From the same 500 specimens no ova of *Clonorchis* were found by the flotation method. These re-

*Contribution from the Division of Parasitology of the California State Board of Health, Berkeley, Cal.

sults subject to question the effectiveness of this method for *Clonorchis sinensis*, and the following experiments were undertaken with the hope of eliminating this element of uncertainty.

The first test consisted in making a careful comparison of the flotation and the centrifuge methods, using for this purpose forty specimens among which there was likelihood of finding some cases of *clonorchiasis*. The specimens were divided, furnishing a part for each method. The procedure followed in the centrifuge method was that employed in the United States Immigration Station Hospital, Angel Island, California, and described by Billings and Hickey.[2] The results of this comparative test may be found in Table I. From these results it will be seen that the flotation method is more critical than the centrifuge method

TABLE I

COMPARATIVE RESULTS IN DETECTION OF OVA IN FORTY SPECIMENS EXAMINED BY BOTH THE CENTRIFUGE AND THE FLOTATION METHODS

POSITIVE FOR	NUMBER OF CASES DETECTED BY THE CENTRIFUGE METHOD	NUMBER OF CASES DETECTED BY THE FLOTATION METHOD
Trichuris trichiura	13	15
Ascaris lumbricoides	10	11
Hookworm .	3	5
Clonorchis sinensis	3	0

for the detection of the ova of the three nematodes found, but it completely failed in the detection of the ova of the trematode, *Clonorchis sinensis*. At the conclusion of the experiment, the sediment remaining in the containers in which the brine had been used, was examined. A large number of ova of *Clonorchis* were present in each of the three cases in which their presence was previously shown by the centrifuge method. The ova had been present, but had not risen to the surface of the brine emulsion.

There seemed a possibility that the age of the ova or the length of time allowed for flotation might be factors in their failure to rise. Some evidence regarding these matters was furnished by experience in the routine examinations in the laboratory. The 500 samples among which the ten cases of *clonorchiasis* were found had been sent to the laboratory in several different lots and had been from one to four days in transit. The specimens used in making the comparison of the centrifuge and flotation methods had been voided within the previous nine hours. These two considerations would indicate that variation in the age of the ova from the time of deposition up to four days following makes no appreciable difference. The time elapsing between the mixing of the specimen and the looping off of the surface, i.e., the flotation time, often varies from forty-five minutes to one hour and fifteen minutes in the making of routine examinations, due to frequent interruption preventing the looping off of the surface at the exact expiration of one hour. So, within these limits it was already evident that the flotation time was of no consequence.

A few simple laboratory tests of a corroborative nature were made possible through the kindness of Dr. J. P. Hickey of the United States Immigration Station, Angel Island, California, who supplied material containing an unusually large number of the ova of *Clonorchis sinensis* and some ova of *Trichuris trichiura*. The first use of this material was made about twenty-four hours after being voided. For the first two experiments (A and B) it was mixed with feces containing ova of the sort recently described by Kofoid[3] as those of a new parasitic nematode of man, *Oxyuris incognita*. These ova, with those of *Trichuris* already in the original material, served as a control on the method. Experiments A and B were identical, being intended as a check, each against the other. In conducting the experiments care was taken to follow closely the description by Kofoid and Barber. Paraffined 2-oz. drug cans served as containers and No. 0 steel wool was used for filtration. A period of fifteen minutes was allowed to elapse before looping off the surface for the first examination. Previous experience had shown this to be the minimum time during which diffusion currents would cease and permit any appreciable stratification to take place. Sampling before such stratification had occurred would be equivalent to mixing the material in water merely, and removing a drop for examination while the material was still in suspension. Following the first examination, the surface was looped off and examined at fifteen minute intervals up to one hour and then at thirty minute intervals until two hours after mixing. This procedure was much simpler than preparing a special sample for each period. Besides, since care was taken to make sure that the entire surface was removed each time, the number of ova found at each examination represented almost exclusively those which had risen during the preceding interval. As a result some evidence was gained regarding the most opportune time for looping off the surface when making routine examinations. This manner of conducting the experiments must be borne in mind when referring to Table II, for in the usual procedure the number of ova

TABLE II

RESULTS OF EXPERIMENTS TESTING THE EFFECTIVENESS OF THE BRINE FLOTATION-LOOP METHOD IN THE DETECTION OF OPERCULATED OVA

FLOTATION TIME	EXPERIMENT A. AGE OF OVA 24 HRS.			EXPERIMENT B. AGE OF OVA 24 HRS.			EXPERIMENT C. AGE OF OVA 24 HRS.		EXPERIMENT D. AGE OF OVA 48 HRS.		EXPERIMENT E. AGE OF OVA 72 HRS.		Experiment with the ova of Pneumonoeces similiplexus. Age of ova, 48 hrs.	Experiment with the ova of Fasciola hepatica. Age of ova, 12 hrs.
The numbers represent the ova detected at each interval.	Clonorchis sinensis	Trichuris trichiura	Oxyuris incognita	Clonorchis sinensis	Trichuris trichiura	Oxyuris incognita	Clonorchis sinensis	Trichuris trichiura	Clonorchis sinensis	Trichuris trichiura	Clonorchis sinensis	Trichuris trichiura		
15 min.	0	2	0	0	2	1	0	0	0	1	0	0	0*	0
30 min.	0	1	2	0	3	0	0	0	0	3	0*	0	0*	0
45 min.	0	2	1	0	0	3	0	1	0	2	0*	0	0*	0
1 hr.	0	1	0	0	1	1	0	0	0*	3	0	0	0*	0
1½ hrs.	0	0	1	0	1	0	0	2	0	4	0	0	0	0
2 hrs.	0	0	0	0	0	0	0	3	0	1	–	–	–	–
No. of ova under 22 mm. coverglass of sediment	216	—	—	180	—	—	680	—	600 to 700		600 to 700		Many distorted	1200

*In these examinations two or three ova were found, not on the surface of the drop, but in the sediment which had settled on the slide.

reported at one hour would be the sum of those reported in this table for the 15, 30, 45 minute and one hour intervals. Experiments C, D, and E were identical with A and B, except that the ova used were progressively older. Table II gives in detail the results for each experiment at the stated intervals.

It will be noted from Table II that not a single ovum of *Clonorchis* was detected by the flotation method. That they were present in enormous numbers is proved by the counts made of the number to be found in a drop of the sediment under a single 22 mm. square cover glass. The lesser number of ova in the sediment in experiments A and B is due to the fact that the material used was mixed with a more than equal quantity of feces not containing the ova.

There are two obvious differences between the ova of *Clonorchis* and those of the other parasites in the detection of which the flotation method has proved so effective. First, the ova have an operculum, characteristic of the ova of most of the trematodes (excluding, of course, Schistosoma). Second, they are of very small size, varying from 23 to 27 microns long by 11 to 14 microns broad. This led to the trial of the method on the operculate ova of two other trematodes. The ova first used were not from a human parasite but from *Pneumonoeces similiplexus*, the lung-fluke of frogs and salamanders. This form was chosen because the material was readily available and because the ova are approximately the size of those of *Clonorchis*, though having a somewhat thinner shell. The ova from two of these flukes, which had been deposited in water, were mixed with human feces in considerable concentration. The remainder of the experiment was conducted the same as those described above. No ova were detected, though many were found in the sediment (see Table II).

Other operculate ova used were those of *Fasciola hepatica*. These were obtained from infected cattle, and were mixed with human feces. The material was then manipulated in the same manner as in the previous experiments. None of these ova were floated to the surface during the entire period of two hours. The concentration of the ova in the material used is indicated by the number found in the sediment after the use of the brine (see Table II).

In most cases, after examining the surface of the drop on the slide, the excess fluid was removed, leaving any sediment which might have settled through the drop. Examination of this sediment in each of three cases revealed two ova of *Clonorchis* and in several instances two or three ova of *Pneumonoeces* were found. These instances are marked by an asterisk in Table II. The presence of these ova in the material looped off is probably explainable by their adherence to debris. Should an ovum become attached to a bit of debris which subsequently floated to the surface, then the ovum would be carried up with it. Both would then be looped off onto the slide. In routine manipulation the wire loop is usually struck sharply against the slide in order to break and release the film which it has transferred. This concussion would in all probability loosen the ovum from the debris, whereupon the former would settle to the bottom of the drop on the slide and completely escape notice in an examination of the surface of the drop. Only the surface of the drop is supposed to be examined in regular procedure.[4]

This explanation is strengthened by the fact that the largest and heaviest ova, those of *Fasciola hepatica* were never found, the next in size and weight, those of *Clonorchis sinensis* were found in only ten per cent of examinations, while the smallest and lightest, those of *Pneumonoeces similiplexus,* were found in the sediment on the slide in eighty per cent of the examinations. This behavior would be logically expected, for small light ova would be carried much more readily than heavy ova by adhering to bits of debris.

DISCUSSION

Kofoid and Barber in their original description of the brine flotation-loop method call attention to its ineffectiveness in the detection of infection with Strongyloides.[5] In the same paper the authors make a tabulation showing the comparative efficiency of this method and the centrifuge method, but in it no ova of trematodes, in fact no operculate ova of any sort, are recorded. However, the following statement occurs somewhat further along. "The ova of parasites such as * * * and of trematodes are floated up by the brine into the surface layer of the pool without distortion or noticeable change in appearance during the usual period of examination" (page 1559). The results reported in this paper make it necessary to qualify this statement with regard to the effectiveness of the flotation method for the ova of trematodes, and subject to question its effectiveness in the case of all operculate ova. In the report made by Kofoid, et al,[6] of the occurrence of intestinal parasites in troops of the United States Army, of a total of 1500 examinations made by this method only one operculate ovum was detected, viz., that of *Diphyllobothrium latum.*[7] However, this is in all probability due to the fact that those parasites which produce operculate ova are very rare in those who have not resided or traveled much outside of the United States.

In the above experiments the failure of the ova to float to the surface of the brine could scarcely be due to their density, for all of them have comparatively thin shells and are probably of less specific gravity than the ova of *Ascaris* or *Trichuris.* It may perhaps be explained by the permeability of the ova. Stephens[8] gives an account of certain yolk granules, not always used up during the development of the embryo, which he believes must serve some other purpose than food supply, possibly that of imbibing water for the use of the embryo. If this is the case then it may be that the brine penetrates the ova of trematodes. But the penetration must needs be very rapid for examinations were made in each experiment within fifteen minutes after addition of the brine. No other direct evidence regarding this hypothesis was gained from these experiments.

A seemingly more plausible explanation of the failure of the flotation method is suggested by the condition of the ova following their treatment with the brine. Invariably, following the use of the brine, ova were found, in which the operculum had become separated from the rest of the shell. Of the ova found in this condition the proportion varies from fifteen per cent in *Pneumonoeces* to fifty per cent in *Clonorchis.* In those ova in which the operculum had not actually opened, the line of attachment was markedly more conspicuous, than in untreated ova, suggesting that it had been loosened. The loosening is probably caused by either osmotic pressure or the variation in pressure between the medium and the contents of the ovum. Apparently the stage of development made no difference in the opening of the operculum, for it occurred in both *Clonorchis* and *Fasciola.* In the former the content of the ovum is a nearly completely developed miracidium while in the latter the embryo is in the early cleavage stages only. Since the efficacy of the flotation method is dependent upon the lighter specific gravity of the ovum as compared with the brine, the loosening of the operculum and consequent entrance of the brine into the ovum defeats the purpose of the method.

The brine flotation-loop method has many advantages over other methods in the saving of time and materials and in the ease of manipulation. However, as shown by these experiments its range of application is limited by the type of ovum. Infections with *Clonorchis* and *Fasciola* are not detected by this method and its effectiveness in the detection of any operculate ova is very doubtful.

REFERENCES

[1]Kofoid, C. A., and Barber, M. A.: Rapid Method for Detection of Ova of Intestinal Parasites in Human Stools, Jour. Am. Med. Assn., Nov. 9, 1918, lxxi, 1557-1561.
[2]Billings, W. C., and Hickey, J. P.: Some Points about Hookworm Disease, Its Diagnosis and Treatment, Jour. Am. Med. Assn., Dec. 23, 1916, lxvii, 1908-1912.
[3]Kofoid, C. A., and White, A. W.: A New Nematode Infection of Man, Jour. Am. Med. Assn., Feb. 22, 1919, lxxii, 567-569.
[4]Kofoid, C. A., and Barber, M. A.: Jour. Am. Med. Assn., Nov. 9, 1918, lxxi, 1559. Note also diagram, page 49, Lab. Methods of U. S. Army, Med. War Manual No. 6, Philadelphia, 1919, Lea and Febiger.
[5]Kofoid, C. A., and Barber, M. A.: Jour. Am. Med. Assn., Nov. 9, 1918, lxxi, 1557.
[6]Kofoid. C. A., et al: Intestinal Parasites in Overseas and Home Service Troops of the U. S. Army, Jour. Am. Med. Assn., June 14, 1919, lxxii, 1721-1724.
[7]This generic name takes precedence over Bothriocephalus, as shown by Magath: The Eggs of *Diphyllobothrium latum*, Jour. Am. Med. Assn., July 12, 1919, lxxiii, 85-87.
[8]Fantham, H. B., Stephens, J. W. W., and Theobald, T. V.: The Animal Parasites of Man, 1916, New York, Wm. Wood and Co., footnote on page 223.

The Journal of Laboratory and Clinical Medicine

Vol. V.   MARCH, 1920   No. 6.

Editor-in-Chief: VICTOR C. VAUGHAN, M.D.
Ann Arbor, Mich.

ASSOCIATE EDITORS

DENNIS E. JACKSON, M.D.	CINCINNATI
HANS ZINSSER, M.D.	NEW YORK
PAUL G. WOOLLEY, M.D.	DETROIT
FREDERICK P. GAY, M.D.	BERKELEY, CAL.
J. J. R. MACLEOD, M.B.	TORONTO
ROY G. PEARCE, M.D.	AKRON, OHIO
W. C. MACCARTY, M.D.	ROCHESTER, MINN.
GERALD B. WEBB, M.D.	COLORADO SPRINGS
WARREN T. VAUGHAN, M.D.	BOSTON

EDITORIALS

The Science of Ventilation and Open Air Treatment

THE well-being of a conscious animal in relation to its environment constitutes the main problem of the study of ventilation. In the case of animals leading an outdoor life, it is a problem of relatively little importance, but for those like man which spend much of their time in confined spaces, it is a problem of great importance, for in them it becomes necessary to determine the limits within which the outside influences may be altered without detriment to health or comfort.

It is often imagined that ventilation is a matter merely of pure air and that it therefore becomes a problem requiring attention only in cases where the air has been polluted by the crowding together of many people. This attitude is a wrong one, for there is very good evidence to show that much discomfort and ill health could be avoided if people understood more clearly the physical conditions of the atmosphere which bear a relationship to the well-being of the body.

When our knowledge of the function of breathing became developed to the extent of showing that an animal requires the oxygen of the air for the living processes of its body, and as a result of these processes that it produces carbonic acid, which is then added to the air, it was natural to suppose that the unfavorable effect of overcrowded confined spaces was due either to the using up of the available oxygen or to a poisonous action of the carbonic acid.

It needs only a few words to point out how utterly erroneous were these earlier explanations. That deficiency of oxygen is no factor is indicated by the facts, first, that this gas is seldom reduced by more than one per cent, even in the most crowded places; and secondly, that people live a normal existence at altitudes at which the oxygen percentage, measured at sea level, is reduced to less than two-thirds the normal.

It is not altogether easy to understand why excess of CO_2 was thought to be responsible for the evil effects of vitiated atmospheres. No doubt the chief reason was that the percentage of this gas is often raised in such atmospheres, but this is nothing more than coincidence, for on the one hand most unsuitable conditions may exist when the percentage of CO_2 is normal, and on the other, air loaded with almost a hundred times the percentage found even in the most polluted atmosphere can be breathed for indefinite periods of time without any unfavorable symptoms.

As a matter of fact, even in the open, we are constantly taking into the pulmonary alveoli large percentages of CO_2, for obviously with each inspiration the first air to be drawn in is that which remains over in the air passage from the preceding expiration. This air contains somewhere about 5 per cent of CO_2, and in quiet breathing it amounts in volume to about one-third of all the air that is drawn in from the outside. This in itself indicates that CO_2 *per se* can not be poisonous, and when we consider further the now well-known fact that a certain amount of this gas in the alveoli is absolutely essential to the well-being of the animal, the whole hypothesis of its toxic action becomes, to say the least of it, absurd. Indeed so important is the presence of this constant amount of CO_2 in the alveolar air that whenever there comes to be a marked increase in the amount of CO_2 in the atmosphere, the breathing becomes greater, so as to ventilate the air sacs more thoroughly, and thus keep the relative amount of CO_2 in them at the normal level. The extent of this increase in respiration is usually so small as to be unnoticed by the individual, and certainly increased breathing is not one of the symptoms of which persons complain who are living in polluted atmospheres.

In face of such evidence, even the most ardent supporters of the theory that the vitiated air owes its evil influence to CO_2, were compelled to abandon their position, but they did not do so without a final attempt to retain for determinations of CO_2 a certain significance in the appraisement of the healthfulness of air. Their new interpretation was to the effect that the CO_2 percentage is proportional to the amount of deleterious organic matter, and for many years this view prevailed. It is still believed by some that an increase from the normal of 3 to 10 parts of CO_2 per 10,000 parts of air indicates a degree of organic pollution which is dangerous to health. More recent work definitely shows, however, that this view also must be abandoned, and there remains for CO_2-analysis only the secondary value that it indicates, in a readily measurable way, to what extent the inside air is being mixed by ventilation with pure air from the outside. However free this dilution may be, the atmosphere may still be deleterious to health and comfort unless certain other properties of it are incidentally altered.

This interpretation of the value of CO_2 analysis naturally leads to a consideration of the next possibility, namely, that the air in confined spaces is contaminated by the accumulation of organic poisons derived from the exhaled air of the persons living in it. It is many years ago now since experiments apparently proving this hypothesis were published. These have been shown to be entirely fallacious, and we need refer to only one group of them here, namely, those that were devised to show that inhalation by one animal of volatile proteins contained in the exhaled air of others caused anaphylactic reactions. As proof for this hypothesis, experiments were performed in which a man breathed through a filter of glass wool (to catch any saliva) into a cooled vessel, and the condensed vapor was then inoculated in appropriate dosage into guinea pigs, so as to sensitize them, and a month or so later the animals were inoculated with a minute trace of human blood serum. The injected animal showed decided symptoms of anaphylactic shock, whereas other animals not previously sensitized were unaffected by the injection of the same amount of serum. Such results taken by themselves did seem to afford substantial support for the new hypothesis, but it is almost certain that they depended on contamination of the condensed vapor by traces of saliva which it is impossible to keep out by any kind of filter. This saliva contains traces of soluble protein (mucin) which had been responsible for the anaphylactic reaction. The symptoms are, however, entirely dissimilar from those of a vitiated atmosphere. Hay fever, some forms of asthma, and the reaction which some persons show when near to horses may be due to anaphylaxis, but the symptoms are not at all like those of persons breathing polluted air.

Once and for all, the toxic theory, as we may call it, both in its new and its old form, is disproved by a very simple series of experiments performed a few years ago by Leonard Hill, Flack and others.[1] These observers kept rats and guinea pigs in deep boxes so that they were huddled together in a very poorly ventilated place, the atmosphere of which indeed often contained 1 per cent of CO_2,—ten times more than the legal limit. The animals lived and thrived for months, although they must have been breathing air which was highly contaminated by the supposed volatile proteins. Not only did the animals show no symptoms while in the box, but they failed to exhibit any anaphylactic reaction when, after some time, they were inoculated subcutaneously with the serum of animals of the other species with whom they had been in cohabitation. This was really a most excellent test of the anaphylactic theory because there are probably no two animals in which anaphylaxis is more pronounced than in the rat and guinea pig. The only things that were found to be of importance in maintaining the animals in a thriving condition were cleanliness and plenty of food.

By an eliminative process we are gradually approaching the correct solution of our problem, but before we proceed to consider this, it may be well to remark that the odor of polluted air has nothing whatever to do with its unhealthy influence, except in so far as it excites disgust and puts one off his appetite. Indeed one very soon becomes so accustomed to these odors that they fail entirely to be sensed after a short period in contact with them. Their influence is entirely psychologic. In many trades and occupations people are constantly exposed to odors that are almost unbearable to one who is unused to them, and these people are perfectly healthy, and indeed do not complain at all of the smells.

We have so far considered in what is approximately their chronologic order the various hypotheses that have been brought forward to account for the harmful influence of vitiated atmospheres. We have done this mainly in order to correct any false conclusions that may still exist in connection with the subject.

And if further evidence be demanded to justify this position, there is one crucial experiment which once and for all shows that changes in the chemical composition of the atmosphere have no relationship whatsoever to the unhealthful influence of vitiated air. This experiment is all the more convincing because it was performed on healthy young men. In its simplest form it consists in crowding as many persons as possible into an air-tight cabinet, provided with an electric fan, and with the necessary apparatus for measurements of the physical and chemical condition of the air. In describing the results of this experiment, I can not do better than quote from Leonard Hill, who, though not the first to perform the experiment, has so greatly extended our knowledge of the science of ventilation during recent years.

"After 44 minutes the dry-bulb thermometer stood at 87° F., the wet bulb at 83° F. The carbon dioxide had risen to 5.26 per cent. The oxygen had fallen to 15.1 per cent. The discomfort felt was great; all were wet with sweat and the skin of all was flushed. The talking and laughing of the occupants had gradually become less and then ceased. On putting on the electric fans and whirling the air in the chamber the relief was immediate and very great, and this in spite of the temperature of the chamber continuing to rise. On putting off the fans the discomfort returned. The occupants cried out for the fans. No headache or after-effects have followed this type of experiment which has been repeated five times." Long before the discomfort had become extreme the oxygen percentage became so low that matches would not light. The disinclination to smoke cigarettes was not noticed until some time after it was impossible to light them.

In other experiments of similar type the person in the cabinet was allowed to breathe outside air through a tube, but with no amelioration of the uncomfortable feeling, or a person outside the chamber breathed for hours the air inside it through a tube without suffering any discomfort. Clearly therefore neither the chemical nature of the air, nor the presence of toxic substances in it, has any relationship to its evil influence. But the experiment is not merely destructive of previously held hypotheses; it also points the way to the true solution of the problem, for it indicates that stagnation of air loaded with moisture has some very close relationship to the discomfort. It shows that a change in the *physical* rather than the chemical properties of the air is the real cause of its deleterious action.

These changes can affect but one function of the body, namely, that of heat dissipation, and by so doing cause disturbances in the mechanism of heat control. This does not necessarily imply that this disturbance is so great as actually to cause an increase in the body temperature, although this is very commonly observed in persons who have been for some time in crowded places, but it interferes with a mechanism which is responsible not alone for proper heat regulation but also for the maintenance of a correct relationship of blood supply to different parts of the body, and for tonic stimulation of the nervous system.[3]

The mechanism by which the body temperature is maintained is in part like that of a radiator, the temperature of which depends, first on the rate at which the furnace is burning and second on the cooling influence of the air in contact with the radiator. The physical properties of the air which determine the cooling are those which influence radiation, conduction and convection. In the animal body, these processes come into play mainly at the surface of the skin, where, however, excessive loss is guarded against partly by the low conductivity for heat of the skin and of the subcutaneous tissue (fat), and partly by the fact that the blood supply to the skin is scanty compared with that of the deeper tissues, so that the blood flowing in the skin has a decidedly lower temperature than that in the tissues a few millimeters deeper. This relationship of superficial and deep temperatures is maintained by the action of vasomotor nerves to the blood vessels, and whenever the body is exposed to warmer air, the vessels of the skin become dilated so as to draft more blood from the deeper to the superficial vessels, causing flushing of the skin. Flushing of the skin is therefore a normal reaction, but at the same time it is a warning that the heat-regulating mechanism is being put on a strain.

But these mechanisms are inadequate to account for all the heat loss, for man can withstand temperatures that are not greatly below those of his body, indeed he can tolerate for some minutes temperatures that are higher. It is recorded, for example, that two observers exposed themselves for a short time in an oven in which a steak was cooking, and it is well known that certain miners work for considerable periods at very high temperatures.

Evidently some other mechanism independent of the cooling effect of air itself, and not acting in the case of a radiator, comes into play. This is evaporation, and it occurs at two places in the body, at the surface of the skin, where sweat is evaporated, and in the lungs where the expired air is saturated with water vapor. The physical factors which control the degree of heat loss by evaporation at these two places, are not precisely the same. In the case of the lungs the inspired air becomes saturated with water at body temperature, and the amount of evaporation necessary to do so depends upon the amount of water already contained in the inspired air, that is, on the *absolute* humidity; the lower this is, the more water will it require to effect saturation.

In the case of the evaporation of sweat, the amount of moisture vaporized from the body depends on the temperature and the *relative* humidity of the atmosphere.

It is in connection with this phase of the subject, more than any other, that many people find it difficult to understand the true significance of relative humidity to the well-being of the body. The difficulty depends on the fact that the relative humidity has an opposite influence at low and high temperatures. In the former case it increases the conductivity of the atmosphere for heat and has a cooling influence, and in the latter it interferes with the evaporation of sweat, and has a heating influence. Below about 65° F. the cooling effect of moist air is prominent because there is little sweating, therefore a cold wet atmosphere is chilling—it conducts heat away. At about 70° F. the cooling effect of air disappears and sweating occurs. The evaporation of the sweat now causes cooling, the degree of which varies inversely with the relative humidity. Between these two temperatures. i. e., 65° and 70° there is a range in which humidity has little influence—a neutral region. The influence of high relative humidity on bodily comfort at temperatures above the neutral temperature becomes very marked indeed; at 85° F. and a relative humidity of 90 per cent, for example, very serious symptoms appear in a few minutes, when there is no movement of the air.

Relative humidity and temperature alone are not, however, the only physical conditions to be considered. Another is *the movement of the air,* for even under the unfavorable conditions just cited, immediate relief is afforded if an electric fan be started, as it will be recalled was the result in Hill's experiment. The movement of the air enables it, though nearly loaded to its full capacity with moisture, to carry away considerable quantities in small loads.

The wearing of clothes greatly affects the rate with which these changes occur. The clothes act as barriers, preventing the movement and exchange of air around the body. The garment next the skin entraps a layer of air which is more or less at the same temperature as the skin, and which soon becomes saturated with moisture at that temperature. Between the inner garments and those over them other layers of air are entrapped, each one being at a somewhat lower temperature and containing less moisture than the one inside. These layers of air, therefore, form stepping stones, as it were, between the extreme conditions next the surface of the skin, and the environment of the clothed body. Obviously if the layers of air next the skin are to be renewed at such a rate that they remain cooler than the skin and unsaturated with moisture, the clothing must be adjusted to suit the outside conditions.

There is every reason for believing that it is because of interference with these processes that improperly ventilated and overcrowded places are uncomfortable. The moisture exhaled and evaporated from the bodies soon raises the relative humidity so that heat loss is retarded from the skin, and the heat that is actually given off raises the temperature so that loss from the body by radiation and convection becomes suppressed. As the temperature steadily rises, the air takes up more and more moisture, with the result that less and less heat comes to be lost from the lungs in saturating the expired air with vapor. The physical conditions of the environment become unsuitable for the physiologic mechanism of heat loss, although meanwhile heat production goes steadily on. The body furnaces are not damped down in proportion as the loss of heat diminishes, and the consequence is a rise in the temperature of the blood—a mild fever. Now it is well known that the cellular activities, which, taken together, make up the life process of the body are extraordinarily sensitive to change of temperature; their chemical activities become interfered with, they demand more oxygen, they fail to get rid of effete products properly, substances which have no action on them under the ordinary conditions of temperature become toxic and so forth. A highly abnormal internal environment therefore becomes created around the living tissues of the body.

But short of a measurable rise in the temperature, improperly ventilated places cause reactions in the human body that are responsible not only for the discomfort which is experienced, but also for a lowering of resistance to infections. These reactions are due in the first instance to alteration in the temperature differences between the skin and the underlying tissues. Normally, as has been remarked before, this difference maintains at the skin a constant stimulation of the thermic nerves, and this stimulation is important in maintaining the tone of the nerve centers. The nerve cells that control the functions of the body do not originate impulses; they only act when other, afferent impulses arrive at them. There are many varieties of stimuli which may excite these afferent impulses, but none more important than those which excite the heat nerves of the skin. This stimulation depends on the rate at which heat is passing through the sense organs (or receptors), in which these nerves terminate. It is necessary to emphasize that it is the rate of change that acts as the stimulus, and this depends on the difference between the deep and superficial temperatures. When the skin vessels become dilated so large a volume of blood reaches the surface that this difference becomes slight, and the thermic receptors are not stimulated. There are many practical applications of these principles; thus it is because of stimulation of the thermic skin nerves that cold baths have a bracing effect, that the open-air treatment, as in tuberculosis, tones up the body and enables it the better to hold its own against the tubercle bacillus, and that sleeping out of doors is the best tonic for maintaining good health. In open-air treatment it is true that the body is closely wrapped up—that is essential—but this does not eliminate the cooling influence, for not only does the cool air play on the exposed face and hands, in the skin of both of which the thermic nerves are very sensitive, but it acts also on these nerves in the skin, under the clothes, for the clothing merely serves to regulate the rate of cooling. This still goes on very much more than it would with much less clothing in an atmosphere that is stagnant, hot, and humid. Open windows in bedrooms are never so healthy as open-air porches, because there is no draft. It is the draft that is important. Naturally it must be regulated so that it is not restricted to one part of the body only—that obviously would introduce conditions to which the body is unaccustomed—it must blow equally all over. There is probably no greater fallacy in popular hygiene than that drafts are dangerous. Like all good and desirable things they become so only when they are improperly used—when a person overheated by being in a hot atmosphere is suddenly subjected to a restricted draft, of course there is danger that the sudden change of conditions, affecting one part of the body only, will cause vascular disturbances that may be undesirable, but if the conditions be properly controlled, drafts are the healthiest stimulants and the best tonics.

This brings us to a problem in ventilation that is attracting very considerable attention at the present time, namely, the relationship between ventilation and infections. It is a common experience not only that ordinary colds, but more serious infections as well, can be directly traced to some unsuitable condition of ventilation; such as sudden exposure to a draft while overheated, or going out into a cold, damp atmosphere from an overheated room. What is the reason for the infection under these conditions? At the outset we must recognize that all these conditions, colds, catarrhs, bronchitis, just like the more acute infectious diseases like diphtheria, pneumonia, cerebrospinal fever, etc., are due to microorganisms, and the question therefore is, why should unfavorable ventilating conditions so frequently be the immediate cause of the attack.

There are two methods by which the infection might occur. First, by a great increase in the number of organisms in the air, and secondly by a lowering of the resistance of the body towards the organisms, which would not then require to become increased in numbers. The former method is usually known as mass infection, and there can be no doubt that it is very common, perhaps, indeed, is the commonest cause for infection. The organisms, of course, come from infected individuals, who add them to the atmosphere in the exhaled air, particularly when this is forcibly discharged as in coughing or sneezing, or even in speaking.

I need recall only a few observations in order to illustrate the importance of this factor. If the mouth be rinsed with a culture of some readily recognizable organism not commonly present in detectable amounts in the atmosphere, and the person, standing in front of a row of Petri dishes, each containing some culture medium upon which the organism will grow, then speaks at ordinary pitch, the plates, after proper incubation, develop colonies of the organism, those nearest the speaker having most, but even those at a distance of several feet also showing them.

A serious problem in zoological gardens has been to keep animals that are highly susceptible to tuberculosis free from this disease. The higher apes, for example, inevitably succumb to it, being infected by the tubercle bacilli exhaled by persons standing in front of their cages, many of whom harbor these bacilli, though they may not show any of the symptoms of tuberculosis. Now it has been found that if glass screens are erected in front of the cages, the animals remain almost free from the disease.

But mass infection does not suffice to explain the cause for the onset of attacks of many conditions that are, nevertheless, fundamentally due to bacteria, such as ordinary colds. These can frequently be traced to some chill, or wet feet, or exposure to sudden change in temperature. In such cases it is believed that the bacteria are present on the mucous membranes of the upper respiratory passages, but that they remain inactive because of the normal protective influences which exist on these surfaces. So long as the blood supply is normal, these protective influences are adequate to protect the body from invasion, but if this should become curtailed, then the bacteria become active and set up pathologic processes. Evidence favoring this view has been obtained by several recent investigators by finding that the blood supply of the upper respiratory passages becomes decidedly curtailed when the surface of the body is cooled. For example Leonard Hill and Muecke[1] some years ago examined with a speculum the mucous membranes of the nose under various conditions, particularly out of doors, and in rooms which were ventilated and heated to an average degree. Out of doors the mucosa was pale and taut, and when touched by a probe did not show any pitting. This is the normal condition. Indoors it was common to find the membrane decidedly swollen, flushed with blood and covered with thick secretion, and when a probe was pressed on it a depression resulted lasting for some time. In one case that was frequently examined during these observations there was a deflected septum which only partly blocked the nasal passage on one side when the person was outside, but which did so completely under unfavorable conditions of ventilation. It is this swelling of the nasal mucosa and probably of that of the cavities which extend upward from it on to the forehead that causes the sense of stuffiness and probably also the headaches which are common in crowded, overheated places.

The conditions found to bring about these changes with greatest certainty
were when the feet were cold and the air round the head was warm, conditions
which are just exactly the opposite of those obtaining out of doors. Here the
head is usually more quickly cooled than the feet because convection currents
of cool air play around it freely, whereas next the ground the air is more stagnant. Besides, if the sun is shining the earth becomes heated by absorbing the
heat. The temperature as registered by a thermometer, either wet or dry bulb,
may be the same at the feet as at the head. It is not this that counts, however,
it is the rate of cooling which is dependent, mainly, on the movement of the air.
Now in a poorly ventilated room, such for example as one heated by a stove, or
even by radiators, and in which there is no movement of air, the feet become
cooler than the head, and it is under these conditions that the nasal membranes
become swollen. It ought to be emphasized that the cause for these changes is
not cold feet alone. It is the combination of cold feet and hot head. Out of
doors, it is well known,, that any one may stand with cold feet for hours without
any risk of catching cold, but then the head is really cooling as fast as the feet,
because of convection currents.

The ideal system of warming a room is to supply radiant heat near the floor
level; open fires, properly flued modern gas fires, and electric heaters at floor
level are the best methods to attain this.

Suppose now the person subjected to conditions which cause the mucous
membrane to become swollen and congested should go outside, then the membrane at once becomes pale because the blood vessels constrict, but for some
time it remains swollen and boggy and continues to show pitting with a probe.
It is while in this state that it offers favorable conditions for the growth of bacteria. The membrane is swollen and covered with secretion, and the blood flow
is cut down. The natural defensive agencies that are normally carried by the
blood do not succeed in combating the multiplication of the bacteria in the swollen membrane. After some time out of doors the blood supply returns because
it is required to warm up the cool air, but this reaction does not occur before
the mucosa has regained its normal condition.*

The protective influence of a rapid blood flow through the nasal membrane
is possibly the explanation of the relative immunity from infectious colds of
those who work in air containing irritating gases, such as workers in various
kinds of chemical factories. Even the irritation set up by coal dust may, by
similar methods, afford some protection against infection by the tubercle haeil-
lus,—for phthisis is relatively infrequent among coal miners. The supposedly
antiseptic action of ozone is probably due to a similar irritating effect. Any
benefit that may be derived from its presence in the atmosphere can not otherwise be explained. It is possible that a useful prophylactic practice to avoid
infection, such as that of influenza, would be to stimulate the nasal mucosa at
intervals by snuff, but this may be an unwise suggestion.

After becoming acclimatized to outdoor conditions, the nasal mucous membrane is in a much more favorable condition to withstand infection than indoors
because of the very rapid blood flow that is necessary in order to supply heat

*The congestion of the mucous membrane brought about by warm moist air does not probably de-
pend on dilatation of the small arteries—entailing increased flow of blood—but rather on dilatation of the
capillaries and therefore a stagnation of blood.

with which to warm up the inspired air. This more rapid blood flow, and the freer flow of lymph which accompanies it, is reinforced by increased secretion, which assists to wash away invading bacteria. Mass infection being equal inside and outside, the animal body can withstand it much less satisfactorily in the former case.

These observations on the reactions of the respiratory membranes to atmospheric conditions have been confirmed by other investigators. Thus Cook[4] caused persons to breathe forcibly through the nostrils onto a mirror surface, and then marked on it with a wax pencil the outlines of the moisture deposited. Although the extent of the outlines varied somewhat with the depth of breathing, they afford a general estimate of the width of the air passages. It was found that there is marked reduction in the nasal air passage in a warm room. Winslow[5] also sums up the observations (150 in number) made on this aspect of the problem, in the following words: "Ordinarily it was found that heat causes a swelling of the inferior turbinate of the nose, tending to diminish the size of the breathing space, increased secretion and reddening of the membranes. The action of cold is, as a rule, just the opposite."

Many other observations bearing on the relationship between chilling and immunity to infection have been recorded, but it would take us beyond our subject to discuss them here. Because of their accuracy and the excellent control of possible fallacies, it is important, however, to say something about the recent investigations of Mudd and Grant.[6] These observers measured the temperature of the mucous membranes of the palate, tonsils, and pharynx by means of thermocouples before and during application to the skin of cold towels, or while cold air from a fan was allowed to play on it. A rise in temperature would indicate that the part had become more vascular, and a fall, the contrary. That this interpretation was the correct one was confirmed by direct inspection of the degree of flushing (redness). It was found that chilling the body surface immediately caused a fall in the temperature of the mucous membranes which could not be accounted for by any accompanying change in blood pressure, or, entirely at least, by changes in respiration or by lowering of the temperature of the blood. The conclusions are "that chilling of the body surface causes reflex vasoconstriction and ischemia in the mucous membranes of the palate, faucial tonsils, oropharynx and nasopharynx."

And now the final question presents itself. What are the ideal conditions of ventilation? It is a most difficult question to answer, and one over which at present several large commissions are at work. Indeed most elaborate experiments have been planned and undertaken to throw light on the question. The observations of the New York Commission on Ventilation, and those conducted by Mr. Watt, in the Graham School in Chicago, are among the most important in this country, and, of course, they interest us much more directly than those conducted on the other side, where the climatic conditions are fundamentally different.

Many of the observations have so far been made on properly selected groups of school children, taught in classrooms with different ventilating conditions. Attention is directed to the general efficiency of the pupils and the condition of their health. The temperature, and the humidity of the air are the physical conditions of the atmosphere which have been more particularly studied, but a great deal more work must be done before any definite conclusions can be offered. It appears, however, that for school room air a temperature of 65-68° F., with a relative humidity of 45-60°/° is the optimum. To maintain these conditions throughout the period a class occupies the room, usually requires, in this country, at least, the addition of a considerable quantity of moisture to the ventilating air. The air of most of our school rooms in winter errs on the side of being too dry, for under these conditions the mucous membranes suffer injuriously. An excellent summary of the various authoritative conclusions with regard to the optimum conditions of ventilation for class rooms is given by Burnham in the Pedagogical Seminary.[7]

Although the present review does not venture to discuss the methods that are employed for the measurement of the various physical properties which have to be considered in gauging its influence on health, or the engineering problem of how ideal conditions may be maintained, it may not be out of place to mention, in connection with the former of these, that the physical property to which most attention should be devoted is the cooling power. This can not be done by reading an ordinary thermometer, for this instrument only registers the temperature of the piece of wood and of the wall against which it is hung. It registers the same whether the air is dry or moist, or whether it is stagnant or moving. Somewhat more information regarding cooling power is afforded by readings of a wet-bulb thermometer, an instrument in which the bulb is kept constantly moist, so that evaporation occurs from it. This evaporation tends to cool the thermometer, in proportion to its rate, and since this is dependent mainly on the degree to which the air can take up more moisture, we can tell by the use of a formula or tables the relative degree of humidity of the air. Still this does not tell us the real degree of cooling which the atmosphere can bring about. It does not adequately register the cooling which is dependent upon movement in the air, the so-called convection currents. To afford this information, Leonard Hill has invented what he calls the Kata thermometer, by which the rate of cooling is directly measured. The instrument consists of an alcohol thermometer with a relatively large bulb, and with the scale registering between 105° F. and 90° F. It is placed in warm water at about the former temperature, and is then removed, and the time required for the temperature to fall from 100° F. to 95° F. is measured by means of a stop watch. This time divided by a factor determined for each instrument, and written on the stem, gives the actual amount of heat in millicalories per square centimeter per second which would be given off from, say the surface of the human body, under similar environmental conditions. Hill and his associates[3] have shown that much important information concerning the cooling power of the atmosphere can be gained in this way, which can not be gained by any other.

REFERENCES

[1] Hill, Leonard, and Muecke, F. F.: Lancet, London, 1913.
[2] Hill, Leonard: Jour. Physiol., 1910, xli, 3.
[3] Hill, Leonard: The Science of Ventilation and Open Air Treatment, Medical Research Committee, H. M. Stationery Office, London, 1919.
[4] Cock, H. Girard: Trans. Am. Laryngol., Rhinol. and Otolog. Soc., June, 1915.
[5] Winslow, C. E. A.: Am. Jour. Pub. Health, 1917, No. 3, p. 157.
[6] Mudd, S., and Grant, S. B.: Jour. Med. Research, 1919, xl, p. 53.
[7] Burnham, W. H.: The Pedagogical Seminary, 1919, xxvi, 311.

—*J. J. R. M.*

Influenza

WITH the increase of influenza once more to epidemic proportions it may be of advantage to review some of the work that has been reported since the epidemic of 1918, concerning the clinical phenomena of the disease. Given a case of illness with sudden onset, prostration, headache and general body pains, with febrile period of fixed duration, and without complications or other causative pathology, such as acute tonsillitis, acute coryza, trichiniasis, accessory sinus disease, etc., and in the absence of an epidemic, one can say that the condition is apparently influenza, but there is no method by which one may prove that it is the same disease as that which caused the pandemic of 1918. There is no one diagnostic sign or group of signs such as we possess in the exanthemata, by which the diagnosis may be finally concluded. It might be helpful to include in the description a statement of its extreme contagiousness and its epidemic propensities. When contagion can be demonstrated it is surely of help in making a clear-cut diagnosis. But there is abundant evidence that in interepidemic cases the contagiousness is by no means as great as during the explosive outbreaks.

Nevertheless, epidemic influenza is a clinical entity caused by a specific organism, and in all probability the interepidemic cases and surely those postepidemic cases which have occurred since the winter of 1919 are due to the same cause. Whether that cause be B. influenzæ or some other unknown virus is not a matter for discussion in this paper.

What is influenza? This question is no easier to answer than is the equally complicated one propounded by Rivers, "What is an influenza bacillus?" It is a disease with certain clinical manifestations as indicated above. Unfortunately similar manifestations may accompany the onset of other infections not influenza. Acute tonsillitis may produce fever, prostration, headache and general body aches. Again, sore throat may be present in influenza, although as a rule, this is mild and the tonsils do not show exudation, ulceration or the intense local inflammation of an acute follicular tonsillitis. Acute coryza is easily distinguished. The absence of systemic symptoms, the more profuse and irritating nasal discharge and the subsequent development of tenacious purulent secretion serve to distinguish it from influenza. In the course of the disease we may through negative findings rule out the other specific infectious diseases. Perhaps the greatest difficulty lies in distinguishing between the mild interepidemic variety and cases of tonsillitis and pharyngitis with constitutional symptoms but without great visible local pathology. Of help here is the delayed return of strength and tonus, the postinfluenzal asthenia which follows even mild infection with the true disease, although even this symptom is less pronounced than during epidemics. In influenza there is no swelling of the lymph glands of the neck as is so often the case in tonsillitis. The presence of leucopenia is a corroborative finding of great value. It has further been found that in the postepidemic cases of 1919 leucopenia has remained characteristic of the disease.[1]

A dusky erythema of the skin, particularly over the face and neck, has been described by Bloomfield and Harrop,[2] an erythema different from the simple flush of fever and not dependent on cyanosis; one which persisted into convalescence and was often followed by desquamation. It is likened in character to that accompanying scarlet fever or urticaria, or following burns. They also describe intense hyperemia of the mucous membrane of the buccal cavity somewhat similar to that seen after the application of a chemical irritant such as adrenalin, and which usually subsided after two or three days. The skin erythema has been described by many writers.[3, 4, 5, 6] The face appears hot and flushed. This, with the conjunctival injection and slight coryza, resembles the appearance of an early measles patient in whom the rash is not yet distinct. At times the influenza rash may be punctate in character. Bloomfield reports that among the postepidemic cases studied the skin and mucous membrane lesions have been present in only slight degree. In them the mucous membrane hyperemia is indicated only by a slight diffuse reddening of the pharynx, pillars and soft palate, and is accompanied by swelling of the lymphoid tissue of the pharyngeal wall.

Hemorrhagic tendency is indicated by epistaxis, hemoptysis, precocious menstruation, profuse bleeding in abortion, and more rarely, hematemesis and purpura.

Arrived at a consideration of those cases which have developed pulmonary symptoms—bronchitis or pneumonia—we are again confronted with an absence of pathognomonic physical signs. One of the most constant and one which aids greatly in establishing the diagnosis, is the unusual degree of cyanosis which is most easily recognized on the mucous membrane of the lips and on the cheeks and ears. This sign comes early, in fact is considered by some to accompany the uncomplicated influenza. We do not know of any work that has been done to determine how early in the disease it occurs. Harrop[7] uses the term cyanosis synonymously with the "dusky erythema" previously referred to. The majority of observers speak of the cyanosis as a manifestation of complicating pulmonary involvement.

The cyanosis exists to an extent out of all proportion to the amount of dyspnea present. In fact in the early pneumonia there is relatively little increase in respiratory rate. The cause of cyanosis has received considerable study. Torrey and Grosh[8] report that a large proportion of their series of cases during the epidemic exhibited clinical signs of pulmonary emphysema. There was an apparent increase in the circumference of the chest during the illness, shallow respiratory excursion, tympany under the sternum, vertebral column and much of the precordium, low standing diaphragm and often bulging supraclavicular fossae. At autopsy the lungs showed well-formed rib markings and emphysematous bullae under the visceral pleura. The lungs could not be collapsed by pressure, and even the apparently solid portions floated high in water. The lung tissue was usually fairly tough at the apices, but extremely friable at the bases where it was easily disintegrated under moderate pressure. Torrey and Grosh conceive of damage to the parenchyma, done perhaps by interference with the normal blood supply by the nodules of peribronchial infiltration, and subsequent rupture of the damaged alveolar walls. Their explanation of the cyanosis, as well as the dyspnea and the epistaxis, is in the pulmonary emphysema which, through increasing the intrathoracic pressure, caused some degree of venous stasis. In support of their theory they state that in those rather frequent cases which developed interstitial emphysema, there was an immediate amelioration of symptoms, with lessened respiratory distress, diminished signs of thoracic inflation, and some lessening of the cyanosis. The fall in intrathoracic pressure following passage of the air into the tissues of the mediastinum lessened, in their opinion, the venous stasis.

Whether or not we accept this explanation for the cyanosis, two facts mentioned by these authors have been established in the experience of many observers during the last epidemic. The pathologists in particular have had opportunity to observe the damaged alveolar walls[9] with frequent emphysematous patches, and all clinicians who have treated any large number of cases can report instances of interstitial emphysema in which the air often passed not only into the upper and lower mediastinum, but up through the fascial tissues of the neck. In extreme cases the emphysema involved the subcutaneous tissue from the region of the eyes downward to the groin. A case reported by Clark and Synnott[10] is of interest in that the discovery of gas in the mediastinal tissues at autopsy explained some very unusual sounds heard through the stethoscope: "over the precordium rales very similar to sounds elicited with moderate pressure of stethoscope over emphysematous cutaneous tissue" were heard.

Kelman[11] observed the frequency of vesicular emphysema which, in her experience, was usually marginal with not infrequent emphysematous bullæ discovered substernally. The roots of the lungs were also quite commonly involved. She also observed the dyspnea and cyanosis which were out of proportion to the amount of lung involvement. Experimenting on rabbits, with artificial pressure inflation of the lungs, she reached the following conclusions: "Increased intrapulmonary pressure causes rupture of some of the superficial distended air vesicles and there is an escape of air underneath the visceral pleura, which is rather firm. The air finds less resistance in escaping underneath the pleura toward the hilus than to break through the pleura. From the hilus it travels along the pleural reflexions over the pulmonary arteries and veins to where it meets the pericardial reflexions over the same vessels, the tissues of the mediastinum, especially the pericardium and pericardial fat, thence it extends to the superior mediastinum and passes downward into the retroperitoneal tissues—the perirenal tissues being most commonly invaded." It may pass on down by the great vessels into the thigh, or superiorly, following the subclavian into the axillary space. That she did not produce cervical emphysema is explained in part by the fact that the neck tissues of the rabbit had been opened for tracheotomy. Kelman showed that in death from anaphylaxis both vesicular and interstitial emphysema may be present. She also showed in living rabbits that emphysema itself was capable of producing dyspnea and cyanosis. She conceives of the vesicular emphysema of influenza as resulting from the strain of coughing on lung tissue damaged by the influenza toxin.

Hoover[12] studied cyanosis and dyspnea in gassed soldiers. The probable cause as described by him might play some part in the cyanosis of influenza pneumonia. Foam in the exudate of the alveoli interferes with the normal transfer of oxygen and carbon dioxide between the alveolar air and the blood. Any portion of the respiratory membrane which is covered by alveolar air foam is deprived of its normal respiratory function, both for the escape of carbon dioxide and for the absorption of oxygen. If a lobe of the lung is filled with this foam, the surface area for gaseous interchange is no longer the very large area of the respiratory epithelium of the lobe, but the cross section of the bronchus leading to the lobe,—the surface area of the foam in the bronchus. Hoover showed that gassed soldiers, whose lungs contained much alveolar foam, when breathing pure oxygen, recovered within a few minutes from their cyanosis but obtained no relief from the associated dyspnea. Within these few minutes the pure oxygen had been well mixed with and absorbed in the alveolar foam, thence gaining access to the blood and relieving the cyanosis. But the concentration of carbon dioxide in the foam remained the same as when atmospheric air was being breathed and the amount in the blood remained unchanged, so the dyspnea persisted. Hoover's work was reported before the epidemic of 1918 but a case described by him may be quoted as an example of the type. "A young man who had bronchitis with an abundance of moisture in his air spaces, had pronounced cyanosis of the lips and fingers. There was only a moderate dyspnea. It did not amount to air hunger. There were no demonstrable areas of consolidation in the lung. * * * He breathed oxygen through the closed system and after he had inhaled it for about three minutes, all traces of cyanosis disappeared. But he breathed with exactly the same rate and volume as when he was breathing atmospheric air."

The oxygen and carbon dioxide content of expired air corresponds to blood content of these gases only so long as the entire alveolar respiratory membrane is functioning properly. When moisture covers portions of the alveoli the gaseous tension of the alveolar air no longer corresponds necessarily to that of the blood, and furthermore the variation may be unequal in the case of the two gases.

That the cyanosis of influenza pneumonia is mechanical rather than biochemical is indicated by the work of Harrop[7] who found that both the oxygen content and oxygen unsaturation of the venous blood showed normal values in both uncomplicated influenza and influenza pneumonia, and particularly by the work of Stadie[13] who confirmed these results and further showed that an increase of cyanosis was accompanied by an increase of unsaturation of the arterial blood. The cyanosis is then due to incomplete saturation of venous blood with oxygen in the lungs. Neither Stadie nor Harrop found any decrease in the oxygen carrying capacity. Methemoglobin formation, if it did occur at all, could not have been present to such an extent as to have been a factor in producing the cyanosis.

A discussion of the clinical phenomena of the disease would scarcely be complete without brief mention of the characteristic lung picture at necropsy. Here at last we may find signs that promise to give as reliable evidence as do Koplik's spots in measles, or rose spots in typhoid fever. The particular lesion has been described by Wolbach,[9] Goodpasture and Burnett[14] and by MacCallum[15] and consists in dilation of the alveolar ducts with a hyaline membrane partially or completely covering their walls and sometimes those of subtended alveoli. These are the pathologic reactions which have been found in no other disease, but other pathologic changes accompany these and are found elsewhere in the lung substance. The other changes are similar in character to those described by MacCallum in post measles pneumonia.

In conclusion we may state that influenza is a disease of unknown or undemonstrated etiology which bears many clinical characteristics analogous to those of measles and kindred exanthemata.

REFERENCES

[1]Bloomfield, A. L.: Medical Clinics of North America, 1919, p. 1635.
[2]Bloomfield, A. L., and Harrop, G. A.: Bull. Johns Hopkins Hosp., 1919, xxxi.
[3]Frankel, B.: New York Med. Jour., 1918.
[4]Conner, Lewis A.: Jour. Am. Med. Assn., lxxiii, 321.
[5]Locke, E. A.: Rönne, G. E., and Lande, H.: Boston Med. and Surg. Jour., 1919, cl, 241.
[6]Cowie, D. M., and Beaven, P. W.: Jour. Mich. State Med. Soc., 1919.
[7]Harrop, Geo. A., Jr.: Bull. Johns Hopkins Hosp., 1919, xxx, 10.
[8]Torrey, R. G., and Grosh, L. C.: Am. Jour. Med. Sc., 1919, clvii, 170.
[9]Wolbach, S. B.: Bull. Johns Hopkins Hosp., 1919, xxx, 104.
[10]Clark, Elbert, and Synnott, Martin J.: Am. Jour. Med. Sc., 1919, clvii, 219.
[11]Kelman, Saral R.: Arch. Int. Med., 1919, xxiv, 332.
[12]Hoover, C. F.: Jour. Am. Med. Assn., 1918, lxxi, 880.
[13]Stadie, W. C.: Jour. Exper. Med., 1919, xxx, 215.
[14]Goodpasture, E. W., and Burnett, F. L.: U. S. Naval Med. Bull., xiii, No. 2, p. 177.
[15]MacCallum, W. G.: Jour. Am. Med. Assn., 1919, lxxii, 720.

—*W. T. V.*

A Medical Man's Opinion Concerning Universal Military Training

I AM often asked whether I approve of Universal Military Training. Under certain conditions I do; under other conditions I do not.

If we are to have Universal Military Training and our sons are to be mobilized and sent to camps in the way that was done in 1917, I am unalterably opposed to Universal Military Training. Under these conditions I would feel that it would be criminal to advise those who have confidence in me to permit their sons to be mobilized and encamped as they were in 1917. At that time it was pointed out to the authorities that the method of mobilization then followed would gather into the camps all infections existing in the areas from which the soldiers came. The drafted men were brought together in villages and cities, they came clean and unclean, bearing the bacteria of all the homes and localities from which they came. In their ordinary clothing they were huddled together until a certain number accumulated, when they were placed on troop-trains and sent to the designated camp. In the fall of 1917 not a troop train reached Camp Wheeler without having on board from one to six cases of fully developed measles.

The men on this train had been en route for from twelve to forty-eight hours. Practically every man on every train, certainly every man in certain cars, had been exposed to measles. To control the disease under these conditions is beyond the power of the most skillful epidemiologist.

In the spring of 1918, several hundred drafted colored men were assembled at Montgomery, Alabama. As in other instances they came in their ordinary clothing, more or less soiled, generally more, bringing the bacterial flora of hundreds of cabins in the State. They were held together until the desired number assembled, then they were placed on troop trains and after a journey of from two to three days reached Camp Custer. Some sixty cases of streptococcus pneumonia were taken directly from the train to the base hospital, and within a month the type of pneumonia throughout the whole division at Camp Custer was changed. Instances of this kind might be multiplied many times. What was the result? This can be ascertained by comparing the death rates from the different infectious diseases in the camps with the death rates in those who remained at home, belonging to the same age group. When we make this comparison, what do we find? The death rate from pneumonia per 100,000 was 9 times greater in the army; from meningitis, 15 times greater; from scarlet fever, 2.5 times greater; from diphtheria 1.1 times greater; from measles 6 times greater; from all causes 1.2 times greater. It must be remembered that tuberculosis was largely excluded. The mortality from this disease was 8 times greater in the civilians of that age group.

If Universal Military Training is to be adopted, the health of those mobilized and called to camp must be so guarded that the death rate must not be higher than among those of the same age group at home. Can this be done? I think that it can, but if it is done, the examination of men to be sent to the camps, their mobilization in their home neighborhood, their transportation, their care after they reached camp must be under the control of our best epidemiologists.

In 1917, army officers stated with truth that the purpose of mobilization is not to make a demonstration in preventive medicine, but to assemble civilians, and to convert them into efficient soldiers as quickly as possible. This explanation was valid at the time, and under the then existing conditions; it would not be valid in peace times. Our unpreparedness in 1917, and the hurried mobilization of troops and their intensive training were absolutely necessary. It was suggested at that time that more sanitary methods of mobilization and handling the drafted men might be put into practice. If we are to have Universal Military Training, the young men of the designated age should be assembled in groups of not more than 30, carefully examined, stripped of their ordinary clothing, barbered, bathed, and put in sterilized uniform, then they should be held in quarantine in some armory hall or in tents or possibly they might be under certain conditions billeted. They should be held for at least 14 days with daily examinations, of course with the exclusion of any infection that might occur during this time. During this period they should receive their vaccinations and at the end of this period each group should be placed in a car, not a troop train, or at least each group should be isolated and sent to the camp. After reaching the camp the isolation of each group should be continued during 14 days longer. This would not mean that they could not be drilled and put through proper exercise during this time. All drilling might be done with the groups while detached; in addition to this the camps must be in perfect sanitary condition. There is no difficulty in securing this. Our camps in 1917 and 1918 were in better sanitary condition by far than the average village or city in the United States. It may be asked whether one has a right to assume that under conditions as just specified our young men could be mobilized without increased death rate. In our larger universities from five to twelve thousand young men and women from all parts of the world assemble every fall without an increased death rate. In my opinion this renders it not only highly probable but quite certain that under proper conditions, mobilization of the young could be practiced without increased morbidity or mortality.

The S. A. T. C. had in it the germ of great possibility of good. It was hurriedly and imperfectly conceived and put into being. The epidemic of influenza came and wrought havoc. The war ended and the people in general are sick of everything military. We will probably continue in this attitude until we are forced to mobilize hurriedly as we did in 1917 with the same great loss of life. I certainly believe that physical training with physical, not military drill, should be introduced into all of our high schools. Every young person attending these schools, girls as well as boys, should undergo a careful physical examination, not a perfunctory one, at least once a year, better twice a year, and all should be drilled, not military drill, but in the most approved forms of physical training. It is to be hoped that our school authorities will appreciate the value of physical training. I would be opposed to military drill in our high schools. Military maneuvers do not furnish the best forms for the physical education of the young. The periodical examinations should enable us to group our young men and women and point out to each what manner of life is best suited to his or her physical condition. Hundreds with incipient tuberculosis go into occupations and professions which hasten the development of this disease. If it had been recognized in its earliest incipiency, the individual might have been guided and instructed in some other vocation, which would have been more suitable to his physical condition. In the past we have waited until the young man has established himself in some trade or profession when he shows signs of developing tuberculosis and we say, he must go and live an outdoor life. The lawyer, the doctor, the manufacturer, the carpenter, after they have established themselves in a special line of work must become a gardener or a farmer. He soon finds that as gardener or farmer he is not a success. He can work successfully only in the trade or profession which he has learned. He goes back to the shop, the office, the counting room, spreads tuberculosis among his fellows, and dies from the disease himself.

I certainly believe in physical preparedness of the race, but attempts to provide for it must be scientific and not haphazard.

—V. C. V.

Raise In Subscription Price

With the February issue of the Journal of Laboratory and Clinical Medicine, the subscription price will be raised to $5.00. As a reason for this increase, we only need to point to the fact that cost of printing and paper, and the making of illustrations, has increased from one hundred to three hundred per cent since the Journal was started four years ago.

The publishers feel that the readers of this Journal prefer to pay an additional cost of two dollars a year rather than have the quality of the Journal lowered in any particular.

Government Needs Physicians

The United States Civil Service Commission announces that a large number of physicians are needed for employment in the Indian Service, the Public Health Service, the Coast and Geodetic Survey, and the Panama Canal Service.

Both men and women will be admitted to examinations, but appointing officers have the legal right to specify the sex desired when requesting the certification of eligibles.

Entrance salaries as high as $200 a month are offered, with prospect of promotion in some branches to $250, $300, and higher rates for special positions.

Further information and application blanks may be obtained from the secretary of the U. S. civil service board at Boston, New York, Philadelphia, Atlanta, Cincinnati, Chicago, St. Paul, St. Louis, New Orleans, Seattle or San Francisco, or from the U. S. Civil Service Commission at Washington, D. C.

The Journal of
Laboratory and Clinical
Medicine

VOL. V.   ST. LOUIS, APRIL, 1920   No. 7

ORIGINAL ARTICLES

NOTE ON SOME RESPIRATORY STUDIES MADE ON LATE STAGES OF GAS POISONING*

BY R. G. PEARCE, M.D., AKRON, OHIO

THE nature of the disability in late stages of gas poisoning is uncertain. The physical examination of the majority of men who complain of symptoms which they believe are due to gas fails to reveal any signs of impairment of their heart and lungs. For the greater part, such patients suffer from subjective symptoms similar to those of the so-called effort syndrome. Three typical cases have been studied from the cardiorespiratory standpoint in my laboratory. I had hoped to extend these studies, but find it impossible to do so, and believe it advisable to present the results at this time.

The first patient studied was a returned British soldier, who was gassed with chlorine very early in the war, and had had a very checkered military and hospital career. When he was first seen by us, some twelve months after he was gassed, physical examination failed to reveal any impairment of his heart and lungs, save some bronchitis. At this time it was a question whether or not he was entitled to a pension. Indeed it was suggested that he was feigning incapacity to escape military service. His chief complaint was inability to work without becoming breathless and faint.

His respiratory exchange, minute volume of air, depth and rate of respiration, tension of carbon dioxide in the alveolar air and that in equilibrium with his venous blood (affluent blood of the lungs), were determined at rest, walking, and running at a dog trot for a short distance; and compared with those of a normal man. At rest practically normal figures were obtained, but on ex-

*From the Cardiorespiratory Laboratory, Medical Service, Lakeside Hospital, Cleveland, Ohio.

ercise his minute volume of air, in comparison with the degree of work done as measured by the oxygen consumption, was greater and out of all proportion to that obtained in the normal being. This superventilation naturally decreased the percentage of carbon dioxide in the alveolar air, but the blood returning to the lungs had a normal or slightly increased tension of carbon dioxide. In spite of this fact, his breathing was labored and fast, and he felt faint. This man was kept under observation for about a year and always gave the same result, save that he gradually developed a more severe bronchitis, together with asthma and emphysema, and finally was advised to go West to a dry climate.

We interpreted the disability in this case as being due to a dissociation between the ability of the blood to obtain oxygen and to rid itself of carbon dioxide. It was thought that the results indicated that the man was able to excrete his carbon dioxide without difficulty, but that he was unable to get enough oxygen. This condition was thought to be due to the presence of bubbles of foam in many of the alveoli, which prevented a free exchange of air while not preventing the free flow of blood through the pulmonary capillaries. The blood passing over these foam-filled alveoli was unventilated and reached the left ventriele in a venous condition. The superventilation present during exercise lowered the carbon dioxide tension in the alveolar air of the functional air sacs, and this blood was superventilated and contained a less than optimal amount of carbon dioxide but a normal amount of oxygen, since superventilation affects little if any the amount of oxygen the blood carries on leaving the lungs. The blood entering the left ventricle therefore would be a mixture of superventilated and underventilated blood. The mixture might have a normal carbon dioxide tension, but would have a subnormal oxygen tension. If the cardiac output were normal the blood returning to the lungs would have a normal carbon dioxide tension but a low oxygen content. In other words, there would be a dissociation between the ability of the blood to get rid of its carbon dioxide and to obtain its oxygen. This condition is analogous to that we have previously pointed out as existing in congenital heart disease, early pneumonias, and foreign bodies in one bronchus, and has been termed by us admixture cyanosis.

Experimental evidence that such a condition might be responsible for this case was found in an experiment performed with Dr. C. F. Hoover on a dog. A tampon made of lamb's wool was introduced into the bronchus of the animal, and the rate and depth of breathing, together with observations on the venosity of the blood, were recorded. It was found that blocking the bronchus of one lobe of the lungs resulted immediately in a quickened and deepened respiration, but in spite of this, blood drawn while the tampon was in place was venous in color. This color immediately disappeared when the tampon was removed. The blood could be made cyanotic or of normal color at will.

Unfortunately for the theory, no definite improvement in the man's condition was found when he was made to work while breathing high pressures of oxygen. In patients suffering from bronchial pneumonia, in which there is a large amount of moisture present, oxygen will relieve the cyanosis but will not affect the respiratory distress. The bubbles of air in the alveoli, being filled with oxygen in this case, oxygenate the alveolar blood but do not decarbonize it; hence the respirations are little if any affected by this form of treatment. In spite of this fact if oxygen want is present in bronchial pneumonias, oxygen therapy is justified in these cases. The improvement in the condition of the cases cited by Barcroft and others, when gassed soldiers are made to breathe oxygen over long periods of time, may be due to an improvement in the tone of the tissues from the increased and more nearly normal oxygen tension of the blood bathing them.

In another case, that of Private R., who was sent to me through the kindness of Capt. F. P. Esselbruegge, of the Convalescent Station, Camp Meade, somewhat different results were obtained. This soldier had been gassed with phosgene and mustard on November 3. After a more or less normal convalescence, he was able to do the ordinary things of life, but found himself unable to exert himself without becoming dizzy and faint. His voice had been affected with mustard and he was unable to articulate well.

He was first seen by me at Camp Meade early in February, when he presented himself for physical examination after he had been marched hurriedly from the barracks to the examining room. He was pale with a bluish tinge, and almost fainted before we could seat him in a chair. On February 26, when he arrived at this hospital, he was able to do the ordinary things all right without discomfort, but any unusual exertion seemed to make him breathless and faint. He did not impress one as being ill, and physical examination was absolutely negative; there was no indication whatever of impairment of heart or lungs. We attempted to determine the nature of his disability by methods similar to those used in the case cited previously.

In these experiments the subject rested or exercised on a rowing machine; he respired through a mask fitted with Geer valves, and expired into a 100-liter spirometer, the excursion of each breath being recorded on a high vertical slow-moving drum. Each expiration was recorded as a vertical and somewhat diagonal line downward; each inspiration as a horizontal line. The stroke was timed by a pendulum and adjusted to give breathlessness at the end of a minute and a half. The number of strokes was recorded by an automatic counter on the machine, and the time determined by a stop watch. The subject seated himself on the rowing machine and at a signal began rowing. At the end of a half minute, one minute, and one minute and a half respectively, on separate tests, he was stopped abruptly and the carbon dioxide tension of the affluent blood of the lungs was determined by a method essentially the same in principle as used by Christiansen, Douglas and Haldane. This method will be described fully in the near future.

Control experiments were made on R.G.P. for comparison.

In the experiments shown in Table I, at the end of a minute Pvt. R. was distressed and complained of dizziness; at the end of a minute and a half he always complained of distress in his stomach, dizziness and shortness of breath. At the end of a minute, and of a minute and a half, it was interesting to note that the pressure of carbon dioxide in equilibrium with the affluent blood of the lungs was

TABLE 1

FEB. 28, 1919. 10:00 A.M.				SUBJECT R. C. PEARCE
	Rest	½ Min.	1 Min.	1½ Min.
Strokes	0	20	40	60
Vol. of air respired	8.1 L.	20 L.	43 L.	69 L.
Corrected Vol. 0° and 760 Min.	7.3 "	18.4 "	37.5 "	60 "
Min. Vol. of air	7.3 "	36.8 "	37.5 "	40 "
Vol. rate per min. at the end of exercise	7.3 "	44 "	52.5 "	74 "
% CO_2 expired air	3.4%	3.7%	4.3%	4.7%
% CO_2 in equilibrium with affluent blood of lungs	7.1%	8.4%	10.4%	11.3%
O_2 absorbed for period	302 c.c.	645 c.c.	1520 c.c.	2800 c.c.
O_2 absorbed per minute	302 c.c.	1290 c.c.	1520 c.c.	1866 c.c.
Pulse rate	90	120	120	130 (irreg.)
Respiratory rate	16	40	40	40
Respiratory quotient	.82	1.05	1.06	1.02
FEB. 28, 1919.				SUBJECT PRIVATE R.
Strokes	0	17	39	54
Vol. of air respired	7.9 L.	21 L.	46 L.	87 L.
Corrected Vol. 0° & 760'	6.9 "	18.1 "	40.5 "	76 "
Minute Vol. of air	6.9 "	36.2 "	40.5 "	51 "
Vol. rate at end of exercise		45 "	60 "	90 "
% CO_2 expired air	3.2%	3.4%	3.6%	3.7%
% CO_2 in equilibrium with affluent blood of lungs	6.6%	8.3%	8.8%	9.5%
O_2 absorbed during period		560 c.c.	1700 c.c.	2800 c.c.
O_2 absorbed per minute	276 c.c.	1120 c.c.	1700 c.c.	1860 c.c.
Pulse rate	80	100	110	110
Respiratory rate per min.	21	46	46	54
Respiratory quotient	.92	1.1	8.6	1.05

not so high as in the case of R. G. P. If Pvt. R.'s limitation of work was determined because of impairment in the ventilatory membrane or because there was an insufficient minute volume of blood passing through the body per unit of time, it would be expected that the tension of carbon dioxide in the affluent blood of the lungs would be abnormally high, but such was not the case. The amount of work he was doing would not normally require a respiratory volume of 87 liters per minute. This is shown (1) by the comparatively low value of the carbon dioxide in the expired air, and (2) by the low value of the carbon dioxide in equilibrium with the affluent blood of the lungs as compared with normal controls; yet, in spite of this, he was cyanotic, dizzy, and in a state of collapse. This experiment suggests that there is some dissociation between the ability of this man to get rid of his carbon dioxide and to receive oxygen from the atmospheric air. Accordingly experiments were devised of a similar nature in which oxygen was breathed in place of air, as follows:

On March 3 Pvt. R. was supposed to row at the approximate rate of 30 strokes per minute, but failed to time himself properly with the pendulum. He was almost in collapse when he finished rowing, and he looked blue. He complained of being dizzy and of having a stomach ache. It was with reluctance that he consented to work again.

He repeated the experiment, but this time the spirometer from which he inspired had been filled with oxygen. When he finished he expressed surprise at the ease with which he had accomplished the work. His pulse rate was 20 beats slower in this case than when air was breathed. He got up immediately and walked over to the faucet to get a drink of water. He was pink in color. The effect of oxygen in causing him to do a greater amount of work was too obvious to be disputed.

The experiment was repeated on R. G. P. In this case a faster rate of rowing was adopted. R. G. P. noted that there was a distinct feeling of comfort while working with oxygen, which was not the case when breathing air. The breaths were more easily taken and the feeling of fatigue following this very extreme exercise was much less. After the exercise with air breathing, the pulse rate was irregular and impossible to count on account of extra systoles. After oxygen breathing, the pulse rate immediately following the exercise was 125 and was free from extra systoles. The results are given in Table II.

TABLE II

MARCH 3, 1919.	AIR BREATHED		OXYGEN BREATHED	
	R. G. P.	Pvt. R.	R. G. P.	Pvt. R.
Time of observation	1′ 30″	1′ 30″	1′ 30″	1′ 30″
Total strokes	51	38	51	41
Vol. of air breathed liters at 0° and 760 min.	62	76.5	56	46.5
% CO_2 expired air	3.7	3.7	4.3	5.2
C.c. CO_2 expired	2300	2980	2400	2450

The marked effect in improving the respiratory picture noted in the case of Pvt. R. was not present in the case of R. G. P. The respiratory quotient was 1.025 for Pvt. R. and .87 for R. G. P. when breathing air. A respiratory quotient over 1. in this case means superventilation.

On the afternoon of March 6, 1919, another experiment was made on Pvt. R. in which he rowed on the rowing machine at the rate of 54 strokes in a minute and a half, in one case breathing air and in the other case breathing oxygen. Some adjustment of the valves in the apparatus had made the work of rowing and breathing somewhat easier than on former occasions. He also had the benefit of six days' exercise. He was in good spirits, and, as he said, feeling extremely well at the time of the experiment.

In the case of air breathing, he expired 77 liters in a minute and a half while making 54 strokes, and the percentage of carbon dioxide in the expired air was 3.7. On this occasion it was not possible to detect cyanosis. He complained of a pain in his side, but had no right heart dilatation as determined by Dr. Hoover.

After a half hour's rest he repeated the experiment, breathing oxygen in this case. He expired 57 liters of air while making 55 strokes in one minute and a half, and the percentage of carbon dioxide in the expired air was 5.2 per cent. He was less out of breath after this experience than on the former occasion, and said that he felt no ill effects whatsoever from the strenuous work; there was a marked difference in his action on the two occasions, although he was unaware of the fact that he had been breathing oxygen in one case and air in the other.

This experiment was repeated on R. G. P., who breathed 62 liters of oxygen while making 54 strokes against 67 liters of air while doing the same amount of work. In the case of oxygen breathing, the expired air contained 5.2 per cent carbon dioxide; whereas it contained 4.8 per cent when air was breathed.

On March 10 a third experiment, similar to those of February 28 and March 6, was performed. In this case Pvt. R. breathed 60 liters of air in rowing one minute and a half, and at the end of this period the affluent blood of his lungs had a carbon dioxide tension in equilibrium with air containing 9 per cent of carbon dioxide. A half hour later he repeated the experiment but breathed oxygen. He breathed 52 liters in one minute and a half, and the carbon dioxide tension of the affluent blood of the lungs at the end of this period was 9.6 per cent, the expired air with air breathing containing 4.5 per cent and with oxygen 5.05 per cent carbon dioxide. On this occasion he said he was more out of breath when he was breathing oxygen than he was when breathing air, but that he performed the work very much more easily than he had at first. He had been required to take rather a large amount of exercise each day in making the tests we required of him, and in our opinion this exercise did him a considerable amount of good; in fact, we do not feel that he was very much below par in his ability to do work.

Inasmuch as Pvt. R. showed a marked increase in efficiency when breathing oxygen over that which he possessed when he was breathing air, it was suggested that we perform some experiments in which he was made to breathe atmospheres containing less than the normal amount of oxygen, in much the same way that aviators are tested in low atmospheres of oxygen by the rebreathing apparatus developed by Yandell Henderson in the aviation service U. S. A. He was able to breathe atmospheres containing 15 per cent of oxygen without any effect on the blood pressure or subjective sensations. The experiment was stopped because he looked blue. Blood counts and hemoglobin estimation showed nothing abnormal.

I can not find any explanation for Pvt. R.'s case. In the beginning, without question, the breathing of oxygen made it possible for him to work much more easily; but the effect soon wore off and he was able to do equally as hard work when breathing air. He received no treatment during his stay at the hospital save the exercise of running on a treadmill or rowing on the machine for brief periods. It is true, though, that he received much more strenuous exercise than he had ever received in camp. This exercise, which necessitated deep breathing, may have done much to relieve the irritation which possibly caused his distress. Oxygen want, due to unequal distribution of air in the lungs, producing an admixture cyanosis similar to that which we have shown may occur in pneumonia, may have been a contributing factor. His individual breaths, however, were too deep to suggest the presence of such a factor. The fact that the respiratory quotients are relatively low during the period of hyperpnea shows that he was keeping in respiratory equilibrium in spite of the abnormally deep ventilation. The improvement may have been simply the result of training and of some increase in his confidence in his ability to work.   I do not believe, however, that Pvt. R.'s case was a so-called neurosis.

The third case appeared to be one of the numerous neuroses which follow gassing.   He was a well-built and well-nourished man of twenty-four.   He had been slightly gassed and had been awarded some disability because of it.   Respiratory studies failed to show anything abnormal in his case.   We found that the suggestion that oxygen was being administered would cut his respiratory volume in half while doing an equal amount of work.   When breathing what he believed was air, he would invariably superventilate his lungs and have a high respiratory quotient and a low pressure of carbon dioxide in the air in equilibrium with his venous blood.   His sensations of dizziness were probably caused by the fact that, thinking he must breathe hard, he overdid the matter and washed out carbon dioxide to such an extent that he became dizzy.

CHEMICAL CHANGES IN THE BLOOD IN DISEASE*

I. Nonprotein and Urea Nitrogen

By Victor C. Myers, Ph.D., New York City

A LTHOUGH the nonprotein nitrogen normally constitutes only about one per cent of the total nitrogen of the blood, nevertheless greater interest is attached at the present time to variations in the bodies which form the nonprotein than the protein nitrogen. This is due largely to the fact that the variations in these nonprotein constituents give us an insight into some of the processes of anabolism and catabolism. The food nitrogen is carried by the blood to the various tissues and the waste nitrogen to the kidneys, directly or indirectly by the same medium. After a meal containing protein there is a temporary elevation in the nonprotein and amino nitrogen of the blood. In diseases of the kidney there may be at first only a slight rise in the uric acid or urea, although in the terminal stages of the disease there is generally a very marked elevation in all the forms of nonprotein nitrogen. The normal range of the various nonprotein nitrogenous components is given in Table I. Data are also included indicating the deviations which may occur in gout, interstitial and parenchymatous nephritis, and eclampsia.

Table I

Nonprotein Nitrogenous Constituents
Mg. to 100 c.c. of blood

CONSTITUENT	NORMAL	GOUT	EARLY INTERSTITIAL NEPHRITIS	TERMINAL INTERSTITIAL NEPHRITIS	PAREN- CHYMATOUS NEPHRITIS	ECLAMPSIA
Nonprotein N	25-30		30-50	to 350		
Urea N	12-15		12-30	300	30-60	10-25
Uric acid	2-3	4-10	3-10	25		
Creatinine	1-2		2-4	35		
Creatine	3-7			30		
Amino acid N	6-8			30	12	4-8
Ammonia N	0.1			1		

The figures for the normal creatine are taken from observations of Denis,[3] those for amino acid nitrogen from Bock,[2] except in the case of eclampsia , where observations of Losee and Van Slyke[5] the recorded. Other data are from our own observations.

The figures for ammonia are very small, but these figures may be taken as the maximal rather than the miminal values. In fact there appears to be some question at the present time as to whether ammonia actually exists in the blood.

The origin and rôle which the various nonprotein nitrogenous constituents play in metabolism, as well as the ease of kidney secretion, obviously greatly influence the content of these substances in the blood, both normally and pathologically. Folin's classic papers on the composition of urine published in 1905,[4] did much to give us a correct appreciation of the significance of the nitrogenous waste products which find their exit through the kidney. He pointed out that the

*From the Laboratory of Pathological Chemistry. New York Post-Graduate Medical School and Hospital.
The introductory paper of this series appeared in the March number of the Journal.

urea and creatinine stood in marked contrast to each other, since the former was largely exogenous in origin, while the latter was almost entirely of endogenous formation. Uric acid stood in somewhat of an intermediate position, being about half endogenous and half exogenous under ordinary conditions of diet.

Regarding the formation of these compounds, the following brief statement may be made. Urea is formed largely in the liver from the ammonia resulting from the deaminization of amino acids set free in digestion, but not of immediate use to the animal organism. Uric acid originates as a result of the enzymatic transformation of the amino- and oxy-purines, in which various glands of the body participate. Creatinine would appear to be formed in the muscle tissue from creatine.

It is of interest to compare the partition of these nonprotein nitrogenous constituents in the blood with the similar partition in the urine. Upon the ordinary mixed diet their approximate distribution in the urine is 85 per cent urea N, 1.5 per cent uric acid N, 5 per cent creatinine N, 4 per cent ammonia N

TABLE II

COMPARATIVE NITROGEN PARTITION OF URINE AND BLOOD
In per cent of total nonprotein nitrogen

FLUID	URIC ACID N	UREA N	CREATININE N	AMMONIA N	REST N
Normal Urine	1.5	85	5	4	4.5
Normal Blood	2	50	2	0.3	46
Blood in Gout and Early Nephritis	6	50	2	0.3	42
Blood in Parenchymatous Nephritis (Nephrosis)	2	55	2	0.3	40
Blood in Terminal Interstitial Nephritis	2 to 3	75	2.5	0.5	20

and 4.5 per cent undetermined N. It is quite natural to expect a somewhat similar relationship in the nonprotein nitrogenous constituents of the blood. The table above discloses quite a different distribution, however. It will be noted that even in normal blood the percentage of uric acid nitrogen is greater, if anything, than in the urine, while the urea is definitely lower, the contrast with the uric acid in the case of the creatinine and ammonia being even more marked. As Folin and Denis[5] have pointed out, the human kidney removes the creatinine from the blood with remarkable ease and certainty, the completeness of the creatinine excretion being exceeded only by the still more complete removal of the ammonium salts. The striking difference between the ability to excrete uric acid on the one hand, and urea and creatinine on the other, is brought out from an examination of the normal concentration of the blood and urine. Judging from their comparative composition, the kidney normally concentrates the creatinine 100 times, the urea 80 times, but the uric acid only 20 times. As the permeability of the kidney is lowered in conditions of renal insufficiency, this becomes evident in the blood, first by a retention of uric acid, later by that of urea, and lastly by that of creatinine, indicating that creatinine is the most readily eliminated of these three nitrogenous waste products, and uric acid the most difficultly eliminated, with urea standing in an intermediate position.[6]

CLINICAL SIGNIFICANCE OF THE BLOOD UREA

Since urea is the chief component of the nonprotein nitrogen, and since its estimation is considerably simpler than that of the nonprotein nitrogen, our attention will be directed chiefly to the urea. Mosenthal and Hiller[7] have made a careful study of the relation of the urea to the nonprotein nitrogen in disease. They point out that the selective action of the kidney maintains the urea nitrogen at a level of 50 per cent or less of the total nonprotein nitrogen of the blood, but that an impairment of renal function, even of very slight degree, may result in an increase of the percentage of urea nitrogen. In advanced cases this may be even higher than the 75 per cent given in Table II.

To give a comparative idea of the values observed for urea nitrogen in various pathologic conditions, illustrative findings are given for a number of different conditions in Table III, the data being taken from actual cases. As will be noted, the conditions in which nitrogen retention may occur are quite

TABLE III

CONDITIONS WITH SIGNIFICANT UREA NITROGEN FINDINGS

CASE	URIC ACID	UREA N	CREATININ	DIAGNOSIS
		mg. to 100 c.c.		
1	15.0	240	33.3	Bichloride poisoning
2	4.5	75	8.5	Double polycystic kidney
3	14.3	263	22.2	Terminal chronic interstitial nephritis
4	9.5	25	2.5	Early chronic interstitial nephritis, died 3 years later
5	8.3	72	3.2	Chronic diffuse nephritis, syphilis
6	2.3	28	1.9	Chronic parenchymatous nephritis
7	11.4	106	6.1	Severe acute nephritis, recovery
8	...	50	2.5	Mild acute nephritis
9	9.7	58	3.3	General carcinomatosis
10	5.5	24	3.3	Carcinoma of larynx
11	9.0	46	2.9	Severe pneumonia, recovery
12	..	43	3.4	Syphilis
13	5.5	44	3.1	Intestinal obstruction
14	..	24	2.2	Gastric ulcer
15	3.3	20	2.9	Duodenal ulcer
16	7.2	18	2.5	Prostatic obstruction
17	..	14	2.0	Myocarditis
18	6.0	18	2.9	Diabetics of long standing
19	8.4	12	2.2	Gout

Strictly normal figures for urea nitrogen may be given as 12 to 15 mg. per 100 c.c. of blood, while figures above 20 mg. on the usual restricted diet of the hospital may be regarded as pathologic.[8]

numerous. Marked urea retention may occur not only in the terminal stages of chronic interstitial nephritis,* but also in such conditions as bichloride poisoning and double polycystic kidney, and in some cases of acute nephritis. In parenchymatous nephritis the findings are comparatively low. Relatively high figures are frequently noted in malignancy, pneumonia, intestinal obstruction, lead poisoning, and sometimes in syphilis and cardiac conditions, although in the last mentioned this may be due to renal complications. In uncomplicated cases of prostatic obstruction the findings do not appear to be much above 20 mg. urea nitrogen. A slight retention is frequently noted in gastric and duodenal ulcer, possibly for the same reason that retention is found in intestinal obstruction.

* For a more detailed discussion of the various factors concerned in some of the conditions, reference may be made to the papers of Farr and Austin,[9] and Tileston and Comfort.[10]

Advanced cases of diabetes frequently show definitely high figures, apparently due in some instances to the high protein diet, in others to a complicating nephritis. The fact that a normal urea is associated with a high uric acid is of practical value in cases of gout not complicated by nephritis. As indicated in Table I, the blood urea is only slightly elevated, if any, in eclampsia. In normal pregnancy, Folin[11] has noted that, strangely enough, the findings are subnormal, figures between 5 and 9 mg. having been observed.

Since urea is largely of exogenous origin, while creatinine is endogenous, it is subject to much greater variation, especially under dietary influences. It is of less prognostic value than the creatinine in advanced cases of nephritis, but a much better guide as to the value of the treatment. In cases of prostatic obstruction[12] the urea is an excellent preoperative prognostic test, much better than the creatinine, for the reason that cases showing creatinine retention already show sufficient urea retention to make them very poor risks. The renal factor can be disregarded when the urea nitrogen is 20 mg. or under, the patient operated on with caution between 20 and 30, while with figures over 30 the outlook is unfavorable. Nephritis in children[13] does not so quickly result in urea retention as in the adult. On this account it is an especially helpful prognostic test in the nephritis occurring in early life.

In conditions showing nitrogen retention there are obviously two lines of attack, (1) to increase the output of the kidneys and (2) to decrease the nitrogen intake, while still maintaining the caloric and other needs of the body. Until quite recently, the first method is the one that has been employed clinically, particularly with the use of such diuretic drugs as the theobromine-sodium salicylate. For some time it has been recognized that in acute cases such drugs were contraindicated, and Christian[14] and his coworkers have further shown that these drugs are of very doubtful value in chronic cases. However, as Foster and Davis[15] have pointed out, some increase in the nitrogen output may be obtained by increasing the fluid intake. That a reduction in the nitrogen intake will reduce the blood retention has been definitely demonstrated, and this is a rational form of treatment which may be employed in almost all cases. In 1913 Goodall[16] reported observations on the favorable influence of a protein-free diet (Folin's starch and cream diet) in chronic nephritis. He found that such a diet could be continuously maintained for periods of from 5 to 10 days without harm to the patient, and further, that such a restriction could be followed by a low protein diet for a considerable period of time, even in advanced cases, without a return of the disagreeable symptoms. Later, Folin, Denis, and Seymour[17] conclusively proved that lowering the level of protein metabolism served to reduce the nonprotein and urea nitrogen of the blood in mild cases of chronic interstitial nephritis. Three years later the dietary end of this treatment was considered somewhat more in detail by Chace and Rose[18] in the wards and laboratory of this hospital. A number of different menus were outlined, the first two of which are given in Table IV. Obviously neither of these should be continued for an extended period.

To illustrate how a reduction in protein intake will lower the urea nitrogen, even in a very severe case of chronic interstitial nephritis, data on J. B. are given in Table V below. Despite the fact that the (endogenous) creatinine could

TABLE IV

TWO DIETS FOR CASES OF SEVERE NEPHRITIS

Juice from 1 lemon, 2/3 cup water, 6 tablespoon lactose, 1 tablespoon cane sugar. Calories, 1,424	Served 4 times a day Ash alkaline	Iron, 0.8 mg.
MORNING	NOON	EVENING
Banana .... 300 gm. Cream .... 100 c.c. Cocoa .... 200 c.c. Calories, 1,585	Cream soup....... 200 c.c. Banana .... 300 gm. Milk .... 200 c.c. Protein, 35.4 gm. Ash, alkaline, 15.6 N	Banana .... 300 gm. Cream .... 100 c.c. Cocoa .... 200 c.c. Iron, negl.

TABLE V

CASE (J. B.) ILLUSTRATING THE INFLUENCE OF A LOW PROTEIN DIET ON UREA NITROGEN IN CHRONIC INTERSTITIAL NEPHRITIS

DATE 1917	URIC ACID	UREA N	CREATININE
	mg. to 100 c.c.	mg. to 100 c.c.	mg. to 100 c.c.
Jan. 5	....	135	9.7
Jan. 9	....	110	12.5
Jan. 16	....	93	9.5
Jan. 30	5.0	48	7.8
Feb. 16	5.4	56	9.1
Feb. 27	7.1	45	7.5
Mar. 6	6.1	49	6.4
Mar. 23	....	40	7.7
Apr. 13	5.9	46	6.4
Apr. 27	....	45	7.5
May 15		33	7.3
May 22		24	7.3
June 5	....	34	6.7
July 17	....	29	6.8

Patient left hospital clinically improved on June 9, returned to work as guard on the subway, but died Nov. 7, 1917.

not be appreciably lowered, the urea nitrogen gradually fell to a level not more than twice the normal.

Some workers have endeavored to obtain more definite information than the blood alone will give regarding the ability of the kidneys to excrete urea, by comparing the urinary excretion with the concentration in the blood. Attention has been given to this particularly by Ambard[19] in France and McLean[20] in this country, who have worked out formulæ to express this relationship. Our own experience with this method has been disappointing in that the results have failed to reveal any added information not given by the blood alone.[21] We have long felt what Folin[11] has recently stated; viz., "The complicated mathematical formulas introduced in connection with the Ambard coefficient do not tend to increase one's confidence in that coefficient. It is difficult to see how square roots and cube roots help to elucidate such a simple metabolism proposition."

During the past year Van Slyke has made an effort to derive a formula which would correctly express the various factors involved, although so far this work has been reported only in a preliminary way.[22]

Obviously if this method of studying the urea excretion is used, it is essential that accurate collections of urine be made for the 60 or 72 minute specimen employed. This can be done if sufficient attention is given to the matter, but practically it seems difficult of execution in most hospitals.

METHOD OF TAKING BLOOD SPECIMENS

For most chemical analyses, blood can best be prevented from clotting by the addition of potassium oxalate. The potassium salt is much to be preferred over the sodium salt on account of its greater solubility. In case it is desired to analyze the plasma instead of the whole blood, this may readily be obtained by centrifuging the specimen. Our method has been to add 2 to 4 drops of 20 per cent potassium oxalate to large neck bottles of about 35 c.c. capacity, and then thoroughly dry these bottles in a hot air oven at a temperature sufficiently high to practically sterilize them. This insures a uniform amount of oxalate in the bottle* in a fairly divided state. The blood should be drawn directly into the bottle and at once gently but thoroughly mixed with the oxalate by rotating the bottle. Occasionally it may be found desirable to draw the blood into a syringe, the barrel of which may be moistened with the oxalate solution.

It is quite essential that specimens be secured under as uniform conditions as possible. Fairly constant conditions are obtained by taking the blood in the morning before breakfast. i. e., after a 12 to 14 hour fast and before any food or fluid has been taken. If dietary treatment is to be instituted (as in cases of gout, nephritis, and diabetes) to be especially helpful, the first specimen taken must precede these dietary restrictions in order that they may give a reliable indication of the influence of the treatment.

The question sometimes arises, how long can a specimen of blood be kept and have the analysis valid. If possible, specimens should always be analyzed the same day they are taken. Where good refrigeration is available, however, specimens can frequently be kept for several days without apparent serious deterioration, but this statement does not apply to specimens sent by mail which are at room temperature for several days. When blood is taken in a sterile oxalated container it may be allowable for such specimens to be sent by mail when analysis is made in 24 hours. Personal experience has shown, however, that such bloods generally show low blood sugars, a very good indication that deterioration has already set in.

METHODS OF CHEMICAL BLOOD ANALYSIS

In hospital work chemical blood analyses are now made so frequently and in such large numbers that it is important that the various procedures should be as simple as possible. As a step in this direction, Folin and Wu[23] have recently devised a system of chemical blood analysis in which a large number of analyses are made on the same protein-free filtrate. With this scheme, it is possible to make very quickly a single or several fairly complete blood analyses. In a hospital laboratory, however, one is frequently called upon to make determinations of such substances as urea, sugar, etc., on a very large number of specimens of blood. The methods we are about to describe appear to fit this second scheme of work. Since this subject is still in its infancy, improvements in technic are

---

*Cummer[32] has recently described a device which may readily be adapted to this work.

almost a daily occurrence. Although chemical blood analysis methods are relatively simple, there are many pitfalls for individuals without suitable chemical training. A physician can not expect that his office girl or nurse can properly manipulate these methods without an appreciation of the chemical factors involved.

ESTIMATION OF NONPROTEIN NITROGEN

The use of acetone-free methyl alcohol was first suggested by Folin and Denis[24] as the protein precipitant in the nonprotein nitrogen estimation. With this precipitant, the results, as Greenwald has pointed out, are somewhat low for the reason that amino acids appear to be partly precipitated. Another objection to the use of methyl alcohol is that some lipoid nitrogen is included in the filtrate. On this account Greenwald[25] suggested the use of trichloracetic acid. Subsequently Folin and Denis[26] recommended the use of m-phosphoric acid, although in their system of blood analysis Folin and Wu[23] use tungstic acid. Folin[27] has stated that he prefers that precipitant which gives the lowest results without lowering the values of any known constituent.

After the removal of the protein constituents it is necessary in any case to carry out a micro-Kjeldahl digestion on the nonprotein nitrogenous material. The ammonia may then be aerated or distilled off and finally estimated either colorimetrically with Nessler's solution or titrated with the aid of 0.01 N acid and alkali. In the recent method of Folin and Wu the digested material is nesslerized directly.

We have found the trichloracetic acid precipitation of Greenwald very satisfactory, although as a protein precipitant, it is mechanically hardly the equal of Folin and Wu's tungstic acid. After aeration we have carried out the final estimation colorimetrically as originally suggested by Folin and Denis.

Method.—Three c.c. of blood are diluted to ten times the volume (30 c.c.) with 5 per cent trichloracetic acid solution. After thorough mixing, it is allowed to stand for thirty minutes, then filtered. With the above treatment sufficient filtrate is generally obtained (20 c.c.) so that duplicate determinations may be made if desired. (In case one prefers the tungstic acid precipitation, the technic of this may be found under the clinical estimation of urea with the Myers' colorimeter, omitting, of course, the urease for this purpose.)

Into a thin glass test tube about 150 mm. in length and of diameter (20 mm.) such that it will readily slip into a 100 c.c. cylinder, are pipetted 10 c.c. of the filtrate, the equivalent of 1 c.c. of blood. Approximately 0.2 gm. of potassium sulphate, 2 drops of 10 per cent copper sulphate solution and 0.3 to 0.5 c.c. of conc. sulphuric acid, all of the highest purity reagents (nitrogen-free), are added and the mixture boiled over a small microburner flame, first gently (to remove the water) and then until digestion is complete, i. e., two minutes after the mixture becomes colorless. The final oxidation may be greatly facilitated by the addition of 1 or 2 drops of hydrogen peroxide. The tube is allowed to cool for a couple of minutes and then about 6 c.c. of distilled water added.

Aeration of the ammonia may be conveniently carried out in the apparatus* (Fig. 1), described by the writer in 1914.[28] This apparatus has two important advantages over that

---

*This aeration apparatus may be very simply constructed provided 100 c.c. cylinders without lips are available. The holes in the ends of aeration tubes, as Folin has pointed out, may readily be made with a platinum wire which is at white heat, provided the glass is only moderately hot. Malleable iron wire works quite as well as the platinum. The cylinders or the apparatus complete may be obtained from the C. M. Sorensen Co., Inc., New York City.

originally suggested by Folin and Denis for this purpose; first, it is not necessary to insert a stopper into a fragile test tube, and second, nesslerization is carried out directly in the second cylinder, which allows a wide range of dilution in contrast to the fixed dilution of a volumetric flask. (The aeration of the ammonia from the urea, described below, is carried out with the same apparatus.)

Into a 100 c.c. graduated cylinder without lip are added 15 c.c. of distilled water and 2 c.c. of 0.1 N hydrochloric acid or 2 to 3 drops of the 10 per cent solution. This is now closed with a two-hole stopper having a glass tube passing nearly to the bottom of the cylinder. The tube is sealed at the lower end, but contains a number of small holes to aid in the complete absorption of the ammonia. The apparatus to connect the pair of cylinders is adjusted, the test tube containing the digested mixture placed in the ungraduated cylinder, 3 c.c. of saturated sodium hydroxide carefully allowed to run down the side of the tube and to the bottom of the acid solution and the stopper quickly inserted. The cylinder containing the digested mixture is connected with a wash bottle containing dilute sulphuric acid so that the incoming air will be completely ammonia-free. The outlet tube in the graduated cylinder is now connected with a suction pump and air slowly allowed to pass through the apparatus, the speed being increased so that at the end of two minutes the air current is as rapid as the apparatus will stand. A series of a half-dozen or more tubes may conveniently be set up in this way. Aeration is complete in 10 to 30 minutes and the apparatus is then disconnected.

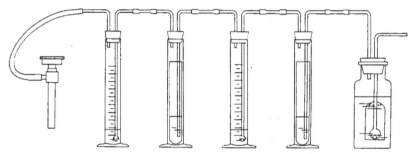

Fig. 1.—Aeration apparatus for nonprotein and urea nitrogen estimation.

Into a volumetric flask of 100 c.c. capacity are pipetted 5 c.c. of ammonium sulphate solution* containing 1 mg. of nitrogen and 50 to 60 c.c. of distilled water are added. Sufficient of the modified Nessler's solution** for the standard and the unknown is diluted about five times with distilled water, and of this about 20 c.c. added to the standard solution, which is then made up to the mark with water. At the same time 7 to 8 c.c. of freshly diluted Nessler's solution are added to the unknown and the volume made up to 25 c.c. in the graduate, unless a high content of nonprotein nitrogen is indicated, in which case more Nessler's solution (up to 25 c.c.) and a dilution to 35, 50, 100 c.c. or even more may be

---

*A standard solution containing 1 mg. of N per 5 c.c. of solution may be prepared by dissolving 0.944 gm. ammonium sulphate or 0.764 gm. ammonium chloride of the highest purity in distilled water and making up to 1,000 c.c.

**Modified Nessler's Solution (Bock and Benedict Formula).—Place 100 gm. mercuric iodide and 70 gm. potassium iodide in a liter volumetric flask and add about 400 c.c. of water. Rotate until solution is complete. Now dissolve 100 gm. sodium hydroxide in about 500 c.c. water, cool thoroughly, and add with constant shaking to the mixture in the flask; then make up with water to the liter mark. This usually becomes perfectly clear. When the small amount of dark brownish red precipitate, which forms, settles out, the supernatant fluid is ready to be poured off and used.

When pure mercuric iodide can not be obtained Folin and Wu have pointed out that metallic mercury and iodine may be substituted. To 75 gm. of potassium iodide and 55 gm. iodine in a 500 c.c. flask add 50 c.c. of water and an excess of metallic mercury, 75 gm. Shake the flask for 7 to 15 minutes or until the dissolved iodine has nearly disappeared. When the red iodine solution has begun to become visibly pale, though still red, cool in running water and continue the shaking until the reddish color of the iodine has been replaced by the greenish color of the double iodide. Now separate the solution from the surplus mercury by decantation and washing with about 400 c.c. of distilled water. Add 500 c.c. of water containing 100 gm. of sodium hydroxide as in the first formula and make up to 1 liter.

needed to make the color of the unknown approximately the same intensity as the standard. This is usually set at the 15 or 20 mm. mark on the colorimeter (Bock-Benedict, Duboscq or Kober). The colors are now matched up, preferably with the aid of a north light.

The following formula may be used for the calculation (applies to all three colorimeters), $\frac{S}{R} \times \frac{X}{100} 1 \times 100 = $ mg. nonprotein N to 100 c.c. of blood in which S represents the depth of standard, R the reading of the unknown, X the dilution of the unknown, 100 the dilution of the standard, 1 the strength of the standard in mg. and 100 the factor to convert the result to mg. per 100 c.c., since the equivalent of 1 c.c. of blood was employed.

ESTIMATION OF UREA NITROGEN

The method for the estimation of urea nitrogen is one that we have constantly employed for the past seven years,[6,27] and although other methods have been tried from time to time, none has been found as expeditious or as satisfactory. With a good preparation of urease the results obtained in the estimation of urea are perhaps the most reliable of any of the chemical blood determinations. The method is based on suggestions of Marshall,[29] of Van Slyke[30] and of Folin.[31]

The apparatus employed for the urea nitrogen estimation is the same as for the nonprotein nitrogen and if desired the two determinations may be run at the same time.

Method.—Into a test tube of the same size as that employed for the nonprotein nitrogen are introduced 1 c.c. of a 5 per cent jack bean urease solution.* Two c.c. of the oxalated blood are now added, preferably with an Ostwald-Folin pipette and the tube (or series of tubes) incubated in a beaker of water at 50° C. for 15 minutes. At the end of this time the aeration apparatus is put in order, 1 to 2 c.c. of amyl alcohol (or 4 to 5 drops of pure caprylic alcohol) are added and then about 4 to 5 c.c. of saturated carbonate. The tube is at once inserted in the ungraduated cylinder, the stopper replaced and aeration carried out for about 30 minutes, the air current being allowed to run slowly at first, but later as rapidly as the apparatus will stand.

The development of the color and comparison in the colorimeter is carried out just as described above, but in making the calculation it should be borne in mind that 2 c.c. of blood have been employed. If it is desired to convert the urea nitrogen into terms of urea, this may be done by multiplying by the factor 2.14.

Where only an occasional estimation of urea is carried out, the aeration procedure may appear a little troublesome. In an attempt to simplify this step we have tried a number of different protein precipitants, but in no case have the results been quite as satisfactory as with aeration. We originally suggested the use of heat and acetic acid together with colloidal iron, but later abandoned this in favor of *m*-phosphoric acid. Picric acid, and a weak acetic acid solution of potassium mercuric iodide were also tried, but recently Folin and Wu's tungstic acid has been employed. This reagent is quite the best protein precipitant that we have used in this connection.

---

*Concentrated preparations of jack bean urease may be obtained on the market (Arlington, Squibb), prepared according to the Van Slyke formula. Folin has pointed out that the keeping power of these preparations is not constant, although we never experienced difficulty with them until quite recently. Folin and Wu suggest the following method of preparation: "Transfer to a 200 c.c. flask about 3 gm. of permutit powder. Wash this by decantation, once with 2 per cent acetic acid, then twice with water. Add to the moist permutit in the flask 100 c.c. of 30 per cent alcohol (35 c.c. of 95 per cent alcohol mixed with 70 c.c. of water). Then introduce 5 gm. jack bean meal (may be obtained from the Arlington Chemical Co.) and shake for 10 minutes. Filter and collect the filtrate in three or four different small clean bottles. Set one aside for immediate use; it will remain serviceable at least 1 week at ordinary room temperature, if not exposed to direct sunlight. Put the others on ice where they will remain good for 3 to 5 weeks."

The blood is digested in the usual way and then diluted 1 to 10 with water and the precipitation reagents. After filtration 5 c.c. of the diluted Nessler's solution are added to 5 c.c. of the filtrate (the equivalent of 0.5 c.c. of blood) and color comparison made in the usual way. Turbidity seldom develops. The results compare favorably with those obtained by the aeration method.

The technic of the method is described below in connection with the simple test tube colorimeter illustrated.

Method.—Into a large test tube (160 x 25 mm.) are introduced 1 c.c. of 5 per cent urease solution or about 0.1 gm. of the dry enzyme. With an Ostwald-Folin pipette 2 c.c. of the oxalate blood (or 1 c.c. if a large amount of urea is anticipated) are now added and the tube incubated in a beaker of water at 50° C. for 10-15 minutes. At the end of this time 14 c.c. (or 15 c.c.) of water are added and 2 c.c. of 10 per cent sodium tungstate, and then while rotating the tube, 2 c.c. of 2/3 N sulphuric acid. Shake vigorously. When a

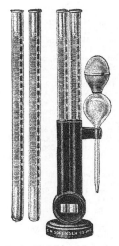

Fig. 2.—Test tube colorimeter.

blood is properly coagulated, the color of the coagulum turns from pink to dark brown. If this change does not occur, the coagulation is incomplete due probably to too much oxalate. In such a case 5 per cent sulphuric acid may be added, a drop at a time, shaking between each addition until the coagulation is complete. If the mixture is now carefully poured upon the double portion of a filter paper just large enough to hold the mixture the filtrate will usually come through perfectly clear, if not; the first portion may be returned to the filter.

Into the left-hand tube of the colorimeter are pipetted 5 c.c. of ammonium sulphate or ammonium chloride solution, containing 0.1 mg. of nitrogen. Two or three c.c. of modified Nessler's solution are now diluted about five times with distilled water to the 10 c.c. mark. This gives a standard 1 mg. N to 100 c.c. in strength. If 0.5 mg. to 100 c.c. dilution is desired, as is generally the case with normal blood, dilute to 20 c.c. with distilled water.

Five c.c. of the blood filtrate are pipetted into the right-hand tube of the instrument and 3-4 c.c. of the diluted Nessler's solution added. (This should be done nearly simultaneously with the addition of the Nessler's to the standard.) The solution should be perfectly clear. Dilution is now made with distilled water, inverting after each addition, until the depth of color is identical with the standard (1 or 0.5 mg. to 100).

For the calculation of the urea nitrogen, the following formula may be employed in which "S" represents the standard and "R" the dilution of the unknown: $\frac{100}{S} \times R \times 200 =$ mg. urea N per 100 c.c. of blood. Since the 5 c.c. of the filtrate employed are the equivalent of 0.5 c.c. of blood, it is obviously necessary to multiply by 200 to obtain the mg. of urea nitrogen per 100 c.c. of blood. With the 0.5 mg. standard and a dilution of 15 c.c. for the unknown the formula would work out as follows: $\frac{0.5}{100} \times 15 \times 200 = 15$ mg. urea N. That is with this scheme the dilution of the unknown gives the mg. urea nitrogen directly.

REFERENCES

[1]Denis: Jour. Biol. Chem., 1918, xxxv, 513.
[2]Bock: Jour. Biol. Chem., 1917, xxix, 191.
[3]Losee and Van Slyke: Am. Jour. Med. Sc., 1917, cliii, 94.
[4]Folin: Am. Jour. Physiol., 1905, xiii, 45, 66, 117.
[5]Folin and Denis: Jour. Biol. Chem., 1914, xvii, 487.
[6]Myers, Fine and Lough: Arch. Int. Med., 1916, xvii, 570.
[7]Rosenthal and Hiller: Jour. Urol., 1917, i, 75
[8]Kast and Wardell: Arch. Int. Med., 1918, xxii, 581.
[9]Farr and Austin: Jour. Exp. Med., 1913, xvii, 228.
[10]Tileston and Comfort: Arch. Int., Med., 1914, xiv, 620.
[11]Folin: Jour. Am. Med. Assn., 1917, lxix, 1209.
[12]Squier and Myers: Jour. Urol., 1918, ii, 1.
[13]Chapin and Myers: Am. Jour. Dis. Child., 1919, xviii, 555.
[14]Christian, Frothingham, O'Hare and Woods: Am. Jour. Med. Sc., 1915, cl, 655.
[15]Foster and Davis: Am. Jour. Med. Sc., 1916, cli, 49.
[16]Goodall: Boston Med. and Surg. Jour., 1913, clxviii, 760.
[17]Folin, Denis, and Seymour: Arch. Int. Med., 1914, xiii, 224.
[18]Chace and Rose: Jour. Am. Med. Assn., 1917, lxix, 440.
[19]Ambard: Compt. rend. Soc. de Biol., 1910, lxix, 411, 506.
[20]McLean: Jour. Exper. Med., 1915, xxii, 212, 366.
[21]Chace and Myers: Jour. Am. Med. Assn., 1916, lxvii, 929; Watanabe: Am. Jour. Med. Sc., 1917, clix, 76.
[22]Van Slyke: Proc. Soc. Exper. Biol. and Med., Dec. 1919.
[23]Folin and Wu: Jour. Biol. Chem., 1919, xxxviii, 81.
[24]Folin and Denis: Jour. Biol. Chem., 1912, xi, 527.
[25]Greenwald: Jour. Biol. Chem., 1915, xxi, 61; 1918, xxxiv, 97.
[26]Folin and Denis: Jour. Biol. Chem., 1916, xxv, 210.
[27]Folin: Harvey Lecture, 1920.
[28]Myers: Post-Graduate, 1914, xxix, 505; also Myers and Fine: Chemical Composition of the Blood in Health and Disease, New York, 1915, p. 9.
[29]Marshall: Jour. Biol. Chem., 1913, xv, 487.
[30]Van Slyke and Cullen: Jour. Biol. Chem., 1914, xix, 211.
[31]Folin: Jour. Biol. Chem., 1912, xi, 527.
[32]Cummer: Jour. Lab. and Clin. Med., 1920, v, 257.

THE HISTOGENESIS OF CARCINOMA IN THE ISLETS OF THE PANCREAS

By E. J. Horgan, M.D., Rochester, Minn.*

THE earliest stages of carcinoma have been found in association with chronic inflammatory changes in many organs of the body; therefore it seemed theoretically possible that similar neoplastic changes might be found in association with chronic pancreatitis. With this idea in mind I examined two hundred and sixty-two pancreases which were removed at necropsy from patients who died with ulcer of the stomach, ulcer of the duodenum, cholecystitis with and without stones, cholangitis with and without stones, and carcinoma of the stomach, liver, gall bladder, and bile ducts. In no case in this series was a definite advanced carcinoma of the pancreas studied, although comparison was made of thirty-six specimens of tissue from late carcinoma with the tissue showing early changes.

In the cases available for study the pathologic condition of the pancreas found in association with those chronic upper abdominal lesions mentioned were acute and chronic pancreatitis, stages of fat necrosis, simple cysts, cyst adenomas, papillary cystadenomas, hypertrophy and hyperplasia in the islets of Langerhans. Of these conditions, hypertrophy and hyperplasia in the islets in chronic pancreatitis were selected as the object of this special investigation. In order to obtain more accurate knowledge which might throw light on the histogenesis of carcinoma of the pancreas, a detailed study of pathologic specimens, grossly and microscopically, was made. This was supplemented by the study of the normal development and structure of the pancreas.

EMBRYOLOGY

The pancreas in man develops from two anlages which appear in the embryo of 3 to 4 mm. in length. The dorsal pancreatic anlage begins as an outpouching on the duodenum, the ventral pancreatic anlage as a grooved bud arising from the common bile duct (Fig. 1). The growth of the dorsal pancreas is more rapid than that of the ventral. The anlages grow separately until they meet posterior to the duodenum where they coalesce and continue development in one mass in the dorsal mesentery. The body and tail grow upward and to the left to lie in the dorsal mesogastrium posterior to the stomach. As the stomach and dorsal mesogastrium change position the pancreas moves within the dorsal mesogastrium until its position is transverse when it becomes firmly fixed to the parietal peritoneum of the posterior abdominal wall. In one embryo,† 26 mm. which I studied, the dorsal and ventral anlages are fused.

The primitive outpouchings are lined with a columnar epithelium similar to that in the duodenum. As the buds grow the epithelium develops branching ducts

*Fellow in Surgery on the Mayo Foundation, Rochester. Minnesota.
†University of Minnesota. Collection No. H29.

ramifying the connective tissue.   The main duct of the dorsal pancreas opens into the duodenum while the main duct of the ventral pancreas opens into the common bile duct at the ampulla.   When the dorsal and ventral anlages unite, the main duct of the ventral pancreas makes a lateral anastomosis into the main duct of the dorsal pancreas.   In this way the main duct of the ventral pancreas with the distal half of the duct of the dorsal pancreas forms the duct of Wirsung, and the proximal half of the duct of the dorsal pancreas is the duct of Santorini. When the embryo is from 26 mm. to 33 mm. in length, and the tail of the pancreas extends well out into the dorsal mesogastrium, branching tubules can be seen throughout the gland.   No acini or islets are to be seen at this stage, and there is no evidence of lobulations.   The connective tissue forms the major portion of the organ.   At the end of the branches of the main duct the tubules have an enlarged bud.   This bud branches and forms new tubules until the acini begin to form by several buds at the tip of each tubule.   After the acini have begun to form throughout the gland the islet cells appear in the connective tissue along the

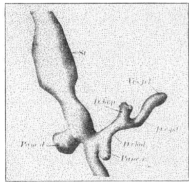

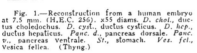

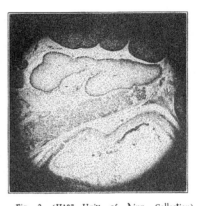

Fig. 1.—Reconstruction from a human embryo at 7.5 mm. (H.E.C. 256). x55 diams. *D. chol.*, ductus choledochus. *D. cyst.*, ductus cysticus. *D. hep.*, ductus hepaticus. *Panc. d.*, pancreas dorsale. *Panc. v.*, pancreas ventrale. *St.*, stomach. *Ves. fel.*, vesica fellea. (Thyng.)

Fig. 2.—(H187 Univ. of Minn. Collection) Microphotograph of pancreas in embryo (158 mm. C. R. Length) showing relation to stomach and left adrenal.

small ducts.   Pearce found masses of cells which he identified as islet cells in an embryo of 54 mm.   In the section of one embryo,* 158 mm. in length, in which I examined the ducts, acini and islets were well developed.   The islets stand out clearly in the loose connective tissue near the ducts.   They are circular masses, the cells of which are not well differentiated.   As the glandular tissue grows into the connective tissue it envelops the islets.   The connective tissue is derived from the mesodermal tissue of the dorsal mesentery (Fig. 2).

HISTOLOGY

The embryology of the pancreas has been sufficiently studied in man and in species of lower vertebrates to establish the fact that all the histologic units develop from the same anlages.

*University of Minnesota, Collection No. 1129.

The pancreas is a 'mixed" epithelial gland composed of three separate and distinct histologic units each made up of differentiated, specialized epithelial cells:

1. The pancreatic ducts (of Wirsung, Santorini, the interlobar and intralobular ducts, and the anastomosing tubules of Bensley).

2. The alveolar glands.

3. The islets of Langerhans (Fig. 3).

The Pancreatic Duct System.—The duct system in the pancreas is made up of one large duct, the duct of Wirsung, and an accessory duct, the duct of Santorini. From these ducts numerous highly branched tubules ramify the organ. The duct of Wirsung passes from the duodenal portion of the organ, where it opens into the ampulla of Vater, to the splenic portion. Throughout its entire length the first division of the tubules opens into it. These primary branches do not enter directly; they pass obliquely through the connective tissue of the duct of Wirsung for a short distance. The terminal branches are rather tortuous;

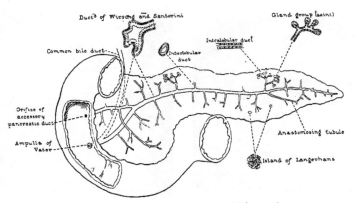

Fig. 3.—Diagram of pancreas showing its histologic units.

Bensley has shown that they have many anastomosing tubules. The main ducts (Wirsung and Santorini) are lined with a single layer of high columnar epithelium on a fine membrana propria; in some sections it is thrown up into folds. In the interlobular and intralobular and anastomosing tubules the epithelium is a single layer of columnar cells, gradually diminishing in height in the terminal branches.

The Alveolar Glands.—Projecting out from the terminal ends of the tubules are the alveolar glands. These are branched tubular glands lined with a single layer of large secreting cells, pyramidal in shape, the apex of which points into the lumen of the acinus; the base, near which is a large circular nucleus, lies on a membrana propria. The cytoplasm is divided into two zones, granular and homogeneous; the granular zone at the apex is made up of the zymogen granules in a faintly staining protoplasm; the homogeneous zone is in the basal portion of the cell. The zymogen granules in the granular layer and the mitochondrial filaments in the homogeneous layer may be studied only by the use of special fixation and staining. The secreting acinic cells receive their blood supply from a capillary network in the membrana propria.

The Islets of Langerhans.—These islets are small circumscribed masses of epithelial cells distributed throughout the entire organ, although they are more numerous in the splenic portion. Most of the islets are spherical, from 0.2 to 0.3 mm. in diameter, but they may be oval in shape. They have no duct connection, either with the pancreatic tubules or with each other, but lie in close relationship to the tubules. The texture of the connective tissue separating them from the acini is very delicate. The arteries supplying the islets form a rich capillary cluster. The vessels do not enter through a hilus. Each islet has a number of small capillaries which pass in from the connective tissue at different points on the surface. The arrangement of the efferent blood stream is the reverse.

The islet cells are of two varieties, A and B. The A cells are the larger; they have a large elliptical nucleus with the chromatin in one or two round

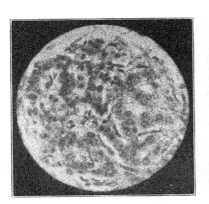

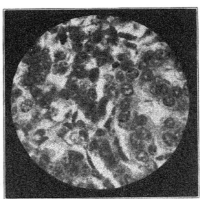

Fig. 4.—(H187 Univ. of Minn. Collection) Microphotograph of islet in embryo pancreas.

Fig. 5.—(11187 Univ. of Minn. Collection) Oil immersion microphotograph of islet cells, embryo 158 mm.

clumps. In the cytoplasm there are many small granules. The smaller B cells are more numerous; they have a central nucleus which is circular and contains a larger amount of chromatin. Their cytoplasm is packed with small granules. These cells may be differentiated from one another and the granules stained only by the fixation and staining methods of Lane. In the sections the cells are seen in irregular masses, in single, or in double cords. They lie in a delicate connective tissue among the loops of the capillary cluster (Figs. 4, 5, 6, 7, 8, and 9).

Blood Vessels.—The blood supply to the pancreas is through the splenic, hepatic, and superior mesenteric arteries. The main trunk of the splenic and hepatic arteries each sends a number of branches. The superior pancreaticoduodenal and the inferior pancreaticoduodenal supply the head with a number of branches. The veins which are tributaries of the portal system follow the arteries.

Lymphatics.—The lymphatics drain into the splenic, anterior, and posterior pancreaticoduodenal groups (Fig. 10).

PATHOLOGY

Technic.—The pancreatic tissue was examined grossly; blocks cut from the duodenal, central, and splenic portions of the pancreas were sectioned and stained for microscopic study. The gross specimens had been preserved in neutral 10 per cent formalin solution. Blocks for microscopic study are preserved in 10 per cent formalin solution, Zenker's fluid with acetic acid, and Bensley's formalin-

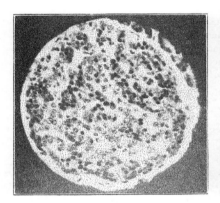

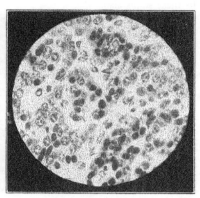

Fig. 6.—(A135776). Microphotograph of islet in an infant aged eight months.

Fig. 7.—(A135770). Oil immersion microphotograph of islet cells in an infant aged eight months.

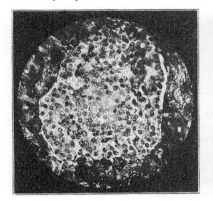

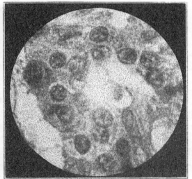

Fig. 8.—(A122722). Microphotograph of islet in pancreas of adult.

Fig. 9.—(A122722). Oil immersion microphotograph of islet in pancreas of adult.

Zenker solution. Blocks from all the specimens which are preserved in for-maldehyde solution were placed in a weak aqueous solution of ammonia for twenty-four hours and a few drops of strong ammonia added to the weaker alcohols when the tissues were being dehydrated; those preserved in Zenker's fluid with acetic acid and Bensley's formalin-Zenker were dehydrated in the usual manner. The blocks were embedded in paraffin and several slides from each block were cut in series for the routine microscopic examination. Additional blocks and sections were cut when needed. A few frozen sections were made. Some sections were stained with Ehrlich's hematoxylin and eosin and Goodpasture's acid polychrome-methylene blue and eosin. Others were stained with phosphotungstic acid hematoxylin and Bensley's brasiline water blue to differentiate the islet epithelium from the acinic epithelium. The blocks of tissue which had been preserved in formaldehyde and treated with ammonia could be differentiated by these stains also.

Chronic Pancreatitis.—Chronic pancreatitis is an almost if not a constant finding in association with gastric and duodenal ulcer; it is most marked, however, in the duodenal portion of the organ. The amount of pancreatic involvement and the degree of inflammatory reaction are dependent on the location and duration of the ulcer and the severity of the acute exacerbations. When the

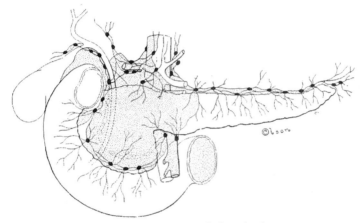

Fig. 10.—Diagram of peripancreatic lymphatic glands.

gastric or duodenal ulcer perforates on to the pancreas and an area of the pancreas becomes the base of the ulcer the marked local pancreatitis which develops gradually changes from an acute to a chronic form (Fig. 11). In addition there is usually a diffuse pancreatitis (Figs. 12 and 13). The pancreatitis is manifested either by a lymphocytic infiltration or by fibrosis extending into the interlobular, interacinar and periductal connective tissue.

Hypertrophy of the Islets Observed in the Series of Cases Studied.—In the microscopic examination of sections of the pancreas from the 262 cases that were selected for this study, hypertrophy of the islets in connection with a chronic pancreatitis was found in 48 cases. When the histories of these 48 cases were examined, two important discoveries were made; first, none of them showed glycosuria in any of the urinalyses of twenty-four hour specimens made while the patients were under observation and examination; second, 79.3 per cent of these were found to be cases in which a gastric or duodenal ulcer was found at operation or at necropsy. In the series of 262 cases which was selected for this study gastric ulcer was found in 71; in seventeen (25 per cent) the islets showed hypertrophy. Duodenal ulcer was found in 61 cases; in nineteen (31 per cent) the islets showed hypertrophy. Gastric and duodenal ulcer were found associated in 11 cases; in two (18.1 per cent) the islets showed hypertrophy. Hypertrophy of the islets was also observed in 6 cases of gastric carcinoma, 2 cases of carcinoma of the rectum, one case of carcinoma of the sigmoid, and 1 case of cyst of the pancreas.

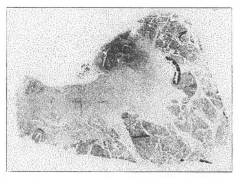

Fig. 11.—(A36163).   Microphotograph of duodenal ulcer perforated onto pancreas, showing marked connective tissue reaction in area of localized pancreatitis.

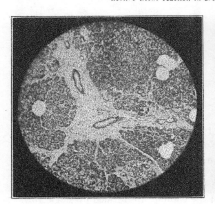
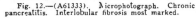
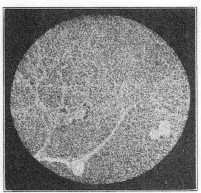

Fig. 12.—(A61333). Microphotograph. Chronic pancreatitis. Interlobular fibrosis most marked.

Fig. 13.—(120520). Microphotograph. Chronic pancreatitis. Interacinar fibrosis most marked.

Hypertrophy of the islets was observed grossly and in section from all portions of the gland.   Grossly the largest ones appeared as creamy white bodies. Microscopically the close relationship of these hypertrophic islets to the ducts was very noticeable.   They varied from slightly above normal to twenty times their normal size, the largest islet measuring 6 mm. in its greatest diameter.

Microscopic Pathology of Hypertrophic Islets.—There is a great variation in the size of the hypertrophic islets; they vary from 0.5 mm. to 6 mm. in diameter.

Most of them are round or oval, on section, although many do not conform to this shape. In a few cases examination of all the sections showed only a few hypertrophic islets in each case; usually they were found in greater numbers. They are found in sections from all portions of the pancreas, but in a few cases all which were observed were in the duodenal portion. Connective tissue in the islets is always increased and the capsule surrounding the islet is always thickened (Fig. 14). Hypertrophic and hyperplastic epithelial cells are found in these islets, and in a few, migration of these hyperplastic epithelial cells takes place; they pass through the three successive stages of neoplasia.

Primary Cytoplasia.*—The arrangement of the cells in the islets in short single and double cordons and masses between the capillary loops is similar to the normal. Most of the epithelial cells of these islets are differentiated; some are hypertrophic and the outline of the cytoplasm in these is not well defined (Fig. 15). These islets have a thickened connective tissue capsule and a diffuse

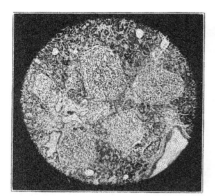

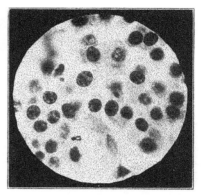

Fig. 14.—(A58947). Microphotograph of hypertrophic islets. Stage of pancreatico-primary-adenocytoplasia.

Fig. 15.—(A116521). Oil immersion microphotograph of hypertrophic islet. State of pancreatico-primary-adenocytoplasia.

fibrosis throughout. They are .5 mm. to 1 mm. in diameter. The capillary blood vessels have slightly thickened walls. No leucocytes or lymphocytes are to be seen nor is there any other evidence of an inflammatory process of the islets except a fibrosis.

Secondary Cytoplasia.—The cordons formed by the epithelial cells are more marked than in the normal islet. Most of the cordons are formed by single rows of epithelial cells, a few by double rows. In the sections these cordons follow the contour of the blood vessels and where the vessels are sectioned transversely the cordons encircle them. The epithelial cells are undifferentiated or partially differentiated. Some of the undifferentiated cells are hypertrophic. The number of epithelial cells has increased markedly, but all the cells are confined within the

*MacCarty's terminology of stages of neoplasia:
Primary cytoplasia = Hypertrophy of regenerative cells plus presence of differentiated cells.
Secondary cytoplasia = Hyperplasia of regenerative cells plus absence of differentiated cells, with or without partial differentiation.
Tertiary cytoplasia = Hyperplasia of regenerative cells plus migration, with or without partial differentiation.

connective tissue capsule (Figs. 16, 17 and 18). Some of these hypertrophic islets with hyperplasia of the epithelial cells are very large (0.6 mm. to 1.5 mm.). The capsule is of dense fibrous connective tissue and fibrosis is diffuse throughout the islet. The capillary blood vessels have increased in proportion to the size of the islets and the vessel wall is thickened. There is no evidence of inflammation except fibrosis.

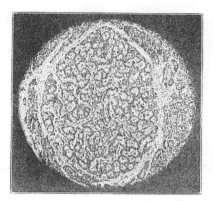

Fig. 16.—(A50276). Microphotograph of hypertrophic islet. Stage of pancreatico-secondary-adenocytoplasia.

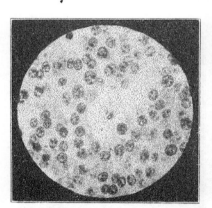

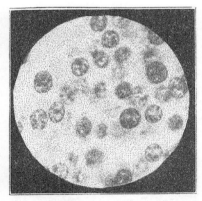

Fig. 17.—(A50276). Oil immersion microphotograph of epithelial cells in hypertrophic islet. Stage of pancreatico-secondary-adenocytoplasia.

Fig. 18.—(A50276). Oil immersion microphotograph of epithelial cells in hypertrophic islet. Stage of pancreatico-secondary-adenocytoplasia.

Tertiary Cytoplasia.—The cordons are not well defined; most of the cells are in masses. The epithelial cells are undifferentiated; some, however, in some islets show partial differentiation. They are hypertrophic and hyperplastic, there being a marked increase in the size and number. In the center of some of the islets there is an area of cellular debris as the result of cellular disintegration; a few nuclei can be identified in this area. Migration of the epithelial cells through the connective tissue may be seen at the periphery. This migration of the epithelial cells is evidence of a carcinoma (Figs. 19 to 24). These islets are very large, the largest being 4 mm. by 6 mm. Proliferation of the connective tissue is very marked throughout the islet and the capsule is thick and densely

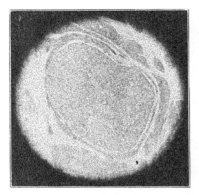

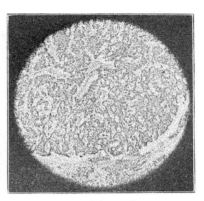

Fig. 19.—(A26398). Microphotograph of islet showing hypertrophic, hyperplastic epithelial cells with migration of these cells through connective tissue capsule. Stage of pancreatico-tertiary-adeno-cytoplasia.

Fig. 20.—(A26398). Microphotograph of periphery of islet showing hypertrophic, hyperplastic epithelial cells with migration of these cells through connective tissue capsule. Stage of pancreatico-tertiary-adenocytoplasia.

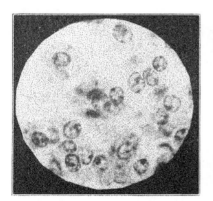

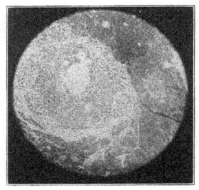

Fig. 21.—(A26398). Oil immersion microphotograph of islet cells showing hypertrophic, hyperplastic epithelial cells. Stage of pancreatico-tertiary-adenocytoplasia.

Fig. 22.—(A50276). Microphotograph of islet showing hypertrophic, hyperplastic epithelial cells with migration of these cells through connective tissue capsule. Stage of pancreatico-tertiary-adenocytoplasia.

fibrous. Bands of fibrous tissue pass out from the capsule of the islet into the interacinar and interlobular connective tissue. The blood vessels are very large, but their size is in proportion to the size of the islet, and their walls are thickened.

DISCUSSION

The islet areas in the pancreas were first described by Langerhans, who considered them to be the end apparatus of nerve fibers. From the collective embryologie, cytologic, and histologic studies of later workers, foremost among them Renaut, Laguesse, Opie, Lane, Lewis, Thyng, Dewitt, and Bensley, it has been well established that the islets are, histologically, a definite epithelial unit of the pancreas developed from the epithelium of the primitive anlages, without duct connection, with a rich capillary blood supply, and a hormone-secreting function.

Hypertrophy of the islets, and adenomas of the islets, are the only conditions reported in the literature which could be considered precancerous. Hypertrophy has been reported mostly in connection with diabetes. It is not characteristic of diabetes, however, neither is it to be found in all cases of diabetes. Nichols, Helmholtz, and Cecil have reported cases of a single hypertrophied islet in the

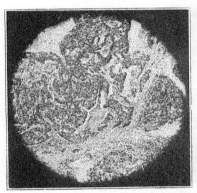
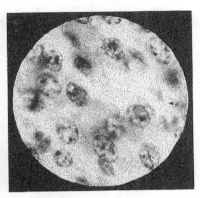

Fig. 23.—(A50276). Microphotograph of periphery of islet showing hypertrophic, hyperplastic epithelial cells with migration of these cells through connective tissue capsule. Stage of pancreatico-tertiary-adenocytoplasia.

Fig. 24.—(A50276). Microphotograph of islet cells showing hypertrophic, hyperplastic epithelial cells. Stage of pancreatico-tertiary-adenocytoplasia

pancreas. Nichols and Helmholtz each considers his case to be an adenoma while Cecil reports his case an hypertrophy of the islet.

After reviewing the literature I find that most writers classify carcinoma of the pancreas either as alveolar or canalicular.

In 1903, Fabozzi reported his study of the pancreatic tissue taken from 5 patients who had died from carcinoma of the pancreas and tried to establish from these the histogenesis of carcinoma of the pancreas. His deduction is that all carcinomas of the pancreas have their origin in the islets. His illustrations are diagrammatic, and his descriptions are not sufficiently conclusive to be accepted by later writers.

It is not reasonable to assume that all neoplasms in a mixed gland, like the pancreas, originate in one only of its three epithelial units. It is more logical to assume that a neoplasm may originate in any one of the epithelial units, the ducts, the acini, or the islets. From a biopathologic point of view the histogenesis of neoplasia of the pancreas should be studied in each of these. Under suitable pathologic conditions, each epithelial unit could be expected to produce undifferentiated cells from its germinative tissue; but the study must be made from the tissues which show the changes antecedent to carcinoma. When neoplasia is

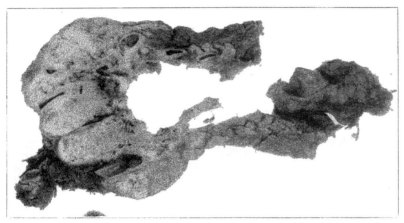

Fig. 25.—(A142013, Aut. 269, 1915).   Advanced carcinoma of pancreas.

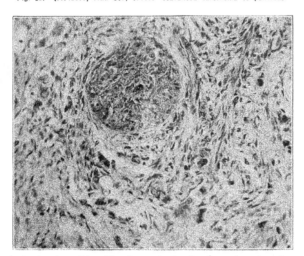

Fig. 26.—(A142013, Aut. 269, 1915).   Microphotograph of section from advanced carcinoma of pancreas showing degenerating epithelial cells in dense fibrous tissue and fibrosis of islet.

well advanced or has caused death, it is impossible to establish the site of origin or the successive pathologic changes from the tissue removed at operation or at necropsy; it is because pathologists have tried to prove the histogenesis from tissue removed at necropsy, after malignancy has caused death, that the histogenesis of carcinoma of the pancreas has not been established (Fig. 25). In a microscopic study of advanced carcinoma of the pancreas we find small masses of cells in the dense fibrous connective tissue. In their form and arrangement they may resemble small ducts, or acini, but if carefully scrutinized they will prove to be groups of degenerating cells. They are epithelial cells, but whether they are degenerating acinic cells or degenerating cells of neoplasia can not be determined (Fig. 26).

The histogenesis of carcinoma of the pancreas must be studied from portions of the pancreas which are too small to be recognized in the gross specimen as carcinoma. For this reason I selected for the study of the early neoplastic changes a series of cases which show chronic inflammation. In the course of the investigation I found a definite hypertrophy and hyperplasia of the islets of Langerhans. This condition was found in about 25 per cent of the cases of

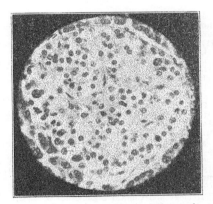

Fig. 27.—(A122622). Microphotograph showing hyalinized fibrosis of islet.

chronic interacinar and interlobular pancreatitis which was associated with chronic gastric and chronic duodenal ulcer. In these hypertrophic islets hypertrophy, hyperplasia, and migration of the cells were observed.

In the hypertrophic islets I found hypertrophic differentiated cells. Accompanying this cellular hypertrophy the connective tissue within and surrounding the islets had increased to protect the adjacent cells from encroachment.

In similar islets I sometimes found also hyperplasia of undifferentiated epithelial cells. These undifferentiated cells, however, are distinctly confined within the dense capsule of the islet.

In some of the hypertrophic islets I found hyperplastic undifferentiated cells migrating through the capsule, a condition which is undoubtedly carcinoma.

These three graphic descriptions apparently represent the stages of neoplasia as described by MacCarty in other epithelial tissues.

Simple fibrosis and sometimes hyalinized fibrosis were the only purely inflammatory reactions found in this series (Fig. 27).

The biologic reactions in the epithelial cells of the islets in the pancreas conform to those that have been observed in epithelial cells in other tissues. Mac-Carty has pointed out that each organ should be studied from the standpoint of each histologic unit; that each histologic unit must be considered alone from the standpoint of regeneration in all its phases; and that each phase should be named with a descriptive term applicable to that tissue; these biopathologic reactions of the epithelium of the islets in the pancreas might then be described as follows:

$$\text{Pancreatico} \begin{cases} \text{primary} \\ \text{tertiary} \\ \text{secondary} \end{cases} \text{adeno-cytoplasia}$$

These descriptive terms are expressive of the successive biopathologic reactions in the regeneration of cells in neoplasia in the islets of the pancreas.

BIBLIOGRAPHY

[1]Bensley, R. R.: Studies on the Pancreas of the Guinea Pig, Am. Jour. Anat., 1911, xii, 297-388: Structures and Relationship of the Islets of Langerhans, Harvey Lectures, 1914-15, x, 250-269.

[2]Cecil, R. L.: On Hypertrophy and Regeneration of the Islands of Langerhans, Jour. Exper. Med., 1911, xiv, 500-519. .

[3]Cecil. R. L.: Concerning Adenomata Originating from the Islands of Langerhans, Jour. Exper. Med., 1911, xii, 595-603.

[4]Dewitt, L. M.: Morphology and Physiology of Areas of Langerhans in Some Vertebrates, Jour. Exper. Med., 1906, viii, 193-239.

[5]Fabozzi, S.: Ueber die Histogenese des primären Krebses des Pankreas. Beitr. z. path. Anat. u. z. allg. Path., 1903, xxxiv, 199-219.

[6]Gelle.: Le cancer primitif du pancréas; étude histologique et physiopathologique, Arch. d. méd. exp. et d'anat, path., 1913, xxv, 1-49.

[7]Laguesse, E.: Le Pancréas, Rev. gén. d'histologie, 1906-8, ii, 1-288.

[8]Lane, A. A.: The Cytological Characters of the Areas of Langerhans, Am. Jour. Anat., 1907, vii, 409-422.

[9]Lewis, F. T.: Development of the Pancreas, In: Keibel, F., and Mall, F. P. Manual of Human Embryology, Philadelphia, Lippincott, 1912, ii, 429-445.

[9a]Langerhans, P.: Beiträge zur mikroskopischen Anatomie der Bauchspeicheldrüse, Inaug. Diss., Berlin, 1869, Quoted by Lane.

[10]MacCarty, W. C.: Pathology and Clinical Significance of Gastric Ulcer, Surg., Gynec. and Obst., 1910, x, 449-462: The Histogenesis of Cancer of the Breast and Its Clinical Significance, Surg., Gynec. and Obst., 1913, xvi, 441-459; The Histogenesis of Carcinoma in Ovarian Simple Cysts and Cystadenoma, Collected Papers of the Mayo Clinic, Philadelphia, Saunders, 1913, v, 380-390; Clinical Suggestions Based Upon a Study of Primary, Secondary (Carcinoma?) and Tertiary or Migratory (Carcinoma) Epithelial Hyperplasia of the Breast, Surg., Gynec. and Obst., 1914, xviii, 284-289; Pre-cancerous Conditions. Jour., Iowa State Med. Soc., 1914-1915, iv, 1-11; The Histogenesis of Cancer of the Stomach, Am. Jour. Med. Sc., 1915, cxlix, 469-476; New Facts about Cancer and Their Clinical Significance. Surg., Gynec. and Obst., 1915, xxi, 6-8; The Biological Position of the Carcinoma Cell, Pan. Am. Surg. and Med. Jour., 1915, xx; The Evolution of Cancer, Collected Papers of the Mayo Clinic, Philadelphia, Saunders, 1915, vii, 903-917; A New Classification of Neoplasms and Its Clinical Value, Am. Jour. Med. Sc., 1916, cli, 799-806; Cancer's Place in General Biology, Am. Naturalist, 1918, pp. 806-818.

[12]MacGrath, B. F.: Cancer of the Prostate, Jour. Am. Med. Assn., 1914, lxiii, 1012-1018.

[13]Opie, E. L.: Disease of the Pancreas, Its Cause and Nature, Philadelphia, Lippincott, ed. 2, 1910, 387 pp.

[14]Pearce, R. M.: The Development of the Islands of Langerhans in the Human Embryo, Am. Jour. Anat., 1902-3, ii, 445-455.

[15]Renaut: Quoted by Lane.

[16]Thyng, F. W.: Models of the Pancreas in Embryos of the Pig, Rabbit, Cat and Man, Am. Jour. Anat., 1908, vii, 505-519.

THE EFFECTS OF HEAVY METAL SALTS UPON A PROTEIN AND THE REVERSAL OF SUCH EFFECTS*

By ROBERT A. KEHOE, CINCINNATI, OHIO

I. INTRODUCTION

IT IS generally held that the toxic effect of the heavy metal salts upon protoplasm is due to the "coagulation" of the proteins, and that this reaction is irreversible. Such a conception necessitates the conclusion that cells and tissues once exposed to the action of the heavy metal salts can not be restored to their normal state, and that death of the affected cells or tissues is inevitable. However, the occasional recovery of a laboratory animal, or an individual, after the administration of an accepted lethal dose of such a toxic salt, suggests that there may be conditions under which the reaction of the heavy metal salts with protein need not be irreversible.

In the treatment of heavy metal poisoning our present methods try, either, (a) to introduce some chemical that will react with the toxic salt and precipitate it in an insoluble or inert form, or, (b) to meet the disastrous effects of such poisoning (as the "acidosis") through the administration of alkalies. It would seem equally wise, if feasible, to attempt to maintain the tissues in their normal physical state in spite of the presence of heavy metal salts, or, if change in physical state has occurred, to try to restore them to normal. The following paragraphs give the results of experiments on protein (gelatin), with this idea in mind. They show that *the coagulation of this material by salts of the heavy metals represents a reversible reaction, in that coagulated mixtures may be brought back into "solution," through treatment with properly chosen lighter metal salts.*

II. EXPERIMENTAL METHODS

By exposing a viscid "solution" of gelatin to low concentrations of various heavy metal salts, we tried to simulate, as nearly as possible, the conditions for heavy metal poisoning as seen in the living organism. The standard gelatin solution used in the following experiments was prepared from a high grade commercial product. Six grams of dry gelatin were added to 300 c.c. distilled water, brought just to a boil, the mixture being stirred until complete solution had been accomplished. When cooled to room temperature, this solution, after several hours, set into a viscid mixture, which, with some difficulty, could be pipetted into test tubes. Preliminary experiments showed the optimal limits of concentration between which satisfactory coagulation of the gelatin could be produced by various heavy metal salt solutions. They also showed that the formation of foam, on mixing the gelatin with the salt solutions, could be avoided and uniform distribution of the two in each other be assured, by adding the salt solutions to the gelatin slowly, while stirring the mixture constantly, by means of the pipette

*From the Eichberg Laboratory of Physiology in the University of Cincinnati, Cincinnati, Ohio.

containing the salt solution. This method was followed throughout all the experiments.

III. EXPERIMENTS

Fig. 1 illustrates the coagulation of gelatin by silver nitrate. Each tube contains 5 c.c. of 2 per cent gelatin, to which there were added, in the case of Tube 1, 5 c.c. distilled water, and into each of the rest, 5 c.c. M/500 silver nitrate. The photograph shows the coagulated gelatin in those tubes to which the silver salt was added, 48 hours later. At this time there were added to Tubes 1 and 2, 5 c.c. distilled water; to Tube 3, 5 c.c. M/3 sodium sulphate; to Tube 4, 5 c.c. M/3 magnesium sulphate; to Tube 5, 5 c.c. M/10 potassium hydroxide. Fig. 2 shows the results 36 hours later. Tubes 1 and 2, it will be observed, are left

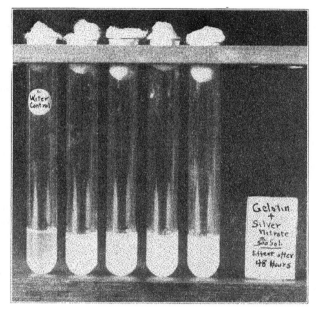

Fig. 1.

unaffected. Compared with the control Tube 2, Tubes 3 and 4 show decidedly less coagulation, while in Tube 5 complete resolution has been obtained.

In Fig. 3 are shown the reversing effects of adding a series of lighter metal salts to a series of gelatins previously coagulated through the addition of 5 c.c. M/500 cupric sulphate, M/1500 ferric sulphate, and M/1000 lead chloride, respectively, to 5 c.c. of 2 per cent gelatin. The reversing agents were added 48 hours after the treatment of the gelatin with the coagulant. The photograph was made 24 hours later. In the cupric sulphate group the concentrations of sodium iodide and potassium hydroxide used were just sufficient to cause a coloring of the mixture without actual precipitation of the colored copper salts. In the lead chloride group the concentration of potassium hydroxide caused a slight precipitation of lead hydroxide, with the formation of the white ring seen near the

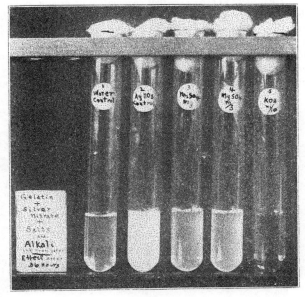

Fig. 2.

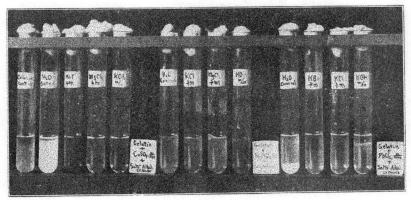

Fig. 3.

upper level of the contents of the tube. In all these tubes the resolution of the original heavy metal coagulum has been obtained, as may be seen by comparison of these tubes with the controls, to which only water was added. In the ferric

sulphate group the results are least distinct, yet, even here, the coagulated material, seen somewhat faintly at the botom of the control tube, is absent in the tubes
treated with lighter metal salts and hydroxide.

It is seen from these experiments that coagulation of gelatin by heavy metal
salts may be reversed by a number of neutral salts of the lighter metals and by
alkali hydroxides. Many salts, other than those indicated in Figs. 1, 2, and 3,
accomplish the same results, and in fact it may be said in general that all salts
or hydroxides of a lighter metal tend to resolve a heavy metal protein coagulum.
Since, however, many of these produce insoluble heavy metal salts, they are not
described in this paper, for the reason that the reversal of coagulation, in the

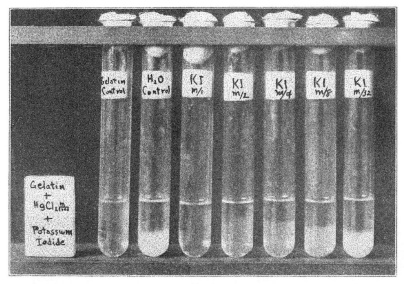

Fig. 4.

experiments described herein, is not a matter of removing the coagulant through
its precipitation. No such direct reaction with the heavy metals is apparent in
the concentrations at which we worked, except in the cases to which special
attention is called.

The importance of the concentration of the salt employed as reversing agent
is shown in Fig. 4. To each of the tubes were added, originally, 5 c.c. 2 per cent
gelatin, and with the exception of the control, to which only 5 c.c. distilled water
were added, each was treated with 5 c.c. M/1000 mercuric chloride. Twenty-
four hours later, 5 c.c. distilled water were added to the first two tubes on the
left (controls), while to each of the others 5 c.c. of potassium iodide solution of
the concentrations M/1, M/2, M/4, M/8, and M/32, respectively. The photograph, taken 24 hours later, shows complete reversal of the mercury coagulation

in the tube to which M/1 potassium iodide was added, less reversal in the next, and so on in decreasing degree to the end of the series.

Fig. 5 shows the results of a similar series of experiments, when 5 c.c. 2 per cent gelatin, treated with 5 c.c. M/1000 mercuric chloride were subjected, 24 hours later, to the action of different concentrations of potassium sulphocyanate. The tube on the left is a control, to which only 5 c.c. distilled water were added, the remaining tubes containing 5 c.c. respectively, 2M, M, M/2, M/4, and M/8 potassium sulphocyanate.

Fig. 6 shows a series of tubes, arranged in the same manner as those in Fig. 5, except that M/200 mercuric chloride was employed as the coagulant.

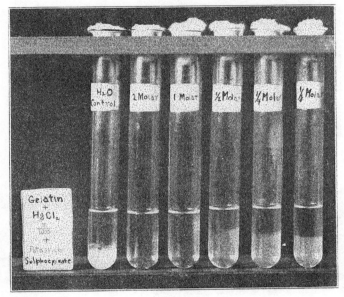

Fig. 5.

While in Fig. 5 both dimolar and molar concentrations of potassium sulphocyanate have brought about complete resolution of the mercury coagulum, in Fig. 6, only dimolar concentration brought about complete resolution. Comparison of corresponding tubes in the two figures shows in every other instance a better degree of reversal in tubes containing the lower concentration of the coagulant.

The speed of the reaction of reversal, and the degree to which it takes place, have been found to depend greatly upon the acid radical of the salt used as the reversing agent. Fig. 7 shows the reversal obtained by a series of potassium salts. Here, to each of a series of tubes containing 5 c.c. 2 per cent gelatin, were added 5 c.c. M/1000 mercuric chloride. To the first were added, 24 hours later, 5 c.c. M/10 potassium hydroxide, and to the others, respectively, from left to right, molar concentrations of potassium sulphocyanate, iodide, bromide, chloride,

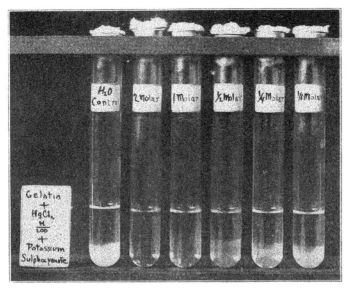

Fig. 6.

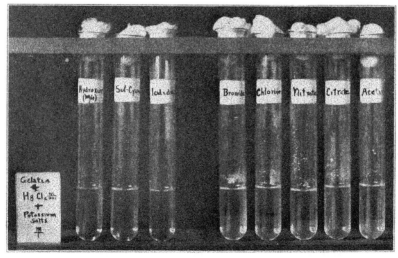

Fig. 7.

nitrate, citrate, and acetate.   Resolution was obtained first in the tube to which the hydroxide was added; next in that of the sulphocyanate, and then in that of the iodide.   All the others were much slower, neither was complete reversal brought about by any of them in the concentrations employed.   Very little difference is observable in the action of the bromide, chloride, nitrate, citrate, and acetate, but they arrange themselves approximately in the order named, the bromide affecting reversal slightly more quickly than the chloride, etc.

The resolution of the coagulated gelatin, under the influence of salts and hydroxides, is hastened by the application of heat to the mixture.   Fig. 8 illustrates this fact.   To each of 3 tubes, containing 5 c.c. 2 per cent gelatin, 5 c.c.

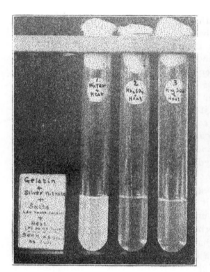 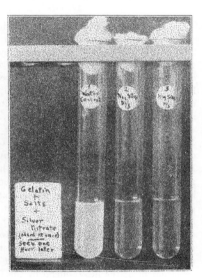

Fig. 8.   Fig. 9.

M/500 silver nitrate were added.   Forty-eight hours later there were added the following: to Tube 1, 5 c.c. distilled water; to Tube 2, 5 c.c. M/3 sodium sulphate; to Tube 3, 5 c.c. M/3 magnesium sulphate.   These tubes were immediately put into a boiling water-bath, and left for 15 minutes.   Upon removal from the bath all were clear, but on cooling gradually to room temperature, the result was as photographed.   Thus the application of heat caused a complete reversal of coagulation in a very short time, while at room temperature such reversal requires from 12 to 72 hours.

We further observed, in the course of the experiments, that the time required for obtaining complete reversal of a heavy metal coagulation, varied greatly with the length of time elapsing between the addition of the coagulant and the addition of the reversing agents, in that the longer this interval of time (up to three days), the longer was the time required for obtaining complete re-

THE JOURNAL OF LABORATORY AND CLINICAL MEDICINE

versal. Coagulation of gelatin by heavy metal salts is apparently a slow reaction, requiring in this case several days to go to completion.

The foregoing experiments have dealt with the *resolution* of gelatin coagulated by heavy metal salts. The experiment illustrated in Fig. 9 shows that it is also possible to *prevent* such coagulation. To 5 c.c. 2 per cent gelatin in each of Tubes 1, 2, and 3, were added, respectively, 5 c.c. distilled water, 5 c.c. M/3 sodium sulphate, and 5 c.c. M/3 magnesium sulphate. Immediately, into each of the tubes were introduced 5 c.c. M/500 silver nitrate. The photograph, taken an hour later, shows coagulation in control Tube 1, and complete inhibition of coagulation in Tubes 2 and 3, no coagulation resulting subsequently.

IV. THEORETICAL CONSIDERATIONS

The belief that proteins, coagulated through the action of heavy metal salts, might by appropriate means be brought back to a state more nearly like that of "normal" protoplasm, was suggested by the analogy which exists between the colloid-chemical behavior of the soaps and that of the proteins, in the presence of various alkalies and salts. It has been found possible to convert the poorly hydrated and insoluble heavy metal soaps into highly hydrated and soluble light metal soaps, by treating the former with the hydroxides, carbonates, or neutral salts of the light metals.[1] Therefore, it seemed reasonable to expect that a similar possibility should exist in the case of the proteins (or protoplasm), coagulated by heavy metals, if such coagulated materials could, in truth, be considered to be metal protein compounds comparable to heavy metal soaps. By such means, insoluble and poorly hydrated heavy metal proteinates, analogous to the heavy metal soaps, might be converted into soluble and more highly hydrated lighter metal proteinates, analogous to the lighter metal soaps. Our experiments justify such belief, so that it seems quite probable that the changes suffered by gelatin, and other proteins,* under the influence of heavy metal salts of low concentration, are due to the formation of particles of poorly hydrated and insoluble heavy metal proteinates; that upon treatment of such heavy metal proteinate, with a salt or hydroxide of a light metal, in proper concentration, a replacement of the heavy metal by the light one results, with the formation of a new compound, a light metal proteinate, more highly hydratable and soluble. The speed and completeness of such a double decomposition, as in all such reactions, are dependent upon the concentrations of the reacting materials, and upon the temperature at which the reaction takes place.

V. PRACTICAL APPLICATIONS

Obviously, the practical application of the facts herein observed, regardless of any theoretical explanation of their occurrence, may well be of importance. If the toxicity of the heavy metal salts is due to the coagulation of the proteins of the body, and if we may restore such coagulated proteins to their former state, by the introduction into the body of proper salts and alkalies, we are thus able to combat intelligently the primary toxic effects of the heavy metal salts.

---

*Incomplete experiments on a protein of the globulin type, casein, indicate that the facts herein observed with regard to gelatin are also true in the case of casein.

The use of neutral salts and alkali carbonates in heavy metal poisoning has been recommended by Fischer,[2] as a means of combating the acid intoxication which is a constant accompaniment of such poisoning. Weiss[3] has reported a number of cases of mercuric chloride poisoning, in which the results of alkaline and salt therapy fully justify their use. MacNider[4] found a marked influence on the part of sodium carbonate, in protecting the kidneys of experimental animals from a degree of damage otherwise the inevitable result of heavy metal poisoning. In these cases, no other end was sought, and no other explanation of results was considered, than that of the neutralization of the effects of a secondary acid intoxication. Doubtless, however, the beneficial effects obtained need not have been due entirely to the overcoming of an "acidosis." They may well, at least in part, have been due to a direct inhibition or reversal of coagulation of the affected body proteins, through replacement of the heavy metal in the coagulated protein by a lighter metal.

I hold that the long-established empiric practice of administering potassium iodide to the victims of chronic lead poisoning,[5] may also be understood in terms of the experiments described above. Any relief of an acid intoxication, by such a neutral salt as potassium iodide, is, of course, out of the question, and the idea that lead is precipitated in insoluble form is negatived by the observation that this heavy metal is eliminated in increased amount, under such therapy. These apparent contradictions are easily explained on the basis of the replacement of the lead, in combination with body proteins, by the lighter potassium. By this means, not only is the coagulated protein brought to a more nearly normal condition, but the combined lead is converted into a diffusible lead salt, easily excreted. Such reversal is accomplished by a concentration of iodide quite insufficient to cause precipitation of lead iodide.

In view of the fact that the presence of sufficiently high concentrations of light metal salts prevents the coagulative action of heavy metal salts upon proteins, the question arises, as to whether the use of potassium iodide, along with mercury and arsenic, in the treatment of syphilis, is a bad or a good therapeutic measure; whether potassium iodide may not inhibit the action of the heavy metal upon the organism of the disease, as well as upon the proteins of the body; or, whether, if used in proper amount, it may not maintain such diffusibility of the heavy metal as to render more easy the attack upon the organism, while at the same time lessening the damage to the tissues of the body.

In the therapy of all heavy metal poisonings, there is a twofold problem, (a) that of combating the primary coagulative effects of the heavy metal upon the body proteins, and (b) that of combating the secondary acid intoxication. The solution of the former problem has been attempted through the precipitation of insoluble salts of the heavy metal. That "insoluble" salts are not without toxic effects, however, is shown by the well-known behavior of such salts as mercurous chloride. It would seem that a better method would be such as would restore the tissues to a more nearly normal state, and, at the same time, release the toxic metal from its combination, converting it into a diffusible salt readily eliminated from the body. Our experiments indicate that such a method is probably feasible, through the use of suitable salts of the light metals. Such salts have the additional advantage of being the best therapeutic agents for the treatment of the secondary acid intoxication.

To bring about the restoration of coagulated tissues, in heavy metal poisoning, a sufficiently high concentration of suitable salts should be obtained in the body at the earliest possible time. The salts which can be introduced into the body and maintained at relatively high concentrations for long periods of time, without damage in themselves, are the salts of sodium and potassium. The salts, which in terms of our experiments, should be most effective, are the sulphocyanate and the iodide, but, since the effect of high concentrations of these salts upon the body is likely to be severe, other salts will probably prove to be of greater practical value. Especially are the bicarbonates and carbonates to be recommended because of their value in neutralizing acids. Such salts should be used, not in the customary doses of a few grains, but in large doses up to the limit of tolerance, if any results in the way of a reversal of coagulation are to be expected.

V. SUMMARY

(A) The coagulation of such a protein as gelatin, under the influence of heavy metal salts, is not an irreversible reaction, but may be reversed through the action of alkalies, or the neutral salts of the alkali and alkaline-earth metals.

(B) Not all salts of an alkali or alkaline-earth metal are of the same value in bringing about such a reversal, there being a marked secondary dependence upon the acid radical combined with the metal.

(C) Reversal of coagulation occurs most readily if the alkali or salt is added *soon* after the mixture of gelatin with coagulant.

(D) The degree and rate of reversal depend upon the concentration of the coagulant and the reversing agent (and upon the temperature).

(E) Coagulation of gelatin, under the influence of heavy metal salts, may be completely inhibited, by the previous or simultaneous addition to the gelatin, of sufficiently high concentrations of alkalies, or the neutral salts of the alkali and alkaline-earth metals.

(F) It is suggested that metal salts react with gelatin to form definite compounds, as do the same metals with the fatty acids to form the soaps.

(G) Suggestions are made as to the treatment of poisoning brought about by heavy metals.

REFERENCES

[1]Fischer, Martin H., and Hooker, Marian O.: Science, 1918, xlviii, 143.
[2]Fischer, Martin H.: Oedema and Nephritis, New York, 1915, ed. 2, pp. 203, 426, 571.
[3]Weiss, H. B.: Jour. Am. Med. Assn., 1917, lxviii, 1618.
[4]MacNider, Wm. de B.: Jour. Exper. Med., 1916, xxiii, 171.
[5]Cushny, Arthur R.: Pharmacology and Therapeutics of the Action of Drugs: Philadelphia and New York, 1915, ed. 6, pp. 524, 657.

THE TUBERCULOSIS COMPLEMENT-FIXATION TEST*

REPORT OF 700 CASES

BY B. STIVELMAN, M.D., BEDFORD HILLS, N. Y.

SO many extraordinary claims have been made for the tuberculosis complement-fixation test in recent years that the impression is conveyed that the
burden of diagnosis has been shifted from the clinician to the laboratory worker.
It has also been stated that clinical activity, as well as the immediate prognosis,
can be determined by means of this test with unprecendented accuracy. To test
the validity of these assertions, we performed the tuberculosis complement-fixation
test in 700 consecutive cases admitted to our sanatorium. We endeavored to ascertain

    1. The diagnostic value of the test.

    2. What light does this test shed on the activity of the process when a diag-
nosis has been made?

    3. The relative value of the test in the different stages of the disease.

    4. The prognostic value of the test.

We used exclusively Miller's bacillary suspension and a similar antigen prepared by the Board of Health of New York City. The efficiency of both antigens
was found to be identical. A Wassermann test was done on all the cases without
exception. All patients were examined roentgenologically and at least by three
clinicians independently. The average stay of all patients was over six months.
In no instance did the laboratory worker obtain information about patients whose
blood was examined.

DIAGNOSTIC VALUE OF THE TEST

Positive fixations were obtained in 26, i.e., 24 per cent of 108 nontuberculous
individuals. It is noteworthy that two of the three cases of pulmonary abscess and
two of the six cases of bronchiectasis gave a positive reaction, thus rendering the
correct diagnosis more difficult. The cases of chronic bronchitis and emphysema
and those suffering from cardiac diseases gave a very high percentage of positive
reactions, but it must be emphasized that all nontuberculous cases were observed
for many months and were subjected to repeated and painstaking roentgenologic
and physical examinations.

Of 592 sera from definitely tuberculous individuals, 310, or 52.4 per cent
gave a positive reaction, and 282, or 47.6 per cent, gave a negative reaction. Over
90 per cent of all the patients with negative reaction were sthenic cases, and the
low percentage of positive reactions could not therefore be ascribed to the exhaustion of the process of antibody formation. Of these 282 patients, 176 had a
positive sputum.

To eliminate as much as possible the personal factor in estimating activity,
we have adopted definite rules as follows: When in a tuberculous patient the
pulse rate rose persistently above 90 in the male and 95 in the female, and was due

*From the Montefiore Home Country Sanatorium, Bedford Hills, N. Y.

TABLE I

NONTUBERCULOUS CASES

	POSITIVE FIXATION	NEGATIVE FIXATION	TOTAL
Abscess Pulmonum	2	1	3
Bronchiectasis	2	4	6
Asthma	1	3	4
Chronic Bronchitis and Emphysema	4	17	21
Cardiacs	4	6	10
Hyperthyroidism	2	2	4
Hysteria		1	1
Syphilis	1	4	5
Malignancy (Gastric)	1		1
Malingering	1	1	2
No definite disease	8	43	51
	26	82	108

to no other ascribable cause, it was judged sufficient to indicate activity. Rectal temperature, rising over 99.8° in the afternoon, was considered to be due to an active tuberculous process. Loss of weight, night sweats, and malaise, even in the absence of fever, signified an active process. Tubercle bacilli in the sputum plus any other constitutional symptoms spelled activity. Patients who coughed and whose sputum was positive for many years, were considered inactive, provided their general condition was good. On the other hand, tuberculous complications in the respiratory, digestive or urinary tracts and frequent hemoptyses, not slightly colored sputum, however mild, were considered as signifying an active process. Dullness on percussion, rales, and abnormal breathing did not influence us to any extent. It is realized that not all observers will subscribe to this description of activity, but our classification is based on these assumptions.

RELATION OF THE TEST TO ACTIVITY OF THE LESION

Of 294 active cases, a positive reaction was obtained in 178, or 60.5 per cent, while of the 298 inactive cases, 132, or 44.3 per cent, reacted positively. (See Table II).

TABLE II

ACTIVITY	NO. OF SERA	FIXATION	SPUTUM
	294	Pos. 178 or 60.5%	$\begin{cases} +163 \\ -\ 15 \end{cases}$
		Neg. 166 or 55.7%	$\begin{cases} +101 \\ -\ 15 \end{cases}$
	298	Pos. 132 or 44.3%	$\begin{cases} +80 \\ -52 \end{cases}$
		Neg. 166 or 55.7%	$\begin{cases} +75 \\ -91 \end{cases}$

RELATION OF THE TEST TO THE STAGE OF DISEASE

The classification of the National Tuberculosis Association was strictly adhered to. Positive reaction was obtained in 49, or 33 per cent of 147 incipient cases; 131, or 52 per cent of 248 moderately advanced cases; 130, or 66 per cent of 197 far advanced cases.

TABLE III

STAGE	ACTIVITY	TOTAL	POS. FIX.	%	NEG. FIX.	%
Incipient	+	21	8	38.1	13	61.9
147	−	126	41	32.5	85	67.5
Mod. Advanced	+	132	67	50.8	65	49.2
248	−	116	64	55.2	52	44.8
Far Advanced	+	141	103	73.0	38	27.0
197	−	56	27	48.2	29	51.8

RELATION OF REACTION TO THE IMMEDIATE PROGNOSIS

Of 258 cases whose tuberculosis fixation was positive on admission, 195, or 75 per cent left the institution in various degress of betterment; while of the 270 cases whose fixation test was negative on admission, 85 per cent left similarly improved. It must be noted, however, that the smaller percentage of recorded improvements in the first group was due to the fact that this group numbered most advanced cases who also gave a positive reaction most frequently.

RELATION OF THE REACTION TO HEMOPTYSIS

Of 108 cases who had pulmonary hemorrhages subsequent to admission, 43 had a negative fixation and 65 a positive fixation. Little importance can be attached to this occurrence since hemoptysis occurs more often in the advanced tuberculous who also give a positive fixation more frequently.

RELATION OF THE TEST TO THE WASSERMANN REACTION

Among the 700 sera tested, 11 reacted strongly positive to the Wassermann test, or an incidence of syphilis of 1.6 per cent. Four of these cases had a positive sputum and a negative tuberculosis fixation test and clinical evidence pointed to the coexistence of both diseases. Four were nontuberculous and gave a negative tuberculosis fixation. One was nontuberculous but reacted positively to the tuberculosis deviation test. The two remaining cases we are satisfied suffered from tuberculosis and syphilis, although this was not bacteriologically proved.

OBSERVATION

1. In attempting this study we endeavored to ascertain the diagnostic and prognostic value of the tuberculosis fixation reaction as well as its relation to active and clinically inactive tuberculosis.

·2· Since 24 per cent of nontuberculous individuals and only 52.4 per cent of the definitely tuberculous give a positive reaction, it would seem hazardous to permit the test in its present stage of development to influence our clinical judgment.

3. The test did not help us in the differential diagnosis of pulmonary diseases.

4. In pulmonary tuberculosis clinical activity could not be diagnosticated from the results of the complement-fixation test.

5. The test sheds no light on the immediate prognosis.

6. We have no reason to believe that a tendency to cross fixation with a Wassermann reaction really exists.

7. The percentage of positive reactions increased as the disease advanced.

The percentage of positive reactions in definitely incipient tuberculous in our series was only 33 per cent. Thus it is seen that where the test could be of greatest assistance it is least applicable.

I wish to express my indebtedness to Dr. S. Wachsmann, Medical Director of the Montefiore Home, New York City, through whose efforts the work was made possible.

LABORATORY METHODS

TRAUMATIC HEMOLYSIS AND THE SYRINGE METHOD OF BLOOD COLLECTION*

By C. E. Roderick, M.D., Battle Creek, Mich.

IN a recent article Olson† condemns the syringe method of blood collection for complement-fixation test because of the large percentage of serums showing hemolysis.

During the past 27 months, we have used the syringe method of blood collection in 14,500 instances and the number of serums showing hemolysis is not more than 2 per cent. I therefore feel that it would not be out of place to state our method of procedure which is as follows:

A 20 c.c. syringe is sterilized in boiling distilled water or by means of a chemical together with a twenty-two gauge needle. The needle is attached to the syringe and the barrel filled with sterile physiologic salt solution made of chemically pure sodium chloride and freshly distilled water, which is then expelled through the needle. The plunger is then worked up and down in order to expel all the saline possible. A very small amount of the salt solution is permitted to remain for the purpose of lubrication, as a glass syringe is more efficient when moist.

The arm of the patient having been cleansed at the bend of the elbow with iodine or alcohol and permitted to dry, and a tourniquet having been properly applied, the needle is introduced, beveled side up, into the vein and about 20 c.c. of blood withdrawn. Half of this quantity is placed in a chemically clean bottle containing a small amount of sodium oxalate to prevent clotting. This portion is used for chemical analysis. The remaining 10 c.c. are placed in a chemically clean, 15 c.c. dry centrifuge tube. The danger of hemolysis from the force of the plunger of the syringe is overcome by first removing the needle and using only sufficient force to empty the syringe *and no more*. Foaming of the blood is to be avoided, but in a number of instances we find the top of the blood column to have a small amount of foam and in very few cases laking could be attributed to this cause.

The blood is sent to the laboratory as soon as possible after collection; more than an hour is seldom required. The serum is separated in most cases by the use of the centrifuge and placed in the ice chest until the time for the test.

A record of the condition of the serum is kept; in less than 2 per cent do we have laking. I have never seen laked blood give a false positive reaction; the

*From the Battle Creek Sanitarium. Battle Creek, Mich.
†Olson, George Manghill, M.D., Minneapolis, Minn., Traumatic Hemolysis and the Wassermann Reaction, The Journal of Laboratory & Clinical Medicine, January 1920. Page 259.

tendency is rather to be anticomplementary. While this latter result is far from satisfactory to both the patient and the doctor, it is not so fraught with danger as is a false positive reaction.

A more common cause of laked blood than the syringe method itself depends upon the preparation of the syringe. The collector will sometimes sterilize the syringe by the use of chemicals and then rinse the syringe in distilled water instead of salt solution, or will boil the syringe and neither dry it nor rinse it in saline. While it is preferable, it is not absolutely essential to have the syringe sterile. It is far more important to have it free from chemicals and dry; or if moist, with salt solution.

CONCLUSIONS

1. The syringe method, having proved satisfactory, is to be recommended.

2. A proper preparation of the syringe and saline solution will overcome the tendency to hemolysis.

A NEW METHOD FOR THE PREPARATION OF CELLOIDIN SACS*

By C. F. ULRICH, M.D., CLEVELAND, OHIO.

ANY ONE to whose lot has fallen the preparation of celloidin sacs will undoubtedly appreciate a method which makes for ease and simplicity in preparation and insures a nonleaking finished product.

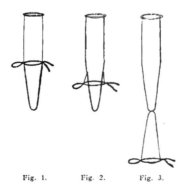

Fig. 1.   Fig. 2.   Fig. 3.

A 20 c.c. conical centrifuge tube, free from scratches or other imperfections in the glass, is thoroughly cleaned and dried. Strong twine is then tied about the base of the conical portion of the tube (Fig. 1). The tube is immersed in celloidin solution, so that the twine is just covered; is quickly removed and

*From the Cardio-Respiratory Laboratory of the Lakeside Hospital, Cleveland, Ohio.

rotated until the odor of ether is no longer perceptible. It is then plunged into cold water.

The upper end of the sac is carefully loosened, and the sac is removed by grasping the twine, drawing it down toward the tip of the tube, and inverting the sac (Figs. 2 and 3).

A NEW QUALITATIVE ALBUMIN TEST

By Hal Bieler, M.D., Twin Falls, Idaho

THERE is a rather interesting test, concerning the type of albumin in the urine of certain cases, showing profound toxemia. Several other laboratory workers, including Dr. R. S. Morris, have noted the reaction, and although the prognostic significance has been realized, the actual chemical nature is none too clear.

The reaction is a color change, affecting any copper hydroxide solution, such as Haines or Fehlings solution. The usual technic of the qualitative sugar test is carried out, the copper solution being diluted to a light blue color and heated almost to the boiling point. Upon addition of one drop of filtered urine, a deep purple color is noticed. It is an interesting fact that blood serum gives the same reaction.

Urines giving this reaction have been from cases of great general intoxication, and great renal protein digestion. Ten cases have been seen by the writer. Five were cerebral hemorrhage cases in coma, three were uremia cases apparently approaching coma, and two eclampsia cases. All but one (eclampsia) case died, and in this one case, convulsions had not as yet occurred, and by a quick Cæsarean section and forced elimination this patient, by a miracle, recovered.

This test increases then, the gravity of the prognosis, almost enough to signify impending dissolution, and should have a laboratory value.

It was noted above that blood serum gives the same reaction. So do also other protein substances when breaking down in the direction of albumoses and peptones—proteins giving the pink Biuret reaction. It is interesting to question whether this protein in the urine is from actual destruction of kidney substance or whether the blood serum is "filtering through." Both are possible.

· For helpful explanatory points concerning this reaction, I am indebted to Drs. A. P. Mathews and Martin H. Fischer, of Cincinnati.

The Journal of
Laboratory and Clinical
Medicine

Vol. V.   APRIL, 1920   No. 7

Editor-in-Chief: VICTOR C. VAUGHAN, M.D.
Ann Arbor, Mich.

ASSOCIATE EDITORS

DENNIS E. JACKSON, M.D.	CINCINNATI
HANS ZINSSER, M.D.	NEW YORK
PAUL G. WOOLLEY, M.D.	DETROIT
FREDERICK P. GAY, M.D.	BERKELEY, CAL.
J. J. R. MacLEOD, M.B.	TORONTO
ROY G. PEARCE, M.D.	AKRON, OHIO
W. C. MacCARTY, M.D.	ROCHESTER, MINN.
GERALD B. WEBB, M.D.	COLORADO SPRINGS
WARREN T. VAUGHAN, M.D.	BOSTON

EDITORIALS

The International Health Board

THERE is no health agency in the world doing better or more effective work than the International Health Board. The purpose of this Board is to demonstrate in different parts of the world the efficiency and value of scientific sanitation and to induce, by practical demonstration, the locality to undertake and continue the work. A brief review of the operations of this Board will, we are sure, be of interest to the medical profession. The work was begun in 1910 and directed to the eradication of hookworm disease in certain southern states. While progress in sanitation during the first six years was extremely slow, for the past four years improvement has been continuous and has steadily gained in momentum. Since 1915 the progress in state and local support has been steady. In 1915 the board was compelled to furnish more than eighty per cent of the money necessary to carry on this work. In 1919 the state boards of health and the counties, seeing the great value of the procedure furnished nearly eighty per cent of the money to continue the work. This indicates that the time will come when state and local authorities, having so valuable a demonstration before them, will proceed without help. In the West Indies the hookworm campaign has extended over British Guiana, Dutch Guiana, Grenada, and many of the West Indian Islands. In Central America it has included Panama, Costa Rica, Nicaragua, Salvador,. and Guatemala. The work in Brazil has met with most encouraging résults. During the current year (1920) the board will expend $200,000 on the work in Brazil, while the federal and state governments have provided $1,150,000. At first the work of the board was limited largely to the control of hookworm disease, but at present malaria is included in the program. It is intended to cover the whole of the great country of Brazil. State departments of health are being established; existing departments are being more effectively organized, and funds are being liberally provided. The work in the federal district is being used as a training center for representatives from the several states and sentiment is being formed for adequate schools to train workers for positions in the public health service. The government of Colombia contributed $6,000 and Ecuador has asked that the work be extended in that country.

In Ceylon, the Planters Association has given hearty cooperation since the work began in 1916. All areas are sanitated in advance of treatment; sanitation has not been effectively maintained but is steadily improving; government and planters are now supplying half the funds for the demonstrations and are maintaining the sanitary organization and follow-up treatment of the infected.

In the Seychelles Islands, the work has been in progress for more than two years. Infection found in the colony was medium; sanitation was practically zero: work was undertaken with the hope of bringing the infection under complete control. The government has given enthusiastic support from the beginning. The infected area has been covered and resurveys are in progress; advance in sanitation has been slow but steady; new sanitary regulations have been promulgated, and the government has undertaken to organize and maintain permanent central supervision.

In 1917 the board provided funds and carried out a survey in Papua for the government of Australia. For a similar demonstration in Queensland, which followed in 1918, the government provided half the funds. In 1918 the board entered into an arrangement for a program in rural sanitation extending over a period of five years and involving the cooperation of the federal and state governments.

The work in Siam was begun in 1917. For 1920 the government has provided an appropriation of $17,000. If the work is to become self-sustaining it must be not only supported by Siamese funds, but it must be directed by trained Siamese physicians. This means that a medical school in which preventive measures are taught should be established in that country. There is now a government school at Bangkok, but it lacks teachers, equipment, and properly prepared students.

. The hookworm work in the Fiji Islands had to be discontinued on account of the necessity of withdrawing the personnel during the war. It is expected that this work will be resumed in the near future. In 1916 the government of Borneo invited the board to cooperate with it in its measures for the control of hookworm disease in that country. This work has been delayed on account of the World War but will be reopened during the present year.

The antimalarial work in different sections of the southern states is being carried on with marked success. Work during the year 1918 in Sunflower County, Miss., covering a selected area of about 100 square miles, with a population of about 9,000, indicated that within a limited area and under average plantation conditions in the Mississippi Delta, malaria may be brought within reasonable control by destroying the parasite in the blood of the hookworm carrier and this at a per capita cost of about $1.08. In this experiment the board furnished the quinine necessary to sterilize the people. In 1919 an attempt was made to extend this work to a population of about 55,000. The people were required to pay for their quinine, and there was no house to house visitation. Frequent experience showed unsatisfactory results. In Hinds County, Miss., an experiment was undertaken in 1918 to test the applicability of antimosquito measures to rural conditions. The results have been encouraging and the work will be continued during 1920. For four years the board has conducted a series of experiments in towns in Arkansas.

The attempt to control malaria by screening alone was made in a small village in Arkansas. The results showed that about 70.6 per cent of the people were kept free from infection at an annual per capita cost, less overhead, of $1.75. The unit of operation was small; the test was conducted for only one year; unfavorable conditions made it necessary to discontinue it for the time being. To arrive at any fair conclusion, it will be necessary to make the tests more extensive, to carry them out under a variety of conditions, and to extend the test under a given set of conditions over a period of at least three years.

A new experiment in dealing with malaria in the South is being tried. This method was devised and used by Dr. Le Prince of the U. S. Public Health Service in Panama. The experiment is relatively simple; involves whitewashing the dwellings (plantation negro cabins) on the inside, drawing a dark line at a convenient height and enlisting the family (preferably the children) in killing the mosquitoes as they collect on the dark band.

Still another method of dealing with malaria in the Delta of the Mississippi is to be tried during the present year. It is generally believed by public health officers that the cost of malaria control by antimosquito measures on plantations in the Mississippi Delta will be prohibitive. The region is low, level, intersected with a patch-work of swamps and bayous; breeding of Anopheles abundant; tenant houses scattered, located mainly along the banks of bayous. The cost of destroying or controlling breeding places for individual houses is prohibitive. By concentrating the houses on a given plantation at a few points selected with reference to control of breeding places would make it possible to control the breeding for a group of houses at a relatively small cost. The feasibility of this plan, so far as concerns the control of malaria, has been demonstrated on the rubber estates in Malaya, by concentrating coolies in lines and clearing the jungle for a given distance around the lines. It is proposed to make a more careful study of conditions in the Delta, to confer with planters as to the feasibility of the project, and if conditions invite, to carry out the experiment on a selected plantation.

Malaria, like hookworm disease, while distributed over a large part of the globe, is in its more serious forms essentially a tropical and semitropical disease. It is a serious menace to life, health, and working efficiency in most of the countries in which the board is engaged in the control of hookworm disease. From many countries requests have been received by the board to extend this work for malaria control to tropical regions. The menace of the infection in many of the countries makes these requests peculiarly appealing. However, the control of malaria under tropical conditions is more difficult than it is in our temperate climate. It is, therefore deemed advisable that before undertaking to conduct any demonstration under tropical conditions efforts be made to adapt working methods to those conditions.

Extermination of yellow fever now seems possible. Until recently, Guayaquil in Ecuador has been the hotbed of yellow fever on the Pacific Coast. General Gorgas has been placed in charge of the sanitation of this city. In December, 1918, there were eighty-six cases of yellow fever in Guayaquil. Since July, 1919, there has not been a case. The study of conditions in Guayaquil has not only led to the eradication of the disease from that city, but has given Noguchi opportunity to solve the riddle of the causation of this disease.

In 1918 an epidemic of yellow fever appeared in Guatemala. This was soon traced down and the disease exterminated. Since that time yellow fever has appeared at Merida, Yucatan, and at various points in Salvador, Nicaragua, and Honduras. It is also known to have recently appeared in Brazil. The Brazilian authorities are apparently undertaking energetic measures for its control and it is believed that these will be successful. Very recently yellow fever has been reported on the west coast of Africa, though there is some doubt about the correct diagnosis of the disease. The board will probably send an expert to that region to investigate and to inaugurate such steps as may be necessary to eradicate the disease.

The board is continuing its antituberculosis work in France. This has resulted in a rapid multiplication of tuberculosis dispensaries. Each dispensary provides the services of one or more physicians. French physicians are aiding in this work and it promises to strengthen the bond of union between the two republics.

The above is a brief and imperfect statement of the work that has been done and is being done under the supervision and direction of the International Health Board. It is far-reaching in its influence. To close a statement of the work of the International Health Board without reference to the splendid school for the training of public health officers established by the board in connection with Johns Hopkins University would not be warranted. This school, under the guidance and direction of that great man in both curative and preventive medicine, Dr. Wm. H. Welch, promises great things for the future of preventive medicine in this country. The annual expenditure of the board amounts to more than $2,000,000, and every dollar is spent in the most efficient and economical way. Some centuries ago, a wise Frenchman said that if the human race is to be brought to physical perfection it must be through the agency of preventive medicine. It is pleasant to recognize Mr. Rockefeller as a follower of that great Frenchman, Descartes. Mr. Rockefeller has shown by the expenditure of his millions his great faith in scientific research and in medicine, both curative and preventive.

—V. C. V.

The Prohibition Experiment

OUR GOVERNMENT is now making the biggest physiologic and psychologic experiment ever made in the history of the world. Instead of employing rabbits and guinea pigs, we are making this experiment on about 110,000,000 human beings. The medical profession must not permit this great experiment, with all its side issues, to escape observation. In different localities different manifestations of the effect of the experiment will be in evidence. No one thinks, at least it is hardly supposable that any one thinks, that everybody will immediately abstain altogether from alcoholic stimulants. In the large number of cases of poisoning by wood alcohol, and possibly in some instances by amylic alcohol, we have a manifestation of the recklessness with which some people follow their tastes even if the taste be a depraved and abnormal one. However, such instances as these should not give us much trouble. The man who will drink wood alcohol is either so ignorant or so thoroughly abnormal on account of his depraved taste that his life can't be worth a great deal to the state. We shall, therefore, not shed any tears over these losses, except in such instances where they fall upon innocent or ignorant companions. The psychology shown in this experiment is well worthy of study.

Up to the present time our observations have been confined largely to those who were most earnest in securing prohibition. It seems that, to the majority at least of those of this class, their success came rather unexpectedly. They had not dreamed that prohibition would be brought about so suddenly, and that the lid would be clamped down so tightly. Among our acquaintances many most estimable men and women belonging to this class, as soon as they saw that prohibition was likely to be a fact, rushed to centers of supply and bought, many of them at fabulous prices, small or large quantities of alcoholic drink. It seems that they had never really convinced themselves that under all conditions they could do without stimulation. They did not know how soon they would have influenza or something else for which whiskey is reputed to be beneficial. It might be asked whether man has ever known or suffered from any ill in which belief in the beneficial action of alcohol has not been expressed, by some one at least. Years ago when alcohol was plentiful and when teetotalers were not so numerous, even the most devout prohibitionists believed that whiskey was a good thing for snake bites, stings of poisonous insects, for rheumatism, for bad colds, for malaria, in fact for most of the ills that human flesh is heir to. It is difficult for us to shake off these old beliefs and their continued influence upon us led the best of us to try to lay in a little stock before the possibility of getting alcoholic drinks was closed off entirely. We need not be afraid that our prohibition friends who have been laying in their supplies are going to be converted into drunkards. Nothing of this kind will happen. There is apparently innate in man a desire to possess that, the possession of which is difficult. We dare say that a close search in the cellars and cupboards of many of our prohibition friends, both male and female, would disclose the hiding places of bottles containing various kinds of liquid refreshment. These people have stored away these bottles, not with the intention of drinking their contents, but simply that they might have something which the ordinary individual does not possess or, at least, has difficulty in securing.

We are sorry to see that the distribution of whiskey is to be placed at the discretion of the medical profession. According to the latest reports, any doctor may under certain forms prescribe whiskey, not more than eight or ten ounces every ten days, for any individual. Now the reputable physician is not going to have anything to do with this matter. It will fall, we predict, largely into the hands of the disreputable practitioner, and that it will be abused there can scarcely be any doubt. We are prohibitionists, but we do not believe that the 110,000,000, more or less, of our people are going suddenly to discontinue altogether the use of alcoholic beverages. If the movement now in force can be carried far enough to do away with the saloon and the excessive drinking which has characterized many classes, it will be a blessing. We are sure that the better class of physicians need no caution as to their prescription of alcohol. So far as we know, the medical profession as a whole, has already repeatedly and plainly stated that alcohol in no form is an essential in the treatment of any disease. Notwithstanding this fact, within the last few months, the public as a whole, has apparently acquiesced in the decision of the government that whiskey shall be used, even quite largely, for medicinal purposes. If physicians find that alcohol is essential or is even beneficial in the treatment of any disease, they should record the observations upon which their judgment is formed and should lay their conclusions before the profession. As we stated in the beginning, it is a physiologic and psychologic experiment on a great scale, and the reactions resulting from this experiment should be observed, recorded, and studied most thoroughly.

—*V. C. V.*

The Toxin-Antitoxin Mixture in Immunization Against Diphtheria

IN the February number of this JOURNAL there appears an editorial expressing caution concerning the administration of this mixture. It was not intended in the editorial to combat or to deny the value of this mixture if properly prepared. Dr. Wm. H. Park, of the Board of Health of the City of New York, has had more experience with this preparation than any one else in the United States. We are glad, therefore, to have his consent to reproduce herewith a letter which he has written to the editor-in-chief. It is as follows:

"I have just read the editorial in your journal. I appreciate the reasons that caused you to write it, but I think that you put too much emphasis upon the dangers. A series of tests just finished in New York yield, I think, the proof that immunity of long duration is offered.

"We have made many studies upon the toxicity of the preparation and find without exception that if the product is properly standardized, it never becomes poisonous; in fact, from month to month it becomes more overneutralized, as the toxin portion of the mixture is less resistant than the antitoxin.

"We have given over 40,000 injections and have never had an accident.

Some 6,000 of these injections were given infants under ten years of age, the amount injected being the same as in older children and adults. Occasionally in older children disagreeable protein reactions occur which give rise to local and constitutional disturbances for several days. We have found that fully ninety per cent become immune after three injections and in those tested after four years this immunity has been found to continue.

"We are so hopeful from these results that we are planning next month to use the Schick test in the pupils of one hundred schools and to urge toxin-antitoxin injections on those giving a positive reaction.

"It is true that in this product we are dealing with a mixture which if improperly prepared might have free diphtheria toxin. If, however, the same precautions are used as with other poisonous drugs there is no reason whatever why any product sent out from a properly officered laboratory should not be entirely safe. Without some form of active immunization it seems impossible to greatly lessen the amount of diphtheria now persisting."

Wm. H. Park,
Bureau of Laboratories, Department of Health,
New York City.

Drainage

A RECENT paper by Horsley[1] on surgical drainage and its biology, calls up a train of thought that leads far beyond the confines set by that author. Horsley calls attention to the fact that the stomach, the rectum, the bladder, and the larynx are able to rid themselves of foreign bodies because they possess a specialized method of protection which depends upon the presence of an anatomic outlet,—by vomiting, by defecation, by urination, and by coughing. These are special examples of the possibilities of drainage which are independent of whatever goes on in the walls of the viscera. In the closed anatomic cavities of the body, as for instance in the peritoneal cavity or in the pleura, attempts may indeed be made to evacuate a foreign substance but such efforts will be not appreciated except as they are indicated by histologic changes which occur in the walls of the cavities. In these walls, as in those of the hollow viscera, there is an outward flow of fluid and this Horsley takes to be the expression of reversal of the circulation. In the pleura or peritoneum the lymph flow is reversed and the lymph is emptied out around the foreign material. A splinter in the finger becomes surrounded by secretions because the lymph flow has been reversed and eventually is freed from the tissues in which it lies and sometimes is evacuated spontaneously. In all such cases in which there is a secretion or excretion produced by a foreign material Horsley believes it is the reversal of the circulation of the lymph or the blood that is the essential condition for healing, or, at least, for the attempt at evacuating the offending noxa. In his own words, "the reversal of the circulation is the chief biologic process by which surgical drainage acts beneficially in solid soft tissue," etc. Surgical drainage

---

[1] Horsley: Journal Am. Med. Assn., 1920, lxxiv, 159.

is merely the surgeon's effort to assist Nature,—which is a good point of view, and one often lost sight of.

But we may question whether this conception (of reversal of the circulation) is based upon facts. Is there such a thing as reversal of the lymph circulation or of the blood circulation? We believe not. Even if there be such a physiologic possibility, as for instance in the pleura, would that necessarily account for the pouring out of lymph? It seems impossible. The lymphatics are not provided with openings. The same is true of the capillaries of the blood circulation. As a matter of fact the entire circulatory system is a completely closed one. The reason why lymph is poured out into cavities or into solid tissues is because the chemical conditions outside the vessels are such that more water is needed there because of chemical changes that have changed the physical and chemical characters of the tissue cells. A need for water always exists outside the vessels and so water is always passing outward. Under abnormal conditions the need is accentuated and therefore is the water-transport. An infection, a trauma, (an infection is a chemical trauma as a rule) changes the metabolism and hastens its rate, in the affected tissues; the intermediate and end-products are formed more rapidly, and these are less rapidly carried away. The walls of the capillaries become more permeable, and instead of mere water transport, there is transport of other materials, such as proteins and cells which filter out, so to speak, through the edematous though continuous vessel walls. Depending upon the degree of the changes in the vascular tissue, serum albumin passes out with the water, if the damage is slight, and we have a serous exudate; or, if the damage is greater, serum albumin and fibrinogen pass out together and we get a plastic exudate. In other words a soluble protein like fibrinogen passes through the vessel walls less easily than does another soluble one. This is evidence of the physicochemical nature of the process and evidence against its purely mechanical nature. Beside, if one needs to flush the body as a whole, which is done with diuretics and cathartics, producing what may be called general drainage, one isn't reversing the whole circulation.

Surgical drainage is a mere mechanical addition to the natural process and being that, one would expect that it would usually be combined with methods which accentuate the normal physical process. From any area of infection, whether it be drained mechanically or not, there is some absorption. Soluble toxins and toxic substances pass into the body, and whatever may be said of the bacteria themselves, these toxic substances can be diluted and washed out— drained out—of the body. We speak of surgical drainage, which is physical. Why not also speak of medical drainage which is fundamentally chemical? Diuretics and cathartics act chemically for the most part, at least that is true of the salines. Both exert enormous flushing action on the body, provided enough water is given with them. In cases of infection in which it is desired to dilute the toxins and wash the tissues a certain result is obtained with a concentrated saline which draws water from the tissues. Thereupon the tissues need more water in order to preserve their normal concentration. Surgical drainage takes care of gross exudates; medical takes care of smaller ones and of the soluble materials absorbed into the body. So, it seems, that to obtain the best results, a combination of the two methods is logical. —P. G. W.

The Treatment of Gonorrhea

DURING the war specialists had abundant opportunity to test the efficiency of various forms of treatment in gonorrhea. In every camp there were hundreds of cases. We shall pass over attempts to treat this disease by vaccines and serums and confine ourselves to antiseptic injections. In some of the camps there was considerable enthusiasm about the results obtained with certain diffusible dyes. When dissolved in water it was found that many of these preparations were highly germicidal, but, unfortunately, when dissolved in urine the germicidal coefficient fell in most instances to a low point. Among all the diffusible dyes tried there were four found to have a high germicidal action in urine as well as in water. These are: malachite green, brilliant green, proflavine, and acriflavine. There was considerable enthusiasm about the last mentioned preparation and it was believed, for a while at least, that the acme had been reached in the search for a chemical agent which would destroy the gonococcus in dilute solutions and would do no harm to the tissue. Experiments showed that acriflavine inhibits the growth of the gonococcus in a dilution of 1-300,000. This is about 600 times the strength of protargol.

More recently, Young, White, and Swartz[1] have reported a preparation which, in their opinion, is far superior to acriflavine. This substance they name mercurochrome, which is a dibrom-fluorescein into the molecule of which an atom of mercury has been introduced. The sodium salt of this compound is the preparation employed and it contains 26 per cent of mercury. According to the authors, the free acid is a red powder, insoluble in water but readily soluble in alkali, forming a fluorescent solution. The salt appears in iridescent green scales. It is slightly hygroscopic and is readily soluble in water. The solution is stable and bears without change exposure to air and moderate heat. Strongly acid urine gives a slight precipitate of the free dye, but in ordinary urine no such change occurs. The solution stains the skin a bright red color, but this is easily removed by washing first with a 2 per cent solution of potassium permanganate and then with a 2 per cent solution of oxalic acid.

In order to determine the penetration of the mucous membrane by this substance, a solution was injected into the bladder of a rabbit. The drug was allowed to remain in the cavity for five minutes, after which it was drawn out and the rabbit quickly killed. Sections made immediately after death showed that the dye had stained the cells of the superficial epithelium and in some places had penetrated even to the muscular coat. Injection of the solution into the ureter showed that the pelvis of the kidney and the renal tubules were stained for a distance from the vertices of the pyramids. Its toxicity was found by experiment upon rabbits and dogs. Intravenous injections of ten milligrams per kilogram, body weight, killed rabbits, but dogs easily tolerated this amount. This seems to justify the authors in claiming that, as used in the treatment of gonorrhea, there is no probability of poisoning the patient. When injected into the genitourinary tract of man there is said to be no sign of irritation. However, if there be a chronic cystitis there may be some complaint of a burning sensation. The authors evidently have gone quite fully into the germicidal action of

[1]Young, White and Swartz: Jour. Am. Med. Assn., lxxiii, 1483.

this agent. They give tables showing the results obtained and make the following statement: "Acriflavine is shown to be much less potent as a germicide in even the most concentrated solutions, if allowed to act on the organisms for one hour or less. It surpasses mercurochrome in the twenty-four hour test, at this time period, appearing to be about four times as effective as the mercury compound. It is hardly logical to judge a local urinary germicide by its action on organisms during such a long period of time; a short period of exposure in the test, on the other hand, approximates clinical conditions. If rapid disinfection is a desideratum, as it seems to be, mercurochrome is superior to acriflavine."

They also state: "The outstanding fact observed on comparing the germicidal values of mercurochrome, acriflavine, protargol, and argyrol, is the rapidity of action of the mercury compound in fairly high dilutions. In one minute it kills B. coli or Staph. aureus in a dilution of about 1:1,000, a result obtained with none of the other drugs even in one hour. In fifteen minutes its effect is nearly as great as in twenty-four hours, killing B. coli in this short time at 1:5,000 and S. aureus at 1:10,000. A few tests were made to learn the minimal time in which a 1:100 solution would sterilize. S. aureus was killed almost instantaneously; that is, as rapidly as we could introduce the drug, withdraw a sample, dilute in water (to dilute the drug out of action in the agar) and plate. This procedure took no longer than ten seconds. The same test on B. coli revealed that a few organisms remained after ten seconds exposure to the drug. Since a 1:800 solution kills this organism in one minute, the time necessary for a 1:100 solution to kill is possibly not more than thirty seconds."

We earnestly hope that these investigators have not been over sanguine in their claims for the new remedy. We have no doubt that it will be tried by many experts along this line and comparisons will be made not only with other dyes, but with the old silver compounds and potassium permanganate solutions. There is an old saying that there is nothing that lies like figures. Every man who has done experimental work no doubt is ready to say that nothing lies like the first experiments a man makes. He is seldom able to confirm them in full.

—*V. C. V.*

The Tuberculosis Problem in England

UNDOUBTEDLY the war has greatly strengthened the tendency to the centralization of authority. This applies not only to military matters, but to economic, social, and public health conditions. In England, a Ministry of Health has been established. The British Journal of Tuberculosis for July, 1919, contains a very interesting symposium on the relation of the Ministry of Health to the tuberculosis problem. We propose to briefly review some of the statements made in this symposium.

Woodhead and Varrier-Jones, the former professor of Pathology in the University of Cambridge and the latter superintendent of one of the best known tuberculosis colonies in England, state that the conditions favorable to the spread of tuberculosis have greatly increased during the war. Soon after war was de-

clared there was a rapid rise in the tuberculosis case-rate not only among soldiers, but among the civil population. This increase in morbidity from this
disease has continued throughout the war period and probably will continue for
some time to come. The new Ministry of Health, no doubt, will be able to deal
with a number of health problems that have long called for attention, but undoubtedly it will have its difficulties. Much good work has already been done
through dispensaries, sanatoria, and colonies. The writers believe that the
Ministry of Health will do well to assist the agencies already in operation rather
than to take over under its control all this work.

Oliver states that the time has not yet come for the establishment of a
tuberculosis department in the state. For the present the prevention and care of
this disease should continue to be a part of the public health service. Hitherto
the treatment of the disease has received the greater part of our energy. The
results of treatment have not been satisfactory. It is true that life has been
lengthened, but this has only given further opportunities for the spread of infection. In the future prevention will occupy a more important place. Control of the milk supply is necessary. In Birmingham the mortality rate has
fallen during the last sixteen years from 0.52 per 1,000 to 0.26. This decline
to one-half the death-rate from all causes does not apply to pulmonary tuberculosis. During the war the incidence and mortality rate of this disease increased.
As housing, feeding, and occupation are three of the circumstances of our social
life under which tuberculosis will have to be tackled, there must be harmony
of action between the Ministry of Health, Municipalities, and Medical Officers
of Health.

Lumsden admits that the war against tuberculosis in Great Britain and
Ireland has been largely a failure and that much public money has been spent
without corresponding results. He believes that the problem of the advanced
consumptive is of the most importance. All cases of open tuberculosis should
be segregated and so placed that the spread of the disease is impossible. He
says: "We have been traveling in a circle—first we send unsuitable cases to
sanatoria, informing the patient we hope to cure him, and we then permit him
to return to his old environment without effort to improve it or to properly
supervise his home and its unhealthy devitalizing condition. Recrudescence or
reinfection commonly occurs, the patient once more becomes a focus of infection for his family and the community, and he returns from the sanatorium for
the tragedy to be played out to its disastrous end. Until this vicious circle is
broken tuberculosis will surely remain with us, and public money will be spent
without any finality being attained. The tragic feature of this urgent and colos-
sal problem is that we now know how the disease can be stamped out, but for
sentimental reasons we lack the pluck to tackle it by putting into force the
necessary machinery. In my humble judgment a thoroughly efficient and strong
tuberculosis department, with all the necessary powers, should be instituted under the new Ministry of Health. Housing, provision of a clean milk supply,
tuberculosis and other dispensaries, school inspection, etc., are all essential factors no doubt, but one of the first efforts should be to secure the segregation or
control of all tuberculous cases of an infectious nature. The disease should be
made compulsorily notifiable, the home should be inspected by the local authority,

and one of the two following courses adopted: (1) Proper sleeping and living conditions established so that infection shall be reduced to a minimum, which we know can be done in most cases with small expense, and generally with the family's cooperation, once the position is made clear to them; (2) If this course can not be accomplished the patient should be compulsorily removed to a home where he can no longer spread his infection."

Hope, a health officer of Liverpool, believes that the Ministry of Health, acting as a central and authoritative body, will link up and make more effective the local agencies. He says: "In dealing with housing, maternity, and infant welfare, pure milk supply, open-air schools, hospitals for advanced cases, industrial colonies, discharged soldiers, etc., the multiplicity of authorities to be considered and consulted has led almost inevitably to some amount of friction and overlapping, with all the resulting waste of effort, time, money, and lives, that such friction and overlapping involve. It is to the new Ministry of Health—which should be able to unify, to direct, to control, and, it may be presumed, will be provided with the necessary powers and money to insure its orders being carried out—that we must look in future for the solution of a problem that is even more urgent now than it was in pre-war days."

Hill, of the London Hospital Medical School, seems inclined to the opinion that insanitary housing is the most important factor in maintaining the high prevalence of tuberculosis. He states that the expectation of life at birth is sixteen years less in insanitary districts than it is in the healthiest communities, while the mortality of children under five years is more than twice as great. He believes that the Ministry of Health must concentrate on the rebuilding of the industrial centers of England, as garden cities, where open-air exercise can balance sedentary indoor work, and fresh, green foods be grown in the gardens and abundantly supplied to the people. At the same time, the children must be educated in the discipline of maintaining their health. He adds that the present conditions of housing and factory life make more sick and inefficient people and kill more than the late war year by year.

O'Donovan, of the Ministry of Munitions, thinks that special attention must be given to the prevention or arrest of tuberculosis among industrial workers. One important thing is the detection of early cases and the prompt attention to such cases. In the interest of the workers and of the community a factory medical service seems to be the only way in which the early detection of phthisis will be practicable in an industrial community. Repeated absences from work should lead to inquiry. The absentees should be sought and it should be ascertained whether their absence is due to failure in health.

Vining, of Leeds, calls attention to the great importance of milk in the spread of tuberculosis in infancy. He thinks that the Ministry can proceed to provide ways and means for the sterilization of milk throughout the country and should insist that every infant be fed upon sterilized milk.

Buckley, director of milk supplies, Ministry of Food, quite naturally emphasizes the importance of milk. He says that about forty per cent of the cattle in England react to the tuberculin test; also that ten per cent of the milk that reaches the large towns contains tubercle bacilli. He says, however, that this does not mean that ten per cent of the cows yield tubercular milk, but since the milk from different animals is mixed he thinks it a fair estimate to say that one per cent of the animals are infected. He calls attention to the fact that manure in stables, even where only a small per cent of the herd may be infected, may contain tubercle bacilli and these find their way into the milk. He says there are two ways of insuring that milk as it reaches the consumer shall not contain living tubercle bacilli. The first is to test every milch-cow with tuberculin and to exclude from the herd all those giving positive reactions. The second method is to properly pasteurize all milk.

Bullock, of St. Leonards-on-Sea, says that the Ministry of Health should insure that a certain proportion of new houses to be built have an open and sunny aspect, and so long as home treatment is applied to the advanced consumptive, at least one sunny room on the ground floor should be available for the patient. He thinks that the inspection of factories should be more stringent and that the provisions against overcrowding, imperfect ventilation, etc., should be more earnestly enforced. In addition to the possibility of infection through milk in childhood, he insists that many poor children do not have enough milk to drink. Of course, the milk should be free from infection, and at the same time there should be enough of it to furnish the child with the proper quantity of food.

Wingfield, of St. Thomas Hospital, advocates placing all matters pertaining to tuberculosis in the hands of the Ministry of Health. At present, tuberculosis sanatoria, hospitals, colonies, etc., are supported and controlled by local authorities. He thinks that all this must pass away. The Ministry of Health must be a strong central body. It should divide the whole Kingdom into areas, each of which must not supply more than 2,000 patients per year. For these units there must be tuberculosis officers, responsible only to the Ministry of Health. This tuberculosis officer must be capable of dealing with all forms of the disease and should have had, previous to assuming his duties, a thorough course of training at some recognized center of tuberculosis work. On him must rest all the responsibility for the work of the district. He should have a definite number of beds for advanced cases, for latent cases, for those who can do some work, etc. No cases should be treated at home. The number of beds should be at least fourteen per cent of all reported cases in the community. The hospital and the sanatorium should be in the same institution. There should be a hospital sorting house in every large town. There should be local homes for advanced cases and these should be attached to each unit. Beds for this purpose will reach two per cent of all patients treated. The patient who has improved in the sanatorium must be taken care of later by the state. This should not be regarded as a charity but as a duty. The Ministry of Health must concentrate on the after-care of patients before all else. If proper after-care was insisted upon now and proper facilities provided for it, the usefulness of our present tuberculosis scheme would increase by ten per cent. The present system of after-care is cumbersome and in actual practice has proved useless.

—*V. C. V.*

Tuberculosis in the French Army During the War

IT will be remembered that in 1917 this country was greatly alarmed by the statement that tuberculosis was vying with the Hun in its deadly warfare on the French soldier. It seems that this alarm came in the first place from French sources. Professor Landouzy, who has visited this country and is more or less well known and appreciated here, estimated the discharges from the French Army from tuberculosis in 1917 at 150,000. In December, 1917, M. Godart stated in the French Senate that the total number of soldiers discharged from the French Army from August 2, 1914, to October 31, 1917, was 89,430. Of these, 70,196 had been discharged prior to March 1, 1916, and they were cases of pre-existing tuberculosis which were accepted for service in 1914 when overthrow of the country was threatened. Later it was shown, especially by Major Rist, that at least forty per cent of these cases had been incorrectly diagnosed and were not tuberculosis after all.

Miller[1] says: "The exact size of the French Army is not public knowledge so that accurate estimate of the meaning of these figures in percentages is not possible, but it certainly could not have been less than 4,000,000 men the first months of the war or less than 3,000,000 in the latter period after March 1, 1916. Upon this basis and accepting the higher figures furnished by M. Godart as official, without consideration of the tremendous reduction which would result from the acceptance of the estimates of Messrs. Sergent and Rist, we may estimate that the maximum amount of tuberculosis necessitating discharge from the army was 1.75 per cent in the early months of the war, when according to general knowledge large numbers of active cases of tuberculosis were mobilized, and 0.63 per cent in the later months of the war after such cases were probably largely eliminated."

According to Bushnell, an average of 0.78 per cent was rejected for tuberculosis in this country. Miller thinks that this indicates, not only that the tuberculosis situation in the French Army was exaggerated, but also that the number of cases developing in the army during active service is not greater than that found in a similar group of men taken from civilian life in America.

—V. C. V

Typhoid Fever in Flanders

GOODALL[1] has given a most interesting account of typhoid fever in Flanders during the fall, winter, and spring of 1914-1915. It seems that this disease was widely prevalent, though not alarmingly so, in Belgium at the time of the German invasion in August, 1914. The people from eastern Belgium fled westward, without adequate supplies of any kind, and even without the necessities of life. Western Belgium is a plain, intersected by rivers, canals and ditches, in all of which the water flows very slowly. This plain is highly cultivated and is manured largely with human excreta. The water-supply in the villages is

[1]Miller, James A.: Am. Rev. Tuber., iii, 339.
[1]Goodall, E. W.: Proc. Roy. Soc. Med., xii, 15.

drawn largely from shallow wells. Wherever this condition exists typhoid fever is endemic. In the fall of 1914, there were four armies in this region—the British, French, and Belgian on one side and the German on the other. The only one of these armies at that time vaccinated was the British, and these soldiers had been vaccinated against only the Eberthian bacillus, while the typhoid fever prevalent at the time was paratyphoid. According to Goodall, there were many thousand cases of typhoid fever among the civilians in the region about Ypres in the fall of 1914. We have no definite information concerning the number of cases in the German Army, but we have intimation that it was quite large. The English took hold of the sanitation of the district positively and most effectively. Orders were issued compelling not only soldiers, but all civilians to be vaccinated. The drinking water was sterilized with chlorin and was dealt out to the population, both military and civil. The value of chlorination of water was apparently demonstrated. At Ypres the water-supply before the war was good. The water tower was not destroyed until the summer of 1915, but in September, 1914, this water-supply was not available because the mains had been broken. The English cleaned a large swimming tank in Ypres, lifted water knowingly polluted from the canals, treated it with chlorin and stored it in the swimming tank, from which it was dealt out to the population. The interesting part of it is that the English cleaned up the region so thoroughly that by the spring of 1915, the epidemic had ceased entirely and there was no return of it at any time during the war. Usually Eberthian typhoid is much more fatal than the paratyphoids, but this was not always the case in the local epidemics that occurred in Flanders. In one hospital the mortality from typhoid fever was 9.7 per cent, while that from paratyphoid in the same hospital was 19.2. Goodall is inclined to attribute the great success that the English had in cleaning up on typhoid fever around Ypres to the sanitary methods rather than to vaccination, because he says that up to that time they vaccinated against only Eberthian typhoid and the typhoid prevalent there was paratyphoid.

It may be interesting to note in this connection that in November, 1914, an epidemic of typhoid fever appeared in the French Army in the region of Belfort. It spread rapidly from the Swiss border to the sea and became alarming in December, 1914, and January, 1915, when it reached a maximum of 7.24 per 1,000. Systematic and thorough vaccination was begun during this period. Typhoid fever rapidly disappeared. Vincent states that had the typhoid rate of December, 1914, and January, 1915, continued during the thirty-eight months of actual hostilities, there would have been in the whole French Army of between four and five million men not less than 1,000,000 cases and 145,000 deaths. He states further that compared with the morbidity and mortality rates in the whole French population before the war, the morbidity from this disease in the French Army during the war was one-seventh and the deaths about one-eighth of what they were in peace times. From August 3, 1914, to September 1, 1917, the French Army Medical Laboratory sent to the front 5,513,073 doses of vaccine.   —V. C. V.

Staining Tubercle Bacilli

GOECKEL[1] has developed a convenient method for concentrating and isolating the tubercle bacilli. It is usual now to treat tuberculous sputum with antiformin, which is a strong solution of sodium hydroxide and sodium hypochlorite. This preparation dissolves the other constituents of the sputum but leaves the tubercle bacilli untouched. Goeckel proposes to substitute for antiformin Rice's Bromine and Alkali Reagent, which is used for determining urea in the urine. Rice's Solution No. 1 consists of:

Bromine	30 gm.
Sodium Bromide	30 gm.
Distilled water	250 c.c.

Solution No. 2 is as follows:

Sodium hydroxide	70 gm.
Distilled water	250 c.c.

The technic of Goeckel is the following: To the sputum or other tissue to be examined add a few c.c. of Rice's Solution No. 2, mix well, and add Rice's Solution No. 1 in successive small portions until a clear fluid is obtained. The use of heat is not necessary. The liquid is diluted with distilled water and is centrifuged at high speed to precipitate the bacilli. These are then washed with two successive portions of distilled water, centrifuging to remove the alkali. The residue is placed on a microscopic slide, fixed with a trace of albumin, and stained.

—V. C. V.

The Treatment of Tuberculosis Cervical Adenitis

ABBOTT[1] holds that in the treatment of this condition we should first attempt to prevent further infection. This can be accomplished, in part at least, by attention to the mouth and throat. Any decayed teeth should be attended to by the dentist. The tooth brush and other methods of cleaning the oral cavity should be resorted to. Hypertrophied tonsils and adenoids should be removed, and any discharges from the nose or ear should be properly treated. The patient, although it is too late to prevent primary infection, should sleep out-of-doors, and have an abundance of properly balanced food. The time-honored syrup of iodide of iron should be tried. In some instances potassium iodide may be of benefit, and according to the author never induces any untoward effect.

Abbott gives first place in the treatment of these glands to tuberculin. He says that he has frequently been consulted by patients seeking to avoid operation, who have patiently plodded the long road of palliative treatment, who have become discouraged and were about to turn to the scalpel as their only hope—he has seen these restored to a perfectly normal condition by the intelligent use of tuberculin. He thinks that tuberculin acts by increasing the formation of

[1]Goeckel, Henry J.: Med. Rec., New York. November 15, 1919.
[1]Abbott, Wilson Ruffin: Am. Rev. Tuber., iii, 175.

fibrous tissue and that this hyperplasia is associated with the protective deposits of mineral salts. In this way progression towards suppuration is arrested and eventually contraction of the fibrous tissues causes a general regression in the size of the glands.

When other measures fail surgical operation should be resorted to. Abbott adds that one should not wait until the glands have broken down, ruptured their capsules and matted together, because by that time the deeper lymphatics will have become involved and the boundaries of the triangle will have been passed. To the reviewer's mind, it seems that trusting to medicinal treatment, whether it be iodide or tuberculin, is in fact delaying too long and that surgical operation should be performed immediately when involvement is confined to the superficial glands.

Abbott is quite sure that, in many instances at least, a cure can be secured by the surgical removal of the infected glands but that this is possible only when the invasion is limited to the triangular area. Moreover, the removal of the infected glands, if done soon enough, will prevent penetration to the deeper lymphatics and possibly the later development of pulmonary tuberculosis. The best results are obtained in children under ten years of age.   —V. C. V.

The Journal of
Laboratory and Clinical
Medicine

VOL. V.	· ST. LOUIS, MAY, 1920	No. 8

ORIGINAL ARTICLES

THE ACTION OF ETHYLENEDIAMINE*

BY HENRY G. BARBOUR, M.D., AND AXEL M. HJORT, PH.D., NEW HAVEN, CONN.

DESPITE the fact that the significance of the amino group in conferring pharmacologic activity has long been axiomatic, our knowledge of the action of the simple amines still remains very incomplete. One of these, ethylenediamine, the subject of this paper, is of interest both as a product of putrefaction, (a homologue of putrescine and cadaverine) and a constituent of certain antiseptics.

Ethylenediamine, $NH_2 . CH_2 . CH_2 . NH_2$, has been known since its synthesis from alcoholic ammonia and ethylene bromide by Cloez, ('53).[1]

Brieger ('83)[2] isolated the base from putrefying fish, and Kulneff ('91)[3] from the gastric contents in a case of pyloric cancer. It has also been obtained by Carbone ('91)[4] from a growth of proteus vulgaris.

The first therapeutic appearance of ethylenediamine was as a constituent of "argentamin" (Schering and Schaeffer, 1894).[5] This antiseptic is a mixture of ten per cent each of silver phosphate and ethylenediamine.

· Other antiseptics containing ethylenediamine are "kresamin," and ·"sublamin," in which it is combined with cresol, and with mercuric sulphate, respectively. Superior tissue penetrating powers are claimed for these preparations. (Schaeffer).[6]

PREVIOUS PHARMACOLOGIC STUDIES

Brieger[7] with "large doses" of the purified hydrochlorid produced in frogs a lethargic condition in which a ready response to stimuli persisted. Mice and

*From the Pharmacological Department of the Yale University School of Medicine, New Haven, Conn. The observations herein reported have been taken from the thesis of A. M. H. presented in candidacy for the degree of Doctor of Philosophy in the Graduate School of Yale University, 1918.
A part of the expenses of the work was defrayed from the Francis E. Loomis Research Fund of the Yale University School of Medicine.

guinea pigs were found less resistant than frogs to the action of ethylenediamine and reacted by a marked stimulation of nasal, ocular, and oral secretions. Dilation of the pupils and exophthalmia were also observed.

Rabbits gave similar results. In a half kilo rabbit Brieger "injected" 0.2 grams of the amine hydrochloride and observed the following symptoms: Hypersecretion from eyes, nose and mouth; pupillary dilation with poor response to light; pulse rate at first accelerated but later diminished; dyspnea; head drawn back in a spasm; marked twitching of the nose. After some hours the respiration returned to normal and muscular depression ensued. The animal made no voluntary movements but had not lost its reflexes. Autopsy findings were negative.

Schaeffer,[8] working with the base, describes ethylenediamine as having too slight a toxicity to interfere with its therapeutic application. He states that rabbits tolerated 0.4 gram of the base "without marked influence upon the health" provided that the concentration of the injected solution was not strong enough to cause corrosion or infiltration. He did not observe the effects upon the secretions and central nervous system noted by Brieger. White mice tolerated 30 milligrams of the diamine, larger doses causing death. Schaeffer apparently employed subcutaneous injections in all of this work.

Desgrez and Dorléans[9] report that ethylenediamine in common with hydrazine and monomethylamine lowers the blood pressure in rabbits and dogs. They claim, however, that large doses (4 mg.) raise the blood pressure in dogs.

In view of the paucity of previous work and the discrepancies between the work of Brieger and Schaeffer it was decided to reinvestigate the action of ethylenediamine. Kahlbaum's hydrochlorid was employed, its purity first being checked by melting point determinations of the picrate. Observations were made upon the toxicity for mice, the central nervous action in frogs, and the effects of single and repeated doses in rabbits. In addition studies were made of the effects upon smooth muscle, as well as on the circulation in anesthetized mammals.

TOXICITY

In rabbits single subcutaneous doses of 0.4 gram per kilo produced no alarming symptoms. Intravenously, however, this dose was fatal to two adult animals; the third recovered after treatment for respiratory failure, while the fourth tolerated a very slow injection.

In white mice, of three which received subcutaneously 12½ milligrams per 20 grams body weight, all survived, while there was but one survivor of three receiving 15 milligrams per 20 grams body weight (Table I). The latter figure equivalent to 0.75 gram per kilo expresses approximately the minimal lethal subcutaneous dose for mice. On the basis of its diamine content the hydrochlorid is therefore four times as toxic by subcutaneous injection as the base.[6] The symptoms noted in mice were depression, cyanosis, and respiratory failure.

TABLE I

MOUSE	WT. (GRAMS)	DOSE PER 20 GRAM WT. (MG.)	FATE
1	19.5	12.5	Recovered
2	19.5	12.5	"
3	16.5	12.5	"
4	20.5	15.0	Dead (60 hours)
5	21.0	15.0	" (100 hours)
6	23.0	15.0	Recovered

CENTRAL NERVOUS ACTION IN FROGS

The lethargic condition described by Brieger was found easy to reproduce in frogs (*R. pipiens*) with about 2 mgms. per gram body weight of the hydrochlorid. Contrary, however, to the impression gained from Brieger's report, the spinal cord becomes depressed as well as the higher centers.

The following typical protocol (Table II) shows the prolongation of the reflex-time. The stimulus employed was 0.5 per cent hydrochloric acid into which the toes were dipped for a distance of 5 mm. The brains of two frogs were pithed and the animals suspended by the lower jaws. One was observed as a control, the other receiving 70 mg. of the diamine in the anterior lymph sac.

TABLE II

PITHED FROGS

TIME	CONTROL FROG NO. 1, 32 GRAMS	ETHYLENEDIAMINE—HCl FROG NO. 2, 34 GRAMS	
1:33 P.M.	————	70 mg. injected	
2:15 P.M.	1.5 seconds	1.5 seconds	
2:45 P.M.	1.5 "	6.0 "	
3:15 P.M.	2.0 "	30.0 "	No response Heart still beating

In experiments upon intact frogs prolongation of the reflex time was always noted before depression of the respiratory movements. Its action therefore conforms in type to that of the methane narcotics (paralysis of cerebrum → cord → medulla).

ACTION UPON RABBITS

The effects of single and repeated injections upon pulse, respiration, temperature, secretions, and general behavior were investigated. Where the injections were repeated daily for ten days, observations were also made upon the amount and character of the urine and the changes in body weight.

All of the rabbits were healthy and were kept upon a quantitative diet of oats, carrots and water, for at least one week previous to the observations.

Large Doses.—Seven rabbits were given ethylenediamine hydrochloride in single doses of 0.4 gm. per kilo. (Nos. 1 to 5 intravenously, and Nos. 6 and 7 subcutaneously.)

Given by vein this dose proved immediately fatal to two animals. A third was saved only by artificial respiration. The other two, and the two which received subcutaneous injections, exhibited certain constant effects. A very brief general depression was observed together with a short lasting increase (approximate doubling) in the number of the respirations. The body temperature, with one exception, was considerably reduced, recovery requiring a number of hours. Neither narcosis nor depression of reflexes was observed.

Secretions.—In spite of careful search the stimulation of lacrimal, nasal or salivary secretions, reported by Brieger, were never observed. Furthermore, a 270 gram guinea pig received subcutaneously 0.1 gram of the hydrocloride* but the only resulting indication of hypersection was a marked diarrhea.

Heart.—The protocols show that ethylenediamine does not affect the pulse rate in rabbits.

Blood.—Rabbit's blood taken shortly after the administration of 0.4 gram per kilo of ethylenediamine exhibits no abnormalities in hemoglobin content or in the appearance of the red blood cells. Methemoglobin is not produced.

Fig. 1.—Action of 10 mg. ethylenediamine hydrochloride upon isolated cat's intestinal muscle suspended in 50 c.c. oxygenated Locke's solution.

Ten mg. diamine added at mark. Cessation of activity and relaxation of tone followed within about five minutes by spontaneous recovery.

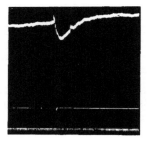

Fig. 2.—Intravenous injection of 10 mg. ethylenediamine hydrochloride 2 kilo rabbit.
1. Blood pressure.   2. Base line zero pressure.   (Injection at the mark.)
3. Time in 5 second intervals.

Local Reaction.—Subcutaneous injections of ethylenediamine hydrochloride in the doses named produced neither abcesses nor other inflammatory reaction at the site of injection.

Intestinal Action.—Diarrhea was noted in every case within a few hours after the administration of ethylenediamine.

In Rabbits 5 and 6 the urine was examined for ethylenediamine by the periodide test of Pohl,''' the results being negative both on the day of injection and the following day in both cases.

Repeated Small Doses.—Two rabbits received subcutaneous injections of 0.1 gm. per kilo daily for a period of ten days. The only significant effect was

*This animal showed marked muscular depression and a 20 per cent increase in the respiratory rate.

the reduction of the body temperature which, as was usual after the larger doses, amounted to 1° C. or more. Both of the animals acquired a tolerance to the temperature reducing effect, the fall becoming less each day until after the fourth day when it was missed altogether.

Other observations upon these animals included the following: A loss of 50 gm. weight in ten days by one animal, the other's weight remaining unchanged. Variations in volume, specific gravity, and cell content of the urine in both cases were within normal limits throughout. The drug never produced albuminuria or glycosuria. Only one of these two animals exhibited diarrhea.

ACTION UPON SMOOTH MUSCLE

A number of strips of excised cat's intestine were tested by the usual method for studying the action of drugs upon smooth muscle. Complete cessation of activity and relaxation of tone was readily produced, recovery occurring spontaneously after a few minutes. Ten and 5 mg., respectively, of the hydrochloride in 50 c.c. of oxygenated Locke's solution sufficed to produce these inhibitory effects. (See Fig. 1.) One mg. was ineffective.

ACTION UPON THE CIRCULATION

Administered intravenously ethylenediamine hydrochloride produces a transitory fall in the blood pressure of anesthetized animals. This action was observed in rabbits, cats, and dogs, confirming the results of Desgrez and Dorléans,[9] and was quite marked even with doses as low as 1 mg. The pressor effect described by these authors in dogs after larger doses was, however, not obtained. The subcutaneous injection of 100 mg. in a 4 kilo dog failed to alter the blood pressure at all. Fig. 2 illustrates the effect of a 10 mg. injection intravenously upon a 2 kilo rabbit under urethane.

Regions of Cardiovascular System Affected.—In many experiments the pulse rate was determined before and after injection. As in the case of the intact animals, no significant change was observed. The blood pressure fall therefore appears to be independent of the heart's action.

It was next attempted to ascertain whether or not the depressor effect is limited to definite areas such as the extremities or the viscera. For this purpose rabbits were anesthetized and the blood supply to various regions excluded by arterial ligation. By clamping the abdominal aorta below the renal arteries, the subclavian arteries, and the unused carotid artery, the circulation in the extremities and part of the head was eliminated. After this procedure (Fig. 3, *y*) 10 mg. of ethylenediamine caused a slightly greater fall in the blood pressure than was produced previous to the ligations (Fig. 3, *x*).

In another rabbit when the mesenteric arteries were ligated the diamine action remained unaltered (Fig. 4). In the same animal later the celiac, mesenteric and subclavian arteries and abdominal aorta were clamped and the drug administered as before. The depressor effect, although somewhat more gradual in onset and prolonged, was still obtained (Fig. 5). The presence of the splanchnic circulation is therefore by no means essential to the diamine effect, in fact the combined response of the vessels of the thorax, the superficial vessels of the

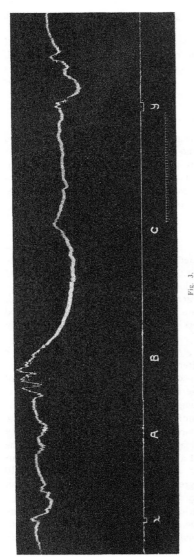

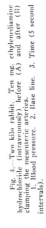

Fig. 3.—Intravenous injection of 10 mg. ethylenediamine hydrochloride in a 2100 gram rabbit before and after exclusion of the circulation of the extremities. 1. Blood pressure. 2. Base line. (Injection marks x and y. A. Aorta clamped. B. Subclavian arteries clamped. C. Timsed carotid artery clamped.) 3. Time in 5 second intervals.

Fig. 3.

Fig. 4.—Two kilo rabbit. Ten mg. ethylenediamine hydrochloride (intravenously) before (A) and after (B) clamping the mesenteric arteries. 1. Blood pressure. 2. Base line. 3. Time (5 second intervals).

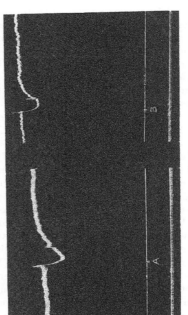

Fig. 4.

upper abdomen, and the vertebrals was nearly as extensive as that of the intact circulation. The depressor action of the drug is thus shown to be independent of any one of the chief regions of the vascular system.

Depression of Sciatic Pressor Reflex.—By an intravenous injection of ethylenediamine in a dog it was found possible to abolish partially for a time the

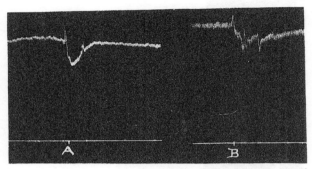

Fig. 5.—Same rabbit as in Fig. 4. Ten mg. ethylenediamine-HCl (intravenously), before (A), and after (B) exclusion of mesenterics, subclavians, and lower abdominal aorta.

1. Blood pressure. 2. Base line.

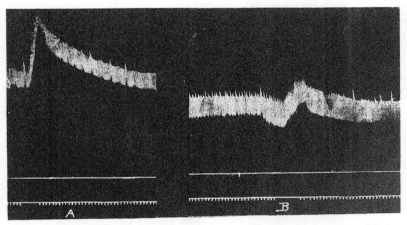

Fig. 6.—Effect of ethylenediamine (intravenously) upon the sciatic Pressor reflex in a 4 kilo dog. A. Effect of stimulation of the central end of cut sciatic. B. Same after injection of 20 mg. ethylenediamine at mark.

1. Blood pressure tracing. 2. Base line. 3. Time (5 second intervals).

sensitivity of the vascular system to reflex stimulation, as the following experiment shows.

The sciatic nerve of a 4 kilo dog under chloretone anesthesia was cut and the central end then stimulated by the induction current. After the resulting reflex blood pressure rise had been recorded (Fig. 6, *A*) 20 mg. of the diamine

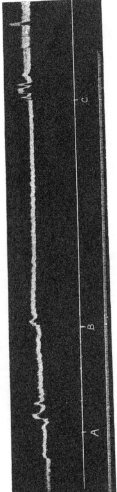

Fig. 7.

Fig. 8.

Fig. 7.—Effect of ethylenediamine hydrochloride (intravenously) on ether ed cat. A, 45 mg. of ethylenediamine-HCl in 3 c.c. saline. B, 3 c.c. saline. C, 45 mg. of diamine in 3 c.c. saline.

1. Blood pressure. 2. Base line. 3. Time (5 second intervals).

Fig. 8.—Effect of intravenous injection of 40 mg. of ethylenediamine hydrochloride in a nembutalized cat.

1. Blood pressure. 2. Base line. 3. Time (5 second intervals).

was injected and the nerve again stimulated with an equal current strength just as the blood pressure was beginning to fall. Only a slight response to this second stimulation was obtained (Fig. 6, *B*). The sensitivity returned after a few minutes and the entire experiment was then repeated with the same result.

Is the depressor action central or peripheral? This is always a difficult point to determine. The question was submitted to two methods of attack: we determined the action of ethylenediamine, (1) after the elimination of the vasomotor centers by pithing; and (2) upon the nicotinized animal.

(1) After elimination of the vasomotor centers by pithing, no fall in blood pressure can be obtained by intravenous injections of the diamine. Three rabbits injected under such conditions gave entirely negative results. Fig. 7 illustrates the effect of two injections of ethylenediamine (and a saline control) in a pithed

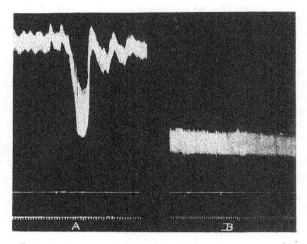

Fig. 9.—Effect of ethylenediamine (20 mg.) on the blood pressure of a dog, before (A) and after (B) nicotinization. Injection at marks.

1. Blood pressure curve. 2. Base line. 3. Time (5 second intervals).

cat, the only responses being slight increases in blood pressure. This type of experiment is unsatisfactory because of the marked circulatory depression produced by the pithing procedure itself. The results indicate, however, that the depressor action of the diamine is a central one.

(2) A number of rabbits were thoroughly nicotinized (until no sciatic pressor reflex could be obtained with maximal stimuli), after which ethylenediamine was impotent to affect the blood pressure. In Fig. 8 is illustrated the effect of an injection of 40 mg. of ethylenediamine in a nicotinized cat. One sees a blood pressure rise similar to that obtained in the pithed cat. A dog also gave a negative result; in Fig. 9 is seen the effect of 20 mg. of the diamine before (*A*), and after (*B*), nicotinization.

In view of the consistent failure to obtain any trace of depressor response to ethylenediamine after decerebration or thorough nicotinization it is concluded that the central nervous system plays at least a large part in the blood pressure reducing effect of ethylenediamine.

CONCLUSIONS

1. Ethylenediamine hydrochloride is a comparatively innocuous substance, the minimal lethal subcutaneous dose for white mice being 15 mg. per 20 gm. body weight.

2. Upon the central nervous system of frogs its action resembles that of the methane narcotics.

3. Rabbits exhibit after nearly fatal intravenous or subcutaneous injections, (0.4 gm. per kilo), a temporary respiratory stimulation and a lowering of body temperature. A slight general depression and transient diarrhea are also produced. Lacrimal, nasal, and salivary secretions are not stimulated. (Contrary to the results of Brieger.)

4. The only constant effect of smaller subcutaneous doses (0.1 mg. per kilo) is the hypothermia. Daily injections render the animals immune to this effect after four days. Continued for ten days such injections have no significant effects upon body weight, kidneys, heart or blood.

5. Ethylenediamine inhibits the activity and relaxes the tone of smooth muscle (isolated cat's intestine).

6. The blood pressure is lowered in dogs, cats and rabbits by intravenous injections of ethylenediamine, 1 mg. often producing this effect. This effect is not of cardiac origin neither is it limited to any particular region of the vascular system. During its exhibition the sciatic pressor reflex is partially abolished.

7. Ethylenediamine fails to lower the blood pressure after pithing or complete nicotinization. Its depressor action is probably of central nervous origin.

PROTOCOLS

Rabbit 1. 850 grams.
Single intravenous injection of ethylenediamine-HCl.
0.4 gram per kilo.

TIME	RESP. PER ¼ MIN.	RECTAL TEMP. °C.	PULSE PER ¼ MIN.
12-12-16			
9:34 A. M.	12	39.0	39
10:38	Injection		
10:41	28		39
11:00	15		
11:20	17	38.6	
2:00[1] P. M.	13	39.0	38
3:00	11	39.3	37
4:00[2]	14	39.5	39
12-13-16			
9:00[3] A. M.	14	39.3	39
12-14-16			
8:30[4] A. M.	14	39.5	39

1. Diarrhea—No other increased secretions. Pupils dilated, poor accommodation. Bright red urine; many r.b.c.
2. Bright red urine—abundance of r.b.c. and albumin.
3. Hematuria, albuminuria.
4. No hematuria, albuminuria.

Rabbit 2. 1990 grams.
Single intravenous injection of ethylenediamine-HCl.
0.4 gram per kilo.

TIME	RESP. PER ¼ MIN.	RECTAL TEMP. °C.
3-26-17		
12:30 P.M.	17	39.0
2:58	Injection	
3:00	Collapse. Resp. failure	Recovery by artificial resp.
3:10	33	
3:45	16	38.3
4:30	13	38.7
7:15	14	38.0
3-27-17		
9:15 A.M.*	16	39.3

*Diarrhea.

Rabbit 3. 1940 grams.
Single intravenous injection of ethylenediamine-HCl.
0.4 gram per kilo.

TIME	RESP. PER ¼ MIN.	RECTAL TEMP. °C.
3-26-17		
12:30 P.M.	10	39.0
3:20 ⎱	Slow injection	
3:25 ⎰		
3:3	20	
3:4	11	38.3
4:3[1]	11	38.1
7:1[2]	12	37.8
3-27-17		
9:15[2] A.M.	8	38.9

1. Slight depression, contracted pupils.
2. Diarrhea.

Rabbit 4. 1185 grams.
Single intravenous injection of ethylenediamine-HCl.
0.4 gram per kilo.
1-15-17   Died during injection.

Rabbit 5. 1105 grams.
Single intravenous injection of ethylenediamine-HCl.
0.4 gram per kilo.
1-15-17   Died during injection.

Rabbit 6. 1510 grams.
Single subcutaneous injection of ethylenediamine-HCl.
0.4 gram per kilo.

TIME	RESP. PER ¼ MIN.	RECTAL TEMP. °C.	PULSE PER ¼ MIN.
1-15-17			
3:55 P.M.	15	39.7	40
4:00	Injection		
4:45*	20	38.9	40
5:15	19	38.5	44
7:15	13	39.0	40
1-16-17			
9:35 A.M.	14	39.8	40

*Diarrhea.

Rabbit 7. 1485 grams.
Single subcutaneous injection of ethylenediamine-HCl. 0.4 gram per kilo.

TIME	RESP. PER ¼ MIN.	RECTAL TEMP. °C.	PULSE PER ¼ MIN.
1-15-17			
4:25 P.M.	10	39.4	42
4:30	Injection		
4:55*	20	39.6	44
5:25	18	39.6	42
7:20	12	39.4	42
1-16-17			
9:55 A.M.	11	39.5	42

*Severe diarrhea.

Rabbit 8.
Subcutaneous injections of ethylenediamine-HCl. 0.1 gram per kilo daily.

TIME	ETHYLENEDIAMINE GM.	RESP. PER ¼ MIN.	RECTAL TEMP. °C.
3-26-17x			
12:30 P.M.		12	39.5
2:45	0.173		
3:45		12	37.9
4:30*		12	38.1
7:15		12	39.6
3-27-17			
9:15 A.M.		14	39.5
2:45 P.M.		12	39.9
3:20	0.173		
4:20		11	38.6
6:45		12	39.3
3-28-17			
3:00		12	39.5
3:25	0.173		
4:30		12	38.8
3-29-17			
1:00		12	39.5
1:05	0.173		
3:00		12	39.3
3-30-17			
12:00		12	38.5
12:15	0.173		
12:30		12	38.6
12:45		10	38.4
1:00		12	38.3
2:00		11	38.7
3-31-17	0.173		
4-1-17	0.173		
4-2-17	0.173		
4-3-17	0.173		
4-4-17x			
11:30 A.M.		10	39.3
11:45	0.173		
12:45 P.M.		11	39.0

*Severe diarrhea.
xWeight first and last days, 1730 gms.

Rabbit 9.
Subcutaneous injections of ethylenediamine-HCl.
0.1 gram per kilo daily.

TIME	ETHYLENEDIAMINE GM.	RESP. PER ¼ MIN.	RECTAL TEMP. °C.
3-26-17*			
12:30 P.M.		12	39.5
2:50	0.178		
3:45		12	38.5
4:30		12	39.0
7:15		12	39.8
3-27-17			
2:45 P.M.		12	39.5
3:25	0.178		
4:20		16 irreg.	39.0
6:45		15	39.8
3-28-17			
3:00		12	39.5
3:30	0.178		
4:30		14	39.3
3-29-17			
1:00		14	39.1
1:10	0.178		
3:00		16 irreg.	39.3
3-30-17			
12:00		14	39.0
12:18	0.178		
12:30		20 irreg.	39:0
12:45		16 "	38.8
1:00		16 "	38.8
2:00		16	39.5
3-31-17	0.178		
4-1-17	0.178		
4-2-17	0.178		
4-3-17	0.178		
4-4-17†			
11:30 A.M.		12 irreg.	39.1
11:45	0.178		
12:45 P.M.		14 "	39.2

*Weight 1780 grams.
†Weight 1730 grams.

REFERENCES

[1]Cloez: "Organische Basen aus dem Chlorethyl." cit. Jahresbericht der Chemie, 1853. p. 468; For Variations in the Method of Preparation see: Hoffmann, A. W.: Ber. d. chem. Gesell., 1871, iv, 666; and Rhoussopoulos, O., Meyer, F., and Kraut, K.: Ann. d. Chem., 1882, ccxii, 351.
[2]Brieger, L.: Ueber Ptomaine, 1883.
[3]Kulneff, N.: Berl. klin. Wchnschr., 1891, xxviii, 1071.
[4]Carbone, T.: Maly's Jahresber., 1891, xxi, 457.
[5]Schering and Schaeffer: Therap. Monatsh., 1894, viii, 354.
[6]Schaeffer, J.: Zeitschr. f. Hygiene, 1894, xvi, 190.
[7]Brieger: Loc. cit.
[8]Schaeffer: Loc. cit.
[9]Desgrez and Dorléans: Comp. rend. Acad. d. Sc., 1913, clvi, 823.
[10]Pohl, J.: "Ueber synthesenhemmung durch Diamine," Arch. f. exper. Path. u. Pharm., 1898, xli, 97.

CHEMICAL CHANGES IN THE BLOOD IN DISEASE*

II. Uric Acid

By Victor C. Myers, Ph.D., New York City

MORE than seventy years ago Sir A. B. Garrod[1] put the subject of the uric acid content of the blood on a definite basis when he identified this substance in the blood of patients suffering from gout, and showed that whereas uric acid was normally present in blood only in traces, it was definitely increased, not only in gout, but also in certain cases of nephritis. He further showed that there is no increase in the blood uric acid in rheumatism, such as is found in gout, and used this as a point of differential diagnosis. No noteworthy advance in this subject was made until Folin and Denis[2] in 1913 introduced their simple colorimetric method for the estimation of this interesting substance. As originally carried out this method was not entirely accurate, but with the modifications since introduced, the method has been considerably simplified and the accuracy greatly improved.

Before considering the results which have been obtained with present methods, further reference should be made to the very interesting work of Garrod, since the general harmony of his conclusions with current views is surprising, when one considers the methods which were then available. It has been suggested that he drew upon his imagination for some of his results, but the correctness of his deductions and the quantitative data which he gives do not support this. This criticism probably originated from the fact that in his later clinical work he endeavored to gauge the amount of uric acid present in the blood by his famous thread test ("uric acid thread experiment").[3] This test was checked against tests where known amounts of uric acid had been employed. In his earlier work, however, the uric acid (or urates) obtained from a given amount of blood, 65 c.c. (1000 grains) was weighed. Such figures as the following recalculated as mg. per 100 c.c. were obtained: in gout, 5, 5, 2.5, 4.5, 3.0 and 17.5; in rheumatism, trace in four and negative in fifth case; in albuminuria, 0.5, 1.2 and 2.7 mg.; and in headache cases, 0.7, trace and 1.0 mg. Sheep and pigeon blood yielded negative results.

The method employed[1] was to evaporate the serum to dryness in thin layers in a water-bath. It was then powdered and treated with rectified spirits, boiled for about 10 to 15 minutes and again treated in the same way. After again washing with spirits, the dried serum was exhausted by means of boiling distilled water, the operation being repeated two or three times, and the watery solutions mixed. The concentrated watery solution was allowed to stand for some hours (forty-eight), when on examination, innumerable tufts of crystals were found deposited on the sides of the vessel, and the surface of the liquid. The crystals were collected, washed with alcohol, and weighed. "These crystals were proved to consist of urate of soda; for crystallized uric acid could be produced from them, and they left an alkaline ash, soluble in water and not consisting of potash."

It is of interest to note that in connection with his later determinations, Garrod writes:[1] "With regard to the weights which have been given, I may observe that in the earlier determinations they doubtless were below the real quantities, a circumstance which arose from the watery solutions of the serum not being sufficiently concentrated, and from sufficient time not being allowed for the deposition of the uric acid. In the experiments

*From the Laboratory of Pathological Chemistry, New York Post-Graduate Medical School and Hospital, New York City.

now made, I do not collect the crystals until forty-eight hours have elapsed. Such slight errors are, however, unavoidable in new investigations on any subject."

In the course of discussions in his several papers and book, Garrod makes many very interesting and pertinent remarks, a few of which will be quoted: "I may remark, that during evaporation of the serum of blood in albuminuria, a peculiar *odor* of urine was frequently detected; this was not observed in healthy serum, or in that taken from gout or rheumatic patients. Some of the coloring matters of the urine seemed, however, to be thrown down with the uric acid in all cases. * * * The results of these experiments on the condition of the blood and urine prove that uric acid is not a product of the action of the kidneys, as is frequently supposed, but that it is merely excreted from the system by these organs. * * * It appears also probable that as, in albuminuria, the 'urea-excreting function' being chiefly impaired, we find a vicarious discharge of this body in the dropsical effusions; so in gout, the 'uric acid-excreting-function' being defective, the chalk-like deposits are produced, by a similar vicarious discharge of urate of soda. * * * Gout would thus appear partly to depend on a loss of power (temporary or permanent) of this 'uric acid-excreting-function' of the kidneys; the premonitory symptoms, and those also which constitute the paroxysm, arising from an excess of this acid in the blood, and from the effort to expel the 'materies morbi' from the system. * * * In conclusion, as we have found that the blood in every patient suffering from genuine gout, contained an abnormal amount of uric acid, and that in acute rheumatism such was not the condition of this fluid; and again, that in all cases which could be traced up to gout (although the symptoms exhibited at the time might not be very characteristic), uric acid was present, whereas it was absent in those cases where no such phenomena could be found, I think we shall in future be justified in considering the condition of the blood as not only most important, but even a *pathognomonic* sign, and one more to be depended on than any of the other symptoms taken separately." In studying the therapeutic action of colchicum Garrod[4] noted no increase in the uric acid output or influence on urea or other solids of the urine, and observed that this drug did not act as a diuretic in all cases, a diminished output of urine sometimes being noted. He did not confine his attention entirely to uric acid for in a study of blood and effused fluids he writes:[5] "Lastly, these effused fluids may be employed, not only to ascertain the existence of uric acid, but likewise of other principles, as urea and sugar, which are contained and can be detected in them."

As noted above, little advance was made from the time of Garrod until Folin and Denis reported their first results[6] on the uric acid content of human blood. In a series of unselected cases they found between 1 and 3 mg. to 100 c.c., the average being close to 2 mg., while in gout their figures varied between 3.5 and 5.5 mg. Somewhat similar increases were observed in lead poisoning and leucemia. Practically no elevation of the uric acid was noted in a series of 11 nephritic bloods with only moderate nitrogen retention, but later they reported data[7] on cases of advanced nephritis in some of which very high values were obtained, up to 10 mg. These latter observations were confirmed by Myers and Fine,[8] who noted very high figures for uric acid in several cases of terminal interstitial nephritis. In one case the uric acid reached the enormous figure of 27 mg. shortly before death (see Table I), while in several cases figures as high as 15 mg. were observed, values much higher than any noted in gout.

The figures which are now regarded as normal for the blood uric acid differ very little from those originally reported by Folin and Denis. Although healthy adults most often yield values between 2 and 3 mg. per 100 c.c. of blood, figures as low as 1 mg. and as high as 3.5 mg. may be encountered in strictly normal individuals, the differences probably depending in part upon dietary factors. High blood uric acids must obviously depend upon either an increased formation or a decreased elimination. In leucemia the first factor accounts for the increase, but high uric acids in most other conditions find a probable explanation on the latter basis. Among these may be mentioned nephritis, acute and chronic (but not parenchymatous), arterial hypertension, lead poisoning, bichloride poisoning, malignancy, acute infections, especially pneumonia, and apparently some cases of nongouty arthritis. Miscellaneous cases illustrating the uric acid findings in most of these conditions are given in Table III of the preceding paper, and in Table II here. Sedgwick and Kingsbury[9] have made the interesting observation that the blood uric acid is high during the first three or four days of life, in harmony with the high uric acid excretion during that period.

NEPHRITIS

It is perfectly logical to expect that high values for the blood uric acid would be found in the last stages of chronic interstitial nephritis, with the consequent accumulation of all the waste products of nitrogenous metabolism. Comparative figures on the blood and urine in one of our first cases[8] are given in Table I. The blood uric acid findings in this case are higher than in any case

TABLE I

COMPARATIVE BLOOD AND URINE FINDINGS IN CHRONIC INTERSTITIAL NEPHRITIS

I. D., female, aged 17

DATE 1914-15	BLOOD ANALYSES MG. TO 100 C.C.				DATE 1914-15	URINE ANALYSES DAILY AVERAGES IN GMS.		
	Nonprotein N	Urea N	Uric Acid	Creatinine		Total N	Uric Acid	Creatinine
Dec. 10	181	139	6.8	10.0	Dec. 18-19	5.57	0.14	0.37
Dec. 21	199	134	12.5	14.5	Dec. 20-23	3.65	0.07	0.29
Dec. 26	244	151	15.4	17.7	Dec. 23-26	3.64	0.16	0.17
Dec. 30	267	170	21.0	16.1	Dec. 26-30	2.91	0.13	0.13
Jan. 4	297	208	27.0	20.0	Dec. 30 to Jan. 3	1.75	0.09	0.15

we have since studied or any elsewhere reported. Indeed, we might have had some doubts about the last findings recorded, were it not that some of the observations were checked in another laboratory. That the retention of uric acid in nephritis results in a fairly even distribution of this substance in the various body tissues has been shown by Fine[10] in tissues obtained at autopsy. The distribution, however, is not quite as uniform as in the case of the urea or even the creatinine, a fact which might be expected from their physical properties.

In 1916 Myers, Fine and Lough[11] called attention to the fact that very high figures for uric acid may be noted, not only in cases of advanced interstitial nephritis, but also in the very early stage of the disease, before a retention of either the urea or creatinine had taken place. It was suggested that, when symptoms of gout were absent, a high blood uric acid might be a valuable early diagnostic sign of nephritis, possibly earlier evidence of renal impairment of an interstitial type than the classic tests of proteinuria and cylinduria.

Subsequently, Baumann, Hansmann, Davis and Stevens[12] took up a study of this question and concluded: "It follows from the above that the uric acid concentration of the blood is a delicate, if not the most delicate, index of renal function at our disposal." More recently Upham and Higley[13] have taken up the renal concentration power for uric acid. It was pointed out by Myers and Fine[14] that under normal conditions the kidney concentrates the uric acid only about twenty times, whereas in the case of urea and creatinine the figures were about 80 and 100, respectively. Upham and Higley have found that in cases free from clinical symptoms of nephritis the concentration power for uric acid was 20 or over, while in cases showing clinical symptoms diagnostic of nephritis, it was 14 or below. In another group of cases showing symptoms suggestive but not diagnostic of nephritis the concentration figure was 18.4 or below.

TABLE II

ILLUSTRATIVE URIC ACID FINDINGS IN NEPHRITIS, LEUCEMIA AND GOUT

| CASE | AGE | SEX | DATE | BLOOD ANALYSES MG. TO 100 C.C. | | | CLINICAL DIAGNOSIS, REMARKS |
				Uric Acid	Urea N	Creat-inine	
1. H. B.	55	♂	3/28/16	6.1	16	2.8	Chronic diffuse nephritis; hypertension.
2. B. D.	25	♀	3/15/16	9.6	19	2.4	Chronic diffuse nephritis; hypertension and edema.
3. D. S.	56	♂	6/ 7/15 7/21/15 9/28/15	7.1 6.6 6.3	16 24 18	2.0 3.3 2.1	Chronic interstitial nephritis.
4. J. J.	65	♂	8/11/15 9/25/15 1/14/16	9.5 8.0 5.0	25 37 37	2.5 2.7 3.9	Chronic interstitial nephritis; died four years later.
5. M. C.	11	♂	6/27/16 7/21/16	8.0 6.3	36 53	2.7 2.9	Chronic diffuse nephritis; improvement.
6. W. C.	49	♂	1/15/16 1/28/16	9.5 2.5	44 19	3.5 1.9	Acute nephritis; acidosis; recovery.
7. F. F.	8	♂	12/18/17 12/21/17 12/27/17	11.4 11.2 5.0	106 93 21	6.1 5.9 4.2	Acute nephritis; suppression of urine; recovery.
8. G. McK.	21	♀	12/ 4/19	9.3	48	13.4	Terminal chronic interstitial nephritis.
9. C. P.	37	♂	3/19/20	7.7	111	21.7	Terminal chronic interstitial nephritis.
10. J. P.	62	♂	4/ 4/16	3.4	28	3.0	Chronic parenchymatous nephritis; died.
11. S. R.	13	♂	8/15/15	10.0	17	2.4	Lymphatic leucemia; died.
12. H. L.	51	♂	3/25/16 4/14/16 5/ 5/16 5/10/16	7.8 6.4 8.2 8.1	12 11 15 15	2.9 2.2 2.3 1.5	Typical gout for 22 years; tophi on ears; severe pains in joints, particularly right big toe; diet purine-free until after second test.

An idea of the uric acid findings in illustrative cases of nephritis may be obtained from Table II. The first two cases show that it is possible to have very high figures for uric acid without any very definite retention of urea. At a later stage in the disease the urea retention becomes definite as is seen in Cases 3, 4, and 5. Acute nephritis may influence not only the uric acid but also the urea and to some extent the creatinine. This is well illustrated by Cases 6 and 7, the first of which showed pronounced acidosis. Note the marked fall in the uric acid following improvement in this case. The nitrogen retention in Case 7 is the most pronounced we have observed with ultimate recovery. The figures on Cases 8 and 9 were obtained in the last stages of the disease, and show a retention of the urea and creatinine as well as of the uric acid. It is of interest regarding the uric acid that early in the disease the values observed may be somewhat higher (7 to 8 mg.) than at a later stage (5 to 6 mg.), due possibly to dietary restrictions, although during the last days of life the amount may be very markedly increased. In parenchymatous nephritis there is very little retention of uric acid.

GOUT AND ARTHRITIS*

Owing to the fact that the tophi found in gout have long been recognized to contain deposits of sodium urate, it is quite natural that the uric acid content of the blood in this condition should possess a special interest. Following the investigations of Folin and Denis a number of different workers took up a study of this question, among whom may be mentioned McLester,[15] Pratt,[16] Fine and Chace,[17] and Daniels and McCrudden.[18] Subsequently Folin and Denis[19] and Fine[20] further discussed this question, while recently McClure in association with several workers[21, 22, 23, 24] has given considerable attention to this subject. His last paper gives an excellent presentation of his own work.[24] Although the method originally described by Folin and Denis[2] yielded fairly satisfactory results when carefully executed, many figures are recorded for the uric acid content of the blood in gout which are open to question. It is possible by dietary restrictions in the purine-containing foods to lower the blood uric acid in gout, but this would scarcely account for the low results reported by some observers, notably some of those of Pratt, and Daniels and McCrudden. The latter investigators reported two cases of gout in women whose blood uric acids were quite normal. It appears rather strange that McClure and Pratt[21] should have thought it wise to omit all reference to work carried out with Benedict's modification of the uric acid method, when they admit that Folin had offered certain criticisms of his own method, their excuse being that the reported figures obtained with the modified method were too high to be compared with those obtained by the use of the original method.

From the normal variations of from 2 to 3 mg. to 100 c.c. of blood, the uric acid may increase to as much as from 4 to 9 mg. in gout, but it does not follow that these uric acid accumulations are infallible signs of gout, since, as noted above, similar uric acid figures may be found in nephritis. This point is well brought out in the table below taken from Fine. A very close

*The author is under obligation to Drs. Fine and Killian for many unpublished observations on uric acid recorded in this paper. He is also under obligation to Dr. Fine, now of the Calco Chemical Company for furnishing the tolysin (neocinchophen) and most of the cinchophen employed in the experiments reported in Table IV.

TABLE III

BLOOD PICTURES IN GOUT AND EARLY INTERSTITIAL NEPHRITIS*

CASE	DATE 1915-1916	AGE	SEX	DIAGNOSIS	URIC ACID, MG. PER 100 C.C.	UREA N, MG. PER 100 C.C.	CREATININE, MG. PER 100 C.C.	PHTHAL-EIN 2 HRS. PER CENT.	SYSTOLIC BLOOD PRESSURE	URINE PROTEIN	URINE CASTS
M. K.	9/3	49	♀	Typical gout	9.5	13	1.1	48	230	+	-
T. B.	10/5	57	♂		8.4	12	2.2	35	164	-	+
H. L.	3/24	51	♂		7.8	12	2.9	59	120	-	-
L. J.	10/6	43	♂		7.2	17	2.4	..	120	-	
C. P.	10/6	45			6.8	14	1.7	..	200	....	....
B. D.	3/31	25	♀	Miscellaneous cases Showing some evidence of early interstitial nephritis — Slight edema	7.7	20	2.6	45	168	+	-
D. S.	6/7	56	♀	Hypertension	6.7	19	2.5	26	185	-	+
E. V.	3/20	14	♀	Endocarditis	6.3	12	3.6	32	120	++	+
H. B.	3/28	55	♂	Incipient nephritis	6.1	16	2.8	57	120	-	+
H. J.	3/23	50	♂	Diabetes	6.0	18	2.9	36	140	+	+
G. C.	3/14	40	♀	Incipient nephritis	5.5	15	2.1	46	147	-	+
M. S.	3/22	46	♀	Gastritis	5.0	12	2.5	52	190	+	-

*Taken from Fine.[20]

scrutiny of Table III does disclose a tendency for the urea and creatinine concentrations of Group 2 to rise above those of Group 1, which are essentially normal, but the differences are slight. Myers and Fine[11] have stated, "The blood pictures in early interstitial nephritis and gout are strikingly similar, particularly as regards the increase in uric acid. In view of the other clinical symptoms in common, it would seem that this similarity must be more than accidental." Fine[20] has raised these questions: "1. Is gout merely a stage in the development of interstitial nephritis, whose further progress may be indefinitely delayed? 2. Is early interstitial nephritis merely potential gout, in which the clinical symptoms may or may not appear? 3. Is the uric acid retention of gout due to the specific condition, *gout*, or to a complicating early interstitial nephritis?" McClure[24] has studied the renal function in six cases of gout in which the clinical diagnosis of nephritis was not justifiable. By means of the phthalein test, nonprotein and urea nitrogen and two-hour renal test, some disturbance of renal function was demonstrated in each case, thus strengthening the general argument given above.

Practically, we may conclude that gout is almost invariably associated with an increased uric acid content of the blood and therefore a high blood uric acid may be of considerable diagnostic value in cases of gouty arthritis, in which tophi containing sodium urate are not already present. It should be borne in mind that cases of arthritis may occasionally show an increase in the uric acid, although this is generally associated with an increased urea and nonprotein nitrogen, thus indicating a complicating nephritis. Such cases of arthritis, however, are the exception rather than the rule. In ten typical cases of arthritis which have come under our observation during the past month the figures for the blood uric acid have ranged from 1.6 to 3.6 mg. to 100 c.c. and all but three cases showed under 3 mg.

INFLUENCE OF DIET AND DRUGS UPON THE BLOOD URIC ACID

That a purine-free diet will definitely, although not markedly lower the blood uric acid in gout is brought out by the observations on Case 12 in Table II, where in the course of about three weeks the uric acid fell from 7.8 to 6.4 mg., but again rose to 8.2 and 8.1 mg. upon the return to a purine diet. A much more pronounced lowering of the uric acid as the result of dietary restrictions may be noted in the first two cases of Table IV.

It has been recognized for some time that the administration of salicylates and cinchophen (2-phenyl-quinolin-4 carboxylic acid) resulted in an increased excretion of uric acid. Recently it has been shown by Folin and Lyman,[25] McLester,[15] Fine and Chace,[17] and Smith and Hawk[26] that the action of cinchophen was accompanied by a marked drop in the uric acid content of the blood and later the same was shown to be true of the salicylates by Fine and Chace[27] and Denis.[28] The action of phlorhizin and the methylated purines on the kidney is probably better known but scarcely as remarkable as that of the drugs mentioned. The action of phlorhizin holds little of clinical interest, and Christian and his coworkers[29] have recently thrown serious doubts on the therapeutic value of methylated purines.

It is now generally assumed that cinchophen and the salicylates induce an increased output of uric acid in the urine and a decreased concentration in the

TABLE IV
INFLUENCE OF DIET AND DRUGS UPON THE BLOOD URIC ACID

CASE	AGE	SEX	DATE	BLOOD ANALYSES MG. TO 100 C.C.			CLINICAL DIAGNOSIS, REMARKS
				Uric Acid	Urea N	Creat-inine	
1. P. P.	28	♂	3/14/16	8.0	20	2.7	Gastric ulcer; diet until 3/17
			3/17/16	6.3	15	2.4	contained broths, but later
			3/28/16	(3.7	20	...	was purine-free.
			4/ 4/16	(3.1	14	1.8	
2. M. S.	46	♀	2/23/16	6.1	12	2.6	Arteriosclerosis, periodic
			3/ 7/16	(3.1	12	2.9	vomiting; diet purine-free
			3/16/16	(3.0	12	2.5	from 2/29 until after 3/16;
			3/23/16	5.0	12	2.5	60 grains of sodium salicyl-
			3/31/16	(1.7	13	3.4	ate 3/27 to 4/2, then purine-
			4/ 7/16	2.5	..	...	free diet.
			4/18/16	5.0	12	2.3	
3. T. G.	46	♂	6/27/16	6.0	17	2.6	Chronic duodenal ulcer,
			7/ 1/16	(3.2	18	1.8	syphilis; purine-free diet 3 days previous to 1st analy- sis; 30 grains of a com- bination of Na salicylate and cinchophen daily for 4 days preceding 2nd analy- sis.
4. M. G.	58	♂	3/26/20	6.0	29	1.5	Chronic interstitial nephritis,
			3/28/20	5.2	29	2.4	arteriosclerosis; 50 grains
			3/31/20	(trace	16	2.0	of tolysin given 3/28 to 4/3.
			4/ 5/20	3.0	24	2.2	
			4/12/20	3.5	18	3.0	
			4/13/20	3.9	15	2.4	
5. M. D.	53	♀	3/16/20	2.8	26	2.6	Neurasthenia, visceroptosis;
			3/18/20	2.8	22	2.6	vegetable diet; tolysin 50
			3/22/20	(trace	13	2.7	grains daily 3/19-22; cin-
			3/25/20	2.6	20	2.4	chophen 50 grains daily
			3/29/20	2.6	19	2.2	4/9-12.
			4/ 9/20	2.8	16	2.4	
			4/12/20	(0.7	13	2.6	
			4/15/20	2.0	17	2.4	
6. G. McK.	21	♀	12/ 4/19	9.3	48	13.4	Chronic interstitial nephritis;
			12/ 5/19	10.4	42	16.8	patient died 12/30; 25
			12/ 6/19	(5.1	52	12.7	grains cinchophen daily
			12/ 7/19	(8.3	45	15.0	12/5-8 with lemonade diet;
			12/ 8/19	(8.1	48	14.3	low protein diet with 25
			12/ 9/19	(5.4	55	12.3	grains of a mixture of
			12/11/19	(7.5	57	12.1	cinchophen and theobro-
			12/13/19	6.1	53	13.0	mine daily 12/9-11.
7. S. H.	37	♂	5/10/15	7.7	76	10.9	Chronic interstitial nephritis;
			5/15/15	(8.0	64	9.6	45 grains cinchophen on
			5/21/15	7.8	53	8.0	5/12 and 13. 60 grains on 5/14; patient died 6/28.

blood (and tissues) by endowing the renal cells with an increased power for eliminating uric acid. The effect of these drugs begins to be manifest nearly as soon as absorption of the drug has taken place and exerts its maximum in-fluence in about one day.

Both of these drugs have marked analgesic effects, as well as that of stimu-lating the excretion of uric acid, and it would appear difficult to decide as to which effect was the more valuable in conditions with high blood uric acids, such as gout. Although the action of these drugs is very similar, cinchophen and neocinchophen, its methyl derivative, have an advantage in that they appear to be free from the toxic influences on the kidney inherent in the salicylates. Tolysin (neocinchophen) is tasteless and is better tolerated by some patients than cinchophen.

The influence of these drugs upon the blood uric acid is shown in Table IV. Case 2 illustrates the effect of sodium salicylate and Case 3 a combination of this drug with cinchophen. In Cases 4 and 5 tolysin was employed, Case 4 showing a high and Case 5 a normal initial uric acid. The control urea nitrogen in both cases was somewhat above normal. In both cases the uric acid was reduced to a quantity too small to estimate, and there was likewise a definite influence on the urea.[30] Cinchophen was subsequently employed in this case with a somewhat less pronounced effect. Fine and Chace[31] have pointed out that in the last stages of interstitial nephritis cinchophen has little influence on the excretion of the uric acid, indicating that the renal cells can no longer be stimulated to increased activity. Cases 6 and 7 illustrate this point, no change in the uric acid being noted in the last of these two cases, even after large doses of cinchophen. We are studying further the comparative action of various drugs in this connection.

ESTIMATION OF URIC ACID

In 1912 Folin and Macallum[32] called attention to the possibilities of the use of phosphotungstic acid in the colorimetric estimation of uric acid, and later in the same year Folin and Denis[2] gave their first description of this estimation as applied to blood. As already pointed out, the results which they first obtained with this method clearly demonstrated the increase in the blood uric acid in gout and lead poisoning[6] and in nephritis.[7] In carrying out these determinations the procedure was to coagulate the blood protein with weak (0.01 N) acetic acid after a 1 to 6 dilution with this solution, filter, wash, evaporate to a very small volume and then precipitate the uric acid with silver lactate, magnesia mixture and ammonia in a small centrifuge tube. (Owing to the presence of phenols in blood it is necessary to separate the uric acid from these color reacting substances.) This was then thrown down in the centrifuge and the precipitate decomposed with hydrogen sulphide. After removal of the excess of hydrogen sulphide, the color reaction was then developed with the special phosphotungstic acid reagent and sodium carbonate.

It could hardly have been expected that such a new method would be perfectly satisfactory in every detail, and in 1915 Benedict[33] introduced certain modifications which did much to increase the accuracy and simplicity of the method. Possibly the greatest source of error was in the decomposition of the silver precipitate with hydrogen sulphide, since low results were obtained, unless considerable care was taken in breaking up the precipitate. For this purpose Benedict employed potassium cyanide, which has proved to be very satisfactory. Other improvements suggested by Benedict were a more dependable standard uric acid solution, the combined use of the silver lactate, magnesia mixture and ammonia into a single reagent and the use of colloidal iron to remove the last trace of protein after coagulation. For this purpose we had been employing alumina cream, and continued to use this in preference to the colloidal iron. Otherwise we at once adopted the suggestions of Benedict. Although this method[11] was somewhat tedious, various checks, which we have made from time to time during the past five years, have led us to believe that it gives perfectly reliable results. A year ago Folin and Wu,[34] in connection with their system of blood analysis, described a method of estimating uric acid directly in the protein-free filtrate obtained after their tungstic acid precipitation without evaporation of the filtrate. Such a procedure obviously greatly simplified the technic of this estimation. In order to secure a permanent standard Folin and Wu have made use of sodium sulphite, which prevents oxidation of the uric acid. As they have noted, the use of this reagent cuts down the peculiar intensification of the blue color obtained by the use of cyanide. They state: "Opinions will doubtless differ as to whether this is an advantage or disadvantage." We are inclined to take the latter view.

In the method described below we have made use of Folin and Wu's new protein precipitant and their lactic acid-silver lactate reagent to precipitate the uric acid, but after the decomposition of the precipitate we still adhere to the suggestions of Benedict. The method as described yields essentially the same results as those obtained with the technic we formerly employed. Fairly satisfactory recoveries of added uric acid may be obtained, provided the proper strength of sulphuric acid has been employed. As Folin and Wu have pointed out, an excess of acid will bring about a precipitation of the uric acid.

Method.—To 5 c.c. of well-mixed oxalated blood in a 100 c.c. Erlenmeyer flask (or 100 c.c. glass stoppered cylinder), add 35 c.c. of water (7 volumes), 5 c.c. of 10 per cent sodium tungstate and then 5 c.c. of exactly 2/3 N sulphuric acid while rotating the flask. Shake thoroughly. (In practice we frequently employ 7 c.c. of blood and in this way rather quickly secure 40 c.c. of filtrate, the equivalent of 4 c.c. of blood. Perfectly satisfactory results may be obtained with 2.5 or 3 c.c., however.) When the blood is properly coagulated, the color of the coagulum turns from pink to brown. If this change does not occur, the coagulation is incomplete, due probably to too much oxalate. In such a case, 5 per cent sulphuric acid may be added a drop at a time, shaking between each addition, until the coagulation is complete. Folin and Wu *caution against* an *excess* of sulphuric acid, since this apparently brings about a precipitation of the uric acid. If the mixture is now carefully poured upon the double portion of a filter just large enough to hold the mixture, the filtrate will probably come through perfectly clear; if not, the first portion may be returned to the filter. To prevent evaporation, a watch glass may be placed over the top of the funnel. It is convenient to filter into a 50 c.c. graduated cylinder.

When the filtration is complete, record volume (ordinarily between 25 and 30 c.c.), and pour contents of cylinder into a 50 c.c. centrifuge tube. Add 5 c.c. of 5 per cent silver lactate solution in 5 per cent lactic acid. After stirring, centrifuge. Pour off and discard supernatant fluid. To the precipitate add about 3 c.c. of 10 per cent sodium chloride in 0.1 N hydrochloric acid* and stir with glass rod. Then add 3 to 4 c.c. of water, 1 drop of 5 per cent potassium cyanide, stir again and centrifuge. This treatment sets free the uric acid from the precipitate. Pour the supernatant fluid into an accurately graduated 25 c.c. cylinder.

Into a similar 25 c.c. cylinder introduce with an Ostwald-Folin pipette 1 c.c. of standard uric acid solution** (contains 0.2 mg. uric acid). Add 4 c.c. of the acidified

*The 10 per cent solution of sodium chloride in 0.1 N hydrochloric acid may be prepared by adding 1 c.c. of concentrated hydrochloric acid to 100 c.c. of 10 per cent chloride solution.
**Benedict's Standard Uric Acid Solution.—This is prepared as follows: Dissolve 4.5 gm. pure crystalline hydrogen disodium phosphate and 0.5 gm. dihydrogen sodium phosphate in 200 to 300 c.c. hot water. Filter and make up to about 250 c.c. with hot water. Pour this warm, clear solution on 100 mg. uric acid suspended in a few c.c. of water in 500 c.c. volumetric flask. Agitate until completely dissolved. Add at once exactly 0.7 c.c. glacial acetic acid, make up to 500 c.c., mix and add 5 .c.c. chloroform. One c.c. of this solution contains 0.2 mg. uric acid. This solution should be freshly prepared every 2 months.

sodium chloride solution and sufficient water to make the volume essentially the same as the unknown. Then add 1 drop of 5 per cent potassium cyanide.

To the standard now add 1 c.c. of the uric acid reagent* and 0.5 c.c. to the unknown, and then 5 to 6 and 3 to 4 c.c. of saturated sodium carbonate respectively. Allow the color to develop for about 5 minutes, then dilute the standard to 20 or 25 c.c., and the unknown, if darker than the standard, to a similar depth of color.

With this technic, fairly deep blue colors are obtained even with normal blood, colors that can readily be matched in the colorimeter. The slight cloud that sometimes appears may easily be separated in the centrifuge. For the calculation the following formula may be used: $\dfrac{S}{R} \times \dfrac{X}{25} \times \dfrac{0.2 \times 100}{B}$ = mg. uric acid to 100 c.c. of blood, in which S represents the depth of the standard (15 mm.), R the reading of the unknown, X the dilution of the unknown, 0.2 the strength of the standard in mg., and B the number of c.c. of blood to which the filtrate employed was equivalent.

ESTIMATION OF URIC ACID WITH THE TEST TUBE COLORIMETER

The technic described above readily lends itself to use with the test tube colorimeter.

Method.—Three c.c. of the well mixed oxalated blood are pipetted into a large test tube or small flask and 21 c.c. of water added. The precipitation of the proteins is now carried out according to the procedure of Folin and Wu, as described above, 3 c.c. each of the sodium tungstate and 2/3 N sulphuric acid being added.

In case it is necessary to add extra sulphuric acid, this should be done carefully as an excess may lead to a precipitation of the uric acid.

To 15 c.c. of the filtrate in a 20 c.c. centrifuge tube† add 2 c.c. of 5 per cent silver lactate in 5 per cent lactic acid. After stirring, centrifuge. Pour off and discard the supernatant fluid. To the precipitate add about 1.5 c.c. of 10 per cent sodium chloride in 0.1 N hydrochloric acid and stir with glass rod. Then add 3 to 4 c.c. of water, stir again and centrifuge. This treatment sets free the uric acid from the precipitate. Pour the clear supernatant fluid into the right hand tube of the colorimeter. Add 1 drop of 2.5 per cent potassium cyanide.

Into the left hand tube of the instrument introduce 1 c.c. of the standard uric acid solution (diluted 1-5, contains 0.04 mg. uric acid). Add 1.5 c.c. of the 10 per cent sodium chloride in 0.1 N hydrochloric acid and sufficient water to make the volume essentially the same as in the unknown. Then add 1 drop of 2.5 per cent potassium cyanide.

To both tubes now add 0.3 c.c. of the uric acid reagent and 2 c.c. of saturated sodium carbonate solution. Allow the color to develop for 3 to 5 minutes, and then dilute the standard to 10 c.c. (20 c.c. if the unknown shows a weak color development) and the unknown to the same intensity of color as the standard, adding the water a drop or two at a time just before the end point in matching colors is reached.

To calculate the mg. of uric acid per 100 c.c. of blood, the following formula may be used, in which S represents the strength of the standard (0.2 or 0.4 mg. to 10 c.c., depending on the dilution), D the dilution in c.c. of unknown required to match the standard, and B the amount of blood employed in c.c.: $\dfrac{}{B}$ = mg. uric acid per 100 c.c. of blood.

If, for example, 15 c.c. of filtrate are used, the equivalent of 1.5 c.c. of blood with a

*Benedict's Modification of Folin-Denis Uric Acid Reagent.—Prepared by boiling 100 gm. of sodium tungstate, 20 c.c. concentrated hydrochloric acid and 30 c.c. 85 per cent phosphoric acid in 750 c.c. distilled water for 2 hours, preferably under a reflux condenser, and then making up to 1000 c.c. with water.

†Cylindrical trunnion cups may be substituted for the conical cups of the ordinary centrifuge. In these, test tubes or special 20 c.c. centrifuge tubes may be employed, and the cups work quite as well for the 15 c.c. conical centrifuge tubes.

standard containing 0.4 mg. diluted to 10 c.c., and the dilution of the unknown required to match the standard is to 17.1 c.c., the formula will work out as follows:

$$\frac{0.4 \times 17.1}{1.5} = 4.6 \text{ mg. to } 100 \text{ c.c.}$$

REFERENCES

[1]Garrod, A. B.: Med. Chir. Trans., 1848, xxxi, 83.
[2]Folin and Denis: Jour. Biol. Chem., 1912-13, xiii, 469.
[3]Garrod: Med. Chir. Trans., 1854, xxxvii, 49; also The Nature and Treatment of Gout and Rheumatic Gout, ed. 2, London, 1853, p. 98.
[4]Garrod: Med. Chir. Trans., 1858, xli, 325.
[5]Garrod: Med. Chir. Trans., 1854, xxxvii, 181.
[6]Folin and Denis: Jour. Biol. Chem., 1913, xiv, 29.
[7]Folin and Denis: Jour. Biol. Chem., 1914, xvii, 487.
[8]Myers and Fine: Jour. Biol. Chem., 1915, xx, 391.
[9]Kingsbury and Sedgwick: Jour. Biol. Chem., 1917, xxxi, 261.
[10]Fine: Jour. Biol. Chem., 1915, xxiii, 471.
[11]Ayers, Fine and Lough: Arch. Int. Med., 1916, xvii, 570.
[12]Baumann, Hausmann, Davis and Stevens: Arch. Int. Med., 1919, xxiv, 70.
[13]Upham and Higley: Arch. Int. Med., 1919, xxiv, 557.
[14]Ayers and Fine: Jour. Biol. Chem., 1919, xxxvii, 239.
[15]McLester: Arch. Int. Med., 1912, xii, 739.
[16]Pratt: Trans. Assn. Am. Phys., 1913, xxviii, 387; Am. Jour. Med. Sc., 1916, cli, 92.
[17]Fine and Chace: Jour. Pharmacol. and Exper. Therap., 1914, vi, 219.
[18]Daniels and McCrudden: Arch. Int. Med., 1915, xv, 1046.
[19]Folin and Denis: Arch. Int. Med., 1915, xvi, 33.
[20]Fine: Jour. Am. Med. Assn., 1916, lxvi, 2051.
[21]McClure and Pratt: Arch. Int. Med., 1917, xx, 481.
[22]Wentworth and McClure: Arch. Int. Med., 1918, xxi, 84.
[23]McClure and McCarthy: Arch. Int. Med., xxiv, 563.
[24]McClure: Medical Clinics of North America, January, 1920, p. 956.
[25]Folin and Lyman: Jour. Pharmacol. and Exper. Therap., 1912-13, iv, 539.
[26]Smith and Hawk: Arch. Int. Med., 1915, xv, 181.
[27]Fine and Chace: Jour. Biol. Chem., 1915, xxi, 371.
[28]Denis: Jour. Pharmacol. and Exper. Therap., 1915, vii, 255, 601.
[29]Christian, Frothingham, O'Hare and Woods: Am. Jour. Med. Sc., 1915, cl. 655.
[30]Myers, Killian and Simpson: Proc. Soc. Exper. Biol. and Med., May, 1920, xvii.
[31]Fine and Chace: Arch. Int. Med., 1915, xvi, 401.
[32]Folin and Macallum: Jour. Biol. Chem., 1912, xi, 265.
[33]Benedict: Jour. Biol. Chem., 1915, xx, 629.
[34]Folin and Wu: Jour. Biol. Chem., 1919, xxxviii, 81.

BACTERIOLOGIC DATA ON THE EPIDEMIOLOGY OF RESPIRATORY DISEASES IN THE ARMY*

By Henry J. Nichols, M.D., Major, Medical Corps, U. S. Army.

ALTHOUGH many investigators have tried to determine the exact route taken by the specific microorganisms of respiratory diseases in passing from one person to another, opinion on this subject is still divided into two more or less opposing hypotheses. According to one, the microorganisms are chiefly air-borne and are inhaled, either at some distance from their source, or usually at short range in the droplets of coughs and sneezes. According to the other theory, the air is practically free of pathogenic microorganisms which settle out quickly or die by drying. The organisms are believed to travel in infected discharges on some intermediate object such as the hands, cups, etc., and then back to the mouth. For brevity, one may be called the direct and the other the indirect method.

I. THE INDIRECT METHOD

The experiences of the war reawakened an interest in the general problem as it affects soldiers, which was brought to a focus by the papers of Lynch and Cumming.[1] These observers presented data, largely statistical, to show that the principal route of travel is "mouth to hand and hand to mouth" through the medium of the dish water in which mess kits are washed. Under direction of Colonel F. F. Russell, M.C., in charge of the Division of Laboratories and Infectious Diseases of the Surgeon General's Office, some work was planned on this subject along with other problems of respiratory diseases. Major Oscar Teague was selected to obtain some actual bacteriologic evidence on the general problem. He made a large number of observations at Camp Meade, Maryland, in December, 1918, and January, February and March, 1919, and made an extensive detailed report to the Surgeon General, which covered a number of points relating to the spread of respiratory diseases. Most of the results of the field work recorded in this paper have been extracted from Major Teague's noteworthy report. The writer is responsible for the general discussion, the work on the antiseptic action of soap and for the conclusions. While the data collected are not considered as at all final or entirely conclusive, they are believed to be of sufficient value to warrant publication, and so far as they go, they support the airborne theory.

ORGANISMS USED—HEMOLYTIC STREPTOCOCCI

The first problem was to find a suitable organism to work with. The search for specific microorganisms with the possible exception of hemolytic streptococci was not considered feasible. It was at first proposed to use some easily recognizable nonpathogenic organism which could be inoculated in the nose and throat

*From the Laboratory of the Base Hospital, Camp Meade, Md.; the Laboratory Service of the Walter Reed Hospital, and the Department of Pathology of the Army Medical School, Washington, D. C.

and then followed on its travels. B. prodigiosus has been considerably used along these lines, but it was soon found that this organism does not parasitize in the nose and throat and disappears a few hours after inoculation. A similar observation has been made by Bloomfield[2] in regard to a pigmented coccus. B. prodigiosus was also found to die on the hands in 10 to 20 minutes. Some further preliminary work was also done with Deneke's vibrio, a black mould, a red coccus, and an orange yeast, but none of these organisms were suitable. Finally, on account of the presence of a large number of throat carriers of hemolytic streptococci and the known viability of these organisms, it was decided to use them. Large numbers of streptococcus carriers were produced in camps in some way, and it was thought that a search for streptococci might throw some light on their epidemiology. The streptococci would also in a measure serve as indicators of the presence of sputum and salivary contamination in the same way that bacilli of the colon group serve as indicators of fecal contamination. Streptococci are not as suitable for this purpose as colon bacilli on account of the difficulty of enrichment, but they seemed the most suitable organisms available.

Some preliminary work was done to determine the length of time streptococci would persist on the hands. A specimen of sputum from a patient who was critically ill of pneumonia, freshly expectorated at 1:35 P.M. was collected in a sterile Petri dish. At 2:15 P.M. a bit of sputum (¼ c.c. to ½ c.c.) was rubbed into a piece of sterile gauze about the size of a handkerchief and the portion of the gauze thus moistened was rubbed over the palmar surface of the tips of all the fingers of O. T. The fingers were then thoroughly wiped with another piece of dry, sterile gauze. The amount of sputum upon the fingers must have been extremely small. At intervals one finger tip after the other was streaked over half the surface of a blood agar plate; the other half was streaked with a platinum loop. Examination of the plates gave the following results:

TABLE I

		NUMBER OF COLONIES OF HEMOLYTIC STREPTOCOCCI
Right hand—5th finger	At once	240
4th finger	½ hour	300
3rd finger	1 hour	187
2nd finger	1¾ hours	19
Left hand—5th finger	3 hours	15
4th finger	4 hours	27
3rd finger	5 hours	44
2nd finger	6 hours	59
1st finger	8 hours	13

These results show that a slight contamination of the hands is detectable for a number of hours. If natural contamination occurs to any great extent, it too should be detectable for some time. A similar experiment made with influenza bacilli in sputum showed that these organisms died in about three minutes. The criterion for hemolytic streptococci was the production of a hemolyzing colony which when picked to broth showed Gram-positive cocci in chains.

The work was carried out on troops of Sanitary Trains at Camp Meade. The throats and tonsils of 318 men were cultured for hemolytic streptococci, and

159, or 50 per cent, were found positive in varying degrees. An effort was then made to trace these organisms in carriers' hands and in their environment. As is well recognized, the crypts of the tonsils are the principal homes of hemolytic streptococci in carriers.[3] The saliva is infected from this source in varying degrees, according to circumstances. In one series of nine carriers the saliva was positive in only three. In another nine cases the saliva was positive in all.

EXAMINATION OF FINGERS

As a control, nine men with positive throat cultures rubbed the index finger back and forth on their lips and then streaked it on a part of a blood agar plate which was more fully spread with a platinum loop. Six of these plates showed colonies ranging from ten to many.

The fingers of carriers were examined in the middle of the morning, (1) by rubbing the index finger of the right hand over part of an agar plate and then spreading by a loop; (2) by washing the fingers in a small amount of salt solution and plating a few drops on agar plates. Out of 159 carriers examined in this way, 27, or 16.9 per cent were positive. More than half of these positive plates showed only a single colony and only five showed more than five colonies.

EXAMINATION OF DISH WATER

The next step was to examine dish water. Dish water was collected from 24 messes after the dinner dishes had been washed. The number of men in these messes ran from 30 to 300. The temperature was not sufficient to kill streptococci—averaging about 38°. One large drop was spread on a blood agar plate. None of these specimens showed any hemolytic streptococci. In eight messes lukewarm water without soap was used by request, and in one of these one colony of streptococci was found and in another two colonies. The antiseptic action of soap will be considered later. Scrapings from dish mop handles showed no streptococci.

HAND SHAKING

Several experiments were made to obtain evidence on the related problem of the importance of hand shaking in the spread of streptococci. (1) A bit of sputum of patient Reid, who was known to harbor hemolytic streptococci in his throat, was taken up on a piece of sterile gauze about the size of a handkerchief and rubbed well into the same. The moistened portion of the gauze was rubbed over the palmar surface of the fingers of O. T. and the fingers were immediately wiped dry with a fresh piece of sterile gauze. After an interval of 45 minutes O. T. shook hands once with McC., who then rubbed the side of his hand over the surface of a blood agar plate. A small sterile cotton swab was moistened with sterile saline, rubbed over the portion of McC.'s hand that came in contact with the fingers of O. T., and streaked over a blood agar plate.

	NUMBER OF COLONIES OF HEMOLYTIC STREPTOCOCCUS
Fingers of O. T. (control)	13
Side of hand McC. No. 1.	0
Side of hand McC. No. 2.	0
Swab	0

(2) A bit of the mixed sputum of Doyle and Clark was taken up on a piece of sterile gauze. The moistened portion of the gauze was rubbed over the palmar surfaces of the fingers of O. T. who twenty minutes later shook hands with McC.

	NUMBER OF COLONIES OF HEMOLYTIC STREPTOCOCCUS
Fingers of O. T. (control)	Numerous
Side of McC.'s hand No. 1.	1
Side of McC.'s hand No. 2.	2
Swab	0

(3) A bit of sputum of patient Meneice, convalescent from streptococcus pneumonia, was taken up on sterile gauze and the moistened portion of the gauze was rubbed over the palmar surface of the fingers of the right hand of O. T. Thirty minutes later O. T. shook hands once with McC.

	NUMBER OF COLONIES OF HEMOLYTIC STREPTOCOCCUS
Fingers of O. T. (control)	about 400
McC. side of hand No. 1.	1
McC. side of hand No. 2.	8
Swab	1

It will be seen from these experiments that few streptococci are transferred in handshaking, and that they reach a part of the hand which does not usually come in contact with the mouth.

POSSIBLE TRANSFER TO THE MOUTH

The final possible step of infecting the mouth from the hands was tested in the following way: Three men on duty in the laboratory of the Walter Reed Hospital volunteered for this experiment. Cultures from their nasopharynx, tonsils and nostrils were negative for hemolytic streptococci on three successive days before the experiment. The tonsils of the two men known to harbor hemolytic streptococci were swabbed and Majors Teague and Simmons and the three volunteers in turn rubbed the index finger over the swabs and immediately afterwards passed the same finger three or four times across the closed lips. The lips (or faces) were not washed during the next five or six hours. The nasopharynx, tonsils and nostrils of the volunteers were cultured almost daily for the next two weeks on blood agar plates; the cultures were negative for hemolytic streptococci.

It will thus be seen that so far as streptococcus carriers are concerned, according to this evidence, they must have been produced in some other way than by "mouth to hand and hand to mouth" method of transferring streptococci through the medium of dish water. Although the fingers can be intentionally contaminated with streptococci by saliva and although the organisms live on the fingers for hours, under ordinary circumstances few streptococci were found on the fingers, and none in the dish water, except when no soap was used. Furthermore, infection of the mouth from infected fingers is not as easy as might be supposed.

As the hand is more generally recognized as a method of spread of causes of intestinal diseases, comparative observations were made, using the colon bacillus group as an indicator of fecal contamination. In order to determine the amount of colon bacillus contamination of the hands of soldiers, 147 men of five field organizations were examined. The tips of the five fingers of the right hand were rubbed together in 5 c.c. of sterile salt solution in a sterile Petri dish, and 3 c.c. was planted in lactose broth fermentation tubes. The work was done indoors about the middle of the morning. After incubation for 48 hours over 20 per cent of gas was considered a presumptive test for the colon group. In a few instances complete identification of the colon group was made. Out of 143 men examined, 42, or 29.4 per cent were found positive. It was thus shown that nearly one-third of these men's fingers carried colon bacilli, presumably of intestinal origin.

The contamination of dish water was then looked into, with the following results:

TABLE II

	DISH WATER USED BY		TEMP.	COLON BACILLI IN		
				1 C.C.	FOUR DROPS	1/100 C.C.
1.	210 men		31	−	−	−
2.	250 "	Soapy	33	−	−	−
		Rinse	37			
3.	200 "	Soapy	36			
		Rinse	37	−	−	
4.	125 "	Soapy	35	+	+	
		Rinse	37	+	+	
5.	250 "	Soapy	31	+	−	
6.	91 "	Soapy	31	+		−
7.	140 "	Soapy	38	+	+	+
		Rinse	41	+	+	+

Table II shows the variation dependent on use of different quantities of water, but even in 1/100 c.c. colon bacilli were present in two out of eleven specimens. In order to compare the number of colon bacilli with that of streptococci more exactly, the following observations were made. The same amount of dish water, four drops, was plated on blood agar and put into lactose fermentation tubes with the results shown in Table III.

TABLE III

	DISH WATER USED BY		TEMP.	PLAIN AGAR COLONIES PER C.C.	BLOOD AGAR OTHER COLONIES H. S.	LACTOSE FERMENTATION TUBE COLON GROUP
1.	210 men	Dish water	31	550	36	0	0
2.	250 "	Wash "	33	3500	many	0	0
		Rinse "	37	40	4	0	0
3.	125 "	Wash "	35	1550	176	0	+
		Rinse '	37	2000	200	0	+
4.	250 "	Wash "	31	6300	338	0	0
5.	91 "	Wash "	31	290	23	0	0
6.	200 "	Wash "	31	900	199	0	0
		Rinse '	37	1500	113	0	0
7.	140 "	Wash "	38	3290	380	0	+
		Rinse "	41	720	290	0	+

In this work no streptococci were found in an amount which gave 4 out of 11 tests positive for colon bacillus.

These data on the colon bacilli show that bacteriologic evidence can easily be obtained to support the hypothesis that the fingers are concerned in the spread of intestinal diseases. Colon bacilli were found on the fingers and in dish water under conditions which showed no streptococci. The inference is that these two groups of organisms and the diseases for which they stand are spread in different ways.

II. The Antiseptic Action of Soap in Dish Water

The antiseptic action of soap in dish water has a direct bearing on the results given above. With the assistance of Captain Stimmel, S. C., a number of observations have been made on various soaps and on dish waters; the effect of different hydrogen-ion concentrations has been considered. Several of the soaps were obtained through the kindness of Mr. Powell of Armour Soap Works. The average strength of soap solution in army messes seems to be about 0.5 per cent, and this strength has been chiefly used in tap water; the organisms were added to a solution of this strength and 0.1 c.c. was spread on blood agar plates after various intervals. Table IV gives some of the typical results:

TABLE IV

SOAP	Organism	½	1	2	5	10	Control	P H	Temperature
Sodium Oleate (Armour)	B. Influenzæ	-	-	-	-	-	In*	8.7	Room
	Pneumococcus	-	-	-	-	-	In	"	"
	Streptococcus pyogenes	-	-	-	-	-	In	"	"
	S. Aureus	In	In	In	In	In	In		
	B. Typhosus	In	In	In	In	In	In		
Sodium Stearate (Merck)	B. Influenzæ	In	In	In	-	-	In	8.2	
	Pneumococcus	In	In	In	In	-	In		
	Streptococcus pyogenes	In	In	In	In	In	In		
	S. Aureus	In	In	In	In	In	In		
	B. Typhosus	In	In	In	In	In	In		
Sodium Resonate (Armour)	B. Influenzæ	-	-	-	-	-	In	8.2	
	Pneumococcus	-	-	-	-	-	In		
	Streptococcus pyogenes	-	-	-	-	-	In		
	S. Aureus	+	+	+	+	+	In		
	B. Typhosus	+	+	+	+	+	In		
Brown Soap (Camp Meade)	B. Influenzæ	-	-	-	-	-	In	8.7÷	
	Pneumococcus	-	-	-	-	-	In		
	Streptococcus pyogenes	++	+	15	-	-	In		
	S. Aureus	In	In	In	In	In	In		
	B. Typhosus	In	In	In	In	In	In		

*In = Innumerable.

The difference in effect of sodium oleate and sodium stearate is brought out, and more particularly the effect of ordinary brown soap, largely sodium resonate, such as is used in dish water in army messes. This soap reduced the number of streptococci from innumerable to 15 in two minutes. Hence, if any streptococci did get from the hands into the dish water they would have small chance to spread further, provided the dish water was soapy. On the other hand, none of the soaps tested killed the typhoid bacillus in 10 minutes. At low temperature, therefore, there is no barrier to the spread of intestinal organisms. The streptococci were killed whether the temperature was 38° or room temperature.

The point was raised by a sanitary inspector whether in a dirty dish water full of grease the antiseptic action might not be lost. To test this idea some boiled mutton fat was added to the soap, but no change occurred, either in reaction or in antiseptic effect. However, it was found that if the reaction of these soaps was changed from about 8.5 to 7 by the addition HCl, their antiseptic action was lost. This result is apparently due to precipitation of the soap from solution. Free alkali apparently plays no part in the antiseptic action as a NaOH solution of P_H 9.6 has no antiseptic effect. But an alkaline solution is necessary and the reading of the reaction of dish waters might be a valuable index for their suitability, as there is apparently enough acid in some dirty dishes to change the reaction and destroy the antiseptic effect. This is seen in the examination of two dish waters as shown in Table V.

TABLE V

SOLUTION	ORGANISM	TIME OF EXPOSURE IN MINUTES AND RESULTS						P_H	TEMP.
		1/2	1	3	5	10	CONTROL		ROOM
Dish Water 242 F.H. Before use	B. Influenzæ	20 colonies	–	–	–	–	In	8.7	
	Pneumococcus	–	–	–	–	–	In		
	Streptococcus pyogenes	18 col.	–	–	–	–	In		
	S. Aureus	In	In	In	In	In	In		
	B. Typhosus	In	In	In	+	+	In		
244 F.H. After use	B. Influenzæ	In	In	In	In	In	In	5.8	
	Pneumococcus	In	In	In	In	In	In		
	Streptococcus pyogenes	In	In	In	+	+	In		
	S. Aureus	In	In	In	In	In	In		
	B. Typhosus	In	In	In	In	In	In		

In the second case the reaction was 5.8 and no antiseptic action occurred. This was an especially dirty water which had been used by a large number of men.

It is well known that certain pure soaps are strongly antiseptic, while others are more or less inert. In general, as Lamar[4] has pointed out, chemical unsaturation, hemolytic activities, and antiseptic action go together. For example, sodium oleate, which in a low dilution kills streptococci rapidly, is hemolytic and chemically unsaturated. On the other hand, sodium stearate is made of a saturated fatty acid and is nonhemolytic and nonantiseptic in similar dilutions.

In addition certain soaps have selective action on certain kinds of bacteria and the possibility suggests itself of special soaps for killing special organisms or of a synthetic soap which will kill a number of different kinds of organisms. Commercial soaps are usually a more or less chance mixture of salts of different fatty acids, or other saponifiable substance, and are not built up from this point of view. Sodium oleate has been used in plates by Avery[5] to inhibit the action of other organisms of the nose and throat and to aid the growth of influenza bacilli. This action is definite in plates, but in solution the oleate seems to kill the influenza bacillus as well as the other organisms. Reasoner[6] has shown that soap solution from Ivory soap and shaving creams have a very rapid solvent effect on

T. pallidum. In case pure soaps are used, sodium oleate shows this effect to a marked degree, but with sodium stearate, very little effect even on motility can be observed after a number of minutes.

As bearing on the problem in hand, it will be seen that the streptococcus is quickly destroyed in the average soapy dish water at ordinary temperature, and it does not seem possible that the few that reach the dish water can survive to pass on to another person. The practical point emerges, however, that the reaction of the dish water should be kept at about a P_H of 8 or over, and that an acid dish water has no antiseptic effect. On the other hand, the ordinary dish washing in the army seems to offer no barrier to the spread of intestinal organisms, and a hot or boiling water is necessary to prevent the possible spread of these organisms.

III. THE DIRECT METHOD

As no bacteriologic data in support of the indirect method of spread of streptococci could be obtained, efforts were made to determine what evidence for the direct method could be obtained.

THE LENGTH OF TIME THAT DROPLETS REMAIN SUSPENDED IN THE AIR

Two men with inflamed throats which culture showed contained numerous hemolytic streptococci went into a quiet room and sprayed their saliva in all directions through partly closed lips for five minutes. They then left the room and a masked observer (T) exposed blood agar plates in sets of three on the floor in the middle of the floor for various periods as given in Table VI.

TABLE VI

LENGTH OF TIME AFTER SPRAYING	TIME OF EXPOSURE IN MINUTES	TOTAL COLONIES	NUMBER OF H. S.
15 min.	15	740	10
30 "	30	1730	8
45 "	30	420	7
60 "	30	310	3
1¼ hrs.	30	180	2
1½ "	30	48	0
2 "	60	130	2
2½ '	30	58	6
3 '	60	84	4
4 "	60	83	5

Thus at the end of four hours streptococci were still settling out of the air. In order to investigate actual conditions of the air, a ward was selected in which there were 20-30 patients, of whom 75 per cent were streptococcus carriers, or cases such as tonsillitis. After the patients had retired, blood agar plates were exposed for three hours on chairs at the foot of the beds. On twelve nights a total of 155 plates were exposed. Nineteen of these, or 12 per cent, were positive for hemolytic streptococci. Since one streptococcus colony was present for every 387 square inches of surface of plates exposed, and the floor space of the ward was about 162 square meters, it follows that about 4000 streptococci settled out of the air in three hours.

A number of other experiments were carried out on the relative size of droplets and other related subjects which will appear elsewhere.[8] As bearing on the so-called successful treatment of contagious diseases in the same ward without cross infection, the point is raised whether the patients are not usually received at hospitals after the very early stages which are probably the most contagious.

DISCUSSION

The interpretation which the writer puts on these data is that streptococcus carriers are not produced by contaminating their mouths with supposedly streptococcus laden dish water, but probably by inhalation. The evidence given above certainly favors this conclusion and if streptococci can be taken as indicators of respiratory organisms in general, the same conclusion holds good for them.

There is of course a large literature on this subject. In place of reviewing this literature and attempting to evaluate it, the writer believes it is more advisable at present to make fresh observations at different angles and to record them for what they are worth.

These data are subject to several limitations. The number of streptococci in carriers may be much less than the number of organisms in the watery discharges of the early stages of respiratory diseases. However, the results would still hold good for streptococcus carriers. Again in the comparison of streptococci and colon bacilli, it is to be remembered that only 50 per cent of the men carried streptococci, some in small numbers, while 100 per cent of persons carry large numbers of colon bacilli. On the other hand, the chances of hand contamination with streptococci are more frequent than with colon bacilli.

More observations can be made to advantage along the same lines and more attention could be paid to the possibility of the presence of agricultural colon bacilli and of streptococci from the stools or air, but it is not believed that more detailed work will materially alter the results.

In regard to the actual program proposed of using boiling wash and rinse water, while it is not believed that this measure will reduce the incidence of respiratory diseases, this work shows the desirability of this measure as a preventative of the spread of intestinal diseases. The necessity for the presence of a sufficient amount of good soap is also emphasized.

If the specific causes of respiratory diseases are spread principally by inhalation, more constant attention must be paid to sanitation (ventilation) and personal hygiene, and the route of spread can frequently be broken. However, in the army, there is a point beyond which such measures can not go. There are times when soldiers must train and fight in common, in spite of the presence of pathogenic organisms in the air. A certain amount of sickness and death from this source is to be counted on, unless the troops have some immunity from previous exposure or unless they can be immunized with specific vaccines.

SUMMARY

1. Hemolytic streptococci were used as test organisms in collecting data on the possible routes of spread of the specific causes of respiratory diseases.

2. No evidence was found to support the theory that these organisms spread through dish water.

(a) Fingers of only 17 per cent of carriers showed streptococci, and only in small numbers.

(b) Dish water showed no streptococci except when no soap was used.

(c) Infection of the mouth did not occur when streptococci were smeared on the lips.

(d) Soapy dish water is antiseptic for streptococci if of proper reaction and made with proper soap.

3. Evidence was found that intestinal organisms can spread through dish water.

(a) Colon bacilli were found on hands of nearly one-third of troops.

(b) They were found in dish water down to 1/100 of a c.c. in some cases.

(c) Soapy dish water has no antiseptic action on colon bacilli.

4. Evidence was also found to support the inhalation theory.

(a) Droplets with streptococci remain suspended for several hours.

(b) The air of streptococcus wards contains streptococci for several hours after men have retired.

5. The use of boiling dish and rinse water is indicated not to prevent spread of respiratory diseases, but to prevent spread of intestinal diseases.

REFERENCES

[1]Lynch and Cumming: Am. Jour. Pub. Health, January, 1919. Military Surgeon, 920,1 xlvi, 150.
[2]Bloomfield, A. L.: Bull. Johns Hopkins Hosp., 1919, xxx. 317.
[3]Nichols and Byran: Jour. Am. Med. Assn., 1918, lxxi. 1813.
[4]Lamar, R. V.: Jour. Exper. Med., 1911, xiii, 1. 374; ibid., xiv. 256.
[5]Avery: Jour. Am. Med. Assn., 1918, lxx, 2050.
[6]Reasoner: Jour. Am. Med. Assn., 1917, lxviii, 73.
[7]Nichols: Ann. Otol., Rhin. and Laryngol., June, 1919.
[8]Teague, O.: Phil. Jour. S., 1912, vii, 137, 157, 255; ibid., viii, 241, Jour. Infect. Dis., 1913, xii, 398.

CHRONIC POISONING FROM HYDROCYANIC ACID

By C. I. REED, A.B., LAWRENCE, KANSAS

A SURVEY of the literature on cyanide poisoning reveals a considerable difference of opinion as to the existence of chronic symptoms in the event of recovery. There has existed a belief that if cyanide poisoning does not produce death within a few hours, there is eventual recovery without any chronic symptoms. It is the purpose of this paper to present a few experimental results on this point.

The greater majority of reports of cyanide poisoning credit patients with complete recovery with no chronic symptoms. Cohen[1] reports a severe case of accidental poisoning from potassium cyanide with complete recovery in a few hours with no chronic symptoms. Wilkes[2] describes the case of a druggist who absorbed hydrocyanic acid through a cut in the thumb, and as a result suffered very severe symptoms for a time but had completely recovered by the next day and subsequently showed no chronic symptoms. Numerous other reports follow a similar history.

On the other hand, Souwers[3] reports having examined a photographer who repeatedly was exposed to a solution of potassium cyanide in the course of his work and who exhibited listlessness, sleeplessness, lumbar pain, loss of appetite, nausea, constipation, chills, dyspnea and slowed pulse. These symptoms abated in a few days after ceasing work but returned on resumption of his occupation. Boddaert[4] observed a man poisoned by habitually eating bread rolls containing extract of bitter almonds, and after some weeks exhibited general lassitude, mental depression, muscular pain and weakness, rise of temperature, slowed pulse and increased susceptibility. (This author does not state how this last manifestation was determined, but one infers that the subject exhibited more severe symptoms on resumption of the habitual diet.) No albuminuria was found. The patient recovered in a few days after changing his diet.

Collins and Martland[5] report peripheral neuritis with eventual recovery as a result of repeated exposure to a solution of hydrocyanic acid of unknown concentration, used by a dishwasher for brightening silverware. Schlegel[6] found experimentally that repeated administration of sublethal doses of cyanides produced chronic cachexia without increased susceptibility.

Koritschöner[7] attempted to treat tuberculous patients with repeated exposures to hydrocyanic acid. Twenty men and ten women were exposed to varying concentrations of the gas every day for six weeks. Seven patients showed chronic intoxication, pharyngeal congestion, itching, salivation, frequent vomiting, progressive decrease in pulse rate, lassitude and drowsiness and finally albuminuria. These symptoms abated in from three to five days after discontinuance of the treatment, but returned upon its resumption.

Twenty patients showed some fever which gradually diminished as the treatment progressed, indicating some degree of tolerance. Pulse and respiratory

* From the Department of Physiology, University of Kansas, Lawrence, Kansas.

rates decreased progressively. Hemoglobin and red cells remained normal. Twenty patients gained weight during the first three weeks, the others losing progressively, but rapidly regaining upon cessation of the treatment. The only symptom constantly noted during exposure was coughing.

This report of pharyngeal congestion constitutes the only instance found in the literature examined of anatomic changes in the respiratory tract resulting from the more common cyanides, though Winternitz[8] states that halogen cyanides produce pulmonary edema and congestion which is quite persistent, but this is evidently due to the halogen radicle.

More recently Fühner[9] has made a rather exhaustive study of chronic cyanide poisoning in connection with the use of hydrocyanic acid vapor as a germicide. He describes the symptoms of acute poisoning as consisting of salivation, metallic taste in the mouth, petechiae on the tongue, reddening of the forehead, general weakness, lowered blood pressure, thoracic muscular pains, general malaise, and vomiting. He further inclines to the view that repeated doses do not produce chronic poisoning but *may* increase susceptibility.

In consideration of this conflicting evidence a few experimental results are here presented. Seven dogs were exposed under constant conditions in an airtight chamber, to sublethal concentrations of hydrocyanic acid vapor, eight times during a pediod of ten days for periods varying from fifteen minutes to two hours.

During exposure, nausea, vomiting, defecation, and urination were constant manifestations, while occasionally there occurred prostration from respiratory paralysis, always with recovery. Respiratory rates were usually increased temporarily and in case of any approach to paralysis, heart rates were increased also but in all cases where the animals remained quiet during exposure there were no changes in either respiratory or pulse rates.

During this period the animals lost from 2 per cent to 11 per cent of total body weight. But most of this loss occurred from the third to the fifth days with no marked change thereafter, while two gained slightly during the remainder of the period. It is also of interest that the two dogs showing the greatest loss of weight did not show any marked symptoms at any time during the exposure except salivation. These facts indicate that, either the loss in weight was due to some unrecognized factor or that there was developed a certain degree of tolerance. Contrary to Fühner's results, there was no evidence of increased susceptibility.

The four dogs showing the greatest loss in weight also underwent progressive decrease in heart rate except a slight transient increase when examined after exposure. There was no marked change in heart rate among the other three. None showed marked cardiac irregularity. Autopsies revealed absolutely normal conditions of the lungs and respiratory tract.

It is regretted that the peculiar conditions under which the experiments were conducted precluded a more detailed study, but the results presented include the more marked gross manifestations. It was not possible to study the metabolism rates or to make any neurologic examinations.

CONCLUSIONS

These results check fairly well with the clinical reports cited, and from the sum total of evidence, it may be concluded that chronic symptoms occur only on repeated exposure, a severe exposure that is not fatal producing no chronic symptoms.

Long exposures to very low concentrations may produce symptoms of poisoning.

According to experimental results there were no manifestations of increased susceptibility but on the contrary some indication of a certain degree of tolerance.

There are no marked anatomic changes that can account for the symptoms; a longer period of treatment may produce changes in the nervous system.

Symptoms of chronic poisoning are those ordinarily associated with general cachexia.

Individual susceptibilities vary over a wide range.

REFERENCES

[1]Cohen: Cited in editorial, Brit. Med. Jour., 1916, p. 464.
[2]Wilkes: Lancet, London, ii, p. 1058.
[3]Souwers: Philadelphia Med. Times, April 27, 1879.
[4]Boddaert: Ann. de la Soc. de Med. Leg. de Belgique, 1897-99. ix-x, p. 238.
[5]Collins and Martland: Jour. Nerv. and Ment. Dis., July, 1908, xxv, No. 17, p. 417.
[6]Schlegel: Inaug. Addr., Berlin, 1891, Cited by Sollman.
[7]Koritschöner: Wien. klin. Wchnschr., 1891, No. 4, p. 91.
[8]Winternitz: Mil. Surgeon, May, 1919.
[9]Führner: Deutsch. med. Wchnschr., 1919, lxv, No. 31, p. 847-850.

INDICANURIA AND ACETONURIA OF GASTROINTESTINAL ORIGIN*

By Eric R. Wilson, A.B., Los Angeles, Cal.

THE analyses of seventy-five specimens of urine of individuals in supposedly normal health on what they considered an average normal diet (the average intake of protein was on questioning found to be high) showed an indicanuria associated with an acetonuria in thirty-six out of the seventy-five specimens examined.

In all cases the urines examined were free from albumin and sugar.

Those specimens showing an indicanuria and acetonuria were all of higher specific gravity and deeper color than the normal urines. Five of the thirty-six cases showed a more or less persistent acetonuria even after the indicanuria had been cleared up by liberal catharsis and diet, extending over a period of from five to thirty-one days.

Each cell shows the three tests in order: ACETONE / DI-ACETIC / INDICAN.

CASE	DAY 1	2	3	4	5	7	14	21	27	31	33
1	+ 0 +	+ 0 +	+ 0 0	+ 0 0	+ 0 0	× 0 0	0 0 0				
2	+ 0 +	+ 0 0	+ 0 0	× 0 0	0 0 0						
3	+ 0 +	+ 0 +	+ 0 0	+ 0 0	+ 0 0	+ 0 0	× 0 0	0 0 0			
4	+ + +	+ + +	+ + 0	+ + 0	+ + 0	+ + 0	+ 0 0	+ 0 0	+ 0 0	× 0 0	0 0 0
5	+ + +	+ + +	+ 0 0	+ 0 0	+ 0 0	+ 0 0	+ 0 0	× 0 0	0 0 0		

+ Positive.
0 Negative.
× Suspicious.

As will be noticed from the above table, three out of the five cases which showed an acetonuria of longer duration than any of the other thirty-six cases cleared up nicely within fourteen days under the administration of alkalies and a somewhat restricted protein diet, while two of the cases seemed to resist treatment. In one case the acetonuria lasted up to the twenty-first day from the time when acetone was first noticed in the urine. The other and most persistent case of this series showed an acetonuria extending over a period of thirty-one days before it cleared up.

It was demonstrated that a prolonged acetonuria, as we believe of gastrointestinal origin, showed a decreased carbon dioxide combining power of the blood plasma. The Van Slyke apparatus and technic were used for this determination.

It was also noticed that in the last two above-mentioned cases the coagulation time of the blood was materially increased from one to three minutes above normal.

The following tests and technic were used.

Acetone: To 10 c.c. of urine in a test tube add about one gram of ammonium sulphate, 2 to 3 drops of a freshly prepared 5 per cent solution of sodium

*From the Department of Pathology, Bacteriology and Laboratory Diagnosis, College of Physicians and Surgeons, University of Southern California, Los Angeles, Cal.

nitroprusside, and 2 c.c. of concentrated ammonium hydroxide which may be stratified or poured on the mixture. The presence of acetone is indicated by the slow development of a permanganate color. The delicacy of this reaction is 1 to 20,000.

Diacetic acid: Arnold's test. Two solutions are kept in stock. One is a 1 per cent aqueous solution of para-amido-acetophenon with 2 c.c. of strong hydrochloric acid in each 100 c.c. of the mixture; the other is a 1 per cent solution of potassium or sodium nitrite. Two parts of the first and one of the second solution are mixed together in a test tube and an equal bulk of urine added, and finally a drop of strong ammonium hydrate. A brown color usually appears in normal urines, but on the addition of several drops of strong hydrochloric acid the color changes to yellow while in a urine containing diacetic acid a purple color develops. Normal urines may show a red color as well as those containing very slight traces of diacetic acid, on shaking, however, the foam will show a violet color when small amounts of diacetic acid are present. This point is particularly emphasized by Waldvogel.

Indican: Obermayer's test. To 10 c.c. faintly acid urine in a test tube add an equal volume of Obermayer's reagent, and about 3 c.c. to 5 c.c. of chloroform. Place the thumb over the mouth of the tube and shake vigorously. On standing a few moments the chloroform will settle and it will assume a blue color, if indican is present. The intensity of the color will vary with the amount of indigo blue which has been brought into solution by the chloroform. Normally, the chloroform should assume only a faint blue color. In other words, normal urine contains a trace of indican.

Bacterial digestion of protein in the intestinal tract is of material pathologic significance, and the one in which we are particulrly interested is that of Tryptophane.

Ten c.c. of a solution of 1% mixture of amino acids with tryptophane predominating in quantity plus five grams of sodium chloride to 1000 c.c. of the mixture was inoculated with 3 loopfuls of a thirty-six hour pure culture of B. coli. Incubated at $37\frac{1}{2}°$ C. for 24 hours at the end of which time the mixture was filtered through two lavers of filter paper and tested for diacetic acid by the Arnold test.
Results: Showed traces of diacetic acid. Showed positive for indole.

Under anaerobic conditions the intestinal bacteria have in general the power of splitting off the amino group, whereas under aerobic conditions they split off the carboxyl group. Under one, the other, or both of these conditions the protein molecule is broken down into more or less toxic substances; viz., indol and skatol, which are partly absorbed by the blood stream as such and their toxicity removed by their combination with sulphuric acid to form sulphates. The aromatic sulphates further combined with the potassium to form ethereal sulphates and as such are excreted in the urine. In the case of tryptophane by the combined action of bacteria it is probably converted into indol-proprionic acid, thence to indol-acetic acid and finally indol and skatol, this is then oxidized, converting these substances into indoxyl and skatoxyl. The indoxyl is excreted in the urine as potassium-indoxyl-sulphate. The indol which is not thus absorbed is excreted by the feces.

It is very probable, therefore, that at a point between the formation of indol-acetic acid and indol and skatol there occurs a process by which diacetic acid is formed and absorbed as such by the blood. The addition of acids to the blood causes their immediate neutralization by one of the buffer salts of the blood, namely, the $NaHCO_3$ and the protein. The buffer substances in the corpuscles may also share in this neutralization of the acid. During this process, however, two important points are to be observed—the appearance of the acid ions and their rate of elimination. It is possible that where an acetonuria has existed or been in progress for any length of time the tissues may develop an abnormal affinity for the H ions, and such we believe, often to be the case.

This affinity would undoubtedly be increased in cases where, for some reason or other, the kidney function has been impaired and elimination delayed, and resist to a greater degree the average therapeutic measures employed in combating an acidosis.

We have lately observed an acetonuria existing with a pronounced indicanuria in colitis, ileo-colitis, and in both staphylococcic and streptococcic cellulitis.

To just what extent, however, an acetonuria of gastrointestinal origin might progress and the effect it would have on the organism as a whole if allowed to continue untreated for any length of time, we are not prepared to say, but we believe that this condition exists and is far commoner than is usually observed.

BIBLIOGRAPHY

Fleescher, E. C.: Calif. State Med. Jour., xi.
Gradwohl and Blaivas: Blood and Urine Chemistry, St. Louis, C. V. Mosby Co., 1917, pp. 59-75, 104-106.
Macleod, J. J. R.: Physiology and Biochemistry in Modern Medicine, St. Louis, C. V Mosby Co., 1918, pp. 499-503. 632, 633.
Matthews, A. P.: Physiological Chemistry, New York, Wm. Wood & Co., pp. 743-748.
Monographic Medicine, New York, D. Appleton Co., 1918, i, 198, 200, 291, 300.
Whitney, J. L.: Arch. Int. Med., 1917, xx.
Wood, F. C.: Chemical and Microscopic Diagnosis, New York, D. Appleton & Co., 1918, p. 553.

ARSPHENAMINE AND NEOARSPHENAMINE

By Wm. A. Smith, Springfield, Ill.

ARSPHENAMINE and neoarsphenamine are two of the most important and most discussed therapeutic agents of the present day. They are striking examples of that newer type of therapy known as chemotherapy, to which we look for great possibilities in the future, in the treatment of infectious diseases. Since there are many phases to this subject, I shall not attempt a complete discussion, but shall limit myself to the main facts in current literature. It might be interesting first to consider briefly the origin and the present supply of these compounds.

ORIGIN

Before the discovery of the causative agent of syphilis, atoxyl was being used in the treatment of trypanosomiasis. Atoxyl is an organic arsenic compound (sodium salt of paraamidophenylarsenic acid) which was introduced by Thomas. When in 1905, Schaudinn discovered that a spirochete was the cause of syphilis, and since the spirochete is closely related to the trypanosomes, atoxyl was promptly taken up in the treatment of syphilis. This was followed in many cases by dangerous reactions in the body, especially blindness. Moreover Paul Ehrlich[1] showed that atoxyl was relatively inactive in the test tube, and he concluded that the atoxyl became a parasiticide in the tissues. This change he thought to be due to reduction of the arsenic from a pentavalent to a trivalent form. This lead him to experiment with allied arsenic compounds. In 1910[2] he succeeded in producing a compound, which was most toxic to the parasite, and least toxic to the human body—combining extreme parasitotropism with a low organotropism. He called this compound salvarsan, but it also became well known as "606," which was his diary number for arsenic compounds. Previous to 1914, all salvarsan came from the Farbwerke-Hoechst Co. of Frankfurt, Germany, where it was made under the supervision of Paul Ehrlich. This firm was protected both by product and process patents. Neosalvarsan, also known as "914" was introduced later; this is a derivative of salvarsan, and in some respects is a more efficient remedy. It also was made only by the above German firm. As a result, the products on the market were fairly uniform in their composition and properties.

PRESENT SUPPLY

During the war, shipments were stopped, and the supply in the United States was exhausted in 1915. Patent protection was withdrawn in the allied countries, and firms in England, France, Japan, and Canada began to manufacture these compounds. After the United States entered the war, the Adamson Bill was passed, granting citizens the right to operate patents owned by enemy aliens. The result was that several products were placed on the market, varying both in their chemical and their physiologic properties. It became necessary to exercise precaution in granting licenses to manufacture these products; for this reason the U. S. Public Health Service defined the properties of good preparations, and the

Federal Trade Commission formulated rules and toxicity tests which must be complied with, or the license of the manufacturer may be revoked. The firms[3] licensed at present are:

The Dermatological Research Laboratories, Philadelphia Polyclinic, whose products are called arsphenamine and neoarsphenamine.

The Takamine Laboratory Co., Inc., New York City, whose products are called arsaminol and neoarsaminol.

The Farbwerke-Hoechst Co., New York City, (at H. A. Metz Laboratories Inc.) whose products are called salvarsan and neosalvarsan.

The Diarsenol Co., Buffalo, N. Y., (Synthetic Drug Co., Toronto, Canada), whose products are known as diarsenol and neodiarsenol.

The product of the Dermatological Research Laboratory was known as Arsenobenzol, and was found to be identical with salvarsan in composition and equal to it therapeutically, by the council on Pharmacy and Chemistry of the A. M. A. Pollitzer[4] even claimed it to be superior to the imported product. This product was made under the direction of Dr. Schamberg, and was the first made in this country.

RULES FOR MANUFACTURE

On March 4, 1918,[3] the Federal Trade Commission adopted certain rules for the manufacture of these products; chief among these are the following:

1. These products are to be named and labeled arsphenamine and neoarsphenamine respectively. (Arsphenamine was also previously called arsphenolamine hydrochloride.)

2. The products are to be sold only in colorless glass ampules, containing an atmosphere of an inert gas.

3. The arsenic content of arsphenamine must be between 29.5 and 31.57 per cent.

4. The arsenic content of neoarsphenamine must be between 18 and 20 per cent.

5. Each lot must be tested for its arsenic content and toxicity.

6. For toxicity tests,[5] at least four or five albino rats are to be used—non-pregnant—weighing 100-150 grams. A 2 per cent solution of neutralized arsphenamine in doses not less than 80 mg. per kg. body weight is injected. It is required that 60 per cent of the animals injected survive at least forty-eight hours. Animals are not to be anesthetized for injection and if more than one rat dies, tests are to be repeated. Special rules are given for feeding and caring for the animals used. Tests are also made on samples submitted, by the U. S. Public Health Service. The Federal Trade Commission can withdraw from the market any lot designated. Detailed records of the tests for each lot are to be kept, and furnished to the Federal Trade Commission.

The maxium tolerated dose of neoarsphenamine must be not below 90 mg. per kg. body weight, with injection of a 2 per cent aqueous solution, intravenously, at the rate of 0.5 c.c. per minute.

Such restrictions have done a great deal to make the products on the market safe for use and have undoubtedly reduced the number of unfavorable reactions following injection.

CHEMISTRY

These products are derivatives of arsenobenzene.

Arsphenamine.[7] Its formula is $C_{12}H_{12}.O_2N_2As_2 .2HCl$

$$CIH.H_2N\underset{OH}{\overset{As==As}{\hexagon}}\quad\underset{OH}{\hexagon}NH_2.HCl$$

Arsphenamine; or dihydroxy diamino arsenobenzene hydrochloride; or para-diamido dioxy arseno-benzol hydrochloride; or 3 diamino 4 dihydroxyl -1 arseno-benzene hydrochloride.

It is prepared from parahydroxy phenylarsenic acid, which is·

$$HO<\text{====}>AsO(OH)_2$$

(a) By addition of nitric and sulphuric acids obtaining a mono-nitro compound—the nitro group being, ortho to the OH group;

$$HO<\overset{NO_2\quad NO_2}{\text{=========}}>As.O.(OH)_2$$

(b) then by reduction with caustic soda, sodium hydrosulphite and magnesium chloride producing arsphenamine. Two molecules of nitro compound produce one molecule of arsphenamine.

Among the reactions are the following:[7]

1. There is no effect with dilute mineral acids (except sulphuric)—unlike neoarsphenamine.

2. With dilute sulphuric acid a yellow precipitate is formed.

3. Concentrated mineral acids (except phosphoric) form a precipitate; in the case of nitric acid, the precipitate dissolves in excess, forming a red solution.

4. Carbon dioxide immediately precipitates arsphenamine from aqueous solutions.

5. Sodium hydroxide forms a precipitate, dissolving in excess.

6. Oxidizing agents as chlorine or bromine water or ferric chloride cause an aqueous solution to become red. (Same as neoarsphenamine.)

7. There are no inorganic arsenic compounds in pure arsphenamine, (or neoarsphenamine) which may be shown by obtaining no precipitate on addition of hydrogen sulphide gas to an aqueous solution. The molecular combination seems to prevent arsenic from combining with the tissues, preventing arsenical poisoning.

Neoarsphenamine.[7] Its formula is

$$NH_2\ OH\ C_6H_3\ As : AsC_6H_3\ OH\ NH(CH_2O)\ OSNa$$

$$H_2N\underset{OH}{\overset{As==As}{\hexagon}}\quad\underset{OH}{\hexagon}NH-CH_2-SO_2.Na$$

Neoarsphenamine, or Sodium 3 diamino 4 dihydroxy-1-arsenobenzene methanal sulphoxylate.

It is prepared by addition of an aqueous solution of sodium methanal sulphoxylate to an aqueous solution of arsphenamine; a precipitate forms, which dissolves in sodium carbonate to form neoarsphenamine.

Among the reactions distinguishing it from arsphenamine, are these [9]

1. Dilute and concentrated mineral acids cause precipitation.
2. Acetic acid, and heat, forms a yellow precipitate, unlike arsphenamine.
3. No precipitate forms with NaOH.

PHYSICAL PROPERTIES[8]

Arsphenamine	*Neoarsphenamine*
A Pale Yellow-microcrystalline hygroscopic powder.	An Orange-yellow, microcrystalline powder, changes to brown in the air.
unstable in the air.	odorless.
odorless.	taste--like garlic.
taste—sour.	Soluble in H_2O, and glycerin (only slightly in alcohol).
Soluble in H_2O, ethyl and methyl alcohol.	
The aqueous solution is greenish yellow and strongly acid to litmus.	The aqueous solution is neutral and yellow, turning brown on exposure to the air.

TECHNIC OF ADMINISTRATION

The preparation of arsphenamine solution is more complicated than neoarsphenamine, as it must be neutralized before injection. The drug is dissolved in cold water, freshly boiled and distilled (hot water is used in the "arsenobenzol" brand) ; this acid solution is then neutralized with 15 per cent NaOH[8]-0.9 c.c. for each 0.1 g. of drug and diluted so as to give a solution containing 0.1 ($\frac{1}{10}$) gram arsphenamine to 30 c.c. of final solution (McCoy[9]). Schamberg[10] states that dilution should be as much as 120 c.c. of water for each 0.6 gm. Guy[11] believes that dilution should be at least 0.1 gram to 15 c.c. of solution. Dilution with freshly distilled water is considered an essential point; to avoid untoward reactions. Injection of the acid solution is very painful and is also responsible for cases of toxicity, so neutralization is important. The solution should always be filtered through sterile cotton to avoid introducing solid particles into the blood.

Authorities agree that the time of injection should be relatively long. Guy[11] states that a dose that may be well borne by animals, when given slowly for 15 minutes, may be fatal when injected in one minute. McCoy[9] states that 2 minutes should be allowed for each 0.1 gm. (30c.c.) injected; thus for an injection of 30- 180 c.c., 2 to 12 minutes would be required. This makes it possible to stop the injection at any moment, if immediate reactions develop. At least on first injections, Bory[12] injects only 1 c.c., then waits 15 seconds and repeats.

Before using any specimen, the ampule should be immersed in 95 per cent alcohol for 15 minutes to detect apertures and cracks.[9] This is because the compound is unstable and easily oxidized by the air. If a breach is discovered, the contents of the ampule are to be discarded.

The gravity method of injection is used in preference to the piston syringe, with more safety to the patient. The drug is administered intramuscularly and intravenously. At first it was given intramuscularly by most physicians, and Leonard[13] still favors this method. The best site for this is at the buttocks. Most writers favor the intravenous method; it is less painful and more efficient. In treating syphilis of the nervous system it has been found helpful to withdraw at the same time a portion of the spinal fluid, so that the drug will reach the nervous system more quickly.

The technic of administering neoarsphenamine differs from that of arsphenamine in several respects. It is more soluble, and gives a neutral solution. Only one ampule should be dissolved at a time, after being tested for cracks, as neoarsphenamine is even more unstable than arsphenamine. Cold, freshly distilled water should be used. McCoy[9] believes 2 c.c. water to each 0.1 gm. of drug should be used. This compound may be injected in a piston syringe, using a very small needle. The injection may be more rapid, McCoy stating that it should be done in not less than 5 minutes, however.

Neoarsphenamine[10] should never be administered unless the solution is brilliantly clear; cloudy solutions produce immediate reactions with syncope a dominant symptom. This action seems to be mechanical.

REACTIONS AND THEIR CAUSE

Unfortunately, the use of these compounds has often been followed by serious reactions, and in a few instances by death. The causes of the reactions have been attributed to different factors in different cases. These are classified by Guy as due to drug toxicity, errors of technic, and a peculiarity of the patient. Some reactions were thought by Danysz to be due to a precipitation of arsphenamine base in the blood stream, owing to the carbonic acid present, since the amount of acid in the blood has a definite relation to the number and severity of reactions. Danysz[11] recommends small initial injections to vaccinate against reactions, by increasing the amount of organic bases in the blood. But this may produce a resistant strain of spirochete, blocking the treatment. It also means a loss of time. Herxheimer reactions have followed small injections, so Danysz's theory is not accepted (Guy). Some cases are due to oxidized products of arsphenamine, which are toxic. Thus ampules should be tested for leaks, and solutions should only be used soon after preparation. Chemically pure NaOH and freshly distilled water are essential.[3] Water containing much Ca and Mg causes more reactions than otherwise. Incomplete neutralization of arsphenamine solutions have accounted for more avoidable reactions than almost any other factor (Pollitzer).[4] The acid solution is 50 to 60 per cent more toxic than the alkaline. Filtration will prevent solid particles from getting into the blood.[5] Different brands of the drug vary in toxicity, and one should observe the directions of the manufacturer of that particular brand being used.[6] Minor reactions might be due to the fact that the lot *just* managed to pass the toxicity requirement. Some reactions are thought to be due to the destruction of enormous numbers of spirochetes, liberating the protein of their bodies in the blood stream and producing anaphylactic reactions. Guy[11] states that Herxheimer reactions are due to the stimulating activity of nonsterilizing doses, and are avoided by a full therapeutic dose. He believes that all other sources must be eliminated before attributing the cause to the drug. Vasomotor reactions occur often while injecting the drug, and these may be controlled by epinephrin, and the injection continued. Guy[11] reports three cases of thrombophlebitis due probably to infiltration of the drug between the coats of vessels. There was pain and tenderness along the course of the swollen and thrombosed vein, with a febrile reaction lasting for 10 to 20 days. The cases recovered, but the hardened and sclerotic vein persisted.

Auer[14] has shown that toxicity is inversely proportional to the acidity and concentration. Either because of the acidity of the injected arsphenamine or because of the increased protein content of the blood of certain syphilitics, an intravascular precipitate forms. This was shown by the fact that the serum of patients contained a substance, which precipitated with arsphenamine *in vitro;* this also probably occurs *in vivo*—causing the symptoms by subsequent vasodilatation, which is controllable by subcutaneous injections of epinephrin (Berman). Some of the symptoms appearing during injection are congestion and swelling of the face, or cyanosis of the face and congestion of the head, oppression of the chest, cough, dyspnea, and pain in the back. These may disappear when the injection is stopped. It has been stated[15] that arsphenamine and neoarsphenamine lead to reduction of the chromaffin tissue in the adrenals, hence to a less epinephrin content in the gland and in the blood—a selective action on the adrenals. Milian[16] objects to giving epinephrin in all cases, as this deprives the physician of a guide to the tolerance of the patient, and there is danger of giving too large a dose. Headache following injection may not be due to toxicity, but lacrimation, watery nasal discharge, and excessive secretion of saliva are signs of an impending "nitritoid crisis" or serous apoplexy. The temperature is a very reliable guide. If it rises above 100.4° F, Milian[16] states it is a sign of marked intolerance, and if it occurs after each dose, the drug should be discontinued. Jackson and Smith[17] recommend the use of tyramin in place of epinephrin as there is less danger of acute heart dilatation and the blood pressure does not rise so high. The effect with tyramin is also more lasting. Toxicity is not due to intermediate products in the manufacture of the drugs, as the Hygienic Laboratory of the U. S. Public Health Service tested these and found them nonpoisonous. These reactions may develop severely in suprarenal conditions (Addison's disease) or a thymolymphatic constitution. Hirano[18] states that the serum of animals injected with arsphenamine or neoarsphenamine contained less vasocontractile substance than normal serum; the content of both adrenals was decreased, the deficiency not being restored. Rieger states that toxic products may arise in the ampule.[19] He believes that arsphenamine insufficiently dried, in six months may develop toxic by-products in the ampule, the amount varying with the time before use. These specimens may pass the biologic test at the time manufactured, and later produce these toxic products. In one specimen, for example, the ampule was sound, but the contents gave a solution of a gun-metal tinge—due to oxidation. (Arsphenamine will shed metallic arsenic when oxidized.) Arsphenamine, after being dried for two hours, contains about 7 per cent methyl alcohol. This alcohol may act on the base in the ampule and methyl arsin accumulate. This injected, will cause nitritoid reactions, even cardiac paralysis may result. Neoarsphenamine, made without the use of methyl alcohol does not have this danger. Some reactions have been clearly due, then, to the drug itself.

Of reactions due to technic, most of the causes have been mentioned. Mauv injections were made too rapidly, too large doses were given, and solutions were incompletely neutralized. Nelkin[20] objects to such high dilution of the drug. He uses 0.6 gm. to 20 c.c. of water and reports no untoward effects. He states that a slow injection is required when a large quantity is given, but otherwise not. He also uses the syringe method, which is more simple and time saving. Guy thinks that injection of a solution too cold accounts for some reactions. Others are due to improper preparation of the patient. He reports 80 cases in all stages of infection, injected without preparation and all developed gastrointestinal reactions. This preparation should include: urinalysis—for evidence of kidney irritation, (one case of death, showed an acute diffuse hemorrhagic nephritis.) A cathartic should be given the evening before, very little food given, and the patient should remain quiet after the injection. All reactions can not be avoided by fixed rules of technic, as no case falls in any well-defined group. Thus different workers have had success with different methods.

Even with the best technic and a comparatively nontoxic drug, reactions will occur, which have their origin in the patient. Guy cites 40 cases in which reactions were due to aggravation of nonsyphilitic pathologic conditions, as bronchitis, bronchopneumonia, and icterus. He also cites two cases due to idiosyncrasy, in which the symptoms were gastrointestinal with signs of prostration. In some cases, the reaction was delayed; injection was followed by no effects up to the fourth day. There was greater prostration in these cases. Reactions are not due to sensitization,[14] since attempts to experimentally sensitize guinea pigs have failed; also because the effects are produced with *one* injection. Incompetent renal, hepatic or pulmonary functions account for many reactions, where the relative functional integrity of organs is upset. If the temperature of a patient is elevated he will not take the drug well. The status of the infection is thought also to influence the reactions. Among the reactions reported, are these:

Neurorecurrence, by Jacobsen,[21] and Berner.[22]

Arsenical eclampsia, by Bory.[12]

Toxic dermatitis, by Nelkin.[20]

Hemorrhagic purpura, by Labbè and Langlois.[23]

(They state that bleeding of gums and nose, and patches of purpura should warn one to stop the treatment.)

Gangrene of the fingers, by Stutter.[24]

Jaundice, by Nagai.[25]

Exfoliative dermatitis with gangrene of toes, by Jones[26]—due to arsenical deposition in the system, causing obliterative arteritis.

Milan[27] thinks that arsphenamine has no affinity for the liver, and that jaundice is due to the action of syphilis; it can best be conquered by pushing the treatment. Sicard[28] disagrees with him, and states that arsphenamine does damage the liver, reflected in the urea content of the blood.

Myocarditis, extensive nephritis (nonsyphilitic) and diabetes are contraindications to arsphenamine.

USE IN THERAPEUTICS

These drugs, while used primarily in syphilis, have been found of value in several nonsyphilitic diseases. Prominent among these are frambesia, relapsing fever and Vincent's angina, all being due to a spirillum. This has led Best[29] to conclude that arsphenamine is specific in diseases caused by any spirillum. Its aid in treatment of amebic dysentery, anthrax and malaria, has led him also to conclude that arsphenamine has curative properties in other diseases where the organism is easily reached, as in the blood and lymph. Brechot[30] reports using neoarsphenamine intravenously, after war wounds, in order to prevent and to cure septicemia, especially acute septicemias without important local lesions. The results were very successful. De Beaurepaire[31] used neoarsphenamine with excellent results in yellow fever. He gave an initial dose, as large as 0.9 g. Head and Seabloom[32] call attention to the fact that syphilis may prolong and delay reparative processes, such as in the lungs of persons having had pneumonia. They cite a case, where resolution was delayed for months. Under arsphenamine treatment, recovery was rapid.

Schamberg[10] states that the best treatment for syphilis is organic arsenicals and mercury. Writers differ in the strength of the dose, the frequency of administration and choice of compound. The trend today, is to make the treatment at first as intensive as is consistent with safety, for the best chance of recovery. The curability of syphilis is directly proportional to the age of the disease.

The first injection kills the mass of parasites, but a few survive and may reinfect the tissues. Mercury is used to avoid tolerance to the drug. Mercury acts slower and longer; thus by combining the two, one gets quick action as well as prolonged action. This is shown by the fact that most of the arsphenamine is excreted in three days, while a sterilizing concentration of mercury is reached only after several days.[1]

Sicard[28] gives neoarsphenamine intravenously in a daily dose of 0.15 g., to a total of 6 to 7 g. in women, and 7 to 9 g. in men. He thus gives 40 to 60 injections in all.

Tauber[33] injects 0.3 to 0.6 gm. every 3 to 7 days, for 4 to 6 injections. Combining this with mercury, he gives no less than three such courses in two months. He points out that congenital syphilis requires longer treatment.

Nelkin[20] gives an average dose of 0.5 gm. to the male and 0.4 gm. to the female. He repeats this weekly for three doses, then two more doses at longer intervals. He gives mercury and iodine between these injections.

In animals[1] a fall of blood pressure follows injections; this has been met with in case of man. Large doses in the rabbit seem to induce nephritis. The after effects in man are usually headache, nausea, vomiting, chills, and often fever. Delbanco[34] used silver arsphenamine in 550 injections with excellent results. Silver has a special affinity for the spirochete, shown by the silver stain. It banished the spirochetes from the primary lesion, as shown by the dark field microscope, and the florid symptoms of the secondary period subsided promptly. He also used mercury with the silver arsphenamine. The advantage of this compound is that the maximum effectual dose is 0.2 to 0.3 g., which is below the threshold of danger, as the arsenic content of silver arsphenamine is only two-thirds that of arsphenamine. He concludes by saying that silver acts chemically as a catalyzer of the arsenobenzol molecule, and biologically as a reenforcer of the specific action of arsenic on spirochetes. Colloidal silver alone has a pronounced action on rabbit syphilis.

The elimination of these compounds has also been observed. Myers[35] states that one-half hour after injecting arsphenamine, 75 per cent of it is fixed in the body cells. Arsenic is found attached to proteins of the plasma and blood cells, even after all free arsphenamine is eliminated.

Arsphenamine[1] appears unchanged in the urine in 5 to 10 minutes after injection, and persists for 5 to 6 hours. Thereafter arsenic is found in urine for several days, as arsenites and arsenates. Less is eliminated in the stools, but it appears there for a longer time. No arsenic is found in any organs after 15 days; 50 to 75 per cent of the arsenic may be regained in the urine. The fate of the remaining 25 per cent is unknown, but appears to be temporarily stored in the liver and bone-marrow. With intravenous injection, the arsenic disappears in 3 to 4 days; with intramuscular injection it disappears from the body in 10 days.

Neoarsphenamine elimination differs from that of arsphenamine in that for the first few hours after injection, formaldehyde appears in the urine. Otherwise it is eliminated in the same manner as arsphenamine.

RELATIVE VALUE OF ARSPHENAMINE AND NEOARSPHENAMINE

I will conclude with a brief discussion of the merits and demerits of each compound. For a long time arsphenamine was used dominantly, but during the war, all treatment at the front, by French, English, American and German doctors was with injections of neoarsphenamine. This must have given better results.

Toxicity—Schamberg[10] showed that neoarsphenamine is two and one-half times *less* toxic for white rats than the arsphenamine from which it is made. Arsphenamine was tolerated at 100 mg. per kg. body weight, while the neoarsphenamine was tolerated at 250 to 300 mg. per kg. body weight. The addition of the formaldehyde sulphoxylate group apparently lessens the affinity for the protoplasm of the parasite, but also lessens the affinity for the body proteins still more. This is due to the closing of one amino group (Schamberg).

Further, arsphenamine in practically all concentrations hemolyzes red blood cells in vitro. Neoarsphenamine does not do so, in any concentration normally used (Schamberg).

The hydrogen-ion content of neoarsphenamine is close to that of the blood; that of arsphenamine, whether alkaline or acid, differs greatly from that of blood. Neoarsphenamine is usually better tolerated than arsphenamine. Milian[10] states that neoarsphenamine never induces nitritoid crises except in extremely predisposed and intolerant persons.

Curative Powers.—Arsphenamine is more curative than the neo-compound. Schamberg[10] found that to sterilize rats experimentally infected with Trypanosome equiperdum (horse syphilis) it took twice as much of the neo-drug as arsphenamine itself. The arsenic content of three parts of neoarsphenamine, equals that of only two parts of arsphenamine.

Schamberg[10] thus concludes, that the arsphenamine is more active therapeutically, but this difference is made up by the discrepancy in tolerated dosage. Nine-tenths gm. of the neo-compound can be given three times a week. Neoarsphenamine creates much less biochemical disturbances in the blood and tissues.

The value of these drugs[1] has been shown by the destruction of spirochetes in the test tube, and also by the fact that this power is greatly enhanced when digested with tissues—inorganic arsenic compounds are presumably formed. We might ask, if these drugs will actually cure syphilis. Authorities differ, but Schamberg[30] has presented an interesting case in support of the curability of this disease. He believes patients treated in the primitive stage intensively may be cured. In this case syphilis was acquired in 1917. The Wassermann was positive. After treatment by neoarsphenamine, the blood gave a negative Wassermann, and the eruption disappeared. In 1919, syphilis was again contracted, a chancre developed at a site different from the first one. The blood now gave a strong positive Wassermann. Schamberg believes the facts warrant the assumption that the first infection had been cured. No immunity was given against the second attack, however. Too much value should not be given to the Wassermann reaction, in deciding the question of curability.

At any rate, under such treatment, if applied early, external lesions disappear; secondary signs, as alopecia, and secondary syphilitic systemic disturbances are prevented.

Tauber[33] crystallizes the view of writers, when he states that "mercury and arsphenamine must be combined in the rational cure of syphilis."

Now that the supply is carefully controlled, and as a result of the investigations as to the cause of reactions, it is hoped that these valuable compounds will be used with better success by the average physician. It might be desirable to further modify them to form a new compound specific for the spirochete pallida. The success of these compounds, on the whole, has given new hope for the cure of all infectious diseases,—by the elaboration of chemical compounds, which will combine a high parasitotropism and a low organotropism in each case.

REFERENCES

[1]Cushny: Pharmacology and Therapeutics, p. 607-609.
[2]Cortlett and Gill: Reference Handbook of Medical Sciences, ed. 3, viii, p. 83.
[3]U. S. Public Health Report, April 12, 1918, p. 340.
[4]Pollitzer: Jour. Am. Med. Assn., July 28, 1917, p. 305.
[5]Guy: Jour. Am. Med. Assn., Sept. 20, 1919, p. 901.
[6]May: Chemistry of Synthetic Drugs, 1918, ed. 2, p. 210.
[7]Myers, C. N.: Qualitative and Quantitative Tests for Arsphenamine and Neoarsphenamine, U. S. Public Health Report, 1918, p. 1003.
[8]Hand Book of Therapy. Jour. Am. Med. Assn., p. 599.
[9]McCoy: Jour. Am. Med. Assn., May 10, 1919, p. 1386.
[10]Schamberg: Jour. Am. Med. Assn., Dec. 20, 1919, p. 1883.
[11]Guy: Jour. Am. Med. Assn., Sept. 20, 1919, p. 901.
[12]Bory: Jour. Am. Med. Assn., May 17, 1919, p. 1498.
[13]Leonard: Jour. Am. Med. Assn., Sept. 27, 1919, p. 1013.
[14]Berman: Arch. Int. Med., Aug. 1918, xxii, p. 217.
[15]Jour. Am. Med. Assn., Nov. 29, 1919, p. 1704.
[16]Milian: Jour. Am. Med. Assn., May 24, 1919, p. 1576.
[17]Jackson and Smith: Jour. Am. Med. Assn., June 14, 1919, p. 1773.
[18]Hirano: Jour. Am. Med. Assn., Aug. 9, 1919, p. 454.
[19]Rieger: Jour. Am. Med. Assn., Aug. 30, 1919, p. 710
[20]Nelkin: Jour. Am. Med. Assn., June 7, 1919, p. 1695.
[21]Jacobsen: Jour. Am. Med. Assn., May 10, 1919, p. 1403.
[22]Berner: Jour. Am. Med. Assn., Sept. 6, 1919, p. 802.
[23]Labbé and Langlois: Jour. Am. Med. Assn., Nov. 22, 1919, p. 1645.
[24]Stutter: Jour. Am. Med. Assn., Nov. 22, 1919, p. 1611.
[25]Nagai: Jour. Am. Med. Assn., Nov. 29, 1919, p. 1727.
[26]Jones: Jour. Am. Med. Assn., Nov. 1, 1919, p. 1359.
[27]Milian: Jour. Am. Med. Assn., Dec. 13, 1919, p. 1858.
[28]Sicard: Journ. Am. Med. Assn., Dec. 13, 1919, p. 1858.
[29]Best: Jour. Am. Med. Assn., Aug. 1, 1914, p. 375.
[30]Brechot: Jour. Am. Med. Assn., July 19, 1919, p. 232.
[31]DeBeaurepaire: Jour. Am. Med. Assn., Sept. 27, 1919, p. 1020.
[32]Head and Seabloom: Jour. Am. Med. Assn., Nov. 1, 1919, p. 1344.
[33]Tauber: Jour. Am. Med. Assn., Nov. 29, 1919, p. 1661.
[34]Delbanco: Jour. Am. Med. Assn., May 31, 1919, p. 1648.
[35]Myers, C. N.: U. S. Public Health Reports, May 21, 1919, p. 881.
[36]Schamberg: Jour. Am. Med. Assn., Sept. 13, 1919, p. 826.

PRIMARY CANCER OF THE LIVER

By I. M. Cohn, Spokane, Washington

PRIMARY malignancy of the liver is a very rare condition. In fact almost every known case has appeared in some medical journal. Many of these cases have been challenged so that the number of instances of this disease is very small.

Maude Slye observed but four cases in 1500 autopsies. While experimenting with mice she made 10,000 autopsies. Twenty-eight showed primary tumors of the liver. Of these only 3 were malignant, one of which produced multiple metastasis in the lung.[1] On the average, it occurs in about 0.1 per cent of autopsies. It is rarer than secondary malignancy. The secondary condition occurs with 20 to 40 times the frequency.[2]

Wheeler reports 15 cases in 5,233 autopsies which were performed at Guy's Hospital in London.[3] Vecchi reviewed 45 cases of so-called primary carcinoma of the liver. Of these he considers only 21 as being correct. The others were doubtful.[4]

The etiology of this disease is unknown. Many theories have been advanced any or all of which may be the direct or indirect cause. The frequency with which the disease is found with cirrhosis of the liver has led many to believe it to be the factor causing the disease. Dickenson reports a case in which the liver was removed from a man with alcoholic habits. It was a mass of cancerous tissue combined with an older coarse cirrhosis.[5] Frequently it has the hobnailed appearance characteristic of cirrhosis.[6] One of the rarest conditions was cited by Hale White. It was the development of a melanotic sarcoma in the liver following cirrhosis. Only three or four cases of primary melanotic sarcoma of the liver have yet been obtained.[7] W. Ford reports a case of a spindle cell sarcoma found in the cirrhotic liver of an alcoholic.[8] In the five cases of malignant adenocarcinoma examined by Muir, all were associated with cirrhosis.[9] Where malignancy of the liver follows cirrhosis, there is no doubt but that the cirrhosis has been a great factor in bringing out the malignancy.[10] All cases of cirrhosis can be considered as potentially malignant, and that cancer is very often the sequela. Some take the view that cirrhosis is the sequela of cancer.

An interesting case is cited by M. DeMassary. His patient was a young French soldier of 25. On autopsy an enlarged liver was revealed. It was syphilitic. The inflammatory reaction set up resulted in cirrhosis, and this in turn gave rise to a malignant carcinoma which caused his death.[11]

Other irritating conditions are important factors in causing the disease. G. Rohdenburg found a round cell sarcoma during an autopsy, the primary nodule being formed about a dead parasite in the liver. There was no doubt but that the parasite was the primary foci.[12] Another interesting case was that of an autopsy on a Chinaman. His liver was covered with carcinomatous masses. On microscopic examination, leprosy bacilli were observed scattered through the stroma of the liver. Previously it was not believed that two such diseases could exist together in the same liver.[13]

Biliary calculi have been associated with carcinoma. There are two views on their relationship. The first, or irritative, theory considers the calculi as the cause of carcinoma. The other, or concentration, theory assumes that the growth causes the calculi. Primary carcinoma arises most frequently in the region of the gall bladder. In most instances gall stones are present, while in secondary carcinoma they are seldom found. The fact that gall bladder cells may show carcinomatous growth in the liver supports the irritation theory. Beadles cites thirteen cases of malignancy, all of which were associated with gallstones. However, these cases may have been confused with primary carcinoma of the gall bladder.[14] A rather far-fetched view is advanced by Fischer. He considers primary cancer of the liver as originating in the biliary passages, as cirrhosis of the liver is present in 85 per cent of the cases of adenocarcinoma of the biliary passages.[15]

Arteriosclerosis has been advanced as a cause. Of the four cases examined by Warner, only one showed evidence of arteriosclerosis. In no instances have vascular changes been proved to be the cause of cancer. Cirrhosis has been the condition most frequently associated with malignancy.[16]

There are three important types of carcinoma of the liver, massive, diffuse, and nodular.[17] The massive type occurs most frequently. It consists of a large carcinomatous mass inside the liver so that the liver tissue acts as a shell for the neoplasm. The tumor cells are usually polyhedral or spheroid. The diffuse type of carcinoma is very rare. In this condition there is an infiltration of spheroidal cells into the liver tissue. The nodular, or multiple primary, carcinoma is more common. It grows rapidly, and quickly degenerates. In this condition the liver has the appearance of being studded with nodes. The cells are polyhedral or spheroidal. Primary carcinoma in a cirrhotic liver is a fourth type, while primary melanotic carcinoma is a fifth type.

Primary sarcomas are divided into five classes similar to carcinoma. Primary massive sarcoma is usually found in the right lobe or pedunculated. The tumor is made up of small round cells, spindle cells and other types. The nodular or multiple sarcoma is made up of spindle, round, irregular or giant cells. In diffuse sarcoma the tumor cells infiltrate both lobes of the liver. Sarcoma also arises in association with cirrhosis. More rarely we have primary melanotic sarcoma of the liver.[18]

A description of a typical sarcomatous liver is described by Delepine.[19] An enlarged liver was removed at autopsy. The surface was nodulated like that of a hobnailed liver. These nodules varied in appearance. Some were white while others were dark brown. A microscopic examination of the tissue revealed considerable changes in the intralobular veins. There was a proliferation of endothelium to the extent of occluding the vessels. Some of these vessels contained golden brown pigment granules and others contained black pigment globules. Ninety per cent of the liver epithelium was destroyed, while many of the remaining cells were pigmented. The larger pigmented nodules were made up of spindle cells.

The tumor is set in action by an irritation of the liver. This leads to a proliferation of endothelial cells in carcinoma, and of connective tissue in sarcoma. The contents of the vessels are replaced by an embryonic tissue similar to that from which blood and blood vessels originate. Along with this is the rapid destruction of normal liver tissue.[19] An examination of the carcinomatous cells show them to be quite similar to hepatic parenchyma. They have a trabecular arrangement, but the cells are larger than normal tissue.[20] The tumor is a direct continuation of normal tissue though it contains many large and irregular cells.[21] In many tumors the cells are bile-producing, as is found in normal tissue.[22] The tumor can be considered as a direct change of liver cells to cancer cells, and a hyperplasia of the new formation.[23] The growth is compensatory and it proliferates by direct extension. It is this factor which gives rise to malignancy.[24]

Metastasis with cancer of the liver comes at a later period than with malignant diseases elsewhere in the body. Neither are the metastases so widespread. The retroperitoneal glands and omentum are frequently involved, but seldom the supraclavicular glands.[25] The lungs are often involved and very rarely the heart.[26]

Primary cancer has a wide variation. It occurs at almost any age in an individual's life. Several cases have been reported in which the disease was present at birth. Pepper reports the case of a baby girl who died with a congenital lymphosarcoma at the age of six and one-half weeks.[27] In this case there was a metastasis to the right suprarenal body. The symptoms were mistaken for congenital syphilis, and only at autopsy was it proved to be a congenital round-cell sarcoma of the liver.[28] Similar cases have been reported in infants by Heaton[29] and Pitt.[30] It may remain latent and not cause death for several years.[31] As a rule, though, it runs a rapid course, death usually occurring within a month after the onset of the symptoms.[32] In these cases of congenital cancer the individual inherits the predisposition to the disease.[33] It occurs more often in the form of a carcinoma than a sarcoma.[34]

In children the disease has been mistaken for intussusception and appendiceal abscesses so rarely does it occur.[35] In most cases the disease is first noticed by an abdominal swelling. A hard lump is felt under the right rib margin. The tumor continues to grow and extends below the rib margin. The enlargement of the liver pushes the other organs to the left. This has often caused it to be mistaken for a cyst and punctures have been unsuccessfully made to relieve the condition.[36] It was only at autopsy that the true character was made out.

The symptoms vary greatly in different cases. Clinically the earliest symptoms are vague gastrointestinal troubles. Sometimes the symptoms of an atrophic cirrhosis predominate. After the tumor develops the patient suffers a loss of flesh, cachexia and digestive disturbances. Icterus is present in 63 per cent of cases; ascites in 58.5 per cent; edema in 41 per cent; splenic tumors in 32 per cent cases and fever in 14 per cent.[37] Eighty-six per cent of the cases are associated with cirrhosis. It is also associated with echinococcus cysts, chronic venous congestion, and tuberculosis of the liver. On the whole it occurs most often when the liver tissue is undergoing regeneration.[38] Emaciation, vomiting, and constipation are symptoms frequently present. The tumor area is usually painful and tender.[39]

The duration of the disease seldom exceeds twelve weeks. If longer, it is more likely to be secondary. The prognosis of the disease is fatal, death almost always results. It is somewhat more common in the male. The family history of the patient is usually negative. Although the liver is usually greatly enlarged it may be smaller in cirrhosis.

A typical case as found in children is cited by Martha Wallstein.[41] A four-month-old baby was brought to the clinic with a history of having vomited for the past three days. On examination, a small lump was noticed under the right lower rib. Further examination produced negative results. During the following two months the child became worse, the abdomen was markedly distended and death resulted at the age of 8½ months. The autopsy revealed a primary malignant sarcoma of the liver. In one case the abdominal swelling continued over a period of eight months.[42] Castle reports a case in which death took place within fourteen days after the onset of the symptoms.[43] An examination of the tumor showed it to be a primary parenchymatous adeno-carcinoma of the liver. Tate reports a similar case in a ten year old girl.[44] Cases are given by Bramwell,[45] Affleck,[46] Roberts.[47] Two cases are reported of boys, one who gave a history of scarlet fever and nephritis,[48] and the other[49] of being kicked in the right side. The symptoms were characteristic. The body was covered with eruptions, the patient became weak and emaciated. Diarrhea and abdominal swelling set in, and the patient died in great pain. On autopsy primary malignant growths were found in the liver.

The cases reported are found at all ages and in both sexes.[50-62] The disease has also been found in mice quite similar to the human form.[63] Very rarely misplaced tissue in the liver may become malignant. In these instances the tumor resembles the tissue from which it is derived. A primary myeloma in the liver was found which had myelogenous functions.[64]

Although this is a very malignant disease, operations have been resorted to with some success.[65] This has been done by cutting the tumor away and scraping out the cavity.[66] In more radical operations the entire affected lobe of the liver has been successfully removed.[67, 68] Where recurrence occurred a second operation was resorted to with more success.[69]

SUMMARY

Occurrence: Very rare.
Etiology:
    1. Irritation of liver cells.
    2. Congenital origin.
    3. Compensatory hyperplasia.

Kind:[3]

1. Liver cells.
2. Bile duct cells.

Symptoms:

1. Cachexia.
2. Anemia.
3. Digestive disturbances.
4. Right hypochondriac pain.
5. Tumor in abdomen.
6. Icterus when bile exits are occluded. 63%.
7. Ascites when lymphatic obstruction occurs. 58%.
8. Edema. 41%.
9. Splenic tumor. 32%.
10. Fever. 14%.

Duration: Fourteen days to a year. Averages six months.

Age: Occurs at any age.

Sex: More common in men.

Macroscopic classification:

1. Nodular—most common.
2. Massive.
3. Diffuse—rare.

Microscopic classification:

1. Simplex.
2. Adenomata.

Metastasis:

1. Liver.
2. Lungs.

Weight: May weigh as much as 267 ounces.

REFERENCES

[1]Slye, M.: Jour. Med. Research, 1915, pp. 171-182.
[2]Rolleston, H.: Diseases of the Liver, pp. 468-484; Trans. of Path. Soc., 1901, p. 203; ibid., 1894, p. 94.
[3]Wheeler, F.: Guy's Hospital Report, 1909, p. 225.
[4]Vecchi and Guerrini: Med. News, 1901, p. 816.
[5]Dickenson: Trans. Path. Soc., London, 1894, p. 87.
[6]Rolleston: Ibid., p. 94.
[7]White, W. Hale: Trans. Path. Soc., London, 1886, p. 272; Albutt's System of Medicine, p. 204.
[8]Ford, W.: Am. Jour. Med. Sc., 1900, p. 413.
[9]Muir, R.: Jour. Path. and Bacteriol., 1908, p. 287.
[10]Rolleston: Brit. Med. Jour., 1901, p. 151.
[11]De Massary, M. and Menetrier, M.: Societe Medicale Des Hopitaux, 1917, p. 1252.
[12]Rohdenburg: Jour. Cancer Research, 1916, p. 87.
[13]Cleland, J. B.: Jour. Tropical Med. & Hyg., 1919, p. 147.
[14]C. Beadles: Brit. Med. Jour., 1895, p. 1164.
[15]Fischer: Jour. Am. Med. Assn., 1904, p. 688.
[16]Warner, F.: Surg., Gynec. and Obst., 1916, p. 417.
[17]Mayo: Keen's Surgery, 984.
[18]Rolleston, H.: Diseases of the Liver, pp. 468-484.
[19]Delepine, S.: Trans. Path. Soc., London, 1891, p. 161.
[20]Weber, F.: Lancet, London, 1910, p. 1066, Proc. Royal Soc. of Med., 1910, p. 147.
[21]McCallum: Text Book on Path., p. 986.

[22]Nair, W.: Jour. Path. and Bacteriol., 1911, p. 389.
[23]Fussel and Kelley: Trans. Assn. Am. Phys., 1895, p. 108.
[24]Wells, G.: Am. Jour. Med. Sc., 1903, p. 403.
[25]Ferranini: Jour. Am. Med. Assn., 1918, p. 1802.
[26]Holsti: Brit. Med. Jour., 1895, epitome, p. 395.
[27]Pepper, W.: Am. Jour. Med. Sc., 1901, p. 287; Philadelphia Med. Times, 1875, p. 666.
[28]Parker: Trans. Path. Soc., 1880, p. 280.
[29]Heaton: Trans. Path. Soc., 1898, p. 140.
[30]Pitt, G.: Trans. Path. Soc., 1898, p 143.
[31]Tooth, K.: Trans. Path. Soc., 1885, p. 286.
[32]Gee, S.: St. Bartholomew's Hosp. Repts., 1877, p. 160.
[33]Neisenbach: Weekly Med. Rept., 1884, p. 433.
[34]Griffith, J. P.: Am. Jour. Med. Sc., 1918, p. 79.
[35]Harge, J. R.: Surgical Clinics of Chicago, 1919, p. 121-125
[36]Pye and Smith: Trans. Path. Soc., London, 1880, p. 125.
[37]Karsner, H.: Arch. Int. Med., 1911, p. 238.
[38]Milne: Jour. Path. and Bacteriol., 1909, p. 348.
[39]Hale, W.: Guy's Hospital Report, 1890, p. 59.
[40]Burt, S. S.: Post-Graduate, 1903, p. 991.
[41]Wollstein, M.: Arch. Pediat., 1919, pp. 268-273.
[42]Freeman: Lancet, London, 1914, p. 157.
[43]Castle, O. L.: Surg., Gynec. and Obst., 1914, p. 477-483.
[44]Tate, M.: Am. Jour. Obst., 1915, p. 637-640.
[45]Bramwell: Lancet, London, 1897, p. 170.
[46]Affleck: Trans. Edinburgh Obst. Soc., 1875, p. 58.
[47]Robert: Lancet, London, 1867, p. 77.
[48]La Page: Proc. Royal Soc. Med., 1912, p. 45.
[49]Lewis: Med. Jour. and Examiner, 1877, p. 325.
[50]Acland, Lancet, London. 1902, p. 1310.
[51]Adami and McCrae: p. 688.
[52]Burnet: Trans. Path. Soc., London, 1885, p. 252.
[53]Travis, C.: Bull. Johns Hopkins Hosp., 1902, p. 108.
[54]Greenfield, W.: Trans. Path. Soc., London, 1874, p. 166.
[55]Legg, J.: St. Bartholomew's Hosp. Repts., 1877, p. 160.
[56]Cruickshank, J.: Jour. Path. and Bacteriol., 1910, p. 282.
[57]Blankingship, A.: Virginia Med. Semi-Monthly, p. 569.
[58]Courmont, J.: Lyon Méd., p. 577.
[59]Bauer, D. J.: Long Island Med. Jour., 1916, p. 341.
[60]Brooks, H.: Memphis Med. Monthly, 1916, p. 272.
[61]Fagge, C.: Trans. Path. Soc., London, 1877, p. 137
[62]Penrose, F.: Trans. Path. Soc., 1885, p. 173.
[63]Itami: Jour. Cancer Research, 1918, p. 275.
[64]Perry, O.: Jour. Med. Research, 1917, p. 171.
[65]Schlimpert: Jour. Cancer Research, 1918, p. 215.
[66]Williams, R.: Lancet, London, 1897, p. 1328.
[67]Keen, W.: Ann. Surg., 1899.
[68]Freeman: Am. Jour. Med. Sc., 1904, p. 611.
[69]Yeomans: Jour. Am. Med. Assn., 1909, p. 1741; ibid., 1915, p. 1301.

THE EFFECT OF TOBACCO ON THE VASCULAR WALL

Tsang G. Ni, M.S., China

THE inhalation of tobacco or injection of nicotine causes a contraction of the artery. This can be shown by the rise of blood pressure. From observations on eight healthy men Lee[1] concludes as follows: In the novice there is always an initial rise of systolic blood pressure. In an excessive smoker the pressure rises and the pulse is unaffected.

The rise of blood pressure may be due either to a change in the heart rate or to the increase in output or to an indirect effect associated with the respiration. Miller, Bruce, and Hooker,[2] from observations on two healthy men, conclude that after smoking (pipe, cigar or cigarette) there is usually an increase in heart rate. Aikman[3] made an experiment on 28 healthy smokers, using a single Turkish cigarette in each case. Of 27 cases, the pulse-rate increased in all but 4, and 16 showed an increase of more than eight beats per minute. Stachelin[4] attempted to ascertain the effect of smoking continued over a period of six months. During this time he smoked six to eight cigars daily, then he abstained from smoking for six months. The pulse rate, as showing by the mean rate on three days was 82 during the smoking period and 75 during the period of abstinence. Similarly the pulse rate after a standard exertion was 157 compared with 124 per minute. Not only was the pulse rate after exertion higher during the smoking period, but it took much longer to return to the normal. This showed that the heart during smoking period was more irritable and its output might be affected. Hesse[5] observed the effect of cigar smoking on 25 subjects, chiefly patients with various chronic diseases. One reading was taken before smoking and one after each cigar. In the majority there occurred an increase in pulse rate, together with a rise of blood pressure. Although experiments have shown that tobacco may affect the heart rate or its output, there are also experiments which appear to prove that the rise of blood pressure may be caused by a vasoconstriction resulting from the inhalation of tobacco.

Aikman[3] observed the effect of cigarette smoking on the pulse rate and blood pressure of 28 subjects, chiefly healthy smokers. In four heavy smokers the pulse rate increased by 40 beats. He noted an initial decrease of 4 to 6 beats in three cases. The rise of blood pressure and the change of pulse rate did not run in the same direction.

Bruce, Miller, and Hooker,[2] studied carefully two healthy smokers and concluded that after smoking there was generally an increase in heart rate. Even when the increase was absent, the blood pressure showed distinct changes. The maximum and minimum presure always rose slightly, the maximum the more, so that the "pulse pressure" tended to increase. This is the case when the rise of blood pressure is caused by a vasoconstriction, therefore the increase in pressure may be independent of the heart rate. Moreover, Lee,[1] studying healthy men, stated that in the case of an excessive smoker the pressure rose and the pulse was unaffected.

John Parkinson[7] made a serious attempt to ascertain the effect of smoking. There was a sudden increase in the average rate during the first half minute of smoking from 80 to 87. No preliminary slowing took place, such as has been described in the case of animals after the introduction of nicotine. In five cases the blood pressure did not rise until ten or more minutes had elapsed. The average diastolic pressure rose gradually. Among the inhalers the average systolic pressure rose 11 mm.; the diastolic pressure rose 6 mm.; the systolic pressure rising more than the diastolic. This shows that the vasoconstriction played an important role in some of his experiments.

The effect of injection of nicotine upon the vascular wall can also be shown by the rise of blood presure. Some writers have thought that the effect of nicotine upon pressure might be indirectly due to the increase in the output of epinephrine. Gley[8] gives a figure showing a rise of pressure from 30 mm. to 140 mm. mercury, following injection of 10 mg. of nicotine into a nine kg. dog with intact adrenals, whereas after the excision of the adrenals, the same dose of nicotine only caused a rise of 24 to about 30 mm. He concludes that the whole pressor effect of nicotine after destruction of the bulbospinal center is due to the increase in the output of epinephrin produced by it. Dale and Laidlaw[9] observed that certain reactions which are elicited by nicotine on the nonpregnant uterus of the cat and in the eye after removal of the superior cervical ganglion are modified when the experiment is made under such conditions that epinephrin can no longer reach these structures from the adrenals. They explain the difference by the hypothesis that the nicotine action is in part due to a stimulation of the adrenals to increase liberation of epinephrin. Cannon, Aub and Binger[10] conclude that "injection of nicotine of small amount (3.5-7.5 mg. in cats) results in augmented adrenal secretion." But such an increase of concentration of epinephrin in adrenal veins is always observed when the blood flow in the cava is slowed from any cause whatever, provided that the epinephrin output continues unchanged or is diminished less than the rate of the blood flow. It is possible that the increase of concentration is owing to the diminution of the rate of blood flow associated with the marked and prolonged fall of blood pressure succeeding the very brief rise.

Langley[11] obtained an excellent rise of pressure when nicotine was injected after the adrenals had been tied off from the circulation. Here, of course, the bulbospinal centers may have participated in the action. It may be assumed that if nicotine stimulates the ganglion cells on the path of the adrenal secretory fibers, or in the absence of ganglion cells on the path of these fibers[12] possibly some part of the medullary cells themselves, an increased epinephrin output may contribute to the rise of pressure. But all the evidence goes to show that even if the output has been proved to be augmented by nicotine and the adrenal blood after being collected for a time is suddenly released, the epinephrin factor in the increase of pressure is far subordinate to the vasomotor factor. It would appear improbable that the excitation of ganglion cells on the cause of vaso-motors should be a negligible factor in the vasoconstriction in comparison with the excitation of the adrenal secretory fibers.

Lauder Bronton[13] has given the following statement: In animals nicotine causes slowing of the heart with enormous rise of blood pressure. The rise of pressure is chiefly due to the contraction of arterioles. This contraction is partly dependent upon the stimulation of the vasomotor center in the medulla oblongata partly also to a local action upon the arterioles themselves, as it is produced by the injection of the drug after the medulla has been destroyed.

As it has been stated that nicotine causes an augmented adrenal secretion, it must have some action on veins. For, as an accepted explanation, epinephrin acts on muscles which are supplied by sympathetic autonomic nerve fibers, and veins receive such kind of nerve fibers. The portal vein receives vasoconstrictor fibers from the splanchnic nerve.[14] The existence of venomotor nerves to the large veins of the neck has been proved.[15] Bancroft[16] made experiments in which it was found that stimulation of the sciatic nerve caused a constriction of the superficial veins of the hind limbs. Moreover it has been described that nicotine does have an action on the vasomotor center.[13] It is not impossible, therefore, that nicotine may act on veins through its own action on the vasomotor center as well as through the action of epinephrin.

The effect of tobacco upon vasoconstriction may be shaded somewhat by the fact that tobacco attacks the hemoglobin. Claude Bernard and Hobert Amory Hare have shown the effect of nicotine, pyridine and gross tobacco itself on the blood. The action consists of attacking the hemoglobin in the red corpuscles of the blood. This fact has been confirmed by Clark, who reports that the hemoglobin content may fall as low as 40 per cent. The largest portion of the oxygen is held in chemical combination with the hemoglobin.[17] In other words, the amount of oxygen in the arterial blood depends upon the amount of hemoglobin there is in one cubic centimeter of blood.[18] When the hemoglobin content falls the oxygen supply is insufficient and certain organic acids, such as lactic acid, may accumulate. Gaskell has shown that acids in slight concentration cause a vascular dilatation. Bayliss[19] has stated that lactic acid or carbon dioxide may act to produce a dilatation. So the vasoconstriction caused by tobacco may be shadowed somehow by its indirect action on the vasodilatation.

CONCLUSION

The inhalation of tobacco causes a contraction of the artery.

The rise of blood pressure after smoking may sometimes be due to a change in heart rate, sometimes due to the vasoconstriction independently.

The injection of nicotine causes a vasoconstriction.

Such vasoconstriction is due either to the augmented adrenal secretion caused by nicotine, or to a direct, local action of nicotine on the vascular wall, or to its action on vasomotor center.

Tobacco affects not only the artery but also the vein.

The effect of tobacco on the vascular wall may be shaded somewhat by its action on hemoglobin and consequently a vasodilatation may come to neutralize its result to some extent.

REFERENCES

[1]Lee, W. E.: Quart. Jour. Exper. Physiol., 1908, i, 335.
[2]Miller, Bruce and Hooker: Am. Jour. Physiol., 1909, xxiv, 104.
[3]Aikman, J: New York Med. Jour., 1915, cii, 891.
[4]Stachelin: Ztschr. f. Exper. Pathol. u. Therap., 1910-11. viii, 323.
[5]Hesse, E.: Deutsch. Arch. f. klin. Med., 1907, xxxix, 565.
[7]Parkinson: Quart. Jour. Med. Oxford, 1913, vii, 42.
[8]Gley: Compt. rend., 1914, clviii, 2008.
[9]Dale and Laidlaw: Jour. Physiol., 1912, xiv.
[10]Cannan, Aub and Binger: Jour. Pharm. and Exper. Therap., 1911-12, iii, 379.
[11]Langley: Jour. Physiol., 1918, iii, 259.
[12]Elliot: Jour. Physiol., 1913, xlvi, 285.
[13]Lauder Bronton: The Practitioner, July, 1905, p. 54.
[14]Mall: Arch. f. Physiol., 1892, p. 409.
[15]Scherrington and Roy: Jour. Physiol., 1890, ii, 85.
[16]Am. Jour. Physiol., 1898, l. 477.
[17]Howell: Physiology, p. 677. Matthews, A. P.: Physiological Chemistry, p. 476.
[18]Mathews, A. P.: Physiological Chemistry, p. 196.
[19]Bavliss: Ergebnisse der Physiol., 1906, v, 319.

LABORATORY METHODS

THE SELECTION OF KIESELGUHR FOR THE FILTRATION OF SERUMS*

By George E. Ewe, Philadelphia, Pa.

IN THE filtration of expensive serums, every possible means of preventing loss must be carefully investigated. One of the avenues of loss is absorption by the filtering medium used to clarify serums.

One of the most commonly employed filtering mediums is kieselguhr. Kieselguhr varies greatly in its power of absorbing liquids. Trials of seven lots of ignited kieselguhr, under precisely the same conditions, showed the following results of relative power to absorb serums:

KIESELGUHR	LOSS OF SERUM
1	2.28%
2	5.7%
3	5.9%
4	2.43%
5	4.3%
6	4.8%
7	2.39%

Therefore, the relative values of these samples of kieselguhr, for the filtration of serum, regarding minimum of loss by absorption, were in the following order: No. 1, No. 7, No. 4, No. 5, No. 6, No. 2, and No. 3.

It is also essential to select kieselguhr which will yield a brilliantly clear filtrate in a minimum of time. The seven kieselguhr samples mentioned above showed great variation in this respect. Table I gives the results of filtration experiments with various lots of serums under exactly the same conditions.

Since the time required for final filtration through a Berkefeld is too short for accurate comparison, only the figures obtained by preliminary filtration through filter paper can be used for comparing the relative value of these seven lots of kieselguhr regarding their ability to produce clear filtrates in a minimum of time. Analyzing the results outlined in the above tables, we find the relative values to be as shown in Table II.

Table II shows the varying ability of different lots of kieselguhr to clarify the same lot of serum. It also shows a fair uniformity in the ability of a particular kieselguhr to clarify different lots of a serum.

Chemical examination of the seven samples in accordance with the tests for kieselguhr in the United States Pharmacopeia yielded the results shown in Table III.

*From the Pharmaceutical Chemical Laboratories of the H. K. Mulford Co., Philadelphia, Pa.

TABLE I

KIESELGUHR SAMPLE NO.	SERUM NO.	MINUTES REQUIRED FOR PRELIMINARY FILTRATION THROUGH PAPER	MINUTES REQUIRED FOR FINAL FILTRATION THROUGH BERKEFELD
1	1	20	3½
	2	21	2
	3	23	1½
	4	20	2
	5	19	2
2	1	55	6
	2	60	5
	3	60	6
	4	120	5
	5	78	5
3	1	35	4
	2	60	2½
	3	120	3½
	4	60	15
	5	66	5
4	1	53	2
	2	47	10
	3	50	5
	4	60	9
	5	50	2
5	1	60	4
	2	18	2
	3	25	7
	4	25	4
	5	25	16
6	1	45	2
	2	37	10
	3	30	5
	4	45	2
	5	50	2
7	1	12	1
	2	15	1

TABLE II

		SERUMS			
	NO. 1	NO. 2	NO. 3	NO. 4	NO. 5
	7	7	–	–	–
	1	5	1	1	1
NO. OF	3	1	5	5	5
KIESELGUHR	6	6	6	6	4
SAMPLE	4	4	4	3	6
	2	2	2	4	3
	5	3	3	2	2

These chemical results do not present evidence of sufficient difference in the ·chemical nature of the seven samples of kieselguhr to account for the variation shown in the value of the samples for the filtration of serum.

Therefore, chemical examination alone seems to present no means of selecting kieselguhr for the filtration of serums.

Microscopic examination did not present a method of comparison for valuation of relative ability of kieselguhr samples for serum filtration.

TABLE III

KIESELGUHR	COLOR	ORGANIC MATTER	LOSS ON IGNITION
No. 1	Yellowish-White	Trace present	11.4%
No. 2	Grayish-White	" "	10.3%
No. 3	" "	" "	10.4%
No. 4	" "		10.4%
No. 5			5.2%
No. 6			10.3%
No. 7	" "	" "	10.9%

So we are reduced to the necessity of actually comparative filtration experiments regarding loss of serum by absorption, rate of filtration, and clarity of filtrate. In addition, chemical examination is necessary in order to insure absence of excessive organic matter and moisture.

Credit is due the Serum Filtration Department of the Mulford-Biological Laboratories at Glenolden, Pa., for conducting the filtration experiments mentioned in this note.

A CONVENIENT STOPCOCK-NEEDLE-CANNULA*

By Paul J. Hanzlik, M.D., Cleveland, Ohio

THE small instrument illustrated in the accompanying figures represents a combination of hypodermic needle and small metal stopcock intended for use as a cannula. The cannula is made by soldering a needle to one end of a simple, one-way, nickel-plated, brass stopcock, with a short tube at the opposite end for admission of the tip of a Luer syringe. The weight of the cannula is about 6 grams.

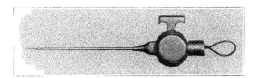

Fig. 1.—Photograph of large size stopcock-needle-cannula; actual size.

I have found the stopcock-needle-cannula very convenient in connection with research and demonstrations for class work, particularly when repeated injections are necessary. The needle portion of the cannula is inserted directly into an exposed vein in the usual way and then secured by a ligature or serrefine clip. For larger veins (saphenous, femoral, jugular, etc.) of larger animals (cats, dogs, etc.) the larger cannula of Fig. 1 is more convenient. For the ear veins of rabbits and guinea pigs the smaller needle-cannula of Fig. 3 is more desirable. This can be securely held in place by means of a small serrefine clip, which encloses the edge of the ear with needle in place.

*From the Department of Pharmacology, School of Medicine, Western Reserve University, Cleveland, Ohio.

The technic of injection by means of the stopcock-needle-cannula is best carried out as follows: Before insertion into the blood vessel, the instrument is filled with normal salt solution (0.9 per cent NaCl) by means of a Luer syringe. This is easily done by turning the stopcock to the transverse position while saline is being forced through. This is done to exclude air and avoid embolus formation. The needle is then placed into position by direct insertion into the vessel and secured by means of a ligature or serrefine clip as described above. The tip of the syringe, which now contains the solution to be injected, is inserted into the cannula and the stopcock quickly opened, and the contents forced in, closing the stopcock (transverse position) when the syringe is emptied. When very small volumes (fraction of a c.c.) are injected, about 1 c.c. of saline should be injected at once in order to wash out the remnants in the needle.

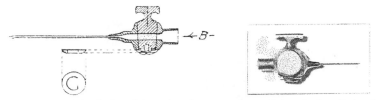

Fig. 2.—Sectional view of large size stop-cock-needle-cannula; actual size; *B*, for insertion of Luer syringe.

Fig. 3.—Photograph of small size stopcock-needle-cannula; actual size; fits Record syringe.

The stopcock-needle-cannula possesses the following advantages: It replaces the more cumbersome glass cannula and burette, with connections. It is nonbreakable. It is serviceable for a wide range of different sized blood vessels, avoiding the maintenance of a large assortment of glass cannulas. It is convenient for making quantitative injections of small volumes of fluid, and small doses of substances, thereby avoiding complications from the injection of additional wash fluid necessary with burettes or other larger apparatus. For instance, in studying the effects of agents on cardiac volume, such a needle-cannula is obviously very convenient, if not indispensable. Larger volumes of fluid can also be injected, since Luer syringes of different sizes fit the instrument equally well.

There is no difficulty with clot-formation in the needle when solutions are injected into the circulation. I have not tried the needle cannula for repeated withdrawal of blood to see whether clot formation would hamper this. However, by insertion of the stiletto this should be easily remedied.

In case the needle should break off, a new one can be easily soldered into the stopcock by a technician of ordinary ability.

The stopcock-needle-cannulas are obtainable from the Geo. H. Wahmann Mfg. Co., 520 West Baltimore St., Baltimore, Md.

I am under obligations to our technician, Mr. M. Dan, for the actual construction of the cannulas here presented, and to Professor T. Wingate Todd for the photographs.

A NEW URINOMETER*

By JACOB ROSENBLOOM, M.D., PH.D., PITTSBURGH, PA.

A T the last meeting of the American Medical Association, there was demonstrated a new urinometer that I devised. The accompanying illustration shows this instrument.† It requires no separate jar, no pouring of the urine back and forth, and can be used when there are only small amounts of urine available.

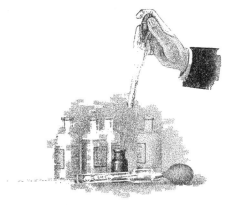

In using the urinometer, one draws the specimen from container by compression of the bulb and the specific gravity is then read off from the hydrometer as in the usual method.

*From the Laboratory of Dr. Jacob Rosenbloom, Pittsburgh, Pa.
†Made by the Scientific Materials Co., Pittsburgh.

The Journal of Laboratory and Clinical Medicine

VOL. V.   MAY, 1920   No. 8

Editor-in-Chief: VICTOR C. VAUGHAN, M.D.
Ann Arbor, Mich.

ASSOCIATE EDITORS

DENNIS E. JACKSON, M.D. - -	CINCINNATI
HANS ZINSSER, M.D. - - -	NEW YORK
PAUL G. WOOLLEY, M.D. - -	DETROIT
FREDERICK P. GAY, M.D. -	- BERKELEY, CAL.
J. J. R. MACLEOD, M.B. - - -	TORONTO
ROY G. PEARCE, M.D. - -	AKRON, OHIO
W. C. MACCARTY, M.D. -	ROCHESTER, MINN.
GERALD B. WEBB, M.D. -	COLORADO SPRINGS
WARREN T. VAUGHAN, M.D. - .	BOSTON

EDITORIALS

The Present Status of Our Knowledge Concerning the Etiology of Influenza

THE medical profession met the great present pandemic of influenza which began in 1915, and has extended to the present day, with no definite information as to the possibilities of a specific method of prevention and therapy. There had been, to be sure, a gradually increasing and an almost settled conviction that the microorganism that Pfeiffer described near the latter end of the last great pandemic of this disease (1892) was really the causative agent involved. It will be recalled that the B. influenzæ was found by Pfeiffer in certain, but by no means all, groups of cases that were to be classed under this malady of many aspects and complications. In subsequent sporadic outbreaks Pfeiffer's bacillus has been found or not as the case might be, success depending in no small measure on the bacteriologic skill involved. This factor of technical difficulty is still of importance in the more recent and otherwise skillful bacteriologic work of the last months. It is, however, by no means sufficient to explain the shifts of opinion and consequent confusion that have arisen concerning the cause of influenza.

Fatal respiratory complications were recognized in the studies of previous influenza epidemics, but it seems certain that they were never so manifest as in the successive waves of the disease that swept the world from 1915 to the present time. The varied bacteriologic causes of the pneumonias that have terminated so many recent cases of influenza have confused the issue as to the primary etiologic agent of the disease itself. It is now apparent that we must separate the primary cause of that prostrating but relatively nonfatal disease known as influenza from its pneumonic sequel of which one or several bacteria may be the cause. It seems now certainly proved that influenzal pneumonias may be produced by several very different microorganisms, among which the most important are the several types of Pneumococci, the Streptococci, both hemolytic and nonhemolytic, the influenza bacillus of Pfeiffer itself, Staphylococci and the bacillus of Friedländer.

The primary etiology of influenza is by no means certain. It is not in the province of this note to attempt to sift in detail the evidence on which the fluctuating scientific opinion in regard to influenza etiology has been based, but to anticipate our argument it may be stated that in the beginning of the present pandemic Pfeiffer's bacillus was generally accepted as the primary cause of influenza, that its etiologic rôle later became rather generally discredited and that finally it would seem in recent months to have regained to a considerable extent its former importance. The data in which these shifts in viewpoint have been founded may now in their salient features concern us.

In discussing the etiology of influenza, attention should again be called to the importance of distinguishing between the microorganisms found in the upper respiratory passages and those detected in the organs, particularly in the pneumonic lungs, of fatal cases. It should further be stated that the difficulty of determining what constitutes a primary pneumonia and what a postinfluenzal pneumonia, still further complicates the question. The organisms found in the upper respiratory passages we may assume represent most nearly the primary causative agent, and those found in the lungs may mean merely secondary invaders.

As a result of a survey of the literature on the bacteriology of influenza the following tentative conclusions may at present be drawn: In the first place, the bacillus of influenza has been found by a large number of observers in the upper respiratory tract of cases of influenza. Among these observers may be mentioned Wolbach,[1] Opie, et al.[2] Medalia,[3] Hickox and Gray,[4] Duval and Harris,[5] Pritchett and Stillman.[6] The percentage of positive results obtained from cultures by these observers varies, but may in many instances approximate 100 per cent. It should be stated that the influenza bacillus has also been found in normal cases by certain observers, notably Opie, et al.[7] in as high as 35.1 per cent normal individuals.

The influenza bacillus is by no means so frequently found in the pneumonic lungs of fatal influenza cases, though by some observers and in some epidemics it has been found there as the predominating organism (Opie, et al.[2]) and (Duval and Harris[8]), and it may unquestionably produce a fatal pneumonia. The blood cultures are almost always negative in such cases (Lamb[9]).

Various other organisms, such as the various types of the pneumococcus, streptococci, Friedländer's bacillus and the like, may be the cause of postinfluenzal pneumonia, and they may also be found in predominating numbers in the early cases in the upper respiratory passages. These findings, however, by no means indicate that any one of them is the cause of the primary disease.

The possibility arises and has been directly asserted by a number, for example by Nicolle and LeBailly,[10, 11] by Gibson and his coworkers,[12, 13] da Cunha, et al,[14] and by Yamanouchi and others[15] that neither the influenza bacillus nor any other organism found in the throat or lungs is the veritable, primary cause of influenza, which in their opinion is a filtrable virus.

As bearing on the etiology of influenza the most important evidence of artificial reproduction of the disease is still in dispute. Many observers have completely failed to produce anything resembling influenza, either in man or in animals by inoculating cultures of influenza bacilli, other bacteria, filtrates from cultures, and also respiratory secretions from influenza cases (Wahl, White, and Lyall,[16] Friedberger,[17] Rosenau,[18] and others).

On the other hand, toxic substances formed by the influenza bacillus have been demonstrated by Parker,[28] by Huntoon and Hannum,[29] and by Albert and Kelman,[30] and lesions in some respects suggesting influenzal processes, have been produced with these toxins by the latter two authors. It has recently been claimed by Blake and Cecil[19] that a pneumonia resembling in all respects influenzal pneumonia can be produced in monkeys by the inoculation of pure cultures, and Davis[20] claims to have produced influenza in man by massive doses of influenza bacillus.

Further evidence bearing on the etiologic role of B. influenzæ is given in numerous reports of the presence of the serum reactions in influenza patients with this microorganism. Agglutinins have been described in influenza cases by Wilson,[21] Fleming,[22] Spooner, Scott, and Heath,[23] Gay and Harris,[24] and Duval and Harris,[25] and fixation antibodies have been described by Rapport[26] and Kolmer, Trist, and Yagle.[27] The question arises as to whether these reactions are etiologically specific or reactions of some nonspecific type.

REFERENCES

[1]Wolbach, S. W.: Bacteriology and Pathology of Influenza Cases, Bull. Johns Hopkins Hosp., 1919, xxx, No. 338.
[2]Opie, E. L., Freeman, A. W., Blake, F. G., Small, J. C., and Rivers, T. M.: Pneumonia Following Influenza at Camp Pike, Ark., Jour. Am. Med. Assn., 1919, lxxii, No. 8, p. 556.
[3]Medalia, L. S.: Influenza Epidemic at Camp MacArthur, Boston Med. and Surg. Jour., 1919, clxxx, No. 12, p. 323.
[4]Hickox, J. A. B., and Gray, Elizabeth: An Investigation of Cases of Influenza Occurring in the Woolwich District during September, October, November, 1918, Lancet, London, 1919, pp. 419-421.
[5]Duval, C. W., and Harris, D. H.: The Role of the Pfeiffer Bacillus in the Recent Epidemic of Influenza, Jour. Infect. Dis., 1919, xxv, No. 5, p. 384.
[6]Pritchett, I. W., and Stillman, E. G.: The Occurrence of Bacillus Influenzæ in Throats and Saliva, Jour. Exper. Med., 1919, xxix, 259.
[7]Opie, E. L., Freeman, A. W., Blake, F. G., Small, J. C., and Rivers, T. W.: Pneumonia at Camp Funston, Jour Am. Med. Assn., 1919, lxxii, No. 2, p. 109.
[8]Duval, C. W., and Harris, D. H.: The Role of the Pfeiffer Bacillus in the Recent Epidemic of Influenza, Jour. Infect. Dis., 1919, xxv, No. 5, p. 384.
[9]Lamb, Frederick H.: Primary and Post Influenzal Pneumonia, Jour. Am. Med. Assn., 1919, lxxii, No. 16, p. 1133.
[10]Nicolle, C. and LeBailly, C.: Quelques notions expérimentales sur le virus de la grippe. Compt. rend. Acad. d. Sc., 1918, clxvii, 607.
[11]Nicolle, C., and LeBailly, C.: Recherches expérimentales sur la grippe. Ann. de l'Inst. Pasteur, 1919, xxxiii, No. 6, p. 395.

[12]Gibson. H. G., Bowman, F. B., and Connor, J. I.: Etiology of Influenza, Brit. Med. Jour., 1919. ii, No. 3038, p. 331.

[13]Gibson, H. G., and Connor, J. I.: Filtrable Virus as Cause of Early Stage of Present Epidemic of Influenza, Brit. Med. Jour., London, 1918, ii, No. 3024, p. 645.

[14]da Cunha, O. M., Magalhães, O., and da Fonseca, O.: Experimental Research on Influenza. Brazil-Medico, Rio de Janeiro, 1918, xxxii, No. 46, p. 377.

[15]Yamanouchi, T., Sakakami, K., and Iwashima, S.: The Infecting Agent in Influenza. An Experimental Research, Lancet, London, June 7, 1919, p. 971.

[16]Wahl, H. R., White, G. B., and Lyall, H. W.: Some Experiments on the Transmission of Influenza, Jour. Infect. Dis., 1919, xxv, No. 5, p. 419.

[17]Friedberger: Med. Verein Greifswald, August 11, 1918.

[18]Rosenau, M. J.: Experiments to Determine Mode of Spread of Influenza, Jour. Am. Med. Assn., 1919, lxxiii, No. 5, p. 311.

[19]Blake, F. G., and Cecil, R. L.: The Production of an Acute Respiratory Disease in Monkeys by Inoculation with Bacillus Influenzæ, Jour. Am. Med. Assn., 1920, lxxiv, No. 3, p. 170.

[20]Davis. D. J.: Successful Human Inoculation with Pure Cultures of Pfeiffer's Bacillus (B. Influenzæ), Jour. Am. Med. Assn., 1919, lxxii, No. 18, p. 1317.

[21]Wilson, W. J.: Specific Agglutinins for Pfeiffer's Bacillus in the Blood Serum of Influenza Patients, Lancet, London, 1919, No. 5014, p. 607.

[22]Fleming. A.: Simply Prepared Culture Mediums for B. Influenzæ, Lancet, London, 1919, ii, No. 4978.

[23]Spooner, L. H., Scott, J. M., and Heath, E. H.: A Bacteriologic Study of the Influenza Epidemic at Camp Devens, Mass., Jour. Am. Med. Assn., 1919, lxxii, No. 3, p. 155.

[24]Gay, F. P., and Harris, D. H.: Serum Reactions in Influenza, Jour. Infect. Dis., 1919, xxv, No. 5, p. 414.

[25]Duval, C. W., and Harris, D. H.: The Role of the Pfeiffer Bacillus in the Recent Epidemic of Influenza, Jour. Infect. Dis., 1919, xxv, No. 5, p. 384.

[26]Rapport, L. H.: The Complement Fixation Test in Influenzal Pneumonia, Jour. Am. Med. Assn., 1919, lxxii, No. 9, p. 633.

[27]Kolmer, J. A., Trist, M. E., and Yagle, E.: Serum Studies on the Etiology of Influenza, Jour. Infect. Dis., 1919, xxiv, 583.

[28]Parker, J. T.: The Poisons of the Influenza Bacillus, Jour. Immunol., 1919, iv, No. 5, p. 331.

[29]Huntoon, F. M., and Hannum, S.: The Role of Bacillus Influenzæ in Clinical Influenza, Jour. Immunol., 1919, iv, No. 4, p. 167.

[30]Albert, Henry, and Kelman, S. R.: The Pathogenicity of Bacillus Influenzæ for Laboratory Animals, Jour. Infect. Dis., 1919, xxv, No. 6, p. 433.

—F. P. G.

Infections and Vaccines

IT IS evident to the observer that vaccines are a very popular form of treatment of infections. It is also as evident that in not infrequent cases the principles of vaccine treatment are hazy in the mind of the physician. The situation is one which causes wonder whether the bacterial substances are being used as a last resort or whether they are being used principally on the chance that they may do good and so save time for the busy practitioner. It seems, therefore, advisable to outline briefly and as practically as possible the principles of vaccine therapy.

In general we may designate a microorganism infectious if it is able to multiply and produce symptoms of disease in the animal body. In order to produce disease it must enter the body, and in so doing it must overcome obstacles, some mechanical, others functional, of the cells and fluids of the host. The rapidity and extent of the invasion depends, in part, on the readiness with which the organism assumes a parasitic existence in the host, the site of entrance into the body, the size of the initial dose, and the resistance of the invader to the attack of the defensive forces of the host. Particular races and strains of an organism may require special qualities by which they are able better to gain entrance to and maintain themselves in a special organ of the host,—"organ affinity;" or during their residence in the host they may be so modified that they are no longer susceptible to the previous lethal action of body fluids,—"serum-fastness;" or they may come to occupy positions of the body relatively inaccessible to the defensive substances of the body. The recognition of these latter factors is of great importance in devising and applying therapeutic measures.

Vaccination has for its aims: (1) The initial increase of resistance of the host so that invasion by bacteria is made more difficult or, in the extreme case (small pox), impossible. (2) To so modify the fluids of the body that once an organism has invaded the body it is not able to survive the condition which discourages parasitism (typhoid). (3) To so modify the fluids that in the case of developed parasitism, the bacteria are eventually killed (furunculosis). It is this latter instance in which we are especially interested at this time.

In considering cases of established infection (parasitism), there are three circumstances to regard: (1) localized infection, (2) general infection, and (3) infection not strictly localized.

In the first case (localized infection) it may be assumed that the reason the infection is localized is that the local (tissue or organ) conditions are such that the growth of the parasites is inhibited to a certain extent because of a locally acquired protective mechanism. That the mechanism is not a general one is shown in certain cases, for instance furunculosis, in which when one or a group of organisms is set free from the original focus a new focus is established in which, as in the first, a local partial immunity or resistance is developed. If, in such a condition, the injection of a substance into the body can cause a sort of mobilization of immunity resources or an increase in the general resistance to the organism concerned in the infection, the local mechanism of defense will be enhanced and the bacteria killed, and at the same time wandering organisms will not find satisfactory conditions for growth and multiplication and will be removed by the destructive cells of the tissues. If we consider furunculosis as a chronic infection associated with a series of acute infections, then what the vaccination does is to immunize prophylactically against succeeding new infections while at the same time assisting in the cure of the old.

In the second case (general infections, especially in streptococcic and staphylococcic sepsis) the use of vaccines has not been brilliant, possibly because the body is already overtaxed with substances of the same character in those injected. The logical conclusion in such cases would be that vaccination is apt to have harmful effects rather than beneficial ones.

In the third case (infections not strictly localized) one is dealing with a group of borderline cases for which it is impossible to formulate any satisfactory rules. In general, Irons says, "the more closely the case approaches a strictly localized infection the more likely it is to prove amenable to vaccines." It is in this group of cases that the possibilities of doing harm by ill advised inoculations are most strikingly evident from a clinical point of view. The delicate balance of aggressive and defensive forces is easily disturbed and an infectious process hitherto confined to one or more foci may be converted quickly into a general infection, temporary perhaps, but accompanied by multiple new metastases.

Theobald Smith commenting upon the general problems of vaccination, says "all parasites tend to increase the resistance of the host in which they live and multiply. Out of this universal fact a number of practical problems arise. In any given disease is it worth while to try to raise this immunity and how much energy will it cost the patient? If worth while, what is the best and most sparing way of raising such immunity artificially? In any localized infection you must ask: Is this a beginning process without attendant immunity, or is it a residual process associated with general immunity? If the latter, then vaccines may be considered safe. In processes associated with fever and bacteriemia science says 'Hands off' until we know whether we have a progressive disease with gradual undermining of the resistance, or a more localized affection in which the excursions into the blood are secondary. Judged from this point of view as well as from the work of the laboratory, we would say that vaccines applied during disease will be rarely, if ever, life saving, but that they may hurry a stationary or languid process which tends toward recovery by bringing into play the unused reserves of the various tissues."

To summarize: Infectious processes in general are suitable for treatment by active immunization, (1) if they are localized, i.e., confined to one or more isolated lesions and are not associated with bacteriemia; (2) if they are more or less chronic.

Vaccines are suspensions of killed bacteria in salt solution, oil, or water, with usually a small amount of preservative, such as phenol or tricresol added.

Autogenous vaccines are prepared from bacteria isolated from the patient who is eventually to receive the vaccine. To quote Irons again. "Assuming that we have a case which clinically is suitable for treatment by active immunization, we may inquire what preparation of bacteria will be most efficient in stimulating the inactive forces of immunity. The researches of recent years indicate that one of the chief elements in the chronicity of an infectious process is a change in the infecting organism by which it becomes less susceptible to the attack of the forces of immunity of the host, and that this bacterial resistance or 'fastness' may be as important as the deficiency in the formation of antibodies of the host. Another similar change in the infecting organism, the acquirement of 'organ specificity' by which through long sojourn in a particular organ of an animal, or series of animals, the invader develops a special aggressiveness for that organ must also be reckoned with. If artificial active immunization is to be effective, it should aim to take cognizance of all, or of as many of these elements as possible, and hence a vaccine should be derived from an organism possessing the properties of those concerned in the infectious process,—an autogenous vaccine."

Stock vaccines are prepared from strains of bacteria isolated at some previous time, and kept in the laboratory in stock. They have no direct biologic relationship with the clinical case in which they are used. The foregoing definition taken with the discussion of autogenous vaccines indicates the reasons for the probable disadvantages of stock vaccines. Nevertheless, there are certain cases in which the stock vaccines are productive of good effects. Wherever this is true, it is also probably true that an autogenous vaccine would be more valuable.

Mixed vaccines are vaccines made of all the microorganisms present in a secretion or in a material. Their value is questionable and their use unscientific. One writer says, the resort to mixed vaccines, particularly to mixed stock vaccines, is either a confession of ignorance of the exact nature of the infection and misapprehension of the principles of immunity or an evidence of indifference and laziness on the part of the physician using them. It were more advisable to use a known unmixed stock vaccine, a carefully studied polyvalent vaccine, or a single purified protein.

Finally and as practically as possible, vaccines (autogenous) seem to be useful in the following infectious disorders:

1. Furunculosis and localized abscesses in soft tissues.
2. Acne vulgaris.
3. Colon bacillus pyelitis and cystitis.
4. Chronic gonorrhea and gonorrheal rheumatism.
5. Chronic bronchitis.
6. Bronchial asthma of bacterial origin.

Vaccines seem to be of little or no value in,—

1. Infection of bone or infections in cavities with rigid walls.
2. Infection of the intestinal tract.
3. Infection of the uterus and adnexa.

Vaccines are contraindicated in,—

1. Acute infections and infectious diseases.
2. Septicemia and pyemia in the acute stages.
3. Malignant endocarditis.

BIBLIOGRAPHY

Irons: Forchheimer's Therapeusis of Internal Diseases, v.
Moody: Jour. Am. Med. Assn., 1920, lxxiv, 391.

—P. G. W.

The Therapeutic Value of Oxygen

THERE is no therapeutic measure that is less efficiently put into practice than the administration of oxygen, and as a consequence, most physicians have little faith in its value. There are several reasons for this state of affairs: in the first place, the physiologic mechanism by which added oxygen could assist in the respiratory functions is not understood; in the second, an insufficient amount of the gas is usually given, and in the third, it is usually given too late.

On the other hand, when oxygen is properly administered in suitable cases before the patient has become moribund, much evidence has accumulated to show that very great benefit indeed results from the treatment, and so far as can be told, a fatal termination is often averted.[1, 2, 3]

In order to understand the physiologic principles involved in this treatment, it is important to remember that although forty to fifty times as much oxygen is combined with hemoglobin as is in simple solution in the blood plasma, yet it is the latter which really diffuses into the tissues. The pressure of oxygen in the plasma, in other words, the diffusion pressure of oxygen, is the determining factor in causing it to permeate the tissues, and whenever this pressure begins to fall under normal conditions, more is added to the plasma by dissociation from the oxyhemoglobin of the corpuscles. The plasma retails the oxygen to the tissues, and the corpuscles are the wholesale warehouses from which the plasma replenishes its stock. The unloading of oxygen from the oxyhemoglobin to the plasma is assisted by various chemical changes that take place while the blood is in the capillaries.

From these considerations it follows that an efficient supply of oxygen to the tissues could be maintained without any hemoglobin if we were to put an excess of the gas into simple solution in the plasma; that is, if enough were forced into solution in the plasma in the lungs so that the tissue requirements could be met without any local addition from oxyhemoglobin. Two experiments may be quoted to show that it is possible to do this.

1. After replacing all the blood from the blood vessels of a frog by artificial plasma (Ringer's solution) the animal can be kept alive for days in a vessel containing pure oxygen (i.e., five times the amount present in air) and during this time the rates of O_2 consumption and CO_2 production are practically the same as normally.

2. Animals (mice) exposed to air containing more than 0.5 per cent of carbon monoxide (contained in coal gas) soon become moribund, because the oxygen carrying power of the hemoglobin is abolished by the formation of carboxy hemoglobin. If the animals are now transferred to pure oxygen under two atmospheres pressure (i.e., ten times the amount in air) they quickly recover, and after leaving them under these conditions for some time, one may then transfer them from the oxygen to air without the toxic symptoms returning. If, on the other hand, they are transferred from the oxygen to air immediately after recovery, the symptoms of asphyxia return and the animal dies.

Both experiments show clearly that if we succeed in getting sufficient oxygen into simple solution in the plasma, the oxyhemoglobin is not necessary to supply the tissues with this gas.

It is evident, therefore, that oxygen administration can be of no avail in poisoning by coal gas or any other substance which destroys the O_2-carrying power of hemoglobin, unless it is forced into the alveoli so as greatly to increase the partial pressure.*

In pulmonary edema, in "gassed" cases, in bronchitis, and in decompensated cardiac cases, oxygen is also of undoubted value, when it is properly administered. Many cases of pneumonia are also benefited by such treatment, but there are others in which the heart is so profoundly affected by toxic substances that oxygen may perhaps be of little use. Evidence of this benefit is afforded by the easier and deeper breathing, the slowing of the pulse, the disappearance of cyanosis and the greater ease and comfort experienced by the patient. Not only do these effects persist as long as the gas is given, and thereby serve to tide over a crisis and permit the natural defensive agencies of the body more successfully to combat the abnormal condition, but they often outlast the administration.

Quantitative evidence that in pneumonia the arterial blood is improperly saturated with oxygen in proportion to the degree of cyanosis, and therefore of the condition of the patient, has been furnished by Stadie.[4] In a normal person

---

*Hemoglobin becomes converted into methemoglobin and incapable of carrying labile O_2 in various types of poisoning, e.g., acetanilide, nitrobenzol.

the arterial blood carries 95 per cent of its full load of oxygen (i.e., it is 5 per cent unsaturated), but in pneumonia it may carry only little over 80 per cent. Meakins[5] has confirmed these findings, and has added most important observations on the effect of oxygen inhalations by the Haldane method. In a case of pneumonia the oxygen unsaturation on the eighth day of the disease was 17.9 per cent. After two hours of oxygen treatment (at a rate of delivery of 2.5 liters O_2 per minute) the unsaturation percentage fell to 9.08, and after eighteen hours (at 1 liter per minute) it was 9.0. The O_2 was then discontinued and in four hours the unsaturation percentage had risen to 15.5. It fell subsequently to 3.05 after twenty-four hours, during which 3 liters O_2 per minute was administered. Shortly after this the crisis occurred. Similar results were obtained in a case of chronic bronchitis, and even in normal men it was found that administration of 3 liters of O_2 per minute for 100 minutes changed the arterial blood from 4.4 per cent unsaturation to 1.87 per cent.

. To explain exactly how the oxygen acts in this group of cases several possibilities must be considered. In the first place we must suppose that the respiratory membrane has become greatly reduced in extent because the alveoli in certain parts of the lungs have become more or less filled with fluid or exudate, although not entirely consolidated. Under these circumstances the blood during the time that it is circulating in the vessels of the affected portion of lung can not be reached by a sufficient amount of oxygen to saturate its hemoglobin fully, because there is an inadequate diffusion pressure of oxygen to penetrate the thick layer of fluid between the alveolar air and blood. So long as the hemoglobin is not fully saturated, the tension of gas in the plasma must become very low, and little can be available for the tissues when the blood arrives at them. When excess of oxygen is breathed, the amount which goes into solution in the fluid will become proportionately raised, so that there will be a much better chance for a sufficient amount to reach the blood so as to saturate the hemoglobin and create a proper tension in the plasma.*

The blood which leaves the lungs as a whole is a mixture of the more or less still venous blood from the affected portions and of arterial blood from the healthy portions, and it may be considered that the mixture is just on the borderline of being adequate to supply the oxygen requirements of the tissues and nerve centers—otherwise the animal could not live. A very little improvement in the oxygen supply will therefore suffice to turn the tide, and it is possible that this may reach it by diffusion through the fluid that has collected in the alveoli. By increasing the pressure of oxygen in the inspired air, more will become dissolved in the fluid (by Henry's law) so that the pressure gradient from air to blood through the fluid will become steeper. But another factor must be considered, namely, that the increased partial pressure in the healthy alveoli has caused more O_2 to go into simple solution in the plasma of the blood circulating in these portions, and although this can not cause the hemoglobin to carry away any greater a load of the gas, yet when this blood is mixed with that from the pathologic lobes, the dissolved oxygen will assist in bringing the hemoglobin up to its proper degree of saturation with oxygen.

*The coefficient of solubility of oxygen in water at 20° C. is 0.34 (i.e. 0.34 c.c. O_2 will diffuse through 1μ (.001 mm.) of water in 1 minute when 1 sq. cm. of the water is exposed to 1 atmosphere of the gas). (Krogh, A.: Jour. of Physiol., 1919. lii. 391.) The amount which will diffuse through fluid is proportional to the thickness of the layer of fluid.

It has been imagined by some that it is useless to give oxygen because the dissociation curve of the blood at varying pressures of the gas shows that even after reducing the partial pressure of oxygen to one half that obtaining in normal alveolar air, the blood still takes up about 80 per cent of its full load. It is argued that it is therefore futile to attempt to increase the oxygen carried by the blood by raising the partial pressure in the air which is inspired into the still healthy alveoli. From what has been said above, however, it is clear that this viewpoint does not take into account two important effects which follow when the partial pressure of the oxygen is increased, namely, that it diffuses much more rapidly through the fluid in the pathologic portions, and that more goes into simple solution in the plasma circulating in the healthy portions.

When the exudation completely fills the alveoli or a portion of the lung completely collapses, the blood ceases to circulate through the capillaries of the affected part, so that all the blood is passing through the capillaries of healthy parts, and the arterial blood may remain of a bright red color. In such conditions it is unlikely that administration of oxygen can be of any value.

The success of treatment with oxygen in suitable cases must depend on several factors, the most important of which are: (1) To get as much of the gas into the alveoli as possible. (2) To start the treatment early before irreparable damage has been done because of anoxemia. (3) To maintain the administration until cyanosis disappears. With regard to the first of these factors, it has sometimes been thought that there is an element of danger in giving too much oxygen. This depends on the observations made by several investigators that animals that have been caused to live in atmospheres containing an excess (80 per cent) of oxygen for some time develop symptoms of pulmonary irritation, leading on to pneumonia.

At percentages just short of this, however, namely, between 60 and 70 Karsner[6] found in rabbits that there was no evidence of pulmonary inflammation even after 11 days continuous exposure. This makes it highly improbable that there could be any danger in man even when the administration of oxygen was pushed to extremes.

The importance of early administration is evident when we realize that the damage of oxygen deficiency on the nerve centers and the tissues usually develops insidiously, and that once started the damage must lead to a progressive deterioration of the vital functions of the body. The respiratory center is among the first to suffer from the anoxemia. The result is shallow and rapid breathing. Such breathing does not, however, properly ventilate the alveoli, so that the anoxemia becomes aggravated, and a vicious respiratory circle becomes established. The defensive agencies of the body against toxins and bacteria are also depressed by the anoxemia so that resistance to the further progress of the disease is deteriorated. It is also possible that prolonged oxygen deficiency, or it may be some toxic substances appearing in the blood as a result, renders the hemoglobin less capable of carrying oxygen by changing some of it into methemoglobin. It is at least significant that this compound is formed in animals after massive injections of streptococci.[7] The maintenance of an adequate tension of oxygen in the plasma by administration of oxygen by the lungs must greatly assist in guarding against these effects.

For similar reasons, the administration should be maintained until all signs of deficient oxidation are removed, the best index of this being the color of the face. So long as there is any anoxemia, this is of a characteristic pale ashen hue, different from that of ordinary capillary congestion.

Regarding *methods of administration*, it may be said at once that the common clinical practice of placing a funnel connected with an oxygen tank in front of the patient's face is worse than useless. At the rate at which the oxygen is usually applied by this method, it is inconceivable how any measurable increase in the percentage of oxygen in the alveolar air could be attained, and if enough gas is turned on really to have some influence, the waste due to diffusion into the air is prohibitive.

Where no special apparatus is obtainable for the administration, the best method is to pass a wide gum elastic catheter into one nostril, through which the gas, after bubbling through water in a flask, is passed as quickly as is comfortable for the patient. The method is rendered much more efficient if the open nostril is closed by the attendant during each inspiratory act. Dr. Rudolf and I have found by this latter method that the percentage of oxygen in the alveolar air can be raised to 35 per cent when the opposite nostril is compressed during inspiration. With the opposite nostril open, this percentage was only slightly raised above the normal.

When special appliances are available, a choice may be made between the mask and valve devised for the purpose by J. S. Haldane,[1] and which was extensively used in the treatment of gassed men, or the hollow tongue depressor of Meltzer.[2] In the Haldane method the oxygen is discharged from a cylinder of the gas, (provided with a reducing valve) through tubing connected with a wide bore T-piece. To one limb of the T a small rubber bag is attached, and the other is furnished with a mica valve and ends in the face mask. The valve does not open on expiration, so that oxygen collects in the bag, and is inhaled on inspiration. The appliance is simple and saves oxygen, but patients not infrequently object to covering up of the face with the mask.

A very satisfactory method is that of S. J. Meltzer, in which a flat metal tube (hollow tongue depressor) is connected by wide rubber tubing to a very easily manipulated respiratory valve, beyond which is a strong rubber bag attached to the rubber tubing coming from an oxygen cylinder. When the valve is in the inspiratory position, the gas passes through the bag into the tongue depressor, when in the expiratory position it fills the bag and none gets beyond the valve. The tongue depressor is inserted in the mouth not much farther than the middle of the tongue, so that there may be no gagging or other discomfort, and the lips are kept closed. The valve is manipulated by the attendant about 10 to 12 times a minute. By this method, with the nose clamped, we have been able to raise the percentage of oxygen in the alveolar to eighty-five.

Of course by far the most satisfactory method is to place the patient in a respiratory cabinet filled with oxygen. Such cabinets are being tried in England, and there is no doubt that they will soon come into frequent use.

REFERENCES

[1]Haldane, J. S.: Brit. Med. Jour., July 19, 1919, p. 64.
[2]Meltzer, S. J.: Jour. Am. Med. Assn., 1917, lxix, 1150.
[3]Rudolf, R. D.: Paper before the Academy of Medicine of Toronto. See Jour. Can. Med.
     Assn., current number.
[4]Stadie: Jour. Exper. Med., 1919, xxx, 215.
[5]Meakins, J. C.: Brit. Med. Jour., March 6, 1920, p. 324.
[6]Karsner, H. T.: Jour. Lab. and Clin. Med., 1917, ii, No. 4.
[7]Peabody, F. W.: Jour. Exper. Med., 1913, xviii, 1.

—J. J. R. M.

The Chemistry and Physiology of Memory

LIPKIN has collected the literature on this subject from which we make the following abstract. The sum total of mental processes which alone is representative of the values that differentiate human existence from that of its humbler associates might be found, upon analysis, to be composed of a group of memory-ideas, through whose coordination and cooperation thought is made effective. No thought is possible which does not derive its material from memory-ideas. No memory-idea is possible which has not at some previous time entered consciousness as a corresponding sensation. Sometime, somewhere, an impulse, that had its origin in an effective stimulus in the external world, entered the brain by way of the sensory paths, produced a sensation, and, though its effects may have long since disappeared from consciousness, left a record which has never been completely eradicated and upon which our thoughts—through our memories—become conditioned. Pillsbury says: "Memory, imagination, reasoning, are limited in the qualities that they make use of to the bare materials of sense. They may recombine them, they may make use of the sense materials in new ways, but they can add no new qualities." Hence, memory resolves itself into the conscious experience of awareness of a group of centrally aroused sensations, sensations already existing in the central nervous system, retained as a result of changes produced in the nerve tissue by some previous stimulation. Explanation of the nature of this retention of memories and their reproduction as well as an analysis of the various factors that go to make up the structures of memory, will be attempted in the following:

Let us assume that we are remembering two simple sensations, one visual—yellow; the other, auditory—middle C. Let us follow these two sensations from their origin to their destination and attempt to arrive at the causes that make recollection of them possible. Waves of light are of different lengths, being composed of vibrations that range from 400 to 800 millimicrons in length. All light waves, the length of whose vibrations does not correspond to that of yellow, which is 554 millimicrons, are absorbed; all others are reflected to enter the eye. These vibrations affect the retina at the rate of 542 trillion times per second. They hit the rods and cones, and thus excite in them a visual impulse. This impulse travels through the bipolar cells, ganglion cells, and along the fibrils of the optic nerve with a velocity of 123 per second. We follow the impulse along the optic tract, and, after partial crossing at the optic chiasm to the external geniculate bodies, where connection is made with a second series of neurons that carry the impulse to the nerve cells of the visual center, which is situated around the calcarine fissure of the median surface of the occipital lobe. Here the impulse excites the nerve cells into activity, resulting in visual sensation.

Sound is composed of vibrations emanating from vibrating medium, as, for example, the vocal cords that are set into vibration when the air passes up the respiratory passage. When middle C is sounded, 132 vibrations reach our ear every second, and set into vibration the tympanic membrane, the hammer, anvil, stirrup, the lymph within the cochlea, and finally the hair-like process of the basilar membrane—18,000 to 24,000 in number, some of which respond in sympathetic vibration with the vibrations of middle C. The sympathetic vibration thus excites the nerve cells of the spiral ganglia into activity and sets an auditory impulse traveling along the auditory nerve. We follow the impulse along the fibrils of the auditory nerve to its connection with a second layer of neurons, either in the ventral root of the eighth nerve or in the tuberculum acusticum, thence to the superior olive lemniscus lateralis, internal geniculate bodies, and finally to the nerve cells of the auditory center in the superior temporal gyrus and the transverse gyri, extending from this into the fissure of Sylvius. Here the impulse excites the nerve cells into activity and the result is an auditory sensation.

In these two illustrations we have two sensations—one produced by the excitation of the nerve cells of the occipital lobe, the other by the excitation of the nerve cells of the temporal lobe. In both cases the sensations were due to the impulses that have reached the brain by way of the visual and auditory paths. Experiments have shown that both impulses are essentially alike in quality; that if the auditory nerve be attached to the eye and the optic nerve to the ear, lightning would be heard and thunder seen, that the particular sensation experienced does not depend upon the stimulus, or impulse, or nerve fibers, but upon the distal nerve ending, whose function it is to excite nerve cells into specific activity. Theories as to the nature of the impulse, or nerve conduction, are enormous, but facts that would substantiate, are neither many nor lacking in contradiction. Doubt as to its being of a chemical nature is derived from the facts that under normal conditions nerve fibers are incapable of fatigue; that no heat is produced as a result of the passage of an impulse, and that there is no conclusive evidence of metabolism. On the other hand, experiments have shown that nerve fibers have become fatigued. Garten has shown that one nerve, the olfactory of the pike, when stimulated by induction shocks, with an interval between the stimuli of as much as .27 seconds, gives evidence of fatigue, since its action current as measured by the capillary electrometer, diminishes in extent quite rapidly and recovers after a short time. It has also been found that, while a nerve deprived of oxygen loses its irritability, this event occurs more promptly if the nerve is constantly stimulated. Tashiro reports that by means of a new method, which is capable of detecting as little as .000,0001 g. of CO_2, he has been able to show that the resting nerve produces CO_2 and that its production is increased two and one-half times when the nerve is stimulated. The assumption, therefore, is that a sensitive and unstable substance existing within the axis-cylinder is upset by the stimulus at the point stimulated, so that the energy thus liberated acts upon contiguous particles, and so the disturbance is propagated along the nerve as a progressive chemical change which may be compared to the passage of a spark along a line of gunpowder. An opposite view is taken in the attempt to prove that the stimulus passing through the nerve fiber is electrical in nature. This would agree with the quickness of recovery from fatigue and the slight evidence of metabolic changes that many observers have recorded as the result of stimulation of nerve fibers. On the positive side it is found that if a cut nerve is connected with its sheath through a delicate galvanometer, an electric current flows from the cut end to the sheath. Furthermore, with a core model consisting of a glass tube with a core of platinum wire and a sheath of solution of NaCl .6 per cent, electrical phenomena can be obtained similar to those shown by the stimulated nerve. If an induction current, serving as a stimulus, is sent into one end of such an artificial nerve, and from the other end two leading off electrodes are connected with a galvanometer, then it can be demonstrated that an electrical charge is propagated along the model at each application of the stimulus. Moreover, such a moving electrical disturbance is the only objective phenomenon known to occur in the stimulated nerve, and it is assumed that it constitutes the nerve impulse. When this electrical disturbance reaches the end organ it initiates the chemical changes that characterize the activity of the organ. Corresponding to the central thread of the core conductor would be the neurofibrils within the axis-cylinder, and to the liquid sheath of less conductive material surrounding the central thread would be the perifibrillar substance. The fact that the rate of propagation of the nerve impulse is 123 meters per second, whereas that of an electric current is 186,000 miles per second, would lead us to believe that the current is not a direct but an intermittent one. Nernst supposes that the electrolytes contained in the axis-cylinder lie within membranous partitions which are impermeable to the passage of certain ions. When an electrical current is passed through a nerve it is conveyed by the dissociated electrolytes and, in consequence of the impermeable character of the septa, there will be a concentration of the positively charged ions on one side of the membrane and the negatively charged on the other. When the concentration of the ions reaches a certain point excitation occurs.

The visual and auditory sensations are now aroused. How are they to be transformed into memory-ideas? How and where are these to be retained? How are they to be reproduced? These are questions for an explanation of which we must turn to the psychologist.

Besides the sense and motor centers, which occupy comparatively small areas of the cortex, there are large areas occupied by cellular and fibrous network which form connections between the various sensory centers. These are called association areas. There are three groups; the frontal or anterior, the median or insular, and the posterior, extending to the occipital lobe and also laterally to the temporal lobes. Their general function is to unite the sense impressions into general knowledge. This function is indicated by the anatomic fact that they are connected with the various sense centers by tracts of association fibers, suggesting a mechanism by which the sense qualities from the separate sense centers may be combined to form a mental image of a complex nature. The posterior area is concerned especially in the organization of the experiences founded upon visual and auditory sensations. The anterior area is especially concerned in the organization of experiences based upon internal sensations. The cortex of Reil is probably a part of the speech area, both on the motor and sensory sides. It is in these association centers that our memory records of past experiences and their connections are laid down in some material change in the network of the nerve cells and fibers. Experiments have shown that lesions in the sense centers or in the association areas connected with the sense centers produce defects of memory corresponding to the sensations which such sense centers normally produce. Auditory aphasia, or loss of power to understand spoken language, is due to injury to the auditory center, or to the immediately contiguous areas of the temporal lobes. Alexia, or loss of power to understand.written or printed language, is due to a lesion involving the inferior parietal convolutions. Olfactory amnesia, or defects in the sense of smell, follow lesions in the distal portion of the hippocampal gyrus. Studies of mental pathology offer adequate proof that memory processes, retention, and reproduction, are dependent upon the sense centers and the association areas connected with them.

It is held by some that memory is a universal function of organized matter. Any change that may be suffered by any substance tends to persist. Every sight and every sound leave impressions on the brain. When subsequently the same or a similar sight or sound is perceived it touches the same spot, as it were, in the brain.

The reproduction or revival of previous impressions may take place by an act of will or by similar impressions or associations of the original impression. When a revival takes place by a repetition of the same sensory impulse we probably have a repetition of the same process in the same nerve elements. When one revives a memory in ideation only, there is also a repetition of the same nerve process in the same nerve elements that took place when the object was originally before the eyes. In addition, we have the laws of association; namely, that memories are recalled by the recurrence of sensations, or revival of memories associated with the original memories, through contiguity, succession, similarity, or contrast.

When we recognize an old memory, we locate it in time and we do this by mentally determining its relation to the present time; in fact, we could have no idea of time if it were not for memory; all would be present; we would have no past, nor could we anticipate the future.

Another conception of the nature of the change induced in nerve cells as a result of previous stimulation has been suggested by Matthews. According to this investigator, there are reasons for believing that when a nerve cell is touched by an impulse a change in its chemical composition or in the arrangement of its molecular structure is produced. An interesting and highly suggestive parallel is drawn by Matthews between the manifestations exhibited by linseed oil and brain cells. One of the chief constituents of the brain cell is cephalin, which contains unsaturated fatty acids of the linoleic acid type. Linseed oil likewise contains linoleic acid. When linseed oil is exposed to light or ultraviolet rays in the presence of air in a closed flask provided with a mercury manometer, for the first twenty-four to thirty-six hours nothing seems to happen. Then slowly the oil begins to oxidize, and it oxidizes at a constantly accelerating pace so that the oxygen is used up in the flask and the negative pressure may be measured by the manometer. It is as though the oil had to be taught by the light to oxidize itself and learns to oxidize better and better. It may be shown that the oil possesses something like a memory. If after sixty hours' illumination, when the oil is oxidizing at a fairly rapid rate, the illumination is discontinued, it will be found that the oxidization no longer waits twenty-four hours before beginning, but the stimulation of the lamp is effective within an hour or more; the oil acts as though it remembered the teaching of a previous illumination, and now oxidizes at a more rapid rate. The processes which the oil undergoes are autocatalytic. They consist in the persistence in the oil of an intermediary catalytic oxidization product. If it were possible that an impulse coming into certain cells caused in those cells the formation of a persistent autocatalytic intermediary oxidization product, a physical basis of memory might be given. However, as it is, our knowledge of the underlying basis of memory is at best imperfect, and only through a continuous and untiring study can we hope to attain a complete solution of this interesting question.   —V. C. V.

United States Civil Service Examination for Bacteriologist, June 22, 1920.

The United States Civil Service Commission announces an open competitive examination for bacteriologist. A vacancy at St. Elizabeth's Hospital, Washington, D. C., at $2,500 a year, with temporary increase granted by Congress of $20 a month, and maintenance, and vacancies in positions requiring similar qualifications, at this or higher or lower salaries, will be filled from this examination, unless it is found in the interest of the service to fill any vacancy by reinstatement, transfer, or promotion.

All citizens of the United States who meet the requirements, both men and women, may enter this examination; appointing officers, however, have the legal right to specify the sex desired in requesting certification of eligibles. For the present vacancy male eligibles are desired.

Competitors will not be required to report for examination at any place but will be rated on the following subjects, which will have the relative weights indicated on a scale of 100: (1) Physical ability, 10. (2) Education, training and experience, 90.

UNDER THE SECOND SUBJECT COMPETITORS WILL BE RATED UPON THE SWORN STATEMENTS IN THEIR APPLICATIONS AND UPON CORROBORATIVE EVIDENCE.

Applicants must have graduated from a recognized medical college, and have had at least five years' bacteriologic and sanitary experience, including experience in the following lines: (a) Performance of autopsies; (b) Wassermann work; (c) Urinalysis; (d) Blood counts; (e) Sputum examination.

Special credit will be given for graduate courses in bacteriology, pathology and general sanitary work in the U. S. Army or in domestic or foreign universities; also for experience in similar work in a hospital for the insane.

Applicants must have reached their twenty-sixth birthday on the date of the examination. Age limits do not apply to persons entitled to preference because of military or naval service.

Applicants must submit with their applications their unmounted photographs, taken within two years, with their names written thereon. Proofs or group photographs will not be accepted. Photographs will not be returned to applicants.

Applicants should at once apply for Form 1312, stating the title of the examination desired, to the Secretary of the Fourth Civil Service District, 8th and E Streets, N. W., Washington, D. C., or to the Secretary of the United States Civil Service Board, Customhouse, Boston, Mass., New York, N. Y., New Orleans, La., Post Office, Philadelphia, Pa., Atlanta, Ga., Cincinnati, Ohio, Chicago, Ill., St. Paul, Minn., Seattle, Wash., San Francisco, Calif., or Old Customhouse, St. Louis, Mo.

Applications should be properly executed, excluding the county officer's certificate, but including the medical certificate and must be filed with the Secretary of the Fourth Civil Service District, 8th and E Streets, N. W., Washington, D. C., prior to the hour of closing business on June 22, 1920.

The Journal of
Laboratory and Clinical
Medicine

| VOL. V. | ST. LOUIS, JUNE, 1920 | No. 9 |

ORIGINAL ARTICLES

BOTULISM FROM CANNED RIPE OLIVES*

By HERBERT W. EMERSON, B.S., M.D., AND GEORGE W. COLLINS, B.S.,
ANN ARBOR, MICH.

A GLASS of succotash and a bottle containing some ripe olives and about 150 mils of olive juice said to have been served at a formal dinner at the residence of Mr. M. W. S., Grosse Point, Detroit, Mich., on October 18, 1919, were delivered to the Hygienic Laboratory of the University of Michigan for bacteriologic examination.

The bacteriologic and chemical examination of the succotash did not show the presence of anything that would cause sickness or death.

The olives had a very good appearance. They were not as dark brown as the average packed ripe olives, and when sliced the interior was quite light in color. There were a few light colored spots on the brown skins of some of the olives. They had a peculiar odor which was not distinctly different from the normal odor of packed ripe olives. The odor was not distinctly suggestive of putrefaction. It was a blend of the normal pleasant, aromatic odor of ripe olives plus the butyric acid odor of rancid butter. This gives a deceptive odor that might not be recognized by a careful housewife or servant.

Small pieces from the surface of the olives, and small pieces from near the pit, likewise samples of the olive juice, were planted in deep tubes of one per cent dextrose agar, that was –0.2 per cent with phenolphthalein. Similar samples were planted in gelatin tubes in 1 per cent glucose bouillon tubes, and in agar and gelatin plates. Some of these tubes and some of the plates were placed in Novy jars and the oxygen removed by using pyrogallic acid and sodium hydroxide solution. Other tubes were overlaid with liquid petrolatum, while a number were left under aerobic conditions. A part of these were grown at room temperature and a part at 37° C. The glucose agar tubes at incubator temperature

*From the Hygienic Laboratory of the University of Michigan, Ann Arbor, Mich.

under anaerobic conditions showed gas bubbles at the end of twelve hours and the agar was markedly fragmented at the end of twenty-four hours. The glucose agar tubes at room temperature and under anaerobic conditions showed gas bubbles at the end of forty-eight hours. Colonies were picked from the agar plates and from some of the gelatin plates at the end of seventy-two hours. Most of the gelatin plates in the Novy jars at the end of seventy-two hours were liquefied and had a very strong butyric acid odor.

The hanging drops of the olive juice and of the suspensions of the picked colonies contained coarse bacilli which were moderately motile and the stained smears showed coarse bacilli with rounded ends occurring singly and in pairs, some with terminal oval spores that were broader than the bacilli. This organism was weakly gram positive. The stained smears of the olive juice showed in addition very many free spores.

The olive juice was found to be very toxic to guinea pigs; 0.1 mil when introduced into guinea pigs' stomachs and 0.1 mil when injected intraperitoneally,

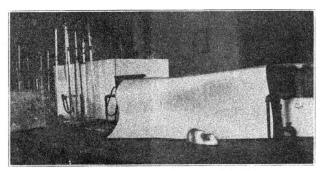

Fig. 1.—Guinea pig 12 hours after 0.1 mil of olive juice.

killed 350 gram guinea pigs in twelve to forty-eight hours. Olive juice filtered through a Berkefeld filter was found to be slightly less toxic than the unfiltered juice. The guinea pigs sometimes vomited a greenish-colored fluid. The saliva was increased. The pupils were dilated. Later the abdomen hung down lower than normal, due to a decrease in the tonicity of these muscles. Later still the head rested on the floor of the cage. The guinea pig usually rested on its abdomen with its extremities extended. The nose and mucous membranes were very cyanotic. The temperature was subnormal. The respiration was abdominal in type, weak, and irregular. (Fig. 1.)

At this time and four days after the samples were received, we reported to Detroit that we had isolated an organism morphologically and culturally like B. botulinus and that the olive juice contained a toxin that killed guinea pigs with symptoms of botulism. That the cases in Detroit were botulism due to the eating of olives containing B. botulinus and the toxin formed by this organism.

These findings were confirmed the next day by Dr. Plinn Morse[1] of Harper Hospital, Detroit, and later by Professor R. Graham[2] of the University of Illinois and by Zoe Northrup Wyant[3] of Michigan Agricultural College.

The Board of Health of Detroit had all the olives of this brand in Detroit collected. A short time later, Commissioner of Health, Dr. Henry Vaughan, notified all the public health officials of the various states and larger cities of the Detroit outbreak and of the brand and serial number of the package concerned. The Bureau of Chemistry Department of Agriculture collected a number of samples of this brand and found some others of the same serial number that contained B. botulinus. They requested that all olives of this pack number be taken at once from the market. This undoubtedly prevented other outbreaks of botulism and saved some lives. One other unfortunate outbreak of botulism at Memphis, costing the lives of six persons, resulted from eating olives from the same source and bearing a closely related serial number. This occurred after the above warning had been given and precautions taken.

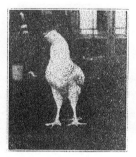

Fig. 2.—Normal rooster.

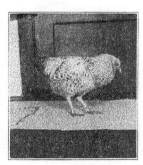

Fig. 3.—Two days after last injection.

EXPERIMENTS ON THE TOXICITY OF THE OLIVE JUICE

GUINEA PIG	WEIGHT	AMOUNT OF OLIVE JUICE	ROUTE	RESULT	TIME
No. 5	620 grams	2.0 mills	Intraperitoneally	plus*	12 hours
No. 6	620 "	2.0 "	stomach	"	36 "
No. 7	400 "	0.5 "	intraper.	"	12 "
No. 8	400 "	0.1	"	"	30 "
No. 9	350 "	0.01 ·	"	"	48 "
No. 10	350 "	0.01 "	"	"	40 "
No. 11	250 "	0.5 filtered	"	"	12 "
No. 12	250 "	0.1 "	"	"	48 "

*Plus means died.

A rooster weighing 2,200 grams was given 0.2 mils intraperitoneally on Monday, October 27. The rooster was apparently normal the following Thursday morning, when it was given 1.0 mil. Thursday night it showed some difficulty in holding its head up. Friday it squatted in the cage all day, appeared tired and sleepy. It would let its head droop and raise it with a jerk and occasionally wiped thick mucus from its mouth. Friday afternoon it grew rapidly weaker and died Friday night.

A second rooster weighing 2,700 grams was given 0.5 mils of olive juice intraperitoneally on Wednesday, November 19. This rooster remained apparently well, and November 27 it was given a second injection of 1.0 mil. There was no apparent change, and December 8 it was given a third injection of 1.0 mil. It began to show symptoms of botulism the next afternoon and these were slightly more marked the next morning. The rooster appeared tired, remained squatting in the cage most of the day. The feathers on its neck were ruffled, its head drooped. It occasionally wiped thick mucus from its mouth, and frequently made peculiar expulsive sounds as if attempting to clear its respiratory tract of this mucus. The symptoms increased very gradually. Respiration became more difficult. The comb, at first bright red, changed slowly to a dark red and then gradually became very cyanotic. The temperature was increasingly subnormal. The limber neck increased. The rooster died Sunday night, six days after the last injection. See Figs. 2 to 8, all taken before the rooster died.

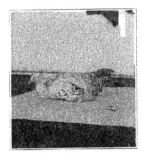 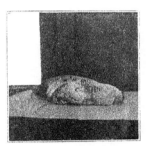

Fig. 4.--Three days after last injection.   Fig. 5.—Four days after last injection.

Cultures of the olive juice in glucose bouillon tubes that had been incubating anaerobically for four days were heated at 60° C. for sixty minutes. Transplants were then made by means of capillary pipettes into nitrated glucose agar tubes. These were incubated for four days in a Novy jar. Then those tubes were selected in which the colonies were sufficiently scattered that one could pick individual colonies.

These colonies were picked up in capillary pipettes and transplanted. Some of the colonies thus selected gave apparently pure cultures of B. botulinus and have been used for toxin production. Other colonies were selected according to the method of Dickson and Burke.[4] The organism growing on glucose bouillon sealed by a layer of liquid petrolatum produced in six days at incubator temperature a toxin, 0.0001 mil of which killed guinea pigs in forty-eight hours.

TOXIN, ANTITOXIN EXPERIMENTS

The toxin in the olive juice was first tested against some antitoxin sent to us by Professor Robert Graham of the University of Illinois.

PIG	QUANTITY OF OLIVE JUICE		GRAHAM'S ANTITOXIN	DATE	RESULT	TIME
1	1.0 mil	plus	1.0 mil	12/1/19	plus	12 hours
2	0.5 mil	plus	1.0 mil	12/1/19	plus	30 hours
3	0.5 mil	plus	2.0 mil	12/1/19	plus	30 hours
4	0.25 mil	plus	2.0 mil	12/1/19	plus	14 hours
5	0.1 mil	plus	1.0 mil	12/1/19	plus	28 hours
6	0.25 mil	plus	none	12/1/19	plus	20 hours
7	none	plus	2.0 mil	12/1/19	neg.	

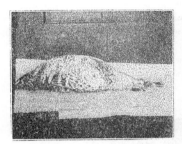

Fig. 6.—Five days after last injection and one day before death.

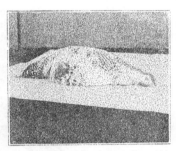

Fig. 7.—Five days after last injection which was one day before death.

The toxin and antitoxin were mixed in a sterile test glass just before it was injected. This antitoxin affords no protection to the toxin in the olive juice.

This antitoxin was similarly tested with the toxin obtained in the bouillon cultures and gave the same results when using the same doses and in doses graded down to about the M.L.D. of the toxin.

The Graham antitoxin was thus tried with the toxin obtained by growing the Nevin strain B. botulinus and found to give marked protection to guinea pigs receiving this toxin-antitoxin mixture. It did not, however, give any protection whatsoever to the toxin obtained by growing the B. botulinus Krumwiede[5] isolated from the olives causing the New York botulism. One often finds guinea pigs receiving the antitoxin-toxin mixture dying before the controls receiving the same amount when the toxin and antitoxin are of different types.

These toxins were next tested in a similar way with antitoxin received from Dr. Buckley and Dr. Giltner[6] Bureau of Animal Industry. This antitoxin gave marked protection to guinea pigs receiving the toxin in the olive juice, the toxin from our culture of B. botulinus, and the toxin from the B. botulinus Krumwiede. It gave no protection to the toxin from the B. botulinus Nevin. The B. botulinus isolated from the Detroit olives and from the New York olives is therefore of the Boise Type[7] or Type A.[8]

There have been five small outbreaks of botulism in the United States in six months, the result of eating ripe olives packed in glass containers. First, the one at Canton, Ohio,[9] costing the lives of seven persons. Second, the outbreak of botulism in Detroit[10] resulting in the deaths of five persons. Third, the cases of botulism near Java, Montana, costing the lives of about six people. Fourth, the outbreak in New York City[11] resulting in six deaths. Fifth,[12] the outbreak in Memphis, Tenn., which added six deaths to the total.

These facts force one to the conclusion that ripe olives as collected at the present time and as processed when packed in glass jars are possible means of spreading widely the toxin of B. botulinus. This menace to life and to health should be removed when this season's ripe olives are packed. The steps necessary can best be accomplished by installing a system of government inspection and supervision under the direction of the Bureau of Chemistry, Department of Agriculture. Such a system of supervision and inspection would be similar to the present federal inspection of slaughter houses and meat packing industry. Such a system, properly introduced and managed, would be, first of all, a protection to the olive consumer. It would also be a marked assistance to the prop-

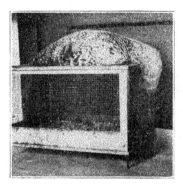

Fig. 8.—Five days after last injection which was one day before death.

erly managed olive packing plant and would be welcomed by it. It would be complained of and disliked only by those attempting to pack and market something that should not be permitted and that might be harmful. That it is quite difficult to kill all the spores of B. botulinus has been shown by the investigations of G. S. Burke.[13]

There is one other group of food canning plants that needs such supervision badly, much more so than do the olive canning plants. These are all the plants canning any kind of fish for the market. We can be justly proud of the federal method of inspection of meat packing plants. It has accomplished much. There is no logical reason why the fish canning plants should not be similarly supervised and inspected.

This report probably does not embrace all of the botulism resulting from canned ripe olives. One must take into serious consideration the large number of deaths reported as due to ptomaine poisoning where the source of the difficulty has not been determined.

SUMMARY

1. There have been at least five small outbreaks of botulism in this country due to the eating of canned ripe olives.

2. Four of these were due to B. botulinus of the Boise Type or Type A.

3. Antitoxin for one type is specific for that type alone.

4. Dickson's work has very recently demonstrated that antitoxin has definite protective value when administered soon after the toxin.[14]

5. This menace to life and health should be removed by adequate government supervision of the plants.

6. This supervision should include the fish packing and canning plants.

7. All plants affected should find such a federal supervision of definite service to the plant.

REFERENCES

[1]Morse: Personal communication.
[2]Graham: Personal communication.
[3]Wyant: Personal communication.
[4]Dickson and Burke: Jour. Am. Med. Assn., Aug., 1918, p. 518.
[5]Supplied to the authors by Dr. Krumwiede.
[6]Supplied to the authors by Drs. Buckley and Giltner of the B. A. I.
[7]Jour. Am. Med. Assn., Sept. 20, 1919, p. 907.
[8]Jour. Bact., iv, No. 5, p. 555.
[9]Public Health Reports, xxxiv, No. 51, p. 2877.
[10]Jour. Am. Med. Assn., lxxiv, No. 2, p. 77.
[11]Jour. Am. Med. Assn., lxxiv, No. 8, p. 516.
[12]Newspaper reports.
[13]Burke: Jour. Am. Med. Assn., lxxii, No. 2, p. 88.
[14]Dickson: Jour. Am. Med. Assn., lxxiv, No. 11, p. 718.

CHEMICAL CHANGES IN THE BLOOD IN DISEASE*
III. Creatinine

By Victor C. Myers, Ph.D., New York City

UNTIL the advent of Folin's colorimetric method for the estimation of creatinine in urine in 1904,[1] we possessed no reliable information regarding this interesting nitrogenous waste product, which in point of quantity is second only to urea. Folin[2] was the first to show that the amount of creatinine excreted in the urine by a normal individual on a meat-free diet is quite independent of either. the amount of protein in the food or of the total nitrogen in the urine, the amount excreted from day to day being practically constant for each individual, thus pointing conclusively to its endogenous origin. He further noted that the fatter the subject, the less creatinine is excreted per kilo of body weight and concluded from this that the amount of creatinine excreted depends primarily upon the mass of active protoplasmic tissue, or, as Shaffer[3] has expressed it, "Creatinine is derived from some special process in normal metabolism taking place largely, if not wholly, in the muscles, and upon the intensity of this process appears to depend the muscular efficiency of the individual." Creatinine is the anhydride of creatine, the chief nonprotein nitrogenous constituent of the muscle tissue of vertebrate animals. That the creatinine of the urine has its origin in the creatine of the muscle would seem obvious on *a priori* grounds, but a definite proof of this hypothesis has been beset with many difficulties. The older observers stated that both administered creatine and creatinine reappeared in the urine as creatinine. When Folin[4] first reinvestigated this question with accurate methods and pure creatine and creatinine, he found that 80 per cent of the administered creatinine did reappear as creatinine, but that when creatine was given in moderate amounts (1 gram to man) it not only failed to reappear as creatinine, but completely disappeared. From this Folin quite naturally concluded that creatine and creatinine were relatively independent in metabolism.

In 1913 Myers and Fine[5] called attention to the fact that the creatine content of the muscle of a given species of animals was very constant (obviously also that of a given animal) and suggested this as a possible basis of the constancy in the daily elimination of creatinine first noted by Folin. Later they pointed out that the creatinine content of muscle was greater than that of any other tissue, and also that in autolysis experiments with muscle tissue the creatine (and any added creatine) was converted to creatinine at a constant rate of about 2 per cent daily, which is just about the normal ratio between the muscle creatine and urinary creatinine. They also found that, when creatine was administered to man or animals, there was a slight conversion to creatinine which corresponds well with the above figure. These facts all go to support the view that creatinine is formed in the muscle tissue from creatine, and at a very constant rate, although no explanation of the physiological significance of this

*From the Laboratory of Pathological Chemistry. New York Post-Graduate Medical School and Hospital. New York City.

transformation can as yet be offered. Excepting possibly the kidney, the muscle normally contains more creatinine than any other body tissue and is followed by the blood, which indicates that after its formation in the muscle the creatinine is carried to the kidney by the blood stream. The only exception to this statement is found in "uremia" where the creatinine content of the blood may slightly exceed that of the muscle.[6]

Folin and Denis[7] were the first to present any very extensive data on the creatinine content of the blood, although almost simultaneously Neubauer[8] reported an observation on a case of "uremia," while Myers and Fine[9] presented several analyses on two cases of nephritis showing marked retention of creatinine. Folin and Denis gave observations on nine cases of "uremia" and were the only observers to give figures for normal human bloods. Shaffer had begun a study of this question some years previously, but unfortunately did not give his protocols[10] until after the appearance of the paper by Folin and Denis. In a preliminary report in 1909 Shaffer and Reinoso[11] stated that using methods which they believed allowed no conversion of creatine to creatinine, they found between 1 and 6 mg. of creatinine per 100 grams of fresh dog muscle, and about 1 mg. per 100 c.c. of serum. Later Myers and Fine took up a study of the creatinine content of muscle tissue and reported some preliminary observations,[12] which confirmed the work of Shaffer and Reinoso. They had described their method[13] but not given their protocols[14] prior to the publication of Folin's simple method[15] for the estimation of creatinine in body fluids and tissues. Essentially the same range of figures was found with the two methods, the findings for various animals and man ranging roughly from 3 to 9 mg. per 100 grams of muscle, excepting instances of impaired renal function.

CREATININE CONTENT OF THE BLOOD

For perfectly normal individuals the creatinine of the blood amounts to 1 to 2 mg. per 100 c.c., the findings for the strictly normal being nearer 1 than 2 mg. As soon as one passes to hospital patients, however, higher values are found. Although the great majority of cases without renal involvement show creatinine figures on the whole blood below 2.5 mg. per 100 c.c., occasionally figures as high as 3.5 mg. are encountered that are not readily explained. It may be noted, however, that a slight retention of creatinine (figures between 3 and 4 mg.) occurs in syphilis, certain heart conditions, sometimes in fevers, and in some cases of advanced diabetes. Creatinine figures above 3.5 mg. are almost invariably accompanied by an appreciable urea retention and this is generally true of those above 3 mg. Many of the cases below 4 mg. show improvement, but with over 4 mg. the reverse is the case. It would appear from this that an appreciable retention of creatinine, i.e., over 4 mg., does not occur until the activity of the kidneys is greatly impaired. That such should be the case it is quite natural to expect, since creatinine is normally the most readily eliminated of the three nitrogenous waste products, uric acid, urea, and creatinine.

CREATINE CONTENT OF THE BLOOD

Normally the creatine content of the blood amounts to from 3 to 7 mg. per 100 c.c., although the amount may be greatly increased in the last stages of nephritis along with other nonprotein nitrogenous substances. The methods for

TABLE I

THE PROGNOSTIC VALUE OF THE CREATININE OF THE BLOOD IN NEPHRITIS*

CASE	AGE	BLOOD ANALYSES MG. TO 100 C.C.		TIME UNDER OBSERVATION	OUTCOME	CASE	AGE	BLOOD ANALYSES MG. TO 100 C.C.		TIME UNDER OBSERVATION	OUTCOME
		Creatinine	Urea N					Creatinine	Urea N		
1	25	33.3	240	1 mo.	Died	44	64	9.7	70	5 mos.	Died
2	39	28.6	186	3 wks.	"	45	30	9.5	140	2 mos.	"
3	53	22.5	106	2 wks.	"	46	51	9.5	89	6 mos.	"
4	37	22.2	262	5 wks.	"	47	69	9.5	89	2 wks.	"
5	34	20.5	152	2 mos.	"	48	..	9.2	54	2 days	"
6	17	20.0	209	1 mo.	"	49	56	9.1	224	2 wks.	"
7	43	20.0	162	4 days	"	50	43	8.8	55	3 wks.	"
8	25	20.0	108	3 wks.	"	51	27	8.3	59	3 mos.	"
9	53	19.8	114	2 wks.	"	52	40	8.3	75	1 yr.	"
10	19	19.2	164	2 wks.	"	53	57	8.2	95	2 wks.	"
11	20	18.9	141	2 wks.	"	54	20	8.0	131	5 days	"
12	30	18.7	68	1 wk.	"	55	50	7.4	81	1 day	"
13	40	18.3	246	2 days	"	56	67	7.1	82	3 mos.	"
14	48	18.1	172	1 wk.	"	57	8	7.0	94	2 mos.	"
15	34	17.6	85	2 wks.	"	58	46	7.0	78	1 wk.	"
16	50	16.7	236	2 days	"	59	64	7.0	128	21 mos.	"
17	33	16.6	182	7 wks.	"	60	60	6.9	97	2 wks.	"
18	42	14.7	170	3 wks.	"	61	43	6.8	105	2 mos.	"
19	39	14.7	148	1 wk.	"	62	47	6.8	77	5 days	"
20	29	14.7	77	2 wks.	"	63	69	6.7	104	2 wks.	"
21	24	14.5	123	2 wks.	"	64	20	6.7	38	3 wks.	"
22	25	14.4	141	2 wks.	"	65	61	6.6	133	2 wks.	"
23	44	13.5	147	2 mos.	"	66	70	6.6	219	3 wks.	"
24	40	12.7	116	3 mos.	"	67	53	6.4	26	8 mos.	"
25	27	12.6	110	3 mos.	"	68	53	6.3	97	1 wk.	"
26	52	12.6	78	5 days	"	69	56	6.2	53	8 mos.	"
27	46	12.5	210	3 mos.	"	70	46	6.2	39	5 wks.	"
28	30	12.5	76	5 mos.	"	71	52	6.2	70	4 mos.	"
29	..	12.5	97	1 wk.	"	72	45	6.1	114	2 wks.	"
30	34	12.5	110	11 mos.	"	73	21	6.1	72	2 days	"
31	38	12.2	72	6 wks.	"	74	8	6.1	106	1 yr.	Recovered
32	51	11.6	57	1 wk.	"	75	60	6.1	41	3 yrs.	Unchanged
33	32	11.5	102	1 wk.	"	76	56	6.0	52	3 mos.	Died
34	8	11.1	90	6 wks.	"	77	59	6.0	169	3 wks.	"
35	41	11.1	91	6 wks.	"	78	21	5.6	70	18 mos.	Recovered
36	36	11.1	139	1 wk.	"	79	50	5.5	62	3 mos.	Died
37	34	11.0	144	2 mos.	"	80	12	5.4	42	4 mos.	"
38	30	11.0	97	3 days	"	81	53	5.3	100	4 mos.	"
39	33	10.7	78	2 mos.	"	82	30	5.3	100	1 mo.	"
40	17	10.2	307	1 wk.	"	83	62	5.3	25	2 mos.	Unchanged
41	26	10.0	112	3 wks.	"	84	29	5.2	65	1 wk.	Died
42	30	9.8	62	7 mos.	"	85	21	5.1	42	5 mos	"
43	78	9.8	60	2 mos.	"						

*Abbreviated from Myers and Killian.[10]

the blood creatine have been less satisfactory than in the case of the creatinine, and furthermore, the information obtained has not been shown to possess any great practical importance.

PROGNOSTIC VALUE OF THE BLOOD CREATININE

In our studies on nitrogen retention[16, 17, 18, 19] it was soon noted that the creatinine of the blood was appreciably increased only after considerable retention of urea had already taken place and the nephritis was rather far advanced.* It was further observed that those cases in which the creatinine had risen above 5 mg. per 100 c.c. of blood rarely showed any marked improvement, and almost invariably died within a comparatively limited time. The only exceptions were

*This point is well illustrated by the data in Table II of the first paper, p. 347.

cases where the retention was due to some acute renal condition. In a recent paper[19] we have discussed in some detail the prognostic value of the blood creatinine* in advanced nephritis and given in tabular form the results we have obtained since 1914. Data on 100 cases with high creatinines were presented, in 85 of which over 5 mg. of creatinine per 100 c.c. of blood were found. The data on these cases are given in abbreviated form in Table I, although for further details reference should be made to the above mentioned paper. As will be noted in the table the data are arranged in order of the magnitude of the blood creatinine, and include figures for the urea nitrogen on the same blood, the time under observation and the outcome of the case. These 85 cases included all the cases with over 5 mg. creatinine which had come under our observation since March, 1914 (to January, 1919), with the exception of three patients we had been unable to trace and who were presumably dead. Of these 85 cases, 81 are known to be dead, one having died (Case 59) since our last report. Of the four cases remaining alive, Cases 74 and 78 suffered from acute nephritis and have apparently recovered. Case 83 we were not able to follow longer than 2 months. Observations on Case 75 have been made at frequent intervals during the past three years. This case has remained nearly stationary for a longer period than any other case which we have encountered. Data on this case are given in Table II. When last seen, however, the patient was definitely worse and the creatinine

TABLE II

INDIVIDUAL OBSERVATIONS ON THE BLOOD OF CASE 75

DATE	CREATININE MG. TO 100 C.C.	UREA N MG. TO 100 C.C.	URIC ACID MG. TO 100 C.C.	CO_2 COMBINING POWER C.C. TO 100 C.C.
1917				
April 24	3.8	28	6.8	
May 8	6.1	41	5.5	50
15	5.2	30	7.7	
22	3.3	28	7.7	
June 1	3.1	36	10.4	
8	4.5	26	....	
1918				
April 2	3.8	57	....	
26	4.5	51	6.7	
1919				
Jan. 19	4.3	64		34
1920				
Feb. 18	7.2	56	5.0	

had risen to 7.2 mg. Even among the cases having very high blood creatinines there were many who were able to be up and about and some who showed considerable clinical improvement. It was in these cases that the blood creatinine gave a particularly good prognostic insight into the true nature of the condition. Case 25 is a good illustration of a patient in the last stages of the disease, but who, nevertheless, was able to be up and about (see Table III). Case 30 illustrates the value of the blood creatinine particularly well.† His blood showed a

*Some attention has been given to the prognostic value of the blood creatinine in nephritis by Rosenberg[29] and by Feigel,[30] although until recently their papers have been unavailable in this country.
†Data on this case are given in tabular form in the second paper of this series (Table V) on nonprotein and urea nitrogen, p. 422.

creatinine of 7.5 mg. when he first came under observation, and although he showed considerable clinical improvement over a period of nearly seven months, still his blood creatinine remained relatively constant, except for a temporary elevation to 12.5 mg. The dietetic measures which were employed to alleviate the nitrogen retention resulted in a gradual reduction of the urea nitrogen from 135 mg. per 100 c.c. to slightly below 30 mg. during this period. Despite his high creatinine (last determination 6.8 mg.), the patient left the hospital feeling well, returned to work as a guard on the subway and did not die until about five months later.

TABLE III
INDIVIDUAL OBSERVATIONS ON THE BLOOD OF CASE 25

DATE 1918	CREATININE MG. TO 100 C.C.	UREA N MG. TO 100 C.C.	URIC ACID MG. TO 100 C.C.	CO_2 COMBINING POWER C.C. TO 100 C.C.
March 12	8.6	97	8.1	31
19	9.4	102	7.0	..
22	12.6	110	...	17
26	12.1	110		28
29	11.9	...		28
April 16	11.2	78		23
30	13.3	81		24
May 7	15.2	76	...	25
24	17.0	148	...	12

This patient was discharged clinically improved on March 30, but came to the laboratory at our request for blood examination on April 16. At this time she apparently felt fairly well. She was readmitted to the hospital on April 27 and died on May 25.

It will be apparent from an inspection of Table I that there is no definite parallelism between the figures for urea and the creatinine. There are several cases with high creatinines in which the urea was not markedly elevated, notably Cases 64, 67, and 70, also Case 30 after prolonged dietetic treatment. Deductions based on the urea nitrogen alone in these cases would obviously have been quite misleading. In contrast to this, a good many cases have been encountered in which there was a marked retention of urea, although the creatinine was practically normal. In most of these cases improvement took place.

Theoretically, the amount of the increase of the creatinine of the blood should be a safer index of the decrease in the permeability of the kidney than the urea, for the reason that creatinine on a meat-free diet is entirely endogenous in origin and its formation (and elimination normally) very constant. Urea, on the other hand, is largely exogenous under normal conditions and its formation consequently subject to greater fluctuation. For this reason it must be evident that a lowered nitrogen intake may reduce the work of the kidney in eliminating urea, but can not affect the creatinine to any extent. Apparently the kidney is never able to overcome the handicap of a high creatinine accumulation. It would seem that creatinine being almost exclusively of endogenous origin, furnishes a most satisfactory criterion as to the deficiency in the excretory power of the kidneys and a most reliable means of following the terminal course of the disease, though it should be noted that urea, being largely of exogenous origin, is more readily influenced by dietary changes, and therefore constitutes a more sensitive index of the response to treatment.

To Folin[20] is due the credit of describing in 1914 the first satisfactory method of estimating creatinine in blood, employing principles similar to his unique quantitative colorimetric method for creatinine in urine, introduced just ten years earlier. It should be noted, however, that in 1909 Shaffer and Reinoso[11] suggested a procedure for the estimation of creatinine in dilute solutions, and with the aid of this method pointed out that normal dog serum contained about 1 mg. of creatinine per 100 c.c. Our first few determinations made on "uremic" blood were carried out following the suggestions of Shaffer and Reinoso. With the publication of Folin's paper we adopted his method for the most part, except that we still continued to carry out the preliminary dilution of the blood with water rather than saturated picric acid solution, for the reason that we regarded this the preferable way of analyzing the whole blood.[21] Hunter and Campbell have made a very careful study of the various factors involved in the estimation of creatinine in blood. Although they originally made their creatinine observations on laked blood, following our suggestion,[22] they have recently obtained[23] data which tend to show that these results are somewhat too high (particularly in normal blood), owing to an interference in the color development on the part of some constituent in the corpuscles. With plasma,* however, the results appear to be approximately correct. Hunter and Campbell plotted time curves for the creatinine color reaction and found that the curve in the case of the plasma followed closely that of the pure creatinine solution, while when whole blood was employed, diluting with saturated picric acid solution according to Folin's technic, there was considerable deviation and that when the corpuscles were laked according to our technic, the deviation was even greater. For a ten minute interval of color development Hunter and Campbell obtained the following results: plasma, 1.06 mg. per 100 c.c.; whole blood not hemolyzed, 1.57 mg.; and whole blood hemolyzed, 1.84 mg. (1.72 mg. at the end of eight minutes). Similar observations regarding the increased color producing effect of hemolyzed blood were made a little earlier by Wilson and Plass.[24] Although, as just indicated, the accuracy of the creatinine estimation in normal blood is probably greater in plasma than in whole blood, the findings with normal whole blood are comparable, and the importance of the above source of error decreases with a rise in the creatinine content of the blood, so that the absolute accuracy of the estimation in whole blood is much greater with pathologic than normal values.

In order to overcome some of the difficulties incident to this determination, other protein precipitants have been tried aside from picric acid. Denis[25] has suggested the use of metaphosphoric acid and apparently obtained quite satisfactory results. In their recent system of blood analysis Folin and Wu[26] employ tungstic acid as their protein precipitant. Both of these methods appear to yield satisfactory results and provide also for a more accurate estimation of the creatine than is possible where picric acid is employed for the precipitation of the

---

*Although it is much more convenient, and desirable from the standpoint of uniformity, to carry out the various blood analyses on whole blood, there are some practical as well as theoretical advantages for making some of the estimations on the plasma. Theoretical reasons for this in the case of the creatinine have been mentioned. There are also theoretical advantages in carrying out the estimation of the sugar and especially the chlorides on the blood plasma. With the Van Slyke apparatus for the CO_2 combining power there are important mechanical advantages in using the plasma, while in the case of cholesterol, the variations are chiefly in the plasma, the corpuscle content remaining fairly constant. For the sake of uniformity most of our work has been done on whole blood, but this plan, as just indicated, is open to certain criticisms, particularly in the case of normal blood.

proteins. In a limited number of creatinine determinations which we have carried out with these methods the results did not materially differ from those obtained with the older method. Disadvantages of these methods are the added steps necessary, and especially the fact that they require a greater dilution of the blood (1 to 12½ and 15 instead of 1 to 5) resulting in a weaker color development. With normal bloods the color development is weak, and yellow colors at best are hard to match. Further dilution also increases the error incident to the sodium picrate. It will thus be seen that the disadvantages of these newer methods about balance their advantages.

One factor of very great importance in the creatinine estimation, no matter what technic is employed, is the picric acid. Before being used for this purpose all picric acid should be tested. Folin and Doisy[27] have suggested a very simple method: "To 20 c.c. of a saturated (1.2 per cent) solution of picric acid add 1 c.c. of 10 per cent sodium hydroxide and let it stand for 15 minutes. The color of the alkaline picrate solution thus obtained must not be more than twice as deep as the color of the saturated acid solution. * * * If the picric acid is unusually pure, the color of the picrate solution will not be more than one and a half times as deep as that of a saturated picric acid solution; i.e., by setting the picric acid solution at 20 mm. in the Duboscq colorimeter, the picrate will give a reading of 13 to 14 mm." They also describe a method of purifying picric acid. As pointed out by Hunter and Campbell[22] saturated picric acid solutions develop a chromogenic substance, on standing exposed to light, an observation we can verify. Therefore, any picric acid solutions used in this connection should be reasonably fresh.

Method.—To 20 c.c. of distilled water in a 50 c.c. centrifuge tube* are added 5 c.c. of the well-mixed oxalated blood (or oxalated plasma). This is then stirred with a glass rod until the blood is thoroughly hemolyzed, after which about 1 gram of dry picric acid (sufficient to completely precipitate the proteins and render the solution saturated) is added. The mixture is thoroughly stirred until it is uniformly yellow and then at intervals for twenty to thirty minutes, after which it is centrifuged and filtered. Sufficient filtrate is obtained for the estimation of both the creatinine and the sugar (also the blood chlorides where 5 c.c. of filtrate are used for the creatinine). To 10 c.c. of this filtrate is added 0.5 c.c. of 10 per cent sodium hydroxide and a similar amount of alkali added to each of three standards (10 c.c. of standard creatinine** in saturated picric acid, containing 0.3, 0.5 and 1.0 mg. creatinine to 100 c.c. of picric acid. A standard is selected which approximates the color intensity of the unknown, and set at the 15 mm. mark. With bloods showing over 5 mg. of creatinine it has been customary to further dilute the blood filtrate with saturated picric acid solution, so that the color when developed closely matches the standard (1.0 mg.), e.g., reads between 12 and 18 mm. with the standard at 15 mm. The colors are compared after they have been allowed to develop for eight minutes.

For the calculation the following formula may be used: $\frac{S}{R} \times S_1 \times D = $ mg. creatinine to 100 c.c. of blood, in which "S" represents the depth of the standard (15 mm.), "R" the reading of the unknown, "S₁" the strength of the standard and "D" the dilution of the

*Large centrifuges which will take 50 and 100 c.c. tubes are unavailable in many laboratories, and the ordinary 15 c.c. conical centrifuge tube can not satisfactorily be used for this purpose, as they are very difficult to clean. In order to adapt the small electric centrifuge to this work, the Sorensen Company, New York City, have prepared a special trunnion cup for their small centrifuge which takes cylindrical centrifuge tubes of 25 c.c. capacity. Although these tubes hold slightly more than 25 c.c., it is best to employ 4 c.c. of blood and 16 c.c. of water in making the determination. For the cup of the Rock-Benedict colorimeter not more than 5 c.c. of filtrate are needed, in which case the color may be developed on this amount of filtrate with 0.25 c.c. of 10 per cent sodium hydroxide, if desired.

**Pure creatinine may be prepared by the admirable method of Benedict.[28] A standard solution of creatinine, 1 mg. to 1 c.c., is kept in 0.1 N hydrochloric acid, and from this the various solutions are prepared with saturated picric acid solution, 100 or 200 c.c. at a time.

blood. For example, with a reading of 15, a standard of 0.3 mg. and a blood dilution of 5 the formula would work out $\frac{15}{15} \times 0.3 \times 5 = 1.5$ mg. creatinine to 100 c.c.

ESTIMATION OF CREATININE WITH THE TEST TUBE COLORIMETER

Method.—The technic is as follows: 3 c.c. of the well-mixed blood are treated with 12 c.c. of water (4 volumes) in a 15 to 20 c.c. cylindrical centrifuge tube (test tube). After the corpuscles have been laked, about 0.5 mg. of dry picric acid is added, and the mixture stirred at intervals with a glass rod until it is a light yellow. When the protein precipitation is complete, the tube is centrifuged and the supernatant fluid filtered through a small filter paper. (Sufficient material is also available for the sugar estimation; see next paper.) To 5 c.c. of the filtrate in a test tube is added 0.25 c.c. of 10 per cent sodium hydroxide and a similar amount of alkali added to 3 standards in test tubes of the same caliber (5 c.c. of each of 0.2, 0.5 and 1.0 mg. creatinine to 100 c.c. of picric acid). At the same time 1.0 c.c. of the sodium hydroxide is added to 20 c.c. of saturated picric acid solution to make a diluting fluid. After 8 minutes have elapsed a standard is selected which is slightly lighter than the unknown. This is poured in the left-hand tube and the unknown into the right-hand tube (the tubes should be perfectly dry). The test tube which held the unknown is now rinsed out with the diluting fluid and the unknown diluted to correspond with the standard. To calculate the mg. of creatinine per 100 c.c. of blood, the following formula may be used, in which "S" represents the strength of the standard (0.2, 0.5 or 1.0 mg. to 100 c.c.), "D" the dilution in c.c. of the unknown required to match the standard, and "B" the amount of blood (1 c.c.) employed in c.c.: $\frac{S \times D}{B}$ less 5 per cent to allow for addition of alkali $=$ mg. creatinine per 100 c.c. of blood, or briefly, since the equivalent of 1 c.c. of blood is employed, multiply the strength of standard by the dilution in the unknown tube and deduct 5 per cent to allow for the addition of the alkali. For example, if the 0.5 standard is used, and the dilution of the unknown is 7.2 c.c., the result would be 3.6 mg. to 100, less 5 per cent, i.e., 3.4 mg.

REFERENCES

[1]Folin: Zeitschr. physiol. Chem., 1904, xli, 233.
[2]Folin: Am. Jour. Physiol., 1905, xiii, 84.
[3]Shaffer: Am. Jour. Physiol., 1908, xxiii, 1.
[4]Folin: Hammarsten's Festschrift, 1906, iii.
[5]Ayers and Fine: Jour. Biol. Chem., 1913, xiv, 9; ibid., 1913, xvi, 169; ibid., 1915, xxi, 377, 383, 389, 583.
[6]Ayers and Fine: Unpublished observations.
[7]Folin and Denis: Jour. Biol. Chem., 1914, xvii, 487.
[8]Neubauer: München. med. Wchnschr., 1914, lxi, 857.
[9]Ayers and Fine: Proc. Soc. Exper. Biol. and Med., 1914, xi, 132.
[10]Shaffer: Jour. Biol. Chem., 1914, xviii, 525.
[11]Shaffer and Reinoso: Jour. Biol. Chem., 1910, vii, (proc.) pp. xiii and xxx.
[12]Ayers and Fine: Jour. Biol. Chem., 1913, xv, 304; Proc. Soc. Exper. Biol. and Med., 1913, xi, 15.
[13]Ayers and Fine: Jour. Biol. Chem., 1914, xvii, 65.
[14]Ayers and Fine: Jour. Biol. Chem., 1915, xxi, 383.
[15]Folin: Jour. Biol. Chem., 1914, xvii, 475.
[16]Ayers and Fine: Jour. Biol. Chem., 1915, xx, 391.
[17]Ayers and Lough: Arch. Int. Med., 1915, xvi, 536.
[18]Chace and Ayers: Jour. Am. Med. Assn., 1916, lxvii, 929.
[19]Ayers and Killian: Am. Jour. Med. Sc., 1919, clvii, 674.
[20]Folin: Jour. Biol. Chem., 1914, xvii, 475.
[21]Ayers and Fine: Chemical Composition of the Blood in Health and Disease, 1915, p. 19.
[22]Hunter and Campbell: Jour. Biol. Chem., 1916-17, xxviii, 335.
[23]Hunter and Campbell: Jour. Biol. Chem., 1917, xxxii, 195.
[24]Wilson and Plass: Jour. Biol. Chem., 1917, xxix, 413.
[25]Denis: Jour. Biol. Chem., 1918, xxxv, 513
[26]Folin and Wu: Jour. Biol. Chem., 1919, xxxviii, 98.
[27]Folin and Doisy: Jour. Biol. Chem., 1916-17, xxviii, 349.
[28]Benedict: Jour. Biol. Chem., 1914, xviii, 183.
[29]Rosenberg: Munchen. med. Wchnschr., 1916, No. 6.
[30]Feigel: Biochem. Ztschr., 1917, lxxxi, 14, ibid., lxxxiv, 264; ibid., 1919, xciv, 84.

HEMOSTATIC AGENTS*

By Herbert C. Hamilton, Detroit, Mich.

THE blood is the agent of metabolism in that it serves as the medium by which nutritive and other substances are conveyed to different parts of the body and waste or noxious substances are removed. The property therefore of remaining liquid in the vascular system is of such vital importance as to overshadow another property that is little appreciated—the property of clotting spontaneously when the blood escapes from the severed vessels either because of wounds or disease. In a few minutes after normal blood has escaped from lacerated tissues it is gradually transformed into a gelatinous mass. It is the formation of this clot that checks the hemorrhage in small injured vessels which would otherwise bleed continuously.

Ordinarily most hemorrhages of moderate degree can be controlled with the usual measures of pressure and dressings. However, even in persons having a normal healthy coagulability of the blood, lacerations of tissue occur in which such ordinary measures of control fail, entailing a great loss of this vital fluid. Instances of this type are hemorrhages due to oozing after tonsillectomies, prostatectomies, nasal operations, and operations in vascular regions. It is evident that an increased coagulability of the blood in these cases is greatly to be desired, since it will increase the automatic control of hemorrhage normally possessed by the organism.

A tendency to hemorrhage due to hemophilia or to hemorrhagic diathesis undoubtedly renders the use of such an agent an indispensable procedure.

The prompt clotting of the blood under normal conditions is apparently due to the fact that the action of antithrombin, maintaining the fluidity in the vessels, is arrested by the fluids exuding from the lacerated tissue. These mix with the blood and initiate the process of clotting.

One of the constituents of the blood immediately concerned in clot formation is fibrinogen which on being subjected to the action of thrombin is changed into an insoluble fibrinous or gelatinous mass called fibrin. The formed elements of the blood become enmeshed in this, and the clot results.

Thrombin as such does not exist in the circulating blood. It is derived from a mother substance conveniently designated as prothrombin, which is quickly changed to thrombin in shed blood by the thrombokinase derived from the blood platelets and the lacerated tissues, in the presence of the free Ca-ions of the serum.

In the normal subject therefore the natural process can be depended upon except when considerable laceration occurs or when it is an internal injury. Under these latter conditions a shortening of the coagulation time is desirable and may even be vitally necessary.

Two substances suggest themselves for the purpose—the thrombokinase that may be derived from blood platelets and from tissue juices, and a substance to neutralize the antithrombin action.

*From the Research Laboratory of Parke, Davis & Co., Detroit, Mich.

The former substance from whatever source derived has been variously named—the term thrombokinase being apparently most appropriate on the theory that the action has the nature of a kinetic function rather than chemical. The sources of thrombokinase are the blood platelets and tissue fluids, while a substance of a similar character known as cephalin is present in the brain. The latter seems to be exceptionally strong in kinetic power but is applicable only for local use because of its waxy insoluble nature.

Thrombokinase is lacking in any specific action to counteract the antithrombin:[1a] it serves only to initiate the change of thrombin from the inactive prothrombin to the active form. The role of the antithrombin therefore seems to be of utmost importance and the minimizing of its power essential in any attempt to shorten the coagulation time of the blood. This may be brought about by the inclusion of a specific antiantithrombin.

There are certain cases, comparatively rare, in which the blood fails to coagulate or in which the process is so slow that a hemorrhage might be fatal before clotting occurs. In these cases it is demonstrated that the equilibrium between antithrombin and prothrombin is at fault, because of an excess of the former or a deficiency of the latter.

The third constituent therefore that should be present in a well balanced hemostatic is prothrombin to restore the balance in the blood.

The substances previously proposed for the control of hemorrhage by changing the character of the blood, are blood serum, both liquid and powder, purified thrombin, blood platelets in both liquid and powder form and brain extract in the waxy form resulting from extraction with ether and acetone. An aqueous suspension has also been prepared by making a salt solution extract. This is for hypodermatic injection.

Freshly prepared blood serum or the powder resulting from a precipitation of the thrombin in an active state has an obvious advantage as an aid in shortening coagulation because in this way active thrombin is apparently made immediately available. Almost equally logical is the use of blood platelets which seem to have a specific action to initiate clot formation.

Both of these classes of coagulants are normal constituents of the blood and both are immediately concerned in the process of clotting—thrombin as the agent which brings about the change of fibrinogen to fibrin, and thrombokinase (from the platelets) because of its observed value in initiating the reaction by which prothrombin takes on the active form of thrombin.

According to Howell[2] and others, cephalin from brain substance is more active in this respect than the disintegrated blood platelets, but such an extract is not well adapted to hypodermic administration and is particularly inadvisable for intravenous use.

No single substance has been suggested which has the power to neutralize or minimize the action of the antithrombin, nor is there available in the above list any true blood coagulant adapted to meet all the necessities of every kind of hemorrhage. Thrombin alone is immediately destroyed by antithrombin; thrombokinase can not act on unreleased prothrombin. Coagulation time may be influenced by any of these agents to a slight extent if the substance is active, is properly applied and is adapted to the particular case, but the highest efficiency is only rarely attainable because one or more of the above conditions is not fulfilled.

There is unquestionably, therefore, a field for a coagulant combining the valuable properties of those mentioned as well as supplying the esential proper- ties which are lacking in the above list.

It should have kinetic power supplied by an active thrombokinase; it should contain prothrombin in case this constituent is deficient; it should have a sub- stance to minimize the action of the antithrombin and thus permit the formation of thrombin. Such an agent is hemostatic serum.[1b]

Hemostatic serum contains prothrombin, antiantithrombin and thrombo- kinase in a physiologically balanced solution with a demonstrated value in short- euing coagulation time when administered by any of the accepted methods. Intravenous administration is naturally the route by which quickest results are obtained.

Various methods have been suggested for standardizing blood coagulants. Of these, local application to a superficial wound and the measurement of the coagulation time of the escaping blood seems least satisfactory. Such a method is logical for adrenalin and substances which act as astringents locally on the tissues; and also for substances such as the insoluble waxy material extracted from brain substance and recommended by Hess the originator[3] for local use only.

There are several reasons why a soluble substance can not be standardized by this method. A liquid is so promptly washed away by the current of blood that it is almost valueless locally unless applied on gauze. It should not be ap- plied by periodic swabbing with a cotton pledget saturated with the agent[4, p. 201] since this retains the fluid and prevents close contact with the wound; it is prac- tically impossible as was attempted by Hanzlik and Weidenthal[4, p. 190] to control conditions in two wounds so that the effect of the coagulant on one of them can be recognized or can be measured quantitatively.

Hemostatic serum requires an appreciable time for activation by mixing with the fresh blood, before it can exert its characteristic property of shortening co- agulation time. Test tube tests, the addition of the agent to blood in a tube, are therefore valueless since this coagulant is exhibited in a stable form which re- quires activation by fresh blood before its peculiar properties become effective. The method of N.N.R.[5] and Howell's method[2] using plasma are of little value for any coagulant, but especially in comparison with the systemic administration of the substance.

The definite results obtainable by systemic administration point to intrave- nous administration as an exceptionally valuable method for purposes of stand- ardization. In order to determine the potency of the agent, its power to decrease the coagulation time of the blood in the living body should always be determined. Such a test can be made an accurate measure of value by establishing a mini- mum standard. There has not been, heretofore, any systematic scheme for standardizing blood coagulants—a fact which accounts, not only for the various attempts to establish values, but also for lack of uniformity in the products mar- keted.

It is not sufficient to find, for example, that a freshly prepared extract of blood platelets is an active coagulant and expect that such an extract will invariably be active and stable. There are too many opportunities for error in preparation or for loss of activity through bacterial or chemical action to assume an activity which it is possible to demonstrate.

There is a tendency to decry the biologic methods of assay on the ground that the action of a therapeutic agent on an animal is no evidence of similar activity on the human. While this argument is illogical in most cases, it can scarcely be even advanced in the case of a blood coagulant. If an agent will shorten the coagulation time of a dog's blood, the blood differing in no essential respect from human blood even to the average coagulation time, there is every reason to expect a similar action in the human. Then further, if clinical tests show almost identical results with those obtained by using the dog as the test animal, every reasonable objection to the biologic test vanishes.

The method of procedure proposed for standardizing blood coagulants of this character by the biologic test is as follows: The dog is anesthetized for convenience of withdrawal of samples of blood and for injection of the coagulant. After complete anesthesia the normal coagulation time is determined. The most convenient and accurate method is to use a sample of about 3 c.c. of blood. A glass cannula is inserted into a carotid artery for obtaining samples of blood. At least three samples should be tested for the normal coagulation time before injecting a coagulant. The blood is drawn into a clean test tube and set in water at 38° to 40° C. It is examined at one minute intervals to observe the first evidence of fibrin formation and the progress of coagulation.

The normal coagulation time for the test animal has been selected as that time when on inverting the tube no fluid blood can be observed. One must be careful that an apparently firm clot is not due to a skin over the surface below which the blood is fluid. It is also advisable to clean out the cannula carefully before drawing the second and subsequent samples of blood in order to prevent particles of clotted blood from getting into the test sample.

If the coagulation time is found to be uniform at 7 to 10 minutes, the coagulant can then be injected into the femoral vein. The first evidence of shortened coagulation time usually does not appear until one-half hour after administering the agent and the maximum effect not before one and one-half hours. Between those periods a sample of blood should be tested every fifteen minutes. This sample is examined to observe the first evidence of fibrin formation, the progress of clotting, and the time when a solid clot has formed which can be shaken and inverted without showing more than a trace of fluid blood.

The different blood coagulants examined have given variable results.[6] Some have appeared to be inactive, while some have shown exceedingly high efficiency. Clinical or other corroborative tests being absent in some cases, one can say only that for shortening the coagulation time of normal blood a combination of the factors concerned in this process seems to be most efficient. While in many cases the coagulation time was shortened to one-sixth or one-eighth of the normal, the average value selected for purposes of comparison is a shortening of the coagulation time to one-third the normal for that animal, the amount injected being 2 c.c. to a 12 kg. dog.

The method here described is an elaboration of an experiment by Howell[2] who tested a sample of cephalin by intravenous administration finding a coagulation time shortened by one-third to one-half the normal for that animal.

Some experiments of Drinker and Drinker[7] might suggest that this method is not applicable because of the tendency of hemorrhages to be self-limiting. The experiments of Drinker and Drinker were carried out very differently, however, since approximately ten times as much blood in proportion to the size of the test animals was used in their experiments as is needed for this method of standardization.

That repeated withdrawals of relatively small quantities of blood do not affect the coagulation time materially has been demonstrated not only intentionally but also involuntarily as when testing a valueless product. From dogs of approximately 12 kilograms weight, 5 c.c. of blood can be drawn repeatedly at 15 minute intervals or less over a period of 1 to 2 hours with no other evidence of disturbance of coagulation time than a slight irregularity. Exceptions occur, however, but it is more common to find a dog which does not react to the standard dose of an active coagulant than to observe a shortened coagulation time with no coagulant injected.

Charts of tests are attached showing these phenomena. Being a physiologic test it is subject to the limitations of the test animal. Not every animal is adapted to this test. In the same way some frogs, rats, guinea pigs, and dogs are necessarily rejected in other physiologic tests because of having exceptionally high or low resistance to the agent.

Animals have been rejected for testing purposes: (1) Because of having too short a normal coagulation time: it should be not less than 6 minutes. (2) Because of some unrecognized factors which influence the coagulation time before the agent is administered. A shortened coagulation time on the second sample of blood to one-third that of the first sample was once observed when not more than 10 c.c. had been withdrawn from a 12 kg. dog. (3) Because of failing to react to an active sample of a coagulant, whose potency had been demonstrated on two test animals.

Three articles have recently appeared on the testing of thromboplastic agents. two[4] of them as to potency and one[8] as to the danger connected with the use of such agents.

In the tests for potency, Hanzlik and Weidenthal[4, p. 206] were unfortunately deterred from applying the most reliable test for such agents, namely, the physiologic test by systemic administration. They incorrectly quote Howell as authority for the statement that hemorrhage itself tends to shorten the coagulation time of the blood. Drinker and Drinker[7] quoted by Howell had shown this to be true but Hanzlik and Weidenthal failed to note that the shortened time in the coagulation after hemorrhage was where the hemorrhage is excessive, as for example, an approximate loss of 20 per cent of the blood at one time, at another 33 per cent, the normal coagulation time being shortened by one-sixth and one-eighth, respectively.

Hanzlik and Weidenthal[4, p. 205] in their experiments observed a shortening in the coagulation time from 9 minutes to 3¾ minute in one case and from 8 minutes to 1¾ minutes in another. No data are included to show the extent of the hemorrhage.

In my own experiments no such procedure was adopted and no such results have been observed. The total amount of blood drawn for observation need not exceed 5 per cent of the total blood, and it is drawn at any one time in an amount not to exceed 0.5 per cent of the total blood. The careful withdrawal of this quantity does not affect the coagulation time.

Tests of thromboplastic agents *in vitro* are always unreliable and not to be compared to the physiologic test. Activity *in vitro* is not sufficient evidence on which to base the conclusion that in the body a similar result would follow, because in the circulating blood conditions are radically different from those in a test tube.

This is well illustrated by Hanzlik and Weidenthal[4] who obtained no satisfactory results from any thromboplastic agent in experiments on the living animal, although some had shown high efficiency when tested *in vitro*.

It should not be overlooked that with few exceptions the thromboplastic agents tested by Hanzlik and his associates have been submitted to the Council of Pharmacy and Chemistry and accepted. Failure, therefore, on the part of these agents to show their expected effects should first be considered from the point of view of the method by which it was attempted to demonstrate their activity.

Scarcely second to this, however, should be the question of whether the nature of the coagulant is such as to be generally applicable for influencing the coagulation time of the blood both in health and disease.

A well balanced agent containing the elements essential for blood coagulation under all conditions and with an efficiency demonstrated on the living animal gives an assurance of value not to be derived from tests on serum or plasma in the test tube.

It is unfortunate that the term "Anaphylactoid Phenomena" should have been used in connection with this third investigation.[8] One might assume this expression to mean phenomena similar to anaphylaxis. "Anaphylaxis is a state of unusual or exaggerated susceptibility to a foreign protein which sometimes follows a primary injection of such protein." (Richtet, 1893.)

The investigators state that these pigs were unsensitized and further show by the experiments that only one dose was injected into each.

This precludes anaphylaxis and we are forced to conclude that nothing resembling an anaphylactic reaction occurred. This conclusion is verified also by the descriptions of the observed reactions which in the case of Coagulen containing no protein or only traces were identical with those from others in which the protein precipitate was unquestionable.

Attention should also be called to the doses used. In the case of hemostatic serum the smallest dose per gm. used by Hanzlik and his coworkers[8, p. 239] was 15 times as large as the maximum dose calculated over a period of 24 hours for a human, while the largest dose used was 80 times as large. Hemostatic serum is recommended in doses of 1 to 2 c.c. to be repeated in extreme cases as often as once in 4 to 6 hours. The largest single dose used in clinical practice is 2 c.c.. which, when calculated as Hanzlik did from the weight of a 60 kg. human, is 0.000033 c.c. per gm. The largest dose used for the pig was 0.016 c.c. per gm. or 500 times the maximum single dose recommended for the human. If there were any lurking danger of anaphylaxis from administration of hemostatic serum or danger of poisoning because of the preservative or any other poison contained in it, certainly a dose of 500 times the maximum single therapeutic dose should have killed the animal. But in their whole series[8] only one animal died within 36 hours. This death was from a brain extract. The others were all killed by a blow on the head, in most cases having shown no serious effects other than those to be expected after an intravenous injection. This speaks well for the safety of hemostatic agents in clinical practice.

Hanzlik and his associates in their conclusions[8, p. 241] fail to make it clear that any one factor was responsible for the observed effects. It is not necessarily the protein content, for one of the agents tested contained practically no protein. Neither is it the preservative, for this same agent contained no preservative but at the same time gave the most pronounced reactions described as anaphylactoid.

It is logical to conclude, therefore, that the method of administration rather than the character of the agent may be responsible for the disturbances noted.

Administered intravenously to guinea pigs few substances fail to produce more or less serious disturbances in the circulation and respiration, such as were observed by Hanzlik and his associates. It is illogical, however, to apply the term "anaphylactoid" to these phenomena because this word calls to the mind of the physician a severe reaction and occasional death from administration of antitoxin to a sensitized patient.

SUMMARY

Without attempting entirely to discredit attempts to estimate the efficiency of thromboplastic agents *in vitro* or by local application to bleeding wounds, a method of a different character is here proposed for the assay of such agents.

The method is logical because it duplicates one of the clinical methods of applying such an agent.

The results of the potency test are conclusive since the action of the agent on the test animal is identical with its action in clinical practice.

Careful observance of certain precautions which have been outlined, such as are necessary in all forms of physiologic testing, makes this method the most dependable for the quantitative determination of the efficiency of hemostatic agents which can be used intravenously.

PROTOCOLS OF TESTS

In the following tables, the first column of figures refers to the time of observation of the sample of the blood.

At the head of the columns that follow is the actual time when the sample of blood is drawn or a sample of coagulant is injected.

The figures below the time are symbols: 1, signifies beginning of fibrin formation; 2 and 3, progressive clotting; 4, solid clot when tube is inverted.

HEMOSTATIC SERUM No. 053129

	9:35	9:43	9:48	9:57	10:05	10:23	10:45	11:02	11:14	Feb. 2, 1920. 11:27	11:29
1.	–	–	–	–	Inj. 2 c.c.	–	1	3	3	4	4
2.	–	–	1	–		1	1	4	3		
3.	1	3	2	1		2	2		4		
4.	2	4	3	2		4	3				
5.	3		4	4		4					
6.	4										

Shortened time from 5 minutes to 1 minute in 1¼ hours.

HEMOSTATIC SERUM No. 051196

Min.	9:56	10:08	10:20	10:22	11:21	11:31	11:44	11:52	11:57	2:15
1	–	–	–	Inj.	–	1	–	3	3	2
2	–	–	–	2 c.c.	--	2	1	4	4	–
3	–	–	–	of	1	3	2			1
4	–	–	–	sam-	2	3	4			2
5	1	–	1	ple	2	4				4
6	2	1	2		3					
7	2	2	2		4					
8	3	3	2							
9	3	3	2							
10	3	3	3							
11	4	3	3							
12		4	4							

Coagulation time reduced from 12 min. to 2 min. in 1½ hours.

TEST OF AN INACTIVE PRODUCT

	1:25	1:33	1:35	2:00	2:16	1:30	2:49	3:00	3:02	3:23	3:51	4:01
1.	–	–	In- ject- ed 2 c.c.	–	–	–	–	In- ject- ed 2 c.c. more	–	–	–	–
2.	1	1		–	–	1	–		–	–	1	1
3.	2	1		–	1	2	1		1	1	2	2
4.	3	2		1	2	3	2		2	2	3	2
5.	3	3		2	2	3	2		3	3	4	3
6.	3	3		2	3	4	3		3	3		4
7.	4	3		3	3		4		4	4		
8.		4		4	4							

COAGULATION TIME

Jan. 6th, 1920.

Dog weighing 8 Kilo not dosed with any hemostatic.

Eleven samples of blood representing about 5 c.c. each time removed to observe any change in coagulation time because of repeated bleedings.

Min.	11:00	11:11	11:19	11:25	11:33	11:47	1:20	1:45	2:57	4:01	4:34
1	–	–	–	–	–	–	–	–	1	–	1
2	–	–	–	–	1	1	1	1	2	1	2
3	1	1	1	1	3	2	2	2	3	2	3
4	2	2	2	2	4	3	3	4	4	3	3
5	3	3	4	3		4	4			4	4
6	4	3		4							
7		4									

COAGULATION TIME

An illustration of one form of failure which occasionally occurs in attempting to test a coagulating agent.

May 21, 1919.

Minutes	10:33	10:43	10.49	10:52	11:48	1:31	2:11	3:00
1.	–	1	1	+	2	1	1	2
2.	–	2	+		4	3	2	3
3.	1	3				4	3	4
4.	2	4					4	
6.	2							
7.	3							
8.	3							
9.	4							

No injection was made into this dog as the coagulation time would not remain uniform at any time.

REFERENCES

[1]Lapenta, Vincent A.: (a) Therap. Gazette, 1919, xliii, 687; (b) ibid., 1918, xlii,.
[2]Howell, W. H.: The Harvey Lectures, 1916-17.
[3]Hess: Jour. Am. Med. Assn., 1915, lxiv, 1395.
[4]Hanzlik and Weidenthal: Jour. Pharm and Exper. Therap., 1919, xiv. 157 and 189.
[5]New and Non-Official Remedies, 1919, p. 121.
[6]Hamilton, Herbert C.: Jour. Am. Ph. Assn., 1919, ix, 118.
[7]Drinker and Drinker: Am. Jour. Physiol., 1915, xxxviii, 233.
[8]Hanzlik, Karsner and Fetterman: Jour. Pharm. and Exper. Therap., 1919, xiv, 229.

ACTION OF CHLORETONE ON ANIMAL TISSUE*

By T. B. Aldrich and H. C. Ward, Detroit, Mich.

TRICHLOROTERTIARY butyl alcohol (chloretone) has a number of properties which make it valuable therapeutically, among which may be mentioned its hypnotic, anesthetic, and bactericidal properties.

It finds its most important use, however, at the present time, as a hypnotic and sedative; but its local and general anesthetic properties must not be lost sight of.

As a general anesthetic for experimental animals, where it is not necessary to recover the animal, it is an ideal general anesthetic, and it is employed for this purpose in many laboratories. When given in small doses prior to general anesthesia with ether or chloroform, in the human, it has been found that the patient requires less ether or chloroform, that the period of excitement is lessened, and that unpleasant postoperative vomiting is often lacking.

As a germicide, its aqueous solution will kill all but the most resistant spore-bearing germs and as a mild local anesthetic it may be employed to advantage in dressing burns, abrasions, cuts, etc.

As an obtundent in dentistry, either alone or in oil, it is ideal, as evidenced by many reports.

The action of chloretone on animal tissue, however, has not been studied to any extent, and it is to this that we wish to call attention.

A number of years ago, it was found that pituitary and adrenal glands when placed in a saturated aqueous solution of chloretone (0.5 to 0.8 per cent) kept indefinitely. In fact, a number of glands in our possession have been kept for over ten years, without any apparent decomposition as evidenced by odor and gross appearance. It was furthermore found that chloretone added to saturation in aqueous solution, would prevent the development of molds and this fact has been made use of in the preparation of aqueous stock solutions of the alkaloids and of solutions of adrenalin, ergot, pituitrin, etc.

It was thought also that the aqueous solution, or a modification of it (physiologic salt solution saturated with chloretone) *might* be of value in the preservation of not only animal tissue, but aquatic specimens (both plant and animal), museum specimens, also material for laboratory class work in high schools and colleges. Histologic studies, as will be cited later, have shown, however, that chloretone can only be employed as a differential preservative: that is to say, a preservative which leaves some tissue elements intact and allows autolysis or other changes to proceed while keeping down bacterial action without the destruction of the active constituents set free. In the investigation of the pituitary glands, for example, the glands as well as the extract may be pre-

*From the Research Laboratory of Parke, Davis & Co., Detroit, Mich.

583

served with chloretone until the finished product is obtained without harm to the active constituent, and it may well be that chloretone will find one of its many uses along this line.

Although the preservative action of aqueous chloretone solution has been known to us and employed by us in the preservation of glands and gland extracts from bacterial decomposition, for a long time, no systematic experimental work has been carried out along this line to show its general action on animal tissue. Our object in presenting this preliminary paper is not to present an exhaustive article, but merely to draw attention to the effect of chloretone in aqueous solution on animal and possibly vegetable tissue.

In order to test the action of a saturated aqueous solution of chloretone on animal tissue, the following organs—brain, heart, kidney, liver, spleen, testicle— were removed as quickly as possible from the animal after death, cut into small pieces and distributed among seven sets of bottles. Each bottle contained about 140 c.c. of saturated solution of chloretone, (0.5 to 0.8 per cent), and was tightly corked to prevent the chloretone from volatilizing. To keep the water and air saturated, a slight excess of chloretone crystals was usually left undissolved at the bottom of the bottle, it being assumed then that the water was sufficiently saturated.

Set "A" was placed in the incubator at 37° C.
Set "B" was placed in the refrigerator at 15° C.
Set "C" was infected with B. proteus and kept at room temperature.
Sets "D," "E," "F," and "G" were kept at room temperature.

A piece of each organ was also placed in each of two bottles, one containing only distilled water and the other 50 per cent alcohol. The sets were examined every few days and the general appearance, odor, change of color, etc., noted.

The gross changes observable after six weeks' exposure to the chloretone solution were as follows: Brain sections appeared unaltered in color but of rather softer consistency.

Heart muscle had lost its normal color, appearing pale even when cut, and more elastic than when fresh.

Kidney segments appeared of a dull uniform yellowish cast as compared to their flesh, dark red, natural color. They were somewhat tough and elastic.

Liver portions presented a rather unusual dull orange-colored appearance confined to the surface, the interior portion retaining the original deep characteristic dark red color. The tissue itself was remarkably soft, flabby, but tough.

Spleen sections retained their original color and appearance although feeling more soft and spongy.

Testicular pieces were apparently unchanged in color or consistency.

When bacteriologic tests were applied at ten day intervals, all bottled lots were found to be sterile.

In three sets molds grew in the culture media but no multiplication had taken place in the preservation bottles. In fact, aside from a rather limited amount of debris arising from occasional handling, the liquid remained clear and bright, the tissues being visibly free from the common signs of decomposition and putrefaction.

In addition to the above records a series of observations* were made upon the histologic changes undergone by the treated tissue. Two samples of material were used (a) liver of dog, which had been kept at 37° in sat. sol. of chloretone in water for 15 days, and (b) bovine suprarenal, which had been kept at room temperature in sat. sol. of chloretone in water for a period of years. Small portions of each tissue were placed in 10 per cent formalin for three days, dehydrated in graded alcohols, cleared in toluol, embedded in paraffin, cut 7 micra thick and stained with Delafield's hematoxylin and eosin. Control sections of formalin-fixed rabbit ovary were stained under identical conditions.

(a) *Dog's Liver.*—The low power section presents a foam-like appearance, due to absence of cytoplasm and nucleus. Only cell membrane remains, staining a grayish-violet, surrounding a clear space. The connective tissue stains a diffuse pink around the larger blood vessels and bile ducts. The fibrils are softened, swollen and edematous. Blood corpuscles are absent.

(b) *Bovine Suprarenal.*—Under the lower power the section may be differentiated into two regions, an outer cortex and an inner medulla. The cortical cells present a greenish-brown appearance and the high power shows the cells filled with coarse brown granules similar in appearance to those seen in formalin preparations. In many cells only faintly stained cell membranes remain. The typical structure of the cortical cells is faintly suggested but not definitely shown.

The medulla presents an appearance similar to that of the cortex. Each cell is distinguishable, however, although the nucleus is absent.

These facts indicate that preservation in chloretone water does not preserve cytological details. The cytoplasm and the nuclear material are completely dissolved. Only the cell outlines are preserved. Connective tissue is altered, swollen. edematous but apparently persists. Certain lipoid granules, characteristic of suprarenal cortical cells, were found present after some years of treatment with chloretone water. This suggests the possibility that specific cell products may be preserved by the chloretone water.

Microscopically there was no evidence of bacterial action in any of the sections examined. They show, however, that the processes of autolysis are not inhibited by chloretone. The resistance of suprarenal lipoidal granules in the face of the generalized destruction of tissue substance is also a noteworthy fact.

The results obtained from our limited study are at first glance distinctly disappointing. Apparently chloretone possesses little value as a fixative of animal tissues. The histologic evidence is conclusive on this point, so far as the selected tissues examined are concerned. This may not prove to be wholly applicable to other tissue on extended study.

But when we consider the greater value of animal tissues as holders of specific principles, we find that this substance does possess in a unique way, what we are pleased to express as differential preservative value. This property, we believe, is capable of being extended to a wide range of practical applications.

The bactericidal action of chloretone is, therefore, of special interest in this connection; since there are but relatively few substances capable of favoring autolysis under ideal conditions.

---

*These observations were reported by C. J. Marinus to whom we wish to express our thanks.

CONCLUSIONS

1. Chloretone in saturated aqueous solution exerts a definite bactericidal action at all temperatures.

2. Chloretone in saturated aqueous solution prevents the development of the common molds.

3. Chloretone solution is not suitable as a fixative for histologic materials.

4. Chloretone in saturated solution while acting as a bactericide, does not inhibit autolytic action as evidenced by our histologic findings.

5. Chloretone solution is a desirable agent for preserving glands and gland extracts from which the active principles are to be obtained.

CLASSIFICATION OF STREPTOCOCCUS*

I. Streptococci Isolated from Normal Throats, Classified by Sugar Fermentations

By Lloyd Arnold, M.D., Nashville, Tenn.

INTRODUCTORY

THE systematic classification of bacteria has been industriously worked upon in recent years. The general biologic relationship between the various varieties of the same strain must be understood before epidemiologic, therapeutic and prophylactic problems can be worked out satisfactorily.

The streptococci were recognized in 1918 as primary and secondary invaders in respiratory lesions, accompanied by a high mortality. On the usual routine laboratory media streptococci were found in the upper respiratory tract of many healthy individuals. There was a very close resemblance between the pathogenic and the nonpathogenic forms. One of the problems of etiology is to determine the number of varieties of the same species of bacteria that are pathogenic and also if there are nonpathogenic forms of the same species.

Systematic observations covering a long period of time and in as many different localities as possible, may help to throw some light on these fundamental problems. It is the purpose of this series of papers to classify by various means the streptococci isolated from several sources. The present paper takes up the classification based on sugar fermentation of strains isolated from the throats of healthy individuals in this locality.

THE OCCURRENCE OF STREPTOCOCCI IN OTHER THAN PATHOLOGIC CONDITIONS

A literature review of the subject is not here given, since the literature has been well summarized by such recent workers as, Holman,[12] Blake,[3] Aschner,[1] Brown,[5] and Gay.[9] The following condensed table shows some more recent observations of streptococcus hemolyticus occurring under normal conditions.

Human	Throat No. Cases	% positive	Investigator
Contact cases	30	50.0%	Greenway, Boettiger and Caldwell[10]
Non-contact controls	14	23.3	Greenway, Boettiger and Caldwell[10]
School children and students	231	25	Sherwood and Downs[23]
Non-infect. diseases	13	100	Lucke and Rea[18]
Normal	24	25	Davis and Pilot[7]
Normal	51	59	Ruediger[21]
Bronchial Asthmatics	50	92	Walker and Adkinson[25]
New recruits		15	Fox and Hamburg[8]
At camp 6 months		83	Fox and Hamburg[8]
New recruits	489	14.8	Levy and Alexander[16]
At camp sometime		83	Levy and Alexander[16]
Discharged from hosp. After measles, etc.		71	Levy and Alexander[16]

*From the City Hospital Laboratory, Nashville. Tenn.

	No. cases	% positive	
Normal	298	23.7	Opie, Freeman, Blake, Small, Rivers[1]
Normal	4415	44.5	Blanton, Burhams Hunter[4]
Normal	61	57	Tongs[24]
Normal	100	55	Levin, Goodman, Pancoast[19]
From body surface of clean individuals 38 cases negative			Schachter[22]
From body surface of filthy individuals	81	10	Schachter[22]
Normal	100	36	Clawson[6]
Nurses	33	21.2	Otteraaen[20]
Students	35	57	Otteraaen[20]

TECHNIC

A report on "Recommendations of the Committee on Standard Routine Method for Isolation and Identification of Hemolytic Streptococci from Throats, Sputa, and Pathogenic Exudates"[13] appointed by the Surgeon-General, outlined a general method which has been followed as far as possible in this work on streptococci in this laboratory in the last year.

MEDIUM

Blood agar: To a 50 per cent fresh beef infusion were added 2.5 per cent agar, 1 per cent peptone and 0.5 per cent sodium chloride. The reaction was adjusted to P_H 7.0 and bottled in 95 c.c. lots, sterilized in an Arnold sterilizer for three successive days. When needed, medium was melted, cooled to 50° C. and 7 c.c. defibrinated human blood added. Seven plates were poured from this amount. It was found advantageous in this climate to use 2.5 per cent agar. The adjustment of the reaction was done according to the method of Barnett and Chapman,[4] taking Kligler's[15] P_H values as our end point. Brom-thymol-blue and phenol-red indicators were found to give a good workable range for general bacteriologic work.

Standard meat infusion broth, adjusted to P_H 7.0: The author found a beef heart peptone infusion can be made using the same technic as the standard beef muscle infusion, except filtration through glass-wool is sufficient to make clear, this does not hold for the beef muscle infusion. This will be dealt with more in detail in a subsequent paper on media for bacteriologic work. With the use of this unfiltered beef heart infusion heavier and quicker growths occurred than on standard beef muscle infusion.

Sugar fermentation medium: Lactose, mannite and salicin were routinely used. Comparisons were run with serum broth (Holman) meat-infusion broth, and the unfiltered beef heart infusion, using Andrade's indicator, the latter was found to give good growths. We agree with Blake that there is little if anything gained by using the serum broth. The results of Holman, Broadhurst and others were verified as to the unsuitableness of sugar-free broth made so by B. coli incubation.

Bile solubility and hemolytic tests were performed as suggested by the committee. We found Holman's[11] cooked meat medium of great value in this work.

The 204 strains isolated, would be classified according to Blake·

117 Streptococcus hemolysans
48 Streptococcus equinus
27 Streptococcus buccalis
 2 Streptococcus fecalis
10 Unclassified strains

The 204 strains classified according to Holman:

Number Strains	Hemolytic Streptococcus	Per cent
75	Str. Subacidus	64.2
26	Str. Equi	22.2
8	Str. Hemolyticus, II	6.8
6	Str. Hemolyticus, III	5.1
1	Str. Anginosus	0.8
1	Str. Hemolyticus, I	0.8

When these strains are compared with Holman's tables, there is a marked absence of streptococcus pyogenes. In fact an outstanding feature is the predominance of the nonlactose fermenters. There have been unusually few cases of acute respiratory diseases in this hospital during the six months this work was being done. This combined with the rigid exclusion of hypertrophied and infected tonsils, also visible tooth infections, may have a bearing on this question. Average throats are not classified as such by Holman, his "Throat (general)" may mean this, but he does not carry this through all his strains tabulated.

Streptococcus subacidus 64.2 per cent seems to run higher than most figures recorded by other workers, comparing nearer with the findings of Floyd and Wolbach. The author has repeatedly tried many strains and found the same results when run alongside fermenting strains as a control. Five strains, after 128 days, were replated, run as nonfermenters.

Number Strains	Nonhemolytic	Per cent
47	Str. Equinus	54.0
11	Str. Mitis	12.7
16	Str. Salivarus	18.4
9	Str. Nonhemolyticus, II	10.3
2	Str. Fecalis	2.3
1	Str. Nonhemolyticus, I	1.1
1	Str. Ignavus	1.1

In all 134 cases were run. Sixty-eight were positive to hemolytic streptococci, making an average of 50.74 per cent. This work was started with only the hemolytic streptococci in view. On the last 56 cases were nonhemolytic types picked, but their occurrence was noticed as running high in the first lot of plates. In these 56 cases, 51 were positive to nonhemolytic streptococci, making 91.0 per cent. In all 204 strains, 117 were hemolytic and 87 were nonhemolytic.

A great deal of the work here cited has been done during the recent epidemic of influenza, and many observations were made at various army camps where an unusually large number of young healthy men were associated together. There has been some work done since this time appearing from time to time, from civilian life. Even under these varied conditions where standard technic was used it has been found that hemolytic streptococcus was present in close to 50 per cent of the average normal throats examined, the variations were not much more than 10 per cent above or below this general average.

In those instances where sugar fermentation was used as a means of further classification, strains isolated from pathologic lesions were being examined Walker and Adkinson show a classification by sugar reactions of strains of hemolytic and nonhemolytic streptococci isolated from bronchial asthmatics, their results run closer to those here recorded than any other observation found in the literature by the author. As mentioned elsewhere, there were noticeably few cases of acute respiratory diseases in this hospital during the time this work was under way. With rigid exclusion of tonsils and teeth infections, the author thinks the strains isolated represent a fair average of the types of hemolytic and nonhemolytic streptococci present in the normal throats in this vicinity.

SUMMARY

In 134 average throats, 50.74 per cent were carriers of hemolytic streptococcus, 91 per cent were carriers of nonhemolytic streptococcus.

One hundred seventeen strains of hemolytic and 87 strains of nonhemolytic streptococci were classified by Holman's classification.

REFERENCES

[1]Aschner: Jour. Infect. Dis., 1917, xxi, 409.
[2]Blanton, Burhams Hunter: Jour. Am. Med. Assn., 1919, lxxii, 1520.
[3]Blake: Jour. Med. Research, 1917, xxxvi, 99.
[4]Barnett and Chapman: Jour. Am. Med. Assn., 1918, lxx, 1062.
[5]Brown: Monograph of Rockefeller Institute for Med. Res., 1919, No. 9.
[6]Clawson: Jour. Infect. Dis., 1920, xxvi, 93.
[7]Davis and Pilot: Ibid., 1919, xxiv, 386.
[8]Fox and Hamburg: Jour. Am. Med. Assn., 1918, lxx, 1758.
[9]Gay: Jour. Lab. and Clin. Med., 1918, 3.
[10]Greenway, Boettiger, Caldwell: Arch. Int. Med., 1919, xxiv, 1.
[11]Hamilton and Havens: Jour. Am. Med. Assn., 1919, lxxii, 272.
[12]Holman: Jour. Med. Research, 1916, xxxiv, 375.
[13]Holman, Avery, Kinsella, Brown: Jour. Lab. and Clin. Med., 1918, iii, 618.
[14]Holman: Jour. Bacteriol., 1919, iv, 149.
[15]Kligler: Jour. Bacteriol., 1919, iv, 35.
[16]Levy and Alexander: Jour. Am. Med. Assn., 1918, lxx, 1827.
[17]Levin, Goodman, Pancoast: Am. Jour. Med. Sc., 1919, clvii, 202.
[18]Lucke and Rea: Jour. Infect. Dis., 1919, xxiv, 533.
[19]Opie, Freeman, Blake, Small, Rivers: Jour. Am. Med. Assn., 1919, lxxii, 108.
[20]Otteraaen: Jour. Infect. Dis., 1920, xxvi, 23.
[21]Ruediger: Ibid., 1906, iii, 755.
[22]Schachter: Proc. Chicago Path. Soc. 10, 301. 1918. Quoted by Davis: Jour. Am. Med. Assn., 1919, lxxii, 319.
[23]Sherwood and Downs: Jour. Infect. Dis., 1919, xxiv, 133.
[24]Tongs: Jour. Am. Med. Assn., 1919, lxxiii, 1050.
[25]Walker and Adkinson: Jour. Med. Research, 1919, xl, 229.

CLASSIFICATION OF STREPTOCOCCUS*

II. Streptococci Isolated from Influenza Throats, Classified by Sugar Fermentations

By Lloyd Arnold, M.D., Nashville, Tenn.

IN February, 1920, we experienced in Nashville a recurrence epidemic of influenza. This communication covers the types of streptococci, based on sugar fermentation, encountered in the throats of patients suffering from "Influenza."

A literature review of the streptococci found in the throats of influenza cases is not attempted in this paper. It was the author's object to ascertain whether the streptococci as a class increased in percentage and whether the types as classified by sugar tests differed from those in normal throats in this vicinity.

The same method of collecting material, identification and other technic was carried out in this work as was reported in a former paper.

EXPERIMENTAL

One hundred sixteen cases, clinically diagnosed as influenza, just entering the hospital were selected for this work.

Fifty-six cases were positive to hemolytic streptococci, making 48.2 per cent positive. One hundred sixteen cases were positive to nonhemolytic streptococci, making 100 per cent positive. Classified according to Holman as follows:

HEMOLYTIC STREPTOCOCCI

NUMBER	CLASS NAME	PER CENT
20	Strept. Equi	35.7
22	Strept. Subacidus	39.3
8	Strept. Hemolyticus, II	14.3
4	Strept. Infrequens	7.1
2	Strept. Anginosis	3.6

NONHEMOLYTIC STREPTOCOCCI

NUMBER	CLASS NAME	PER CENT
66	Strept. Equinus	34.74
48	Strept. Salivarius	25.26
44	Strept. Mitis	23.15
26	Strept. Ignavus	13.70
6	Strept. Fecalis	3.15

Classified according to Blake as follows:

HEMOLYTIC STREPTOCOCCI

NUMBER	CLASS NAME	PER CENT
56	Strept. Hemolysans	48.2

NONHEMOLYTIC STREPTOCOCCI

NUMBER	CLASS NAME	PER CENT
92	Strept. Equinus	48.42
92	Strept. Buccalis	48.42
6	Strept. Fecalis	3.16

*From the City Hospital Laboratory, Nashville, Tenn.

DISCUSSION

The percentage of hemolytic streptococci (50.74 per cent) in normal throats, recorded during October, November, and December, 1919, and the percentage (48.2 per cent) found during the recurrent epidemic of influenza do not show much difference. The types as classified by sugar fermentations run very close together in the two series. A postepidemic series is now being run in this laboratory, and the types so far observed run close to the preepidemic and epidemic strains already recorded. The same comparison holds for the nonhemolytic streptococci. There certainly was not present in the throats of patients suffering from an attack of influenza in February, 1920, in Nashville, streptococci of the hemolytic or nonhemolytic types that differed from the strains isolated and studied by the fermentation tests, from normal throats during a period three months prior to the epidemic.

ON THE USE OF TETHELIN IN A CASE OF MULTIPLE BEDSORES

By Dr. Hampden Carr, Adelaide, South Australia

THE accompanying notes are presented as affording an instance of successful treatment by tethelin, a lipoid prepared from the anterior lobe of the pituitary body,* of a case of delayed or arrested healing which yielded no response to any of the customary procedures. I am indebted to Dr. F. S. Scott for his permission to publish these notes upon his patient, whom I attended for him during his absence from this city. I saw the patient, Mrs. H., for the first time on the 16th of October, 1919. The history of the case prior to that date is as follows:

The patient was admitted to Parkwynd Hospital, Adelaide, on August 31, about thirty days after she had been confined by a midwife in a lying-in home. She was in a semiconscious condition, features pinched, wan, could not bear to be touched or moved, temperature 101°, pulse 104. Urine, sp. gr. 1.025, acid in reaction, containing no sugar or albumin.

On September 2, the patient was curetted. The contents of the uterus were offensive. Posterior culdesac opened, seropus evacuated and drained. Patient complained of pain in both shoulders. Temperature 103°. Hot douches were administered.

On the following day the patient complained of pain in the left arm, temperature varied between 100° and 103°. On the fourth the left arm and shoulder was swollen and very painful. On the sixth, rigor after douche. Patient complains of back feeling sore; no pressure marks; taking very little nourishment; looking very ill; temperature 102°.

September 7. Rigor this morning; arms and legs very painful; patient is turned frequently from side to side, no pressure marks.

September 10. Back looking red, being rubbed with spts. meth. and zinc oxide ointment.

From the seventeenth to the twenty-fifth this condition remained unchanged. Patient taking scarcely any nourishment, feet and legs swollen. No power of movement in body or legs.

On the twenty-sixth a pressure mark about 1½ inches in diameter appeared on the lower part of the back. The area was quite black. The surrounding parts were well rubbed and the pressure marks treated as above.

September 27. Patient being turned every two hours. Each time of turning shows marks of pressure.

September 28. When turned this morning after sleeping in one position for three hours a large pressure mark was found on the right hip. Patient lying on air pillows all the time.

October 1. On the right hip a deep and sloughing wound. A new pressure mark has appeared on the back above the old one. Patient lifeless and apathetic; moans when moved. Temperature 102°, pulse 126.

*Robertson, T. Brailsford: Jour. Am. Med. Assn., 1916, lxvi, 1009. Barney, E. L.: Jour. Lab. and Clin. Med., 1918, iii, No. 8.

593

October 4. A new pressure mark on the left hip. Other wounds very painful; temperature 100°.

October 6. Patient has been turned on her face to relieve back and hips. After two hours in this position the left crest of the ilium had a long pressure mark. Temperature 102°.

October 7. Another pressure mark on left hip. Wounds on back and

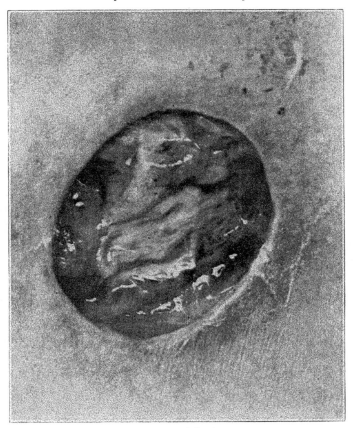

Fig. 1.—Ulcer on hip before treatment.

right hip discharging profuse amount of offensive matter. These are being dressed with eusol. No desire for food, legs stiff and useless.

I saw Mrs. H. on October 16. She had a continuous discharge and was being douched daily. I gave her an intrauterine douche and found that the uterus was involuting well. I dressed the wound on the hip with eusol, employing Dakin's method of continuous irrigation. Temperature 99°, pulse 116.

October 23. Three pressure marks now appeared on the left side, looking angry, with black slough. The patient was placed in a suspension bed to relieve the pressure on back and buttocks. Temperature 99°, pulse 120.

This appeared to be a suitable case for the employment of tethelin, and, acting upon the advice of Professor Robertson, on October 28 we applied the tethelin (Mulford), incorporated in a lanoline base, to those bedsores from

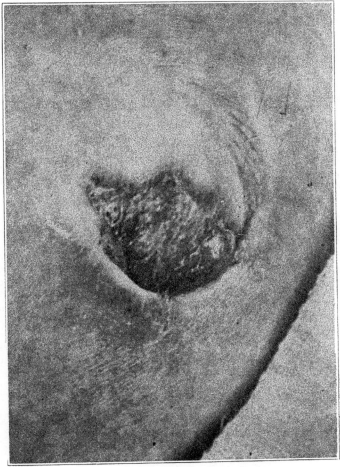

Fig. 2.—Ulcer of hip at conclusion of treatments.

which the sloughs had separated. The remaining bedsores were still treated with eusol and antiphlogistine. On the same day the accompanying photograph (Fig. 1) was taken of the largest sore upon the right hip.

On October 29 and 31 tethelin was applied to the wounds on the back and right hip, antiphlogistine being still applied to the left hip. The wounds treated with tethelin looked decidedly cleaner, and from this date until November 26, the wounds were dressed every forty-eight hours with tethelin in lanoline base, the wounds progressively improving. Her position was changed every two hours, alternating between an ordinary bed, air pillows and suspension. Temperature did not rise above 99°. Patient still very much depressed.

On November 26 I found that the wound on the right hip was not progressing so well. The skin had become undermined all round the wound to the extent of an inch. I injected tethelin in aqueous solution hypodermically into the healthy tissues all round the wound, but the patient bore it so badly that I did not repeat this treatment, reinstituting the former dressing.

On December 2 I found the patient looking brighter and taking an interest in outside affairs. She also took nourishment better. The swelling of the legs had subsided, although they were stiff and sore. The treatment was continued, temperature normal.

December 20. The patient continued to make good progress. The wounds looked healthy and were healing well. She began to regain strength and to help herself a little.

January 8. The patient stood upright for the first time, very stiff and shaky, but otherwise well. The wounds were looking well and the accompanying photograph (Fig. 2) was taken of the wound on the hip.

In this case tethelin undoubtedly acted as a stimulant to the granulation of the wounds. No improvement was exhibited until it was applied, and within a few days after application the wounds became, in each instance, healthy granulating sores.

Owing to the patient's extreme depression and the toxic condition the final recovery was, however, slower than one would have liked. On March 5, 1920, after the patient had been at home for six weeks she had gained strength considerably, has put on weight, and is getting about with the aid of a stick. The ulcers are now all practically healed, a mere pin-point on two ulcers remaining unhealed. The necrosis of so much tissue has left depressed scars which are otherwise healthy.

I am indebted to Sister Fry of Parkwynd Hospital for her careful notes of this case and also for the excellent nursing given during the long and critical period of the illness.

ANAPHYLAXIS AND ALLIED PHENOMENA IN RELATION TO DISEASE*

By T. Harris Boughton, S.M., M.D., Akron, Ohio.

THE term anaphylaxis was introduced by Richet[1] in 1898 to describe a condition of increased susceptibility to a toxic protein (eel serum) but has later been extended, as a result of the work especially of Arthus[2] and Theobald Smith, to include the toxic action of nontoxic proteins. Probably the first recorded observation on anaphylaxis is one by Jenner in his *Inquiry into the Causes and Effects of Variolæ Vaccinæ*, in 1798. He found that quite regularly in persons who had had either cowpox or smallpox previously the inoculation of variolous matter produced only "a tingling sensation" and "an erysipelatous look appearing on the skin near the punctured parts" but it "died away in a few days without producing any variolous symptoms." In a footnote to Case 4 he says, "It is remarkable that variolous matter, when the system is disposed to reject it, should excite inflammation on the part to which it is applied more speedily than when it produces the smallpox. Indeed it becomes almost a criterion by which we can determine whether the infection will be received or not. It seems as though a change which endures through life had been produced in the action or disposition to action in the vessels of the skin; and it is remarkable, too, that whether this change has been effected by the smallpox or the cowpox, the disposition to sudden cuticular change is the same on the application of variolous matter."

Magendie[3] in 1839 (injecting egg albumen into dogs) and Flexner[4] in 1894 (injecting dog serum into rabbits) recorded typical instances of experimental anaphylaxis, but these early observations were apparently lost sight of, and the phenomenon was rediscovered, and was experimentally analyzed by Arthus,[5] Pirquet and Schick,[6] Wolff-Eisner,[7] Otto,[8] Rosenau and Anderson,[9] Vaughan,[10] Gay and Southard,[11] Besredka.[12] and since 1908 by a large number of observers.

The typical anaphylactic experiment is too well known to warrant repetition. Suffice it to say, however, that while the typical experiment results in definite shock or death following the second injection of a protein, yet we recognize many irregularities in the reaction. For instance there are great individual variations in the response of different animals to the experiment, so that it is extremely difficult to put this work on a definite quantitative basis further than to establish maximums, minimums, and averages. Thus I have had a group of four guinea pigs of the same size and all treated in the same way, and following the second injection, one died promptly; one had a severe reaction, but recovered; one had a mild reaction; and one had no reaction at all. I have had one lot of pigs in which it was difficult to produce a distinct shock without killing the animal, and a year later, another lot of pigs in which it was difficult to produce a fatal shock by the same methods. One pig, after surviving a shock, will be completely refractory to later injections of whatever size. An-

*From the Department of Pathology of the University of Illinois, College of Medicine, Chicago, Ill., and the Laboratory of Pathology, City Hospital, Akron, Ohio.

other pig, under the same conditions, after surviving a shock, will succumb the next day to a dose of the same size. One animal, if injected at weekly intervals, will become completely refractory and never develop anaphylaxis, while another, under similar conditions, will develop fatal anaphylaxis after the third or fourth injection. We should expect, and, indeed, we do find as great if not greater variations among human beings in the clinical conditions that we ascribe to anaphylaxis. And these great individual variations that exist in the type of reaction must be borne in mind if the full clinical significance of anaphylactic states is to be appreciated.

Anaphylaxis manifests itself in one or both of two ways—local and general. In the general reaction we may have either increase or decrease in temperature, a fall in blood pressure, cyanosis, delayed coagulability of the blood, leucopenia, dyspnea, pain in chest or head, dizziness, convulsions, and unconsciousness. In the local reaction, we see evidences of vasomotor disturbance—hyperemia and edema, and sometimes vesicle or pustule formation, as in urticaria, angioneurotic edema, and the local manifestations of serum disease, and in such clinical tests as the Schick, Pirquet, Calmette, luetin, and the various protein skin tests used in asthma, eczema, and related conditions.

The phenomenon of anaphylaxis is very highly specific, but not absolutely so. Thus an animal sensitized with the serum of one species may react partially to the serum of a closely related species. This has also been shown by Wells and Osborne[53] to be true of the isolated proteins of wheat and barley. This corresponds to group agglutination in bacteriology, and to that elusive form of partial immunity to one infectious disease that sometimes seems to follow recovery from another infectious disease (as seen particularly by the statistical method in public health studies).

The term "anaphylaxis" has been objected to since it implies the direct opposite to immunity, whereas it might better be said to include immunity. The term "allergy," which was introduced to indicate a state of altered immunity, is undoubtedly better, but has not been generally adopted in this sense. and has been used by some writers to indicate the altered immunologic state existing in infections as distinguished from that produced by nonorganized proteins, and by others to indicate congenital hypersusceptibility. The term "protein intoxication," while expressive and definite, is cumbersome. The original expression of Richet is no more misleading than any of the substitutes suggested, and has the sanction of age and custom. It is simpler to make a slight change in the interpretation of a word than to change the word completely.

THEORIES

The various theories evolved to explain anaphylaxis may be grouped into two classes: the humoral and the cellular. One group of the supporters of the humoral theory have held that the reaction, which took place in the blood stream, was essentially of the nature of an antigen-antibody reaction. The work especially of Doerr and Russ[13] lent great weight to this conception. The work of Vaughan and Wheeler[14] was of especial importance as providing a definite and demonstrable chemical explanation of the phenomena. They believe that the first injection of protein stimulates the production of a specific lysin capable of splitting the protein molecule into a toxic and a nontoxic portion, and that on the second injection this splitting takes place very rapidly, and the liberated toxic fraction produces the symptoms of shock. Every true protein investigated by Vaughan was found to be capable of being split by chemical means into a toxic and a nontoxic fraction. The toxic fraction when injected into animals produces symptoms similar to anaphylaxis. The writer[116] has found that repeated injections of this toxic fraction into animals produce histologic lesions similar to those of chronic anaphylaxis. It has been shown, however, by Manwaring, Kusama, and Crowe[15] and others that the toxic fraction is derived not from the splitting of the injected antigen, but from the splitting of the serum proteins of the individual.

Another group believe that while the reaction takes place in the blood stream, yet it is not so specific in nature as the antigen-antibody assumption would necessitate, since the reaction (or at least a very similar reaction) can be elicited by nonspecific substances. Jobling and Peterson[16] showed that during anaphylactic shock there was a marked increase in serum ferment, and in the end-products of protein disintegration, and a decrease in the serum antiferment. They believe that the injection of protein stimulates the production of a nonspecific proteolytic ferment which, following the second injection, splits the serum proteins, and liberates their toxic fraction. Friedberger[17] noted that the injection of inert substances, such as kaolin, was followed by anaphylactic symptoms, and Jobling and Peterson[18] found almost the same serum changes following kaolin injections as in typical anaphylaxis, and concluded that the kaolin by adsorption removed the antiferment and allowed the native serum ferment to split off the toxic fraction from the serum proteins.

Novy[19] has taken the middle ground between these positions. He believes that the toxic substance, anaphylatoxin, is produced by an "inducing body" which is itself the result of antigen-antibody union. The specificity of the reaction, then, concerns the production of this inducing substance, and not the production of the anaphylatoxin. Very diverse substances such as bacteria, starch, kaolin, agar, peptone, organ cells or extracts, and even distilled water are also able to act as "inducers" or accelerators of this reaction by which the matrix of the poison is broken down, and the poison liberated. Novy was able to produce a typical shock by the injection of agar, even so small an amount as 9 milligrams of dry agar per kilo of guinea pig proving fatal. He calls attention to the fact that this dose is less than that of most pathogenic bacteria, and suggests that the results of bacterial injections may depend on the physical effect of bacteria on the serum colloids.

Schultz[20] showed that the excised smooth muscle of a sensitized animal is hypersensitive, and the work of Pearce and Eisenbrey,[21] Dale,[22] Weil,[23] and Coca[24] has supported and extended his original findings, and lent great weight to the contention that the seat of the reaction in anaphylaxis is in the body cells and not in the blood. Undoubtedly the last word has not been said, but the acceptable theory that explains anaphylaxis must take into account these various apparently contradictory findings.

It is probable that in immunity, as we ordinarily understand the term, at least in acquired immunity, we are dealing with a process of the same nature as anaphylaxis. It is probable that an antibody, perhaps a ferment, increased in amount by the process of immunization, acts upon the toxic substance to break it down into simpler nontoxic fractions. Such a ferment may be specific, or more probably be nonspecific (complement?) but activated or liberated by a specific factor. This process may be conceived of as one stage in anaphylaxis.

PASSIVE ANAPHYLAXIS

The phenomenon of passive anaphylaxis was first described by Gay and Southard,[25] and later in the same year by Otto.[26] If a guinea pig is injected with horse serum, and after he is sensitized his serum is withdrawn and injected into a normal pig, the second pig now becomes sensitive to horse serum, and develops an anaphylactic shock on the first injection. In the earlier experiments it was thought necessary to wait fifteen to twenty-four hours before the second pig became passively sensitized, but Doerr and Russ, and Friedmann later showed that if the amounts of guinea pig serum and horse serum were rightly proportioned, an immediate reaction could be obtained. A female pig thus passively sensitized may transmit this sensitization to her offspring.

ANTIANAPHYLAXIS

If an animal responds to a second injection of a protein with a typical nonfatal anaphylactic shock, he is usually refractory to subsequent injections of the protein. This condition is called antianaphylaxis, or desensitization, and may persist for a few months in guinea pigs. If an animal is injected with a protein, and then before sensitization is complete (say about the sixth or seventh day) he is injected with a fairly large dose of the same antigen, he then becomes refractory without ever having been sensitive. If an animal has been sensitized to a certain protein, he can also be desensitized by injecting a small dose of the same protein—a dose too small to produce shock. He then becomes entirely refractory to subsequent doses that would otherwise have proved fatal. It is also possible to desensitize animals nonspecifically. If an animal be injected with horse serum, and after sensitization is complete he be given an injection of egg albumen, he will now be found partially desensitized, and a subsequent injection of horse serum may produce a mild shock, but will not kill him. Injections of many other proteins and of peptone are able to desensitize more or less completely. Many drugs have been used, such as ether, chloroform, chloral, atropine, urethane, paraldehyde, but while they may mask the symptoms, or delay death, they do not prevent death. When an animal is rendered antianaphylactic by any of the methods mentioned, this refractory condition may persist for some time, but will eventually disappear, and the animal become sensitive again. If blood is withdrawn from a refractory animal, and the serum injected into a normal animal, that animal may become more highly sensitized than when injected with serum from a sensitized animal. No theory yet advanced accounts satisfactorily for all of the known facts of antianaphylaxis.

BACTERIAL ANAPHYLAXIS

Since anaphylaxis has been shown to depend upon sensitization to proteins and to nothing else, and since bacteria contain 50 to 80 per cent of protein and protein derivatives, this phenomenon has been offered as an explanation of bacterial disease. Vaughan has shown that the bacterial proteins may be split chemically to yield his protein poison, and that properly spaced injections of killed pathogenic or nonpathogenic bacteria may produce typical anaphylaxis in guinea pigs. The "endotoxin" of Pfeiffer then would correspond to the toxic fraction split off from the protein molecule. The characteristics of bacterial disease—the period of incubation, the sudden onset of the symptoms, the fever, the skin eruption, the crisis, the subsequent immunity—all have their counterpart in experimental anaphylaxis. The immunity against certain infections that may be conferred by injecting bacterial vaccines has its counterpart in desensitization.

RELATED PHENOMENA

There is a group of phenomena that are closely related to anaphylaxis. Biedl and Kraus,[27] Arthus,[28] DeWaele,[108] and others have shown that injections of peptone produce in animals symptoms very similar to anaphylaxis. It produces in dogs the same fall in blood pressure, delayed coagulability of the blood, and leucopenia, and in guinea pigs the same bronchial spasms. Injections of peptone into sensitized animals produce some degree of desensitization toward the specific protein used. I[29] have shown that the histologic lesions produced in guinea pigs by repeated injections of peptone are closely similar to those in chronic anaphylaxis. Phillippson[30] noted that a solution of peptone applied to the scarified skin produces local urticarial wheals similar to those found in anaphylactic states. Vaughan[107] noted a similar action of his protein poison.

Witte's peptone contains variable amounts of toxic secondary proteoses and of peptone. Pullitzer[31] in 1885 first separated the proteoses from the peptone, and studied their physiologic action. Grosjean[32] in 1892 isolated the individual proteoses and studied their effects when injected into animals. The effects of proteose intoxication have since been investigated carefully by Thompson,[33] Chittenden, Mendel, and Henderson,[34] Underhill[35] and others. Injections of proteoses into the blood stream of dogs produce rapid and marked fall of blood pressure, delayed coagulation, increased lymph flow, narcosis, and other toxic symptoms and some immunity (tolerance) for later injections. DeKruif and Eggerth[36] have shown that the toxic principle of Witte's peptone easily passes membranes that hold back all of the anaphylatoxin, hence "peptone" or proteose intoxication is probably not identical with anaphylaxis. Injections of toxic proteoses, however, have been used in the treatment of infectious diseases in the hope of producing a condition similar to anaphylaxis, and thus benefiting the clinical condition.

Barger and Dale[37] and Kutscher[38] simultaneously but independently discovered the physiologic activity of histamine. This substance is β-imidazolylethylamine, and is produced by the decarboxylation of histidine. Its action has been further studied by Dale and Laidlaw,[39] Ackermann and Kutscher,[40] Barbour,[41] Oehme,[42] and Jackson and Mills.[43] Its effects on blood pressure and on smooth muscle are very similar to those found in anaphylaxis, and Barger and Dale have suggested that histamine may be a factor in producing the symptoms of anaphylaxis. Eppinger,[44] and Sollmann and Pilcher[45] found that the local application of histamine in high dilution to the human skin produces redness, swelling, and an urticarial wheal. I[46] have found that repeated injections of histamine in animals produce histologic lesions somewhat similar to those found in chronic anaphylaxis. Barger and Dale[47] have recovered histamine from intestinal mucosa. Berthelot and Bertrand,[48] Mellanby and Twort,[49] and Jones[50] have described methods of isolating an organism (B. aminophilis intestinalis) from feces which is able to produce histamine from histidine, and Koessler and Hanke[51] have found that the B.eoli can do the same thing under proper conditions. Dale and Laidlaw[52] have pointed out certain similarities in the action of histamine to the manifestations of surgical shock, and have suggested that the ease with which surgical shock is brought on by traumatizing the intestine is related to the histamine content of that organ. Histamine acts partly as an endothelial poison relaxing capillaries and increasing their permeability. I have found definite histologic evidence of endothelial damage. Locally applied, it produces an urticarial wheal similar to that seen in local anaphylaxis. But a sharp blow on the skin may produce the same wheal. A definite relationship may be perceived between anaphylactic shock and surgical shock, though this relationship may extend no farther than a similarity of mechanism.

CLINICAL CONSIDERATIONS

One of the best known and most important manifestations of anaphylaxis, serum disease, has been well described by Pirquet and Schick,[54] Axenow,[55] Weaver,[56] Bokay,[57] Schultz,[58] Goodall,[59] Davidson,[60] and others, and is too well known to require further description. Most of the reported cases have been due to horse serum injected for curative purposes. Netter,[61] however, has reported the case of a child with poliomyelitis who developed serum disease after the second injection of human serum. There were joint pains, elevated temperature, and rash; the child recovered.

Within recent years several diseases, previously little understood, have been explained as due to anaphylaxis. As a result of the work especially of I. Chandler Walker,[62] and others, about 50 per cent of cases of bronchial asthma have been shown to be due to anaphylaxis, and the specific protein to which the patient is sensitized may be determined by skin tests. These proteins are classified as those from (1) animal hair (horse, cat, rabbit); (2) foods (eggs, meat, milk, etc.); (3) bacteria; and (4) pollens. Sometimes an individual may be sensitized to several different proteins, and the degree of specificity involved is often remarkable. Thus an individual may be sensitized to horse hair protein, but not to horse serum protein, or to only a single protein of horse hair, and not to the others. Hay fever is anaphylaxis induced by pollens.

Most cases of urticaria are known to have a very definite relation to anaphylaxis as shown by Strickler,[63] McBride and Schorer,[64] Schwann,[65] Widal,[66] and others. Blackfan[68] found positive cutaneous reactions with egg white, cow's milk, and human milk in 22 of 27 cases of eczema. Strickler[69] obtained endermic reactions with foods in 20 per cent of cases of eczema, and White[70] found that nearly 50 per cent of his eczema cases reacted to foods. The same phenomenon of protein sensitization has been found to be at the bottom of certain cases of angioneurotic edema. This condition has also been shown to have a definite hereditary tendency, though the exciting cause may be different in related individuals.

Idiosyncrasies against certain foods such as shell-fish, eggs, strawberries, etc., are also evidences of anaphylaxis. This has been discussed by Talbot.[106] It is probable that in those individuals who show such sensitization, the course of digestion is somewhat abnormal or that the intestinal mucosa allows the absorption of certain products of protein digestion that are ordinarily excluded. In some cases, drug idiosyncrasies are also due to anaphylaxis.

Sensitization to foreign proteins occurs in some cases through inhalation. This is especially true in hay fever, and in asthma due to animal hair. In some cases, as in foods, sensitization occurs by way of the intestinal tract, though the exact mechanism is not known. In cases of serum disease the sensitization may probably occur by either of these routes (inhalation of horse hair and skin secretions, or ingestion of horse meat) or by direct inoculation (anti-toxin). The duration of sensitization is variable: in many cases it appears to persist through life, but occasionally it disappears spontaneously.

If human beings could be desensitized as readily as laboratory animals it would be of enormous clinical importance. Deaths from anaphylaxis are occasionally reported (I[71] have reviewed this literature elsewhere) and many of these could be prevented if we could safely and surely desensitize patients who are likely to develop anaphylaxis following serum injections. Besredka[72] devised a method which he called the method of "doses subintrantes" by which he hoped to render serum injections completely safe. He injected sensitized guinea pigs with several doses of horse serum beginning with a dose too small to produce symptoms, and rapidly increasing the size of the injections until within a few hours the animal could safely withstand a dose of 40 to 200 times the fatal dose for sensitized control pigs. All of Besredka's animals, however, were sensitized with a small dose of antigen. If an animal has been sensitized with a large dose of protein, a large dose is required to desensitize him—a dose, indeed, larger than the fatal dose for an animal sensitized with a minimum dose of antigen. This method is therefore impractical unless we know the size of the sensitizing dose, and in human beings this is almost never possible. Moreover, as Weil[73] has pointed out, this repetition of preliminary doses does not always produce desensitization, but some animals respond to successively increasing doses with symptoms of successively increasing severity, and eventually death. Netter,[74] Grysez and Dupuich,[75] and Doerr[76] have reported similar observations in patients. Because of the uncertainty of the method itself, and because of the marked variations in their manner of response which many individuals show, this method of desensitization, as a clinical procedure is practically useless.

Another method of desensitization has been employed with greater success. If an individual sensitized against a certain protein receive injections of a very dilute solution of the protein at intervals of a few days, and the amount injected be cautiously increased, the individual may become entirely refractory, and this refractory condition may last for a long time. This method has been worked out in great detail by Walker[77] in the treatment of asthma, and is applicable also to such chronic conditions as eczema and food sensitization.

This is essentially the method that is used in the administration of vaccines for chronic infections, with the exception that the bacterial protein injected is primarily toxic. Injections of killed bacteria in the treatment of infectious disease were used empirically before our ideas on immunity were at all definite, and long before the nature of anaphylaxis was appreciated. It has never been possible to explain either the good results or the frequent disappointments met with in the use of bacterial vaccines in the treatment of disease, on the basis exclusively of immune antibodies produced, since the patient may be better when those antibodies detectable in the test tube are low, or he may be worse when the antibodies are high. All that we know of bacterial vaccines in disease, and of anaphylaxis tends to support the contention that injections of dead bacteria when they produce any effects at all, produce anaphylaxis, or desensitization, which, as we have seen, should be considered as one phase of anaphylaxis. (The injection of dead bacteria for prophylactic purposes, as in the antityphoid inoculation, should be considered an exception to this statement, for here we are dealing with specific easily demonstrable antibodies.) The mobilization of the serum ferments, and the elevation of temperature (frequently seen in bacterial injections, and obtainable by very small doses of simple proteins[67] are evidently a means of defense. There is no reason to think that there is any difference whatever in the anaphylaxis produced by different proteins. If these assumptions are true (that vaccines act by inducing anaphylaxis, and that the nature of anaphylaxis does not vary with the inducing protein), then it is not necessary to use cultures of the specific infecting organism, and it is possible that any foreign protein or protein derivative that will produce a mild anaphylactic shock will accomplish as much good as can be accomplished by bacterial injections. It may easily be that bacteria represent a type of protein that is more readily acted upon, and hence more "stimulating" than are unorganized proteins or protein derivatives. Not all strains of bacteria produce equally satisfactory vaccines for clinical use. There is some evidence that a particular strain of bacteria that produces good results when injected as a vaccine in one case may produce just as good results in other cases regardless of the type of infecting organism. Of course the problem of dosage, and of the degree of the anaphylactic shock desired, as well as variations in the susceptibility of different patients make the whole question very uncertain, and emphasizes the fact that this procedure (the injection of bacteria or of proteins) is still almost wholly empirical.

In support of the view that anaphylaxis therapeutically induced need not be specific, it may be mentioned that many observers have reported good results by the use of nonspecific vaccines, especially in typhoid and arthritis, but also in a variety of infections including puerperal sepsis, gonorrheal complications, asthma, influenza, pneumonia, and some skin diseases. Rumpf[78] in 1893 treated typhoid fever with a vaccine of B. pyocyaneus, and in the last four years Luedke,[79] Kraus,[80] Miller and Lusk,[81] Culver,[82] Engman and McGarry,[83] Cowie and Calhoun,[84] Roberts and Carv,[85] Cowie and Beaver,[86] Snyder,[93] Reibmayr,[104] Dansyz,[105] Cadbury[117] and many others have reported good results from the use of nonspecific vaccines.

Less favorable testimony, however, is at hand. Sholly, Blum, and Smith[87] in pertussis, Whittington[88] in typhoid fever, and Bumpus[89] in prostatic cases found that though their cases seemed at first glance to do well, a careful analysis showed that they did not do quite so well as the cases that received no vaccine.

A partial explanation of these diverse results is found in the work of Herrmann[90] who showed that in rabbits "sensitized" (immunized) to streptococcus or meningococcus, a definite liberation of specific opsonins and agglutinins followed the injection of foreign proteins (human serum and ascitic fluid), but similar treatment of typhoid sensitized rabbits gave no results. But on the other hand, Dunklin[91] found that injections of proteose in typhoid immune rabbits produced an increase in the antibodies of the serum. Jobling and Peterson[92] showed that in animals, injections of bacteria, of kaolin, and of protein split products are followed by mobilization of serum protease, and this presumably might aid in the destruction of bacteria, and would explain some of the good results obtained by nonspecific means.

Since nonspecific vaccines have given good results in many cases, it is only a step to the use of simple toxic proteins. Matthes[93] in 1894 found that injections of secondary proteose produced about the same results as tuberculin. Luedke[79] in 1915 treated typhoid fever successfully by means of injections of secondary proteose. With the same substance good results were obtained in typhoid fever and arthritis by Miller and Lusk,[81] in arthritis and other complications of gonorrhea by Culver,[94] in arthritis, gonorrheal epididymitis, and in erysipelas by Jobling, Peterson, and Manier.[95] Beebe[96] used a protein prepared from the seeds of millet and alfalfa in the treatment of arthritis, and Brooks and Stanton[97] used 'hemoprotein" from ox-blood in the same condition, both with success. Nolf[98] found good results in the treatment of a variety of infections with intravenous injections of Witte's peptone. Baldwin and L'Esperance[99] found that injections of typhoid bacteria produced improvement in tuberculous guinea pigs, but Krause and Willis[100] found that animals receiving repeated injections of egg white were less resistant to subsequent injections of tuberculous material, and repeated anaphylactic shocks had no effect on the course of an established tuberculosis. Peterson[118] has pointed out that resistance to tuberculosis depends more on the ferment-antiferment balance than on specific immune factors, and that therefore appropriate nonspecific therapy might be expected to produce better results in tuberculosis than that calculated to increase specific immune antibodies. Wells[101] obtained good results in the treatment of influenzal pneumonia by injection of the residue left after the alcoholic extraction of typhoid bacilli, and Lamb and Brannin[102] in the same condition used a variety of antitoxic serums, and the bacterial filtrates of organisms commonly found in influenza and pneumonia, but they "make no great claims for this treatment." This diversity of methods and of results shows the condition of uncertainty that exists with respect to nonspecific protein therapy. All writers agree, however, on one point, and that is that the administration of foreign proteins by the intravenous route is potentially highly dangerous, and must be performed with great care. Thomas[103] says he knows of several deaths due to the unskillful use of this method.

Passive anaphylaxis is of some practical importance clinically. Ramirez[109] has reported the case of a man who acquired horse asthma (was passively sensitized to horse hair protein) by receiving a blood transfusion from an asthmatic. This constitutes a new hazard in transfusion cases. DeBesche[110] records two cases of horse asthma and one of cat asthma in which guinea pigs were passively sensitized by injections of patient's serum, and later killed by injecting the specific antigen. Bruck[111] had a similar experience with the serum of patients sensitized to pork and to iodoform. Schloss,[112] working with the serum of a patient sensitized to egg, and Koessler[113] with the serum of hay fever patients, obtained the same results. It is possible that this reaction might be of diagnostic value in some cases. Of course the skin test is much simpler, but it is not completely reliable, for cases have been found in which anaphylaxis developed after the administration of therapeutic serums, even when the skin test was negative for horse serum.

The frequency with which vaccines and other foreign proteins are being injected today for the treatment of all manner of diseases makes it appropriate to inquire whether there may be any harmful results aside from the immediate effects of the injection. Longcope[114] has shown that repeated anaphylactic shocks in animals produce degenerative and inflammatory changes in kidney, liver, and heart. I[115] have obtained similar results, and have further shown that there is a distinct degenerative change in the arteries in many organs. Just how far these results are applicable to human beings has not yet been determined, though I have studied one case of anaphylaxis[116] in which the microscopic findings were very similar to those of experimental anaphylaxis in animals. It is well to remember that protein therapy is still in the experimental stage, that it is a potent instrument for harm, and that at least a few deaths are traceable to its injudicious use.

REFERENCES

[1]Richet and Hericourt: Compt. rend. Soc. de biol., 1898, l. 137.
[2]Arthus and Breton: Compt. rend. Soc. biol., 1903, lv. 1478.
[3]Magendie: Vorlesung ueber das Blut, 1839.
[4]Flexner: Med. News, 1894, lxv, 116.
[5]Arthus: Compt. rend. Soc. biol., 1903, lv, 817.
[6]Pirquet and Schick: Wien. klin. Wchnschr., 1903, xvi, 758. Die Serumkrankheit, Franz Deuticke, Leipzig, 1905.
[7]Wolff-Eisner: Ztschr. f. Bakteriol., 1904; Berl. klin. Wchnschr., 1904, xli, 1105, 1131, 1156, 1273.
[8]Otto: Das Theobald Smithsche Phaenomen, v. Leuthold Gedenkschrift, i, 1905.
[9]Rosenau, M. J., and Anderson, J. F.: Hygienic Lab. Bull., 1906, No. 29, ibid., 1907, No. 36; ibid., 1908, No. 45.
[10]Vaughan, V. C.: Jour. Infect. Dis., 1907, iv, 476.
[11]Gay, F. P., and Southard, E. E.: Jour. Med. Research, 1907, xvi, 143; ibid., 1908, xviii, 407; ibid., 1908, xix, 1, 5, 17.
[12]Besredka: Ann. de l'Inst. Pasteur, 1907, xxi, 384, 777, 950. Compt. rend. Soc. biol., 1907, lxii, 1053; ibid., 1907, lxiii, 294; ibid., 1908, lxv, 478.
[13]Doerr and Russ: Ztschr., f. Immunitat., 1909, ii, 208.
[14]Vaughan and Wheeler: Jour. Infect. Dis., 1907, iv, 476.
    Protein Split Products, Philadelphia, 1913, Lea and Febiger.
[15]Manwaring, W. H., Kusama, Y., and Crowe, H. E.: Jour. Immunol., 1917, ii, 511.
[16]Jobling and Peterson: Jour. Exper. Med., 1915, xxii, 401; Bull. Johns Hopkins Hosp., 1915, xxvi, 296.
[17]Friedberger, E., and Kumagai, T.: Ztschr. f. Immun., Orig., 1912, xiii, 127.
    Friedberger, E., and Tsuneoka, K.: Ibid., 1913, xx, 405.
[18]Jobling and Peterson: Jour. Exper. Med., 1915, xxii, 590.
[19]Novy, F. G.: Jour. Infect. Dis., 1917, xx, 490.
[20]Schultz: Jour. Pharm. and Exper. Therap., 1910, i, 549, ibid., 1910, ii, 221.
[21]Pearce and Eisenbrey: Trans. Congr. Am. Phys. Surg., 1910, viii.
[22]Dale, H. H.: Jour. Pharm. and Exper. Therap., 1913, iv, 167.
[23]Weil, R.: Jour. Med. Research, 1913, xxvii, 497; ibid., 1914, xxx, 299.
[24]Coca, A.: Ztschr. f. Immun., 1914, xx, 622.
[25]Gay, F. P., and Southard, E. E.: Jour. Med. Research, 1907, xvi, 143.
[26]Otto: München. med. Wchnschr., 1907, liv, 1605.

27Biedl and Kraus: Wien. klin. Wchnschr., 1909, xxii, 363.
28Arthus: Compt. rend. l'Acad. de Sc., 1909, cxlviii, 999, 1002.
29Boughton, T. H.: Jour. Immunol., September, 1919, iv, No. 5.
30Phillippson: Gior. ital. d. mal. ven., 1899.
31Pullitzer: Jour. Physiol., 1885, vii, 283.
32Grosjean: Arch. de biol., 1892, xi, 381.
33Thompson: Jour. Physiol., 1896, xx. 455.
34Chittenden, R. H., Mendel, L. B., and Henderson, Y.: Am. Jour. Physiol., 1898, ii. 142.
35Underhill, F. P.: Am. Jour. Physiol., 1903, ix, 345; Jour. Biol. Chem., 1915, xxii, 465.
36DeKruif, P. H., and Eggerth, A. H.: Jour. Infec. Dis., 1919, xxiv, 505.
37Barger, G., and Dale, H. H.: Proc. Chem. Soc., 1910, xxvi, 128.
38Kutscher: Zentralbl. f. Physiol., 1910, xxiv, 163.
39Dale, H. H., and Laidlaw, P. P.: Jour. Physiol., 1910, xli, 318.
40Ackermann and Kutscher: Ztschr. f. Biol., 1910, liv. 387.
41Barbour, J.: Jour. Pharm. and Exper. Therap., 1912. iv, 245.
42Oehme, C.: Arch. f. exper. Path. u. Pharmacol., 1913, lxii, 76.
43Jackson, D. E., and Mills, C. A.: Jour. Lab. and Clin. Med., 1919, v, 2.
44Eppinger, H.: Wien. klin. Wchnschr., 1913. xxiii, 1414.
45Sollmann and Pilcher: Jour. Pharm. and Exper. Therap., 1917, ix, 309.
46Boughton, T. H.: In press.
47Barger, G., and Dale, H. H.: Jour. Physiol., 1910, xli, 499.
48Berthelot and Bertrand: Compt. rend. de l'Acad. de Sc., 1912, cliv, 1643, 1826.
49Mellanby, E., and Twort, F. W.: Jour. Physiol., 1912, xlv, 53.
50Jones, H. M.: Jour. Infect. Dis., 1918, xxii, 125.
51Koessler, K. K., and Hanke, M. T.: Jour. Biol. Chem., 1919, xxxix, 539.
52Dale, H. H., and Laidlaw, P. P.: Jour. Physiol., 1919, lii, 355.
53Wells and Osborne: Jour. Infect. Dis., 1913, xii, 341.
54Pirquet and Schick: Die Serumkrankheit, Franz Deuticke, Leipzig. 1905.
55Axenow: Jahrb. f. Kinderh., 1913, lxxviii. 565.
56Weaver, G. H.: Arch. Int. Med., 1909, iii, 485.
57Bokay: Deutsch. med. Wchnschr., 1911, xxxvii, 9.
58Schultz: Berl. klin. Wchnschr., 1914, li, 349, 401.
59Goodall: Jour. Hyg., 1907, vii, 607; Brit. Med. Jour., ii, 1359.
60Davidson: Glasgow Med. Jour., 1919, xci, 321.
61Netter: Compt. rend. Soc. de Biol., 1915, lxxviii, 505.
62Walker, I. C.: Jour. Med. Research, 1917-8, xxxv, xxxvi, xxxvii.
Jour. Am. Med. Assn., 1918, lxx, 897.
63Strickler, A.: New York Med. Jour., 1916, civ, 198.
64McBride and Schorer: Jour. Cutan. Dis., 1916, xxxiv, 70.
65Schwann, A. W.: Jour. Am. Med. Assn., 1915, lxiv, 737.
66Widal, F.: Bull. et mém. Soc. méd d. hôp. de Paris, 1914, xxxvii. 256.
67Friedberger: Deutsch. med. Wchnschr., 1911, i, 61; Ztschr. f. Immun., 1911, Orig. x, 216.
68Blackfan, K. D.: Am. Jour. Dis. Child., 1916, xi, 441.
69Strickler, A.: Jour. Am. Med. Assn., 1916, lxvii, 70.
70White, J. C.: Jour. Am. Med. Assn., 1917, lxviii, 81.
71Boughton, T. H.: Jour. Am. Med. Assn., Dec. 27, 1919, lxxiii.
72Besredka: Ann. de l'Inst. Pasteur, 1910, xxiv, 879.
73Weil, R.: Jour. Med. Research, 1913, xxix, 233.
74Netter: Bull. et mém Soc. méd. d. hôp. de Paris, 1912, xxxiii, 401.
75Grysez and Dupuich: Ibid., 1912, xxxiii, 374.
76Doerr in Kolle and Wassermann: Handbuch der Pathogenen Mikroorganismen. 1913, p. 1082.
77Walker, I. C.: Arch. Int. Med., 1918, xxii, 466.
78Rumpf, T. R.: Deutsch med. Wchnschr., 1893, xix, 987.
79Luedke, H.: München, med. Wchnschr., 1915, lxii, 327.
80Kraus, R.: Wien. klin. Wchnschr., 1915, xxxviii, 29.
81Miller, J., and Lusk, F.: Jour. Am. Med. Assn., 1916, lxvi, 1756; ibid., 1916. lxvii. 2010; ibid., 1917, lxix, 765.
82Culver, H.: Jour. Am. Med. Assn., 1917, lxviii, 362.
83Engman, M., and McGarry. R.: Jour. Am. Med. Assn., 1916, lxvii, 1741.
84Cowie, D. M., and Calhoun, H.: Arch. Int. Med., 1919, xxiii, 69.
85Roberts, D., and Cary, E. G.: Jour. Am. Med. Assn., 1919, lxxii, 922.
86Cowie, D. M., and Beaver, P. W.: Jour. Am. Med. Assn., Apr. 19. 1919, lxxii. 1117.
87Scholly, A. I., Blum, J., and Smith, L.: Jour. Am. Med. Assn., 1917, lxviii, 1451.
88Whittington, T. H.: Lancet, London, 1916, i, 759.
89Bumpus, H. C.: Jour. Am. Med. Assn., 1918, lxxvi. 213.
90Herrmann, S. J.: Jour. Infect. Dis., 1918, xxiii, 45.
91Dunklin: quoted by Jobling and Peterson: Jour. Am. Med. Assn., 1916, lxvi, 1753.

[92]Jobling and Peterson: Jour. Am. Med. Assn., 1915, lxv, 515.
[93]Matthes, M.: Deutsch. Arch. f. klin. Med. 1894, liv, 39.
[94]Culver, H.: Jour. Lab. and Clin. Med., 1917, iii, 11.
[95]Jobling, Peterson, and Manier: Arch. Int. Med., 1917, xix, 1042.
[96]Beebe, S. P.: Med. Rec., New York, July 21, 1917, xcii.
[97]Brooks, C., and Stanton, F. M.: New York Med. Jour., 1919, cix, 452.
[98]Nolf, P.: Presse Méd., Feb. 24, 1919, xxvii, 93; Jour. Am. Med. Assn., Nov. 22, 1919,
    lxxiii, 1579.
[99]Baldwin, H., and L'Esperance, E.: Jour. Immun., 1917, ii, 283.
[100]Krause, A. K., and Willis, H. S.: Am. Rev. of Tuberculosis, 1919, iii, 153.
[101]Wells, C. N.: Jour. Am. Med. Assn., 1919, lxxii, 1813.
[102]Lamb, F. H., and Brannin, E. B.: Jour. Am. Med. Assn., Apr. 12, 1919, lxxii, 1056.
[103]Thomas, H. B.: Jour. Am. Med. Assn., 1917, lxix, 770.
[104]Reibmayr, H.: München. med. Wchnschr., 1915, lxii, 610.
[105]Dansyz, J.: Presse méd., 1918, xxvi, 367.
[106]Talbot, F. B.: Med. Rec., New York, 1917, xci, 875.
[107]Vaughan, V. C.: Jour. Am. Med. Assn., 1916, lxvii, 1559.
[108]De Waele: Bull. Acad. roy. de méd. de Belg., 1907, xxi, 715.
[109]Ramirez, A. A.: Jour. Am. Med. Assn., Sept. 27, 1919, lxxiii, 984.
[110]DeBesche, A.: Jour. Infec. Dis., 1918, xxii, 594.
[111]Bruck: Arch. f. Dermatol., 1909, xcvi, 241.
[112]Schloss: Am. Jour. Child. Dis., 1912, iii, 341.
[113]Koessler, K.: in Forschheimer's Therapeusis, v, p. 671.
[114]Longcope, W. T.: Jour. Exper. Med., 1913, xviii, 678.
[115]Boughton, T. H.: Jour. Immunol., 1916, i, 105; ibid, 1917, ii, 501; ibid., 1919, iv, 213.
[116]Boughton, T. H.: In press.
[117]Cadbury, W. W.: China Med. Jour., May, 1919, xxxiii, 213.
[118]Peterson, W. F.: Arch. Int. Med., 1918, xxi, 14.

LABORATORY METHODS

THE SELECTION OF SUGARS FOR BACTERIOLOGIC WORK*

By Peter Masucci and George E. Éwe, Philadelphia, Pa.

ONE of the minor effects of the Great War was to cut short supplies of sugars, used in bacteriologic work. It was not long, however, before American chemists arose to the occasion, and sugars of excellent quality were placed upon the market.

Most of the sugars were quite the equal or superior of the imported products, but considerable variation was noted and it soon became evident that careful bacteriologic and chemical control of supplies was necessary in order to insure satisfactory materials. It is hardly necessary to dwell at length on the very great importance of the purity of sugars and other carbohydrates used in culture media for the differentiation of bacterial strains. The fallacy of using sugar broths without first freeing the media from the muscle sugar usually present in the broth, and the practice of adding serum to media to aid growth are two of the most familiar examples to the bacteriologist of the absolute necessity of getting rid of traces of foreign sugars. Both ordinary bouillon and serum contain sufficient dextrose to give rise to enough acid to render the use of such differentiating media worthless. It is therefore just as important to use pure sugars not only free from inorganic impurities, but also free from other sugars. Much valuable work pertaining to the action of bacteria upon specific carbohydrates has yielded contradictory results due mainly to use of impure sugars.

The following requirements for sugars for bacteriologic work are offered as tentative and are the result of a considerable research with the sugars named.

PURIFIED DEXTROSE—BACTERIOLOGIC DEXTROSE

Dextrose for bacteriologic work should be as free from impurities as it is economically possible to make it. The more likely impurities are organic coloring matters, chloride, sulphates, alcohol, heavy metals, insoluble matters, and excessive moisture and ash.

Some of the dextrose offered for 'bacteriologic dextrose" is not satisfactory from the standpoint of impurities; some lots contain as much as 0.36 per cent chlorides and 1.5 per cent ash. The presence of excessive sulphates, coloring matters, and alcohol makes cloudy solutions. An investigation of the various market offerings of bacteriologic dextrose indicates that the following requirements are commercially attainable without adding excessively to the cost of the

*From the Pharmaceutical Laboratories of the H. K. Mulford Co., Philadelphia, Pa.

product; dextrose conforming to these requirements is generally satisfactory as bacteriologic dextrose and conformance with these requirements should be insisted upon:

Color.—Pure white.

Ash.—Unweighable (less than 0.0005 gm. per 1 gm. sample).

Moisture.—(Loss at 100° C.) :—Not more than 10 per cent of sample.

Alcohol.—1 gm. of sample plus 5 mils water, plus 1 mil potassium hydroxide test solution should give no stronger iodoform-like odor than a blank.

Heavy Metals.—A 1:20 solution should not change color when warmed with an equal volume of hydrogen sulphide test solution.

Sulphates.—A 10 per cent solution should yield not more than a negligible turbidity with barium chloride after addition of dilute hydrochloric acid.

Chlorides.—A 10 per cent solution should yield not more than a negligible turbidity with silver nitrate, after addition of dilute nitric acid.

Solution and Color.—A 50 per cent solution in water should be practically colorless and free from any cloudiness.

Reaction.—A 10 per cent solution of dextrose should have a reaction of P_H 4.0-5.0 (C_H 1.0×10^{-4} to 1.0×10^{-5}). When the solution is boiled to drive off the carbon dioxide and cooled the reaction should be P_H $6.8 - 7.0$ (C_H $+ 1.6 \times 10^{-7}$ to C_H 1.0×10^{-7}) or practically neutral. If the solution is not neutral on boiling and subsequent cooling, then there are present free dissociated acids, which, of course, are not desirable.

Behavior on Autoclaving.—On autoclaving a 10 per cent dextrose solution for 30 min. at 120° C. the reaction should not be lower than P_H 4.0. This does not change on boiling and subsequent cooling and is apparently due to the oxidation of dextrose to some organic acid. There should be no change in color in the solution.

PURIFIED LACTOSE—BACTERIOLOGIC LACTOSE

Lactose is used extensively by bacteriologists in media for the differentiation of bacterial groups. Its use in lactose broth, Russel Medium, Endo Medium, Krumwiede Triple Sugar Agar, etc., as a differential sugar for members of the Typhoid-Colon group, shows the great role it plays; obviously lactose used for this purpose must be free from even traces of foreign sugars and must not contain any free dissociated acids which would hydrolyze the sugar on autoclaving, to dextrose and galactose. The presence of the latter sugars in lactose would give erroneous fermentation results and render the work worthless. Examination of lactose for bacteriologic work presented evidence of the necessity of carefully applying chemical and bacteriologic tests to insure a satisfactory product.

Bacteriologic lactose should answer the following chemical requirements:

Color.—Pure white.

Ash.—Unweighable (less than 0.0005gm. per 1 gm. sample).

Moisture.—Not more than 5 per cent.

Alcohol.—When 1 gm. of lactose is dissolved in 5 mils of water, and 1 mil of potassium hydroxide test solution and 1 mil of iodine test solution are added in the order named, no iodoform-like odor, which is stronger than that produced in a blank test, should be noticeable.

Sulphates.—A 10 per cent aqueous solution after addition of dilute hydrochloric acid should not yield more than a negligible turbidity with barium chloride test solution.

Chlorides.—A 10 per cent aqueous solution, after addition of dilute nitric acid. should yield not more than a negligible turbidity with silver nitrate.

Reaction.—A 10 per cent aqueous solution should behave similar to that of dextrose already mentioned. The presence of free dissociated acids is far more important than in dextrose, for in an acid solution when autoclaved at 120° C., lactose is hydrolyzed to dextrose and galactose.

Behavior on Autoclaving.—A 10 per cent solution of lactose when sterilized at 120° C. for 30 min. should not show an acid reaction greater than P_H 4.0. On boiling and subsequent cooling the reaction does not become neutral but remains acid, thus showing that the sugar has undergone some change. The solution, however, should not show the presence of dextrose.

Dextrose in lactose is determined by fermentation tests as follows:

A. Menstrum sugar free broth (broth free from muscle sugar by fermentation with B. coli) titrated to P_H7.6. Add 0.5 mil of a 0.02 per cent solution phenol red (phenolsulphonephthalein) and 0.5 mil of a 0.02 per cent solution of brom cresol purple (dibromorthocresolsulphonephthalein). Fill into fermentation tubes and sterilize. Add to the broth in a sterile manner, 3 mils of a 10 per cent solution of lactose, previously sterilized for 15 minutes at 100° C.

B. Mix, and for trace of dextrose in lactose, inoculate with B. paratyphoid B.

Examine tubes after 24 hours, 48 hours. and one week for:

1. Acidity as indicated by change of color of indicator. The actual hydrogen-ion concentration may be determined colorimetrically by Clark and Lubs method.

2. Gas production.

C. Uninoculated controls are to be kept at incubator temperature at same time.

Lactose free from dextrose should not show any acid production. and. of course. no gas.

PURIFIED INULIN—BACTERIOLOGIC INULIN

Inulin broth is of considerable diagnostic value in the differentiation of pneumococci and streptococci. As is well known the inulin is fermented by typical pneumococci but not by the streptococci. Inulin is very easily hydrolyzed by mineral acids and converted into levulose. Unless extreme care is taken to prevent this during its manufacture, inulin will contain sufficient levulose to render its value as a diagnostic agent for pneumococci and streptococci worthless. Therefore, inulin intended for bacteriologic use should be tested carefully for the presence of levulose. This is done exactly in the same manner as already described for lactose. The same medium and the same organism are used. Inulin broth free from levulose should not show any acidity or increase in hydogen-ion concentration when inoculated with B. paratyphoid B.

Inulin for bacteriologic use should also pass the following chemical requirements.

Color.—Pure white.

Ash.—Not more than 0.3 per cent.

Moisture.—(Loss of weight at 105° C.) : not more than 10 per cent.

Solubility at 15° C.—One part should be soluble in about 130 parts of water at 15° C. when an excess is shaken with water at that temperature for six hours. It is much more soluble in hot water and does not readily separate when hot concentrated solutions are cooled. It must be completely soluble in an excess of hot water.

Optical Rotation.—When a 10 per cent hot aqueous solution is filtered and cooled to 25° C., its optical rotation should be not less than minus 6° in a 200 m. tube.

The tests for the presence of alcohol, heavy metals, sulphates, and chlorides are the same as those outlined for dextrose and lactose.

As a matter of interest the results found upon analysis of a lot of inulin bought on the market for bacteriologic work, which failed to answer the requirements outlined above, is herewith reproduced :

Ash.—2.9 per cent.

Moisture.—14.7 per cent.

Solubility at 150° C.—Soluble in 42.5 parts water. Color of 10 per cent solution—pale yellow.

Optical rotation of 10 per cent solution in 200 mm. tube : minus 5.9°.

Alcohol.—Large quantity.

Heavy Metals.—None.

Suphate.—Large quantity.

SUMMARY

The necessity of testing sugars intended for bacteriologic purposes is brought out. Both chemical and bacteriologic tests are required in order to insure a satisfactory product. It is hoped that the methods described will be of use to bacteriologists, for much work has been made valueless where results depended on fermentation tests, in which impure sugars were used.

A SIMPLE APPARATUS FOR OBTAINING BLOOD SAMPLES

By Paul G. Woolley, M.D., Detroit, Mich.

THE accompanying cut illustrates in diagrammatic cross section a very simple apparatus for obtaining blood for Wassermanns or for other purposes. It consists of an ordinary centrifuge tube with a two hole stopper (rubber or cork), a bit of glass tubing bent at right angles, and an 18 gauge, 5/8 inch hypodermic needle. The needle is placed in one of the openings in the rubber stopper, and the glass tubing is passed through the other. The whole affair is then assembled and is ready for sterilization in the autoclave.

This apparatus is merely a modification of similar ones in wide use, one of which has been described recently by Owens and Martin[1]. The advantage

[1]Jour. Am. Med. Assn., 1920, lxxiv, 98.

of the one we describe is that all of the parts are stock in any laboratory and that when it is assembled it is tight, and by attaching a piece of rubber tubing to the glass tubing, suction can be applied. For those who like vacuum tubes, this one has the advantage that immediately the vein is punctured the blood can be seen in the tube and then suction can be applied. Also repeated punctures can be made if that becomes necessary. In other words there is no danger of losing the vacuum, a danger that is always present when one uses a one-stemmed container. Very frequently the blood will flow freely into the tube without the production of a negative pressure. The glass tubing may, therefore, be looked upon as an emergency attachment. The only virtue in the direct insertion of the needle in the stopper, instead of connecting it by means of rubber tubing, is that the centrifuge tube makes a convenient handle for it, and, therefore, a shorter needle can be used.

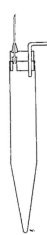

If one desires larger blood samples (for chemical analysis) than can be contained in the ordinary 15 c.c. centrifuge tube, the larger, i.e., 50 c.c., tubes can be used in exactly the same way, and if one uses the larger centrifuge tubes that are made with necks, the stoppers (that fit the smaller tubes) are interchangeable.

LANGE REACTION IN ENCEPHALITIS LETHARGICA*

By I. C. BRILL AND R. L. BENSON, PORTLAND, OREGON.

THE purpose of this report is to call attention to the similarity in the gold chloride reactions on the spinal fluids of a number of cases positively diagnosed as encephalitis lethargica. This series includes thirteen cases in which the diagnosis was definitely established, and in which the spinal fluid was obtained blood-free and in all respects suitable for the Lange test.

Case 1—	A. D.	1223210000
Case 2—	B.	1112100000
Case 3—	Mrs. B.	0122100000
Case 4—	S.	0012210000
Case 5—	L. R.	0123321000
Case 6—	E. E.	0011210000
Case 7—	I. S.	0112211000
Case 8—	H.	0011000000
Case 9—	P.	1112220000
Case 10—	J.	0012331000
Case 11—	E. B.	0122100000
Case 12—	Y.	0012210000
Case 13—	L. H.	0122321000

*From the Pathological Laboratory, University of Oregon Medical School, Portland, Oregon.

Of these cases, six were studied clinically by us, and all of the gold chloride tests were performed by us. Those not seen clinically by us were suspected as cases of this disease by going over our series of Lange tests. In each instance the diagnosis was afterward confirmed by the clinical record obtained from the physician in charge. Four of the cases died, but only one came to autopsy.

In general it is obvious that the reaction occurs in the zone usually designated as the tabetic zone. It is noticeable further that the reaction is weaker than the usual luetic curve.

Since compiling these records we have observed that a similar reaction was noted by Bassoe[1] and Barker.[2]

It is not intended to make the Lange reaction appear as an absolute diagnostic feature of encephalitis lethargica. We are aware that such a weak curve in the luetic zone may be obtained in other conditions, as, for example, brain tumor. It is hoped, however, that the reaction may prove of value as an additional laboratory test in cases where the clinical symptoms point to the diagnosis of lethargic encephalitis.

Note.—We are indebted to Drs. L. Selling, A. Rosenfeld, C. U. Moore, and M. K. Hall for the clinical records on these cases which we have not seen clinleally.

REFERENCES

[1]Bassoe, Peter: Jour. Am. Med. Assn., April 10, 1920, lxxiv. 15.
[2]Barker, Cross, and Irwin: Am. Jour. Med. Sc., February, 1920.

The Journal of Laboratory and Clinical Medicine

Vol. V.	JUNE, 1920	No. 9

Editor-in-Chief: VICTOR C. VAUGHAN, M.D.
Ann Arbor, Mich.

ASSOCIATE EDITORS

DENNIS E. JACKSON, M.D.	- - CINCINNATI
HANS ZINSSER, M.D.	- - - NEW YORK
PAUL G. WOOLLEY, M.D.	- - DETROIT
FREDERICK P. GAY, M.D.	- - BERKELEY, CAL.
J. J. R. MACLEOD, M.B.	- - - TORONTO
ROY G. PEARCE, M.D.	- - AKRON, OHIO
W. C. MACCARTY, M.D.	- ROCHESTER, MINN.
GERALD B. WEBB, M.D.	- COLORADO SPRINGS
WARREN T. VAUGHAN, M.D.	- . BOSTON

EDITORIALS

Fatigue of the Nervous System

PIERSON has collected the literature on this subject from which we make the following extract: Lee has defined fatigue "a depression of physiologic activity." In the case of muscles and gland cells this depression has been studied, but when one comes to the nervous system he finds no general agreement among investigators as to the histologic or chemical changes present in fatigue. The question of the relative importance of the areas of the brain, of the centers in the medulla, of the ganglion cells, of the nerves, and of the synapses, in the production of the common symptoms, remains unanswered. Mosso has well said that what may constitute excess for some may be only an agreeable stimulus for others. Such divergencies may be explained by primary differences in the quality of protoplasm, by the psychic attitude towards the task in hand, and by the effect of training. In general, however, the patient who is suffering from fatigue of the nervous system complains of inability to keep the attention fixed, of impairment of the memory, and of failure to grasp new ideas. Physical and mental work become abhorrent and are accomplished only with effort. There may be psychic instability, depression, morbid fears, suspicions, hallucinations, and increased irritability and sensibility, especially to noises. When activity is continued to exhaustion marked physical symptoms appear, motor restlessness, a loss of physical resisting power, a decrease in body weight, a failure in strength, pain in the back of the head, and nervous dyspepsia. The individual feels sleepy, but is tortured by insomnia. The sleep may resemble stupor. Hunt has observed in an officers' training camp that under severe mental strain certain men develop symptoms of early paresis, pupillary changes, tremors, and disturbances of articulation. With rest these symptoms generally clear up. Continuous overtaxing of the nervous system may lead to sclerosis of the brain or may dispose to serious diseases, such as Bright's disease and tuberculosis. It may even precipitate certain forms of insanity.

The physiologist has added to the clinical picture certain specific signs and has found for many of them explanations. To the more copious flow of blood to the brain caused by vasoconstriction in other parts of the body, Mosso attributes the weak pulse, the hot head, the blood-shot eyes, and the cold extremities, which so often accompany excessive mental activity. Close observation has shown a rise in temperature accompanying excessive intellectual effort. The action of the heart may become irregular and increase in rapidity. The respiration becomes shallow and fast at first, with two to four extra respirations per minute. Later it becomes deeper, and in excessive fatigue slower and shallower again. In physical fatigue, on the other hand, the pulse is accelerated and the respiration deep. The curve of mental fatigue probably differs from that for physical fatigue, since Taylor finds that the former comes on more slowly, while Levy observed that cortical fatigue appears early and progresses rapidly in contrast to muscular fatigue, which is long delayed.

It is necessary to go further and to seek in the changed chemistry and histology of the fatigued nervous tissues an explanation of the symptoms. Mosso attributed the headache of nervous exhaustion to the accumulation of the decomposition products of the nerve cells. He believes that, though the fatigue is confined to certain regions of the brain, the toxic substances formed may be distributed and give rise to the general symptoms. So complex are the causes which lead to fatigue of the nervous system that it is difficult to indicate specifically the part played by each of the elements; cortical nerve cells, nerve centers in the medulla, spinal nerve cells, synapses and motor end plates in the final result, and to separate fatigue of the nervous system following fatigue of other tissues, especially muscle, which is primary.

How far fatigue is localized in any one area of the brain is not definitely known, although the fact that change from one type of mental work to another is restful would indicate that fatigue effects may be local. That the centers may be overtaxed has been given as a possibility by Mills and by Mosso, both of whom protest against children's doing gymnastic work to relieve brain fatigue. Lee, however, infers that, like the nerves, the centers are highly resistant to fatigue and any unfavorable change they undergo in excessive activity is compensated for by increased anabolism. It will be seen that there are two views as to the roles of the central and the peripheral nervous system in fatigue. Lee's contention is that the brain and spinal cord, like the nerve fibers, are highly resistant to fatigue—a contention based on the fact that the central nervous system controls the activities of the organism and is most resistant of all tissues in many diseases and in starvation. Mental fatigue is probably peripheral in origin. On the other hand, Mosso claims that the central nervous system is the first to fatigue and that from the central nervous system fatigue proceeds to the periphery. He believes that all fatigue, muscular as well as nervous, represents the exhaustion of the nervous system.

That the nerve fiber itself is not easily subject to fatigue is agreed. Halliburton and Bowditch found nerves still resistant after experiments lasting for fifteen hours. The fact that muscle ultimately ceases to respond to successive stimuli sent through its nerve, though it is still irritable to direct stimulation, has led men to believe that it is not the nerve but the nerve ending which has become fatigued. As in the fatigue caused by voluntary contractions, that element which weakens first may be the motor end plate in the muscle, the synapsis, or the spinal nerve cells.

So far as the nerve cells themselves are concerned, we have evidence of morphologic changes in fatigue. The only exception is found in the sympathetic system where nerve impulses do not seem to be able to bring about fatigue. The only change after excessive activity is a slight diffuse blue staining of the cell substance. Some of the earliest work was done by Hodge, who described the changes due to fatigue as seen in the spinal and ganglion cells of the frog, the cat, and the dog.

Hodge found the following changes in the nucleus: (1) Size decreases. (2) Outline becomes irregular and crenated. (3) The open reticular appearance is lost and the substance stains more deeply.

In the cell protoplasm, Hodge found the following changes: (1) The protoplasm shrinks slightly in the spinal ganglia and vacuoles appear. (2) In the cerebrum and cerebellum the cells shrink considerably and the pericellular lymph spaces are enlarged. (3) The power to stain and to reduce osmic acid is lessened.

Dolley noticed the irregularity of the cell tissue in fatigue and the large amount of cytoplasm as compared with the size of the nucleus. He emphasizes the importance of the changes in the amount of chromatin in the nucleus, describing it as disappearing first from the cytoplasm. Next it is used up in the cytoplasm, whereupon there is a further discharge from the nucleus. Last of all, the karyosome is used up by diffusion into the cytoplasm. The cell, having lost all of its basic chromatin, is exhausted. This disorganization may be temporary or permanent, even leading to the death of the cell. These results have been little questioned except by Kocker, who found no constant deviation from the normal in the histologic structure of nerve cells that had been active. Marui also calls attention to the shrinking of the fatigued nerve cell and its nucleus and to the chromatolysis of the Nissl substance. He makes a distinction between the turgescence of the cell and the nucleus in overactivity and their shrinkage with exhaustion. He adds that the nucleolus in fatigue may be swollen or shrunken and irregular in outline. Moreover, he demonstrates the importance of the synapse, describing the appearance of ameboid glia cells in the pathologic nutrition conditions of fatigue as an indication of catabolism in the synapse. The reticular glia structure of the synapse is broken up and ameboid cells showing fat drops are set free.

It is generally admitted that we have no data on the chemical changes in mental fatigue. One may imagine that in fatigue certain toxic products, such as cholin and neurin, will be split off from the lecithin, which are so abundant in nervous tissue. Legrende says: "Animals kept for a long time from sleeping show the presence in their blood, cerebrospinal fluid, and brain tissue, of a poisonous property, causing somnolence in other animals." This can not well be cholin or any similar substance, for it does not filter, is insoluble in alcohol, and is destroyed by heating to 65° C. In exhaustion of the motor nerve cells of the spinal cord caused by strychnine, we find the cells showing a diffusion of the blue stain used due to the solution of the basophile granules by an acid formed in the fatigue process. The cells of the posterior root ganglion, on the other hand, do not stain diffusely and do not give an acid reaction to litmus. Chemistry has also been called upon to explain the fact that a nerve deprived of oxygen fails in a short time to respond to stimuli. Ordinarily, it is supposed that oxygen enough is present to oxidize the fatigue substances formed. Verworn made the experiment of replacing the blood in a frog by a gas-free salt solution. Convulsions were produced by the administration of strychnine and the circulation of the solution stopped. The excitability soon lost, reappeared when the circulation was restored—a result apparently due to the washing away of fatigue products.

Totally different is the suggestion that the enormous increase in conduction in the nervous system, which appears in nervous breakdown, follows from the action, of adrenalin centrally or at the synapsis. Experimental verification is lacking for this, as well as for the statement made by Mosso that in cerebral exhaustion the blood carries albuminous matter from the muscles to the brain.

It seems evident that further progress in the study of fatigue is most likely to come under the province of chemistry. The importance of this subject grows day by day on account of the increasing conviction that there is some relation between nervous fatigue and the industrial diseases.

—V. C. V.

Encephalitis Lethargica

SO MUCH has recently been written in the newspapers about the appearance of sleeping sickness in various parts of Europe, and even of the United States, that the League of Red Cross Societies has deemed it advisable to call attention, through its Bulletin, to a few of the striking features of the disease, and to some of the popular misconceptions concerning it.

"In the first place," says the Bulletin, "the name 'sleeping sickness' should not be applied to it as this name should be used only in connection with the African sleeping sickness—a disease of absolutely different cause although resembling in some of its clinical features certain aspects of the disease now so much talked of in Europe.

"This disease is absolutely different in origin and for that reason the name used to describe it should be 'encephalitis lethargica' the name given to it by Von Economo when he first described it in Vienna in 1917, although it is probable that the disease has been present in sporadic form and not recognized before his description. Subsequent to Von Economo's report, cases were noted in various portions of Austria and Germany, and by Netter in France, while in 1918 a fair number of instances of the disease were described in England and America. After a cessation of a number of months there has recently been again a quite marked outbreak of 'encephalitis lethargica,' in England, America, France, Scandinavia, Central Europe, Spain, Italy—even in Switzerland; but as before, the cases are comparatively few in number although very widely distributed, and do not at all present the usual picture of a marked epidemic.

"While there are a few cases of great mildness and a few others of fulminating severity, the majority of the cases present a fairly clean cut clinical picture, with, as their striking triad of symptoms, fever, of greater or less extent; paralysis of certain cranial nerves, notably those of the eyes and eyelids, so that ptosis or drooping of the lids is especially common; and a striking tendency to sleep, which is usually progressive, so that it is not unusual to find patients constantly in a coma. They often can be aroused by loud shouting and are frequently relatively clear mentally after being awakened, but they usually relapse into a state of somnolence almost immediately. The disease often ends fatally but recovery is by no means uncommon. Regarded at various times and by various observers as due to food poisoning, or as representing an unusual form of poliomyelitis or other similar disease, the general belief at the present time is that 'encephalitis lethargica' is an independent disease of infectious origin.

"The fact that it is frequently present at the same time and in the same localities wherein epidemic influenza abounds, while at first causing many investigators to believe that the diseases are definitely related, is now explained by most authorities on the basis that the diseases both develop under the same conditions but are independent. Whether an abnormal physical or mental condition consequent upon the war may be a factor one can not say, though there are a few who believe that an increased susceptibility or lowered resistance due to these causes plays a distinct role. The studies done upon these cases seem to show that the disease really represents an inflammation of certain portions of the brain and nervous apparatus, although the exact cause of this inflammation has not been determined. Recently a filterable virus has been obtained from the mucous membrane of the nose and throat of certain cases dying of the disease, and this virus seems to be able to reproduce in monkeys and in rabbits symptoms and lesions similar to those found in human beings. These same observers, by special methods of culture, state that they have been able to grow an organism which they believe is the cause of the disease, which requires an especially refined technic and which differs from others heretofore described.

"At the present state of our knowledge therefore, it would seem that 'encephalitis lethargica' is met with over a widespread area, but that it is only mildly epidemic, and that it is slightly if at all contagious in the usual acceptance of this word; that individual susceptibility seems to play a distinct role in its incidence and possibly many persons harbor the causative virus or microorganism, probably in the nose and throat without showing any symptoms whatsoever; that no causal relationship between it and epidemic influenza has yet been demonstrated; and that its main symptoms are fever, paralysis of certain muscles of the eye; and sleepiness.

"With 'encephalitis lethargica' occupying such a prominent position in the press, it is obvious that many treatments should have been suggested but at the present writing there is no recognized, specific treatment which offers any real hope of cure. After all, this is what would be expected in the case of a disease, the exact nature of which, as well as its method of propagation and dissemination, is still unknown, although it is probable that the infection is first localized in the nose and throat. On the other hand recent work gives us the hope that before long our knowledge will be increased, and one has a right to look for a possible and rational cure in the comparatively near future."

—*American Red Cross News Service.*

The Frontiers of Thought

THE urge for knowledge concerning the mechanical cause and reason for everything is inborn. All of us are philosophers of greater or less degree. However, we have so far failed to discover the "final cause" by a consideration of material nature or natural laws or by reflective judgment. Experimentation has revealed to us some of the characters of material and dynamic nature, but it has failed to explain the intimate nature of the living processes and of the adaptation which the organism has made to its environment.

Physiologic thought of the latter part of the nineteenth century was predominately mechanistic. This was the period when many new fields of physiology were being investigated by experimental methods which were relatively simple, and the great harvest of facts gathered, led us to hope that the secret of the universe would be discovered. As science developed the methods employed to elicit new facts became more and more involved and less possible to control. It was this fact that led Haldane, in his Harvey Lecture of 1916, to decry mechanistic physiology as an instrument to interpret the living in terms of physicochemical laws and to urge the establishment of a new physiology which concerns the study of normals. Physiology as a means of determining the essential nature of the life process or teleology appeared to him impossible.

Recently one of our most eminent physiologists, Dr. L. J. Henderson, has given us an essay on the "Order of Nature[1]" in which he presents the problem of adaptation in a simpler manner than do earlier writers. He does not complicate the problem with the riddle of life, but limits it to a physicochemical discussion, and in so doing stimulates new interest in the question of the world's evolution. He shows that beneath the organic structures and functions lie the molecules and their activities, which have moulded the process of evolution, and in turn shaped environment.

In an earlier work (Fitness and Environment[2]) Henderson called attention to the efficiency by which the physicochemical properties of the primary constituents of the environment made the world and living things stable, durable, and complex, yet adaptable. In this essay he elaborates on this idea and more rigorously discusses the importance of the three elements, hydrogen, carbon and oxygen, for the process of cosmic evolution, and by eliminating all biologic theories and principles rests the conclusion on the secure foundation of pure science.

He proceeds by making a careful scientific examination of the properties and activities of the three elements and then reviews these with the hope of throwing new light on the question of evolution and of the origin of the teleologic appearance of nature. Although he believes that these questions are insoluble, except through an impossible description of all the details of the evolutionary process, he sees in the total of the properties found in the elements hydrogen, carbon, and oxygen and in the compounds they form, sufficiently diversified and available properties to provide a most remarkable group of causes for the teleologic appearance of nature. And if these causes be considered along with the natural laws, and the characteristics of the solar system and the incomprehensible origin of life he believes that an intelligent although incomplete account of the orderly evolution of the diverse forms of nature may be had.

This order or pattern in the properties of hydrogen, carbon, and oxygen and their compounds, especially water and carbon dioxide, when considered along with time becomes related to evolution, because the unique ensemble of properties they possess makes the fittest ensemble of characteristics for a durable mechanism. Henderson says, "No other environment, that is to say, no environment other than the surface of a planet upon which water and carbon dioxide are the primary constituents does or could so highly favor the widest range of durability and activity in the widest range of material systems,—in systems varying with respect to phases, to components and concentrations."

The physicochemical properties of these elements and their compounds, which make possible this optimal environment and material for growth Henderson believes can not be due to blind chance, and must be due to the operation of natural laws which in some way connects these elements. He fears that the discovery of the explanation of the phenomena is improbable, and if forthcoming would avail little, for a more complex problem would still remain. This is "How does it come about that these many unique properties should be favorable to the production of systems and therefore to the evolutionary process." The connection existing between the properties of these elements appear best explained as being due to a preparation for the process of evolution, i.e., it resembles adaptation. The properties of the elements antedated the evolution of the planet, nor can he imagine an evolution of these properties due to evolutionary process.

Henderson believes that any other distribution of properties among the elements would greatly restrict the possibility of multiplication of systems, and the possibility is negligible that conditions equally favorable to the production of diversity in the course of evolution should arise without relevant cause. The process of evolution consists in increase in the diversity of systems and activities, the production of much from little. It must be that the same relevant causal connection exists between the properties of the elements and the freedom of evolution. The possibility that this relationship is due to chance is only a remote mathematical possibility.

It is on these grounds that Henderson believes that the elements themselves are teleological. In the properties of these three elements we find a special case in which the characters of material nature have been made available by the laws of nature for a hypothetical final cause. However, can a final cause be postulated?

On this point Henderson says, "The relationship between the numerous properties of hydrogen, carbon and oxygen, severally and in cooperation (relatively to the same relation between the elements and the necessary conditions of existence of systems in respect to diversity and durability as these conditions are defined by exact analysis) is not contingent. In other words the statistical probability that this connection has a relevant cause, i.e. relevant to the evolutionary process, is greater than the statistical probability which we can reasonably demand or generally realize in the establishment of the principles and facts of science.

This essay takes us to one of the frontiers of thought beyond which we can not hope to pass. It reduces the question of evolution and adaptation to the simplest problem possible at present, and leaves us with the necessity of accepting the properties of material nature as being teleologic.

REFERENCES

[1]The Order of Nature, Harvard University Press, 1917.
[2]Fitness of the Environment, Harvard University Press, 1913.

—R. G. P.

Lethargic Encephalitis

IT is, Flexner* says, of more than ordinary interest that within the last dozen years, at least two epidemic diseases, affecting chiefly the central nervous system, have prevailed widely in Europe and America. The first is poliomyelitis; the second is lethargic encephalitis. Concerning the one considerable is known for it has been studied in many epidemics, and it has served as the subject of many extensive if not exhaustive laboratory researches. About it a voluminous literature has grown. Concerning the other but little is known. It is, at least so far as America is concerned, a very recent disease. Perhaps it is not a relatively new disease, but at least it is only within the past two years that it has attracted attention, and has been widely distributed.

It appears that the first cases of lethargic encephalitis recognized in the United States appeared during the winter of 1918-19. Never before so far as is known had the disease been observed in America. These first cases were related epidemiologically, says Flexner, to an outbreak which occurred in Vienna and neighboring parts of Austria during the winter of 1916, but because of the war conditions, knowledge of these Austrian cases did not reach the United States, and it was not until the disease had appeared in France and England in the early months of 1918, that definite attention was attracted to the disease which reached America a year later.

*Jour. Am. Med. Assn., 1920, lxxiv, 865.

The history of epidemic encephalitis prior to the Vienna outbreak is wrapped in obscurity. The earliest account of a similar symptom-complex has to do with an epidemic in the region about Tübingen in Germany in 1712. Later, in 1890 accounts of a diesase known as *nona*, prevailing in the territory bounded by Austria, Italy, and Switzerland, appeared in the papers of that region, particularly in the lay press. But these older reports, of 1712 and 1890, are not sufficiently concise to differentiate the disease, though the symptoms taken together with the geographical distribution of the cases suggest the identity of the reported disease with that which now prevails in widely separated parts of the world. In other words it seems now that the present widespread epidemic had its starting point in the *nona* region, which accordingly may be, as Flexner suggests, the endemic home of epidemic lethargic encephalitis.

In Austria and England the disease was first mistaken for an expression of food intoxication or of botulism. One reason for such an error was the general state of food conditions, due to the blockades. These conditions placed an emphasis upon food and everything related to it, and a state of mind that related everything abnormal to food. Another reason lay in the early third nerve paralysis which is also an early symptom in certain forms of food poisoning. But bacteriologic studies have shown that B. botulinus is not the cause. Epidemiologic studies have shown that it is not food which is the immediate cause. Anatomic studies of cases in Austria, England, France and the United States have discovered a concordant and consistent pathologic picture which forms the present basis for the conception that lethargic encephalitis is not a form of food poisoning, but is a distinct disease.

The anatomic lesions are apparently confined to the central nervous system, and particularly to the brain in which they seem to occur by choice in the gray matter at its base. While the gray matter elsewhere may be involved and while lesions may be found in the cortex and in the cerebellum, the structures particularly involved are those about the third ventricle, the aqueduct of Sylvius and the lateral ventricle and optic thalamus, and the pons and medulla. The spinal cord is variously affected. The lesions themselves consist of cellular aggregations about the blood vessels, cellular infiltrations in the nerve tissues themselves, small, often microscopic hemorrhages, and edema of the tissues. The characteristic cells of the lesions are mononuclears. Polynuclear cells are infrequent. The lesions in their best developed form are definitely related to the symptoms.

The outstanding feature of clinical cases is the lethargy, which gives the disease its common name, and which is progressive in character. This symptom appears in three-fourths of all the cases. It may appear suddenly but usually it is gradual in its onset. Symptoms referable to meningeal irritation may be present, but these are slight, as a rule. The spinal fluid is clear, the number of cells rarely reaches 100 (average 10 to 20) and the globulin content is only a little or not at all increased. Kernig's sign is rarely present. Paralyses are uncommon, but rigidity or spasticity of the extremities is far from uncommon. The duration of the stupor is variable. It may last a few days, weeks or months, and still end in recovery. The mortality ranges, according to different reports, from 20 per cent to 40 per cent.

It is probable, Flexner thinks, that, since knowledge of the disease is still very restricted and incomplete, and diagnosis therefore still in its beginnings, many of the milder cases (abortive or ambulatory) are overlooked or given other names and interpretations, thus making it impossible at present to arrive at an accurate estimate of the distribution, prognosis, and mortality. It is also true that many cases in which lethargy is a prominent symptom, are mistaken for lethargic encephalitis. The chief causes of death have been intercurrent pneumonia and paralysis of the respiratory center.

In explanation of the lethargy it has been suggested that it is of toxic origin. Flexner, however, believes that it is due rather to mechanical influences. It is known that sensory stimuli from the organs of special sense pass to the cortex by way of the thalamus. If, therefore, the thalamus is the seat of infiltrative lesions, the sensory pathways are apt to be partially or completely blocked and the response of the individual to his surroundings will be slowed in proportion to the blocking. In this disease the interruption of the sensory paths is never absolute, and patients can be roused, though oftentimes with difficulty.

On various sides the question of the relationship of lethargic encephalitis to influenza has been raised—this especially in America where the appearance of the diseases coincided more or less closely, or at least when the appearance of the former disease followed so closely on the heels of the latter that the suggestion of cause and effect seemed exceedingly reasonable. It is not generally believed, however, that the diseases are etiologically related. On the contrary, it is felt that the reason for the epidemiologic relationship lies in the fact that influenza reduces the resistance of the individual to a point at which the other disease can gain a foothold in the body. The same explanation of the effect of food in predisposing to the disease has been put forward. The earlier cases in Austria (1916) coincided, not with influenza, but with hunger and other byproducts of war. Nevertheless the Tübingen epidemic of 1712, and the "nona" of 1890 were closely related to outbreaks of influenza. If in truth this newer encephalitis should happen to be found definitely associated with influenza, then we will be confronted with a very nice etiologic problem which can be settled only after the cause of each disease is known and the two compared. It may be, for instance, that encephalitis is a true expression of influenzal infection in an individual who, normally immune to influenzal inection, has had his immunity reduced by environmental factors. At the present there is no numerical relationship between the extent of influenza and encephalitis.

There seems to be no doubt, at least the appearances give every suggestion, that lethargic encephalitis is an infectious disease. Also the scanty experimental work done on transmission adds confirmatory evidence. But even at that the total evidence is too slight to make for certainty. The assumption of infection as a working hypothesis is the one that leads in the direction of increased knowledge and is the one which should impress physicians and sanitarians and stimulate them to careful and exact studies. The most important cases are undoubtedly the abortive and ambulant cases, and these are all too infrequently recognized. They are the ones (compared with typhoid and poliomyelitis) which are the chief means of transmission and spread of the disease.

—P. G. W.

Variations In Wassermann Reactions

IT HAS been the custom at the Psychopathic Department of the Boston State
Hospital to have Wassermann reactions done at two different laboratories.
This has been done to safeguard the patients against erroneous conclusions based
on one test, and to obtain information which would be valuable in estimating the
laboratory results, i.e., to make interpretations more exact. The results of this
comparative work in 3000 cases is given in a recent article by Solomon.

First as to methods: One laboratory uses three cholesterinized antigens of
different sensitiveness to check each positive reaction. The other uses, in addition to cholesterinized antigen, an acetone-insoluble antigen. Whenever possible, those cases in which the reports from the two laboratories did not agree were
retested, on the assumption that possibly a technical error was the cause of the
variation. Usually in such cases the reports agreed after the first test. In some
cases in which one laboratory made the test many times with consistently positive results for ten, fifteen, or more times, a negative reaction would suddenly
crop out and be followed in subsequent tests by a series of positives. Solomon
seems to believe that this may have been due to error in technic, though he ven-
tures the possibility of a change in the patient's serum, "a condition which is not
so very likely, and which at any rate is not explicable." (One wonders whether
Solomon can explain the Wassermann reaction itself.) However that may be,
the total number of variations between the reports for the two laboratories was
6.56%, but this includes those cases reported positive, moderately positive, or
doubtful by one laboratory, and negative by the other. In cases reported positive
by one laboratory and negative by the other, the variation was 4.0% which represents a figure of 1.4% positive in one laboratory and 2.6% in the other. In the
cases known to be syphilitic there were 35 reports that did not agree. Of these
20 were reported positive by laboratory 'A" and negative by laboratory "B."
Fifteen were reported negative by laboratory "A" and positive by "B."

Some of the cases, says Solomon, reported positive by one laboratory and
negative by the other were known to be syphilitic so that the negative reaction
was the incorrect one. In other words in some cases the Wassermann reaction
furnishes a result that is of no immediate value in a case. It is a symptom
which may be laid aside if it be negative, which means that the Wassermann
reaction is a symptom which when definitely present is of value. A strongly
positive reaction (sometimes designated as 100% inhibition of hemolysis, or four
plus) probably means syphilis, but a negative reaction does not exclude it. The
varying reactions between a strongly positive and a negative one may or may not
mean syphilitic infection and a true interpretation in each case must be left
to the clinician who has all the data upon which to base a diagnosis. The serum
of certain individuals, perhaps of all, may contain at times substances which produce false positive reactions. Serum which has stood at a high temperature, especially when it is not sterile, may give false positives. In the case of one of the
laboratories mentioned by Solomon, often the blood did not reach the laboratory
for three or four days. The records of this laboratory were not as good as those
of the other. Then also mercury and salvarsan both lead to false negative reactions and it is believed that a negative reaction on cases which have been under

treatment is of value only when it has obtained six weeks or more after the termination of the medication.

It seems to be the consensus of opinion that the original Wassermann technic using the anti-sheep system gives, taking it by and large, the most reliable and constant results. There are many modifications, some of which give remarkable sensitivity. According to Kolmer, these give from 2% to 8% negatives; from 3% to 10% false positives and that with them at least 2% to 10% of human sera can not be used to make the test without further modification in technic.

BIBLIOGRAPHY

Solomon: Jour. Am. Med. Assn., 1920, lxxiv, 788.
Kolmer: Am. Jour. Syph., 1919, iii, 541.

—*P. G. W.*

The Early Diagnosis of Pulmonary Tuberculosis

IT would seem that now is a good time, two years after a thorough effort by expert diagnosticians to eliminate pulmonary tuberculosis from upwards of four million of the young manhood drawn to the country's service to evaluate the possibility in physical examination of the early diagnosis of this disease. Those who worked on Tuberculosis Boards for the War Department soon realized that there were many divergent views among expert examiners as to what physical signs determined the presence of active or even manifest disease.

French,* in England, a well-known diagnostician, asks this question: "Can you, from physical examination of the chest diagnose early phthisis, that is to say, phthisis in its earliest stages?" His own answer runs: "Personally I think that you can neither diagnose it nor exclude it by physical examination alone when it is *early*; you may suspect it, but of all the methods of diagnosing phthisis *early*, I consider that physical examination of the thorax is the least certain. *Early* phthisis is generally diagnosed by the discovery of tubercle bacilli in the sputum, examination of the latter having been suggested by the symptoms. When there is impairment of percussion note at one apex in front or behind, or when there are definite crepitations at one apex, the phthisis has generally been present for some time; or it may have been present formerly, then become quiescent, and now active again. I believe that phthisis in its beginnings can not be diagnosed from physical signs, notwithstanding all that one hears about the refinements of percussion and auscultation. I am sure that those who rely mainly on physical signs, diagnose phthisis which does not exist and may miss phthisis that is present. Again and again one has met with patients whose sputum has been found to contain tubercle bacilli, but whose chest signs are such that if they were mixed with a dozen healthy men without the fact being known they would not be picked out as the phthisical cases by physical examination alone."

From pathologic knowledge of the development of tubercle and from clinical and x-ray experience, two types of pulmonary tuberculosis have been differentiated. The "open" (tubercle bacilli usually present in sputum), alveolar or parenchymatous type, in which the disease is present in the lung tissue itself,

*French: Guy's Hospital Gazette, London, 1918.

and the "closed" (tubercle bacilli rarely present in the sputum), peribronchial type associated with definite hilus lesions. Such types are considered to conform in a general way with the open and closed types of tuberculous joint disease. The French school (Rist and Sergent) deny that any recognition of pulmonary tuberculosis can be made before the finding of tubercle bacilli in the sputum. Unfortunately the peribronchial or closed type yields practically no or few physical signs and roentgenologists can not as a whole be relied upon to make a definite diagnosis of active disease in this type of case. There is no question that comparisons of serial x-ray plates over many months does offer a means of determining what may be termed the "subterranean" spread of tuberculosis.

From the nature of the disease and of its progress we can never expect to elaborate any fixed program for early diagnosis and certainly, as French points out, no one sign can be depended upon. French continues: "There is one physical sign which, though it is not pathognomonic, is, nevertheless, so important that it should always arouse suspicion of phthisis and lead to testing of the sputum; and this is a physical sign not of percussion or auscultation, but of inspection; namely, local wasting of the tissues above and below one clavicle in front or in one supra-spinatus region behind. I am not speaking of a general attenuation of the frame, because every thin person with prominent clavicles and "salt-cellars" above them has not got phthisis. I am referring to local wasting or hollowness on one side when it is compared with the condition of the other. This local wasting is not due to local retraction of the chest wall or to the loss of underlying bone tissue; it is a dwindling of the bulk of the upper part of the pectoralis major and of the subcutaneous tissues, and it is comparable, I think, with the wasting that occurs in that part of the limb which is immediately above a joint that is diseased or injured. The exact reason for this one does not know, but one assumes in a vague way there is some reflex neuro-trophic influence at work. So in the case of recent and active tuberculous disease of the apex of one lung there seems to be, temporarily at any rate, a neuro-trophic reflex which causes local atrophy of the chest wall muscles in the corresponding region." French warns, however, that one must not diagnose phthisis simply when there is this local wasting, the sign being suggestive only and not conclusive.

Pottenger claims to be able to feel the changes in the muscles that this author sees, but careful observers do not agree either that these changes are constant or that they are indicative of an early lesion; or that they are unaccompanied by other signs of greater reliability. We saw many cases exhibiting this sign in soldiers who had been the victims of pneumonia. It is certainly well worth while for clinicians to carefully note the occurrence of this sign, and it must be remembered that the profession has not yet reached the point where a careful, accurate, physical examination of the chest is the rule. In pulmonary tuberculosis we treat symptoms and not signs, and we must cultivate among ourselves and our patients an attitude which will permit of an adjustment of environment before tuberculosis is allowed to become manifest. Especially those who belong to tuberculous families or who have been associated in childhood with tuberculosis "carriers," should be carefully watched. Probably over 30 per cent of cases of pulmonary tuberculosis coming under observation belong to this class. When possible, a yearly examination at least by x-ray and clinical means should be arranged.   Repeated and thorough examinations of even minute quantities of sputum—a patient often being unconscious that he has any—is of paramount importance.   There is great necessity for proper observation and differential diagnosis—especially from cases of hyperthyroidism—in many patients with indefinite or no physical signs, with no cough or sputum but who present slight evidence of chronic toxemia, malaise and occasional rise of temperature, the latter especially in women before the menstrual period.   Theoretically, from the spread of tuberculosis through the lungs from some definite deposit, probably at the hilus, we should be able to predetermine the candidate for pulmonary disease.   In practice, however, we can not do so any more than we can foretell what individual may succumb to any other bacterial disease.   Up to date it is impossible to measure immunity and to estimate accurately what conditions or environments will eventually lead to active pulmonary tuberculosis.

It is not to be wondered at therefore that in the examinations of upwards of four million men, many cases of pulmonary tuberculosis were overlooked and many others soon to become actively diseased were not recognized.

—*G. B. W.*

Typhoid-Paratyphoid Relationships

DURING the first half of the World War the reports from French and Italian observers regarding typhoidal and allied infections concerned themselves in great part with studies of the paratyphoid fevers.   At that time vaccination was made as a rule only against B. typhosus.   Individuals protected against this organism succumbed to invasion by either B. paratyphosus A or B. paratyphosus B.   So in the allied armies the paratyphoid fevers tended to play the dominant role, with the typhoid bacillus causing a relatively small proportion of the cases.

By contrast, the members of the American Expeditionary Forces, vaccinated against all three types showed among the cases that did become infected a much higher proportion of straight typhoid fever.   In a reported series of 314 cases 270 were infected with B. typhosus, 23 with B. paratyphosus B and only nine with B. paratyphosus A.   An additional twelve were classed as "paratyphoid, type undetermined."

The consensus of opinion among foreign observers has been that vaccination against B. typhosus, while protecting against that organism, exerts no protective influence against the para forms.   Some, indeed, call attention to a notable increase in the actual number of cases of paratyphoid fever above that for the troops in prevaccination days.   Attempts have been made to explain this as a predisposition to such infection resultant on the vaccination.

Rist suggests another interesting explanation.   He thinks that in the vast majority of instances of typhoid infection there has been a multiple exposure, exposure to all three of the organisms, and that the disease is usually manifested by infection with the most virulent.   So, in the straight typhoid vaccinated, when dual or triple exposures occur it is the para form which infects.   The proof of such a condition of multiple exposures would require more time than was at the disposal of the observers during the activities of the war.   It is readily seen that should an individual become heavily infected with B. typhosus and mildly with one of the para organisms or vice versa the work of isolating a great number of colonies from the stools or blood in pure culture and following the cultural characteristics of each would be no inconsiderable task.

A few chance observations have given substance to Rist's hypothesis. Such is the report by Galeotti and Bruno of one case in which both B. typhosus and an atypical B. paratyphosus were isolated from the blood of one patient. Bernard and Paraf discovered in the course of routine examinations of thirty patients one case of double blood infection (para A and B) and one case with para B in the blood and para A in the stool. Three per cent of their cases then were infected with two types and three per cent were shown to be infected with one type while carrying an additional type in the intestinal tract. Mixed exposure or infection was discovered in over 6 per cent of cases with no more careful or detailed work than is used in the routine laboratory examination. Were attention directed especially to this phase of the problem, the percentage might conceivably be markedly increased.

We have personal record of another such case in an American soldier in France who on the tenth day of his illness gave a positive blood culture for B. paratyphosus B and on the following day a positive stool culture for the para A organism. This relationship is more important than the reverse would be,—para A in the blood and para B in the stool,—because the latter is supposed to exist frequently in the alimentary tract without causing harm.

One further item of importance is the fact that rarely have there been widespread epidemics in which only one of the types of germs was present. This is particularly true in armies where the exposure is indiscriminate. For epidemics traceable to a single first case the above statement does not always hold. But as a rule where one type of organism is found one may be confident of finding a few or many cases infected with the other two.

Study of the clinical symptoms is usually insufficient to correctly distinguish the different forms of infections. Certain characteristics are found to apply more to one than to another when studied statistically in large series, but individual cases are often indistinguishable. For diagnosis recourse must be had to bacteriologic examination, and it may be that more detailed work on these lines will confirm Rist's hypothesis at least in so far as it applies to individual cases or epidemics where the exposure has been as nondescript as it usually is among troops stationed in a highly polluted area. —*W. T. V.*

The Mechanism of Respiratory Infection

IN a recent editorial we discussed under the title of "The Transmission of Respiratory Infection" recent investigations into the modes of conveyance of the virus of infection from one individual to another. Consideration was given chiefly to the means whereby the virus is conveyed to the individual and to the fate of the organism from the time it reaches the mouth or nose until it is eliminated or invasion takes place. The third phase of the "infection cycle," the manner of actual invasion of the virus into the body claims present attention.

In another editorial we have presented the two prevailing views as to the site of invasion of the tubercle bacillus in cases of pulmonary tuberculosis.

Bacteria may for convenience be divided into three groups; saprophytic bacteria which live on inorganic and dead organic pabulum; parasitic which require living tissues for their existence; and pathogenic which while usually also parasitic, possess the further ability to invade the tissues of the living host and cause disease. Parasitic bacteria may by this classification be said to include the organisms normally found on the skin and mucous membranes of animals. These exist in complete harmony with the host and as a rule do not produce disease. Under certain circumstances, as by implantation through a cut or wound, or following a lowering of the general resistance, they may invade the tissues and, interfering with the well being of the host, cause disease. These are the "opportunist" organisms of Theobald Smith. The type of disease caused by such temporary pathogens as the staphylococcus, streptococcus viridans, etc., is not constant and may involve different tissues of the body in different cases.

The true or habitual pathogens on the other hand usually invade some one tissue by predilection and produce a fixed type of disease. For the continued life cycle of the habitual pathogens three phases must be accomplished. They must be able to effect an entrance into the tissues of the host, must be able to multiply temporarily therein and finally must be able to escape in order to enter another host. It is in great part this last power that renders these bacteria so much more highly infectious than the last class considered. A streptococcus may enter through a skin wound and produce widespread disease and even death, but it can not secure a ready means of escape from the body. Failing in this we may consider such opportunists as dying with their hosts.

In the absence of a portal of exit, other things being equal, the more virulent the organism the less dangerous it is to the community, for, having killed its host, it also must die. Thus we see the cause of Pasteur's failure to exterminate the rabbits of Australia. There are many races of the bacillus of rabbit septicemia. The one which is found as an opportunist, normally, on the mucous membranes of the rabbit is an organism of low virulence. Pasteur felt that by inoculating with a race of very high virulence the disease might spread throughout the rabbits of the continent. Some of these organisms are so virulent that implantation in the merest scratch of the skin results in death within twenty-four hours. But this portal of entry was artificial and no means of escape had been perfected. And so the rabbits inoculated died and with them the organisms perished.

Transfer to a new host may be artificially made and then the disease is repeated, often becoming more severe. Such was the case with surgical erysipelas in the days before improvements in aseptic technic. The actual procedure corresponded to the present laboratory trick of enhancing the virulence of a comparatively avirulent organism by animal passage. Portals of invasion and of escape were artificially provided.

Some habitual pathogens enter and escape by means equally complicated. Without the mosquito, malaria becomes nonexistent. Bubonic plague is in an analogous class. In the pneumonic form of plague, on the other hand, the germ has perfected much more ready means of escape and the disease can here persist in the absence of the rat and the flea.

We now see that just as habitual pathogens possess a highly specialized affinity for certain tissues, so also the manner and site of primary tissue invasion vary with different members of this group. Those bacteria which possess a preference for the tissues of the respiratory tract are among the most highly contagious in part at least because there is here provided an easy portal of escape. There are several ways in which the pneumococcus might gain entrance to the lung tissues. The simplest and most direct is through the air passages by aspiration. Such infection may occur with aspiration of foreign bodies, or following impaired function of the protective ciliated epithelium, damaged by cold or by chemical irritant. Postoperative pneumonia is often quoted as an example but postoperative pneumonia was a well-known condition before the days of anesthesia. Pneumonia after "gassing" exemplifies the effects of chemical damage to the ciliated epithelium while foreign body aspiration results in direct mechanical implantation of the bacteria within the smaller bronchi. Infection by way of the lymphatics, perhaps from the tonsils, is a possibility. It has also been suggested in view of the frequent finding of pneumococcus septicemia early in pneumococcus pneumonia that the process may be primarily a blood infection with the local condition developing secondarily.

Blake and Cecil have recently succeeded in producing lobar pneumonia in monkeys with all four types of pneumococci. The disease in these animals corresponded both clinically and pathologically with the disease in humans. The complications were the same. Through their work we have approached nearer to an understanding of the mechanism of invasion, although several steps still remain unexplained.

These workers, using doses of pneumococci varying from 1 to 0.000001 c.c. of an 18 hour broth culture, injected the organism intratracheally into thirty-seven normal monkeys and produced the disease in thirty-two. Killed cultures of the organism and sterile broth injected in the same manner produced no ill effects. From their work they conclude that the germs must penetrate to the larger bronchi before they will produce disease. Inoculation of the nose and throat with Type I pneumococci produced a carrier condition which lasted as long as one month but did not result in infection. Six monkeys were exposed to infection in a monkey sick with Type I pneumonia. One of the six contracted the same disease. Blake and Cecil do not attempt to explain why or under what circumstances the organism will pass from the upper air passages where it is only potentially harmful to the lower tract where it nearly invariably produces disease. They assume that this passage does occur through the lumen of the trachea and bronchi.

Müller produced aspiration pneumonia in rabbits after vagotomy. He found that within six hours after the operation bacteria-laden saliva had reached the terminal bronchioles. Within an additional two hours there was evidence of active bacterial infection. We may conceive of the impairment of function which permits this downward invasion in pneumonia as resulting from mechanical or chemical causes as previously suggested or from nervous causes—impairment of the reflex protective mechanism.

That the infection is not primarily one of the blood stream is shown by further experiments by Blake and Cecil. In no case were they able to produce pneumonia by subcutaneous or intravenous inoculation of virulent pneumococci.

The animal died of pneumococcus septicemia and the lungs showed no evidence of special involvement even under microscopic examination. This was true both for normal monkeys and for monkeys whose resistance to pneumococcus infection had been previously increased with pneumococcus vaccination. Furthermore they demonstrated infection of the blood stream within from 6 to 24 hours after intratracheal injection, frequently before clinical evidence of pneumonia or elevation of temperature had developed. This spread to the blood stream took place evidently from the bronchi. The blood usually became sterile at some time before crisis.

The determination of the probable site of actual tissue invasion was made by inoculating a monkey intratracheally with a large dose of pneumococci and sacrificing the animal three hours later. The authors conclude from their studies that the pneumococcus primarily invades the lung tissue at some point or points near the root of the lobe. Penetrating the epithelium of the larger bronchi at this point the process extends peripherally as an infection of the interstitial framework of the lungs, ultimately reaching the tissue forming the walls of the alveoli. Spread takes place in the tissue itself and in the lymphatics. At the stage just preceding exudation into the alveoli the walls of the bronchioles and alveoli show leucocytic infiltration, vascular engorgement and invading pneumococci. At this stage there are few or no organisms in the alveolar spaces. Following exudation the organisms are present in the exudate and diminish in numbers in the interstitial tissue. Those in the exudate are often phagocytized or stain poorly. Blake and Cecil do not claim to have proved definitely that pneumococci do not primarily penetrate through the lumen into the bronchioles and alveolar spaces, but their observations show no support for such an assumption.

By what manner of reaction do the tissues resist this invasion? The leucocytic infiltration in the infected tissue has been referred to. In a monkey killed three hours after intratracheal injection this process was already well advanced in the peribronchial tissues around the hilum. It represents the attempt on the part of the host to combat the invasion at the point of entrance. Phagocytosis was also observed early. In the blood a preliminary leucocytosis began within six hours and reached its apex within twenty-four to forty-eight hours. This, like the septicemia, was often well developed before clinical evidence of pneumonia or elevation of temperature had occurred. There appears to be an initial intense stimulation of the bone marrow and the leucocytes available at the onset of the disease are transported "bodily" from the bone marrow to the lungs. In the severe cases with overwhelming septicemia the fall in leucocyte count progressed without subsequent rise, immature white cells appeared in the blood,—occasionally also nucleated red cells and, at atopsy, the bone marrow was frequently almost entirely devoid of polymorphonuclear leucocytes. In favorable cases the leucocyte count again rises and at the same time the septicemia commences to diminish, the blood usually becoming sterile several days before crisis.

The serous exudation into the alveoli appears to be an inflammatory reaction to infection of the tissues themselves, and we suggest that it may be visualized as comparable to the serous exudation of acute coryza, an infection higher in the same respiratory tract.

With the influenza bacillus Blake and Cecil obtained rather different results. Without going into detail as to the actual site of invasion of the organism they report a series of twenty-two monkeys inoculated in the upper respiratory tract, in the nose or the nose and mouth, and in every instance the animal came down with a disease clinically and pathologically similar to influenza in man. Five developed as complication an acute sinusitis and two developed bronchopneumonia. In these the lung picture resembled exactly that described for influenza, and B. influenzæ was recovered in pure culture from the lungs. Ten monkeys were inoculated intratracheally. Seven developed the same form of pneumonia, two developed tracheobronchitis without pneumonia, and one resisted infection. In two cases the infection spread to the upper respiratory tract producing coryza and frequent sneezing.

If we assume that these findings indicate B. influenzæ as the cause of influenza we must conclude that the mechanism of infection is different from that in pneumococcus pneumonia. The mechanism which prevents the pneumococcus from descending to the lower respiratory tract is not as successful in influenza. The difference appears to be that influenza is primarily an upper respiratory tract disease. After it has caused its damage there and has lowered the general resistance, B. influenzæ, or some other organism, penetrates much more easily beyond the barrier into the lower respiratory tract. These organisms then invade very much as before, producing at first an interstitial infection evidenced as bronchopneumonia.

From the nature of the disease a great deal is known concerning the manner of invasion of the diphtheria bacillus. On the other hand very little is known of the mechanism in the exanthemata, particularly measles.

There is much yet to be learned concerning the mechanism of respiratory infection.

BIBLIOGRAPHY

Blake, F. G., and Cecil, R. L.: Production of Pneumococcus Lobar Pneumonia in Monkeys, Jour. Exper. Med., 1920, xxxi, 403.
—Pathology and Pathogenesis of Pneumococcus Lobar Pneumonia in Monkeys, ibid., p. 445.
—The Production of an Acute Respiratory Disease in Monkeys by Inoculation with B. Influenzæ, Jour. Am. Med. Assn., 1920, lxxiv, 170.
Kendall, A. I.: Saprophytism, Parasitism and Pathogenism, Boston Med. and Surg. Jour., 1913, clxix, 741.
Smith, Theobald: Some Problems in the Life History of Pathogenic Microorganisms, Am. Med., 1904, viii, 711.
Vaughan, W. T.: The Transmission of Respiratory Infection, Jour. Lab. and Clin. Med., 1920, v, 330.
Vaughan, W. T.: The Pathogenesis of Pulmonary Tuberculosis, ibid., p. 340.

—*W. T. V.*

Note to the Editor

Richmond, Va., May 3, 1920.

To the Editor:

The editorial in the Journal of Laboratory and Clinical Medicine of April, 1920, on pages 466 and 467, refers to my paper, "Surgical Drainage from a Biologic Point of View," which appeared in the *Journal of the American Medical Association*, Jan. 17, 1920. The editorial writer takes exception to the expression "reversal of the lymph circulation" that I used to describe what appears to be the chief biologic process by which drainage acts beneficially in solid soft tissue and in endothelial cavities.

The wording of this phrase is unfortunate, but I believe the editorial writer and I are in accord concerning the facts involved. I fully appreciate the impossibility of any real reversal of blood circulation and in other communications I have attempted to demonstrate that a vein and its contributing branches would not function as an artery when an arterial current is turned into the vein.* It was at one time, however, rather generally held that the blood circulation could be reversed in this manner.

By the phrase "reversal of the lymph circulation" I did not mean reversal in a physiologic sense, that is, a complete change in the direction of the lymph current within its normal channels. The facts that confront us in surgical drainage, which is a pathologic condition, are well illustrated by a splinter in the finger around which lymph is continually poured until the offending splinter is removed. When the splinter is removed, drainage ceases. These phenomena are well known and require no demonstration. We have, then, the pouring out of lymph or serum which appears to be an effort at extrusion of an irritating foreign substance. This lymph which is poured out for days or weeks probably comes partly from injured lymph channels and lymph spaces in the tissue, and partly through uninjured walls of the lymph channels, which become more permeable, as explained in your editorial.

These facts, I take it, will be accepted. The moot point is whether this process can be called reversal of the lymph circulation. I used the words 'reversal of the lymph circulation" because it seems to me that the current of lymph or serum continually poured out to the surface of the skin for days or weeks constitutes in a sense a circulation of lymph. This current, if it rises to the surface of the body and appears on the skin or mucous membrane, is not in the direction of any known normal lymph current and probably is a reversal, or at least a deflection, of the direction of the adjoining normal lymph currents. Then, too, this phrase seems to emphasize a phenomenon that many surgeons apparently ignore. The phrase "outpouring of lymph" occurred to me, but this suggests an almost instantaneous process, or at least one that covers a very short space of time.

It may also be objected that "lymph" is used in a rather loose sense. I have employed it as describing in a general way the thin, clear fluid that is found in the lymph channels and spaces of the body and that infiltrates the tissues in edema. In order to describe the phenomena of drainage it appears to be necessary to use the words lymph or serum to include such fluids.

Respectfully,

—J. Shelton Horsley.

*Horsley and Whitehead: Jour. Am. Med. Assn., March 13, 1915, pp. 873-877; Horsley, J. S.: Ann. Surg., March, 1916, pp. 277-279.

The Journal of Laboratory and Clinical Medicine

| VOL. V. | ST. LOUIS, JULY, 1920 | No. 10 |

ORIGINAL ARTICLES

LEUKOPLAKIA OF THE PELVIS OF THE KIDNEY—A STUDY IN METAPLASIA*

By DeWAYNE G. RICHEY, M.D., PITTSBURGH, PA.

THE following study of leukoplakia has been made with more particular reference concerning its development in the pelvis of the kidney as well as offering certain features which suggest some of the underlying factors having to do with the process of metaplasia. We recognize in metaplasia, "the postnatal production of specialized tissues from cells which normally produce tissues of other orders," embracing both a morphologic and functional change in the cells and is an adaptation on the part of the cells to an altered environment. It would appear that this conversion to another form of cell does not occur directly but is brought about only by a preliminary reversion to a vegetative type of cell or, where the mother cells are present, by the development of cells modified by their surroundings. Metaplasia occurs both as a physiologic process and as a result of certain pathologic conditions, the latter involving repeated insults to a tissue over an extended period of time. In either event, the tendency is the formation of more highly specialized tissues from less highly specialized ones, although the reverse may occur. True metaplasia undoubtedly has its limitations, being governed by certain rigid laws and must not be confused with such phenomena as heterotopia, heteroplasia and anaplasia. While tissues of mesoblastic origin lend themselves more readily to metaplastic transformation than those of epiblastic or hypoblastic origin, nevertheless, innumerable examples have been encountered where structures which are normally of the stratified squamous, transitional, cuboidal or columnar type have assumed characteristics of keratinizing stratified squamous epithelium.

Such terms as cornification, keratinization or epidermization which have been applied to metaplasia of epithelial tissues to the stratified squamous character, as

*From the Magee Pathological Institute. Mercy Hospital, Pittsburgh, Pa.
Read before the American Association of Pathologists and Bacteriologists, April, 1920.

635

a rule, denote a degree of the same process and when the change has become sufficiently prominent to admit of recognition as a pearly, opaque, firm plaque, it is called leukoplakia. Although leukoplakia is more commonly encountered on the tongue and the buccal and esophageal mucous membranes, it is by no means unknown on the surfaces of other viscera and its occurrence along the urinary tract has been noted by several observers. In 1914, Beer collected from the literature forty-five instances of leukoplakia as found along the urinary tract, of which ten occurred in the pelvis of the kidney, supplementing two of his own. To his series can be added those cases described by Rokitanski, Orth, Epstein, Marchand and Pollack.

The present case of leukoplakia occurred in the pelvis of the right kidney which has been removed at operation by Doctor J. J. Buchanan from a man, age 43, who, for twenty-two years, had experienced periodic paroxysms of pain following injury to the back. The seizures would begin high in the right lumbar region and radiate to the genitalia. They would recur two or three times a year, last from several minutes to three hours and were invariably severe. Albumin, pus, blood and mucus were found in the urine from the right kidney. Culture from this urine yielded B. coli communis and B. acidi lactici.

The right kidney weighed 110 grams and was considerably distorted. The lower two-thirds of the kidney was quite healthy, while the upper third of the organ was so cavitated that only a narrow rim of the original renal substance remained. The cavities varied in size from a small marble to a large walnut and communicated freely with the pelvis. A remarkable appearance was noted in connection with the larger cavities at the upper pole. These cavities were lined by a white, silvery, finely wrinkled membrane, looking not unlike the delicately corrugated skin of the scrotum of infants. The surface of the membrane was firm and unbroken, as it extended in fine processes upon the injected walls of the lesser cavities. The pelvis, in the remaining portion of the kidney, showed a similar metaplasia which continued downwards along the tract of the ureter so that it resembled the streaks of leukoplakia seen at the lower end of the esophagus. There was no evidence of calculus or caseation within the organ.

Microscopic section of the kidney substance proper showed some normal portions, and varying stages of obliteration of the glomeruli and tubules by fibrous connective tissue which was, in places, densely infiltrated with lymphoid and plasma cells. Sections taken through the wall of the pelvis and ureter showed the lining to consist of a thick layer of stratified squamous epithelium, presenting a large amount of keratinization on the free surface. The epithelial covering was undulating in character and, though uniform in distribution, was uneven in thickness, varying from ten to eighteen cells in depth. In the intermediate zone, where the cells were polyhedral in shape, definite intercellular bridges were noted, as seen in the prickle cell layer of the epidermis. No membrana propria could be demonstrated, the deepest layer of the epithelium resting directly upon a bed of granulation tissue, into which it exhibited no tendency to invade. The supporting muscle bundles had been extensively fragmented by a replacement fibrosis. The pathologic diagnosis was chronic suppurative pyonephrosis and ureteritis; leukoplakia of pelvis of kidney and ureter.

Metaplasia, as indicated by Orth, entails a transformation of one well-characterized tissue into another equally well-characterized but morphologically and functionally different tissue. Such a conversion occurs through the mediation of cells which are not completely differentiated, so that, as Schridde says, the formative cells of the growing layers of any kind of epithelium, or their immediate daughter cells, may abandon their specific attributes and revert to cells which have all the powers of differentiation possessed by the embryonic cells from which the epithelium developed. Such cells may form any type of epithelium but their power of differentiation is limited to the epithelial tissues and does not include transformation to connective tissue or endothelium. Even Ribbert, the chief antagonist of the theory of metaplasia, in considering the replacement of columnar by squamous epithelium in the submaxillary duct refers to an "innate tend-

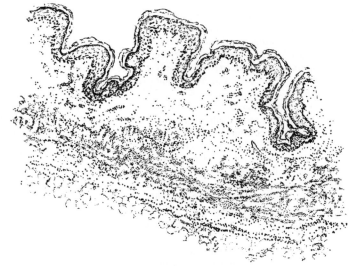

Fig. 1.—Leukoplakia of pelvis of kidney.

ency" on the part of this epithelium, a derivative of squamous epithelium to form squamous epithelium and admits the same for like changes in the urinary passages under altered conditions, concluding that only tissues, while externally different, which possess the same histogenic capacities can undergo metaplasia one into another. Consequently with the knowledge that mesothelium may resemble epiblastic derivatives more than other mesoblastic tissue and that the "histogenic capacities" of cells are brought out by their environment, we do not hesitate to explain leukoplakia of the renal pelvis and ureter upon the theory of metaplasia, as a histogenic transformation induced by the alteration of environment wrought by a long-standing inflammatory process with a resultant change in morphology of the cells from the normal transitional to stratified squamous epithelium even to the formation of a superficial layer of keratin, a quality, which as Wells points out, might be interpreted as an intrinsic chemical alteration in the cells, due to abnormal stimuli.

It will be remembered that the lining of the pelvis and ureter of this kidney had been exposed to chronic inflammation, with repeated losses of the original epithelium, destruction of the basement membrane, and formation of granulation tissue attended by a slowly progressive fibrosis, all of which materially altered the normal biologic conditions of the cells. Haythorn, in studying metaplasia of columnar to stratified squamous epithelium occurring in the bronchus, found that this transformation was present in those places where the basement membrane was absent and we concur with this author that as a result, the mucosa, in its altered surroundings, being destroyed beyond hope of specific regeneration, sought to protect itself with the best reparative cells it could produce in its exhausted state.

The findings in our own laboratories coincide with those reported by Braasch, that, with dilatation of the chronically inflamed pelvis and ureter, limited proliferation and cornification of the mucosa is often seen. Until this process is sufficiently advanced so that it can be recognized in the gross as a definite whitish patch, it is not leukoplakia, but represents only a stage in the process. Although leukoplakia of the renal pelvis and ureter, indicated above, is not rare, it is less common than in the lower urinary passages. It is associated with chronic forms of irritation, as nephrolithiasis and inflammatory processes, either pyogenic or tuberculous. Halle mentions the high coincidence of leukoplakia and calculus, believing, however, that mechanical irritation is not the direct cause, but is secondary to the new conditions arising in chronic inflammation. Just why certain types of mechanical injury or infection do not always cause leukoplakia and why this condition is occasionally, though rarely, observed without the evidence of previous irritation, is, of course, hard to explain. While there is the possibility of some predisposition in the cells of the part, there is also the likelihood of an underlying general disturbance, as the frequent coincidence of syphilis and leukoplakia buccalis in inveterate smokers or of leukoplakia of the esophagus in chronic alcoholics.

In one of the cases reported by Bcer and one by Baselin, it was possible to diagnose the condition by the presence in the urine of pearly white membranes, resembling paraffin shavings. In most instances, though, the cholesteatomatous transformation was not suspected until the kidney was examined at operation or necropsy. The clinical manifestations of leukoplakia are usually those of the underlying factor, but the passage of desquamated epithelial plaques has been known to give rise to typical attacks of renal colic. It is reasonable to suspect, in a certain percentage of cases of long-standing pyelitis, which are not amenable to appropriate treatment, that cornification or leukoplakia of the pelvic mucosa has occurred.

That leukoplakia may be the predecessor of carcinoma is indubitable. Osler states that 20 per cent of leukoplakia of the tongue become carcinomatous, while Albarran, Barker, Ewing and others indicate that leukoplakia in any organ should be watched carefully for malignancy, often being, in the absence of early carcinoma, very suspicious of precancerous changes. Morris collected 27 cases of tumors originating in the kidney pelvis, of which 10 were malignant, while recently, Kretschmer was able to gather 43 instances of nonpapillary carcinoma of the renal pelvis, including 21 of apparent transitional or squamous type. The former author states that the most frequent form of carcinoma is transitional or squamous cell, pointing out that long-standing irritation may lead to the transformation of the renal epithelium to an epidermic character, with a resultant leukoplakia which may be the starting point of squamous cell cancer.

In conclusion, therefore, it is clear that leukoplakia of the pelvis of the kidney and ureter is a pathologic entity which seeks logical explanation on the basis of true metaplasia, entailing a transformation from the normal transitional epithelium, even presenting a superficial layer of keratin. It would appear that the absence of a demonstrable membrana propria, as noted by Haythorn, plays an important role in the metaplastic process by permanently altering the environment of the lining cells. The loss of the basement membrane is the outcome of repeated insults wrought by long-continued trauma, either inflammatory, mechanical or both. It is possible that a certain number of cases of pyelitis are refractory to appropriate treatment as a result of leukoplakia of the pelvic mucosa. As in the buccal cavity, bronchi, esophagus, gall bladder, urinary bladder, prostate, fundus uteri and elsewhere, leukoplakia of the renal pelvis and ureter may be a potential site for subsequent malignant metamorphosis.

The author acknowledges his indebtedness to Professor Oskar Klotz for the many valuable suggestions offered during the preparation of this work.

BIBLIOGRAPHY

Adami: Principles of Pathology, 1908, i, 591 and 643.
Adami and McCrae: Textbook of Pathology, 1912, p. 202.
Adami and Nicholls: Principles of Pathology, 1911, ii, 818.
Barker: Practitioner, London, 1914, xciii, ii, 157.
Beer: Am. Jour. Med. Sc., 1914, cxlvii, 244.
Braasch: Jour. Am. Med. Assn., 1919, cxxiii, 733.
Cabot: Modern Urology, 1918, ii, 453.
Ewing: Neoplastic Diseases, 1919, p. 537.
Haythorn: Jour. Med. Research, 1912, xxvi, 523.
Kretschmer: Jour. Urol., 1917, i, 405.
Fuetterer: Lubarsch-Ostertag Ergebnisse, 1903, ii, 715.
MacCallum: Textbook of Pathology, 1919, p. 183.
Morris: System of Medicine (Allbutt and Rolleston), 1908, iv, i, 719.
Osler: Modern Medicine, 1908, v, 66.
Satani: Jour. Urol., 1919, iii, 253.
Wells: Chemical Pathology, 1918, p. 285.
Young and Davis: Jour. Urol., 1917, i, 17.
Ziegler: General Pathology, 1908, p. 314.

CHEMICAL CHANGES IN THE BLOOD IN DISEASE.*

IV. Blood Sugar

By Victor C. Myers, Ph.D., New York City

THAT blood may contain a sugar-like substance was first recognized in 1775 by Dobson, although it was not until seventy years later that its presence in normal blood was discovered by the noted French physiologist, Claude Bernard, who made many of our classic observations on carbohydrate metabolism. By means of his sugar *piqûre* he first noted the connection between hyperglycemia and glycosuria (glycuresis). It remained for Lewis and Benedict[1] in 1913 to introduce a colorimetric method for blood sugar estimation so simple that it could readily be employed for clinical as well as scientific purposes. Earlier in the same year Bang[2] had described a very ingenious method requiring only two to three drops of blood, but the fact that it was a gravimetric-volumetric procedure precluded any very extensive clinical application.

Stimulated by these methods many studies dealing with the sugar of the blood have appeared during the past seven years, while previously to this time Bang[3] had written a very interesting monograph under the title "Der Blutzucker." Obviously reference can be made here only to a few of these papers.**

If we may rely upon the findings with the Benedict method, the blood sugar of the normal human subject falls somewhere between 0.09 and 0.12 per cent, on the average being 0.10 per cent. There are a considerable number of miscellaneous hospital cases, however, which show blood sugars of 0.12 to 0.14 per cent. These figures represent observations made in the morning previous to the intake of any carbohydrate. After a meal rich in carbohydrate there may be an appreciable rise in the sugar content of the blood, while after the intake of even moderately large amounts of glucose, the hyperglycemia may be sufficient to induce a slight temporary glycosuria (glycuresis).†

Conditions of hyperglycemia are much more common and of greater clinical interest than those of hypoglycemia, owing primarily to the fact that diabetes belongs to the former group. Among other conditions which frequently show a moderate hyperglycemia are nephritis and hyperthyroidism. Hypoendocrine function would appear to result in hypoglycemia, and comparatively low blood sugars have been observed in myxedema, cretinism, Addison's disease, pituitary disease and other less clearly defined endocrine conditions such as muscular dystrophy.

*From the Laboratory of Pathological Chemistry, New York Post-Graduate Medical School and Hospital, New York City.

**Among these should be mentioned the papers of Hopkins,[4] Geyelin,[5] Hamman and Hirschman,[6] Denis, Aub and Minot,[7] Mosenthal, Clausen and Hiller,[8] Janney and Isaacson,[9] Bailey,[10] Williams and Humphreys[11] and Allen, Stillman and Fitz.[12]

†As it is now generally recognized that sugar is present in normal urine (to the extent of about 0.05 to 0.20 per cent), the term glycosuria is somewhat of a misnomer. It implies no more than glycemia does in the case of blood. We might speak of a hyperglycosuria in the same way that we refer to a hyperglycemia, or better employ the term "glycuresis" suggested by Benedict.[13] This would indicate an increase in the sugar content of the urine to the extent that it could be detected by ordinary qualitative tests, and not a new appearance of sugar.

RELATION OF GLYCOSURIA TO HYPERGLYCEMIA AND THE THRESHOLD POINT

All forms of glycosuria are accompanied by hyperglycemia, if we except the glycosuria produced by such substances as phlorhizin and uranium, and the analogous clinical condition, "renal diabetes." In mild cases of diabetes the hyperglycemia is not excessive, generally 0.2 to 0.3 per cent, although in severe cases figures up to and even above 1.0 per cent have been obtained. The normal threshold of sugar excretion (i.e., the point of glycuresis) is about 0.16 to 0.18 per cent. With blood sugar concentrations of 0.15 to 0.20 per cent the appearance of sugar in the urine is apparently dependent on whether or not diuresis exists, glycosuria appearing especially in the latter case. When the threshold point has been passed, however, the overflow of sugar into the urine may continue until the concentration in the blood has fallen nearly to normal. Mild cases of diabetes usually have a normal threshold, although some severe cases apparently have a lowered threshold, increasing the severity of the condition. Ordinarily in the early stages of the disease there is a fairly direct relationship between the hyperglycemia and glycosuria. In the later stages of the disease, however, cases are frequently encountered with marked hyperglycemia and only slight glycosuria, showing that the threshold point has been raised. The cause of glycosuria in "renal diabetes" is obviously due to the reverse condition, viz., a threshold point below the level of the normal blood sugar.

DIASTATIC ACTIVITY AND HYPERGLYCEMIA

In 1917 Myers and Killian[14] described a simple method of estimating the diastatic activity of the blood and called attention to the fact that conditions of hyperglycemia were associated with an increased diastatic activity, and suggested that this might be the important factor in the production of the hyperglycemia in both diabetes and nephritis. The increase in the diatase of the blood in nephritis finds probable explanation in the decreased excretion of diastase in the urine, now well known in this condition, although a satisfactory explanation of the increased activity in diabetes is not so readily given. De Niord and Schreiner[15] have noted the exception that diabetics who are also syphilitic do not show a high diastatic activity. Table I gives values for blood sugar and diastatic activity in normal individuals, diabetics, nephritics, and illustrative endocrine cases. It will be noted that with the three normals the diastase was 16 and 17 and the blood sugar 0.1 per cent. Cases 4 and 5 are especially interesting, both being physicians whose blood diastase was estimated incidentally to other tests. High diastatic activities being observed, a history of so called "alimentary" glycosuria was elicited in each case. Of the diabetics, Case 7 was on a rigidly restricted diet throughout the period of observation. This serves to explain the comparatively low figures for blood sugar with the high diastase figures, while, on the other hand, the high diastatic activity affords an explanation as to why the restriction in the diet was unable to bring the blood sugar down to normal The improvement in Case 8 was very rapid as is evident by the marked drop which occurred in both the diastatic activity and the sugar in six days. The parallel fluctuations in the diastase and urea in Case 9 would suggest that the increased diastatic activity in nephritis is a retention phenomenon. Hyperfunction on the part of

TABLE I

DIASTATIC ACTIVITY OF THE BLOOD IN NORMAL CASES, DIABETES, NEPHRITIS, ENDOCRINE
CONDITIONS AND CARCINOMA OF THE PANCREAS

CASE	AGE	SEX	DIASTATIC ACTIVITY	SUGAR	UREA N	CO$_2$ COMBINING POWER	REMARKS
				PER CENT	MG. TO 100	C.C. TO 100	
1. J. K.	25	♂	17	0.10	15		
2. A. L.	27	♂	17	0.10	14		Normals
3. R. H.	28	♂	16	0.10	14		
4. E. H.	36	♂	34	0.16	13		Glycosuria noted on one occasion, slight proteinuria.
			29	0.11	12		
5. Z. D.	53	♂	29	0.12	13		Glycosuria noted on two occasions.
6. F. P.	51	♂	74	0.55		54	
			47	0.28			
7. F. M.	26	♂	59	0.17		49	Diabetes, Case 7 being on a rigidly restricted diet during this period.
			44	0.16		56	
			43	0.17			
			39	0.18			
			41	0.20			
8. L. M.	62	♀	42	0.26			
			24	0.12			
9. J. B.	34	♂	32	0.14	60		
			32	0.14	62	32	
			41	0.16	135		
			38	0.16	110		Nephritis
10. J. M.	41	♂	30	0.16	47	47	
11. C. G.	24	♀	24	0.13			Hyperthyroidism
12. J. S.	24	♂	10	0.09	13		Addison's disease
13. T. L.	43	♀	45	0.15			Carcinoma of the pancreas
14. D. N.	63	♂	45	0.14			

the ductless glands appears to result in an increase in the blood diastase and hypofunction in the reverse effect, as shown by the data on Cases 11 and 12.

RENAL DIABETES

So-called "renal diabetes" has been the subject of considerable discussion since Lépine in 1895 postulated the existence of this rather interesting condition in which the glycosuria is actually the result of renal disease, and not due to hyperglycemia as in diabetes. Some thirty cases have now been recorded in the literature, although the condition is probably not as uncommon as this number might imply. A few of these cases have shown definite evidence of renal disease

TABLE II

OBSERVATIONS ON RENAL DIABETES

CASE	AGE	SEX	DATE	SUGAR OF BLOOD	SUGAR OF URINE	REMARKS
				PER CENT	PER CENT	
1. A. B.	31	♀	8/25/15	0.09	1.3	Renal diabetes, diet low in carbohydrate on first test, regular diet on second test.
			10/13/16	0.11	4.5	
2. P. L.	10	♀	5/12/16	0.12	1.2	
			8/ 7/16	0.14	0.4	Cases of parenchymatous nephritis with fairly constant mild glycosuria.
3. J. P.	62	♂	8/27/15	0.18	0.6	
			5/29/16	0.15	1.1	
4. C. M.	54	♂	4/27/15	0.19	1.1	
			12/ 7/15	0.17	0.3	

aside from the glycosuria, but some would appear to be entirely free from the symptoms ordinarily associated with disease of the kidney. Renal diabetes has often been compared with phlorhizin glycosuria, demonstrated by von Mering in 1886, in which condition we have glycosuria without hyperglycemia. Some of the cases, however, appear to find a more direct analogy in the glycosuria of uranium nephritis, in which there is only a mild glycosuria, with a normal or nearly normal glycemia and a constant proteinuria. Data on four cases which might be put in the category of renal diabetes are given in Table II. The first of these was a very typical case of renal diabetes. Bailey[16] has already presented a report of this case (1) and also Case 3 with a general discussion of this subject. The slight glycosuria in the last three cases was associated with parenchymatous nephritis and was quite independent of the mild hyperglycemia found in the last two cases. From the above discussion it is apparent that a satisfactory diagnosis of renal diabetes cannot be made without a knowledge of the blood sugar. Now that this determination may be so easily made it seems probable that many cases presenting a history of a low grade glycosuria but without the classic symptoms of diabetes mellitus, will be definitely recognized as cases of renal diabetes.

DIABETES MELLITUS

Since the glycosuria of diabetes mellitus is dependent upon hyperglycemia, it is apparent that this latter condition is more fundamental than the glycosuria. Glycosuria is evidently only a safety factor, and the internist in applying his dietetic treatment should endeavor primarily to relieve the hyperglycemia; although in so doing he relieves the glycosuria, he should be finally guided by the concentration of sugar in the blood. In the early stages of the disease the glycosuria is an excellent index of the hyperglycemia, but when the threshold point has been raised, as for example in diabetes associated with chronic kidney disease, the disappearance of sugar in the urine is a rather poor guide to the glycemia. As will be observed in Table III, blood sugar figures of 0.2 to 0.3 per cent, and

TABLE III

INFLUENCE OF NEPHRITIS UPON THE EXCRETION OF SUGAR IN DIABETES

CASE	AGE	SEX	SUGAR OF		SEVERITY OF NEPHRITIS	CASE	AGE	SEX	SUGAR OF		SEVERITY OF NEPHRITIS
			BLOOD	URINE					BLOOD	URINE	
			PER CENT	PER CENT					PER CENT	PER CENT	
1	63	♀	0.19	0	++	11	53	♂	0.37	1.7	++
2	47	♂	0.22	0	++	12	35	♀	0.38	6.2	?
3	53	♂	0.24	1.7	+	13	48	♀	0.39	2.2	++
4	57	♀	0.24	5.0	++	14	30	♂	0.42	5.0	?
5	27	♀	0.31	6.0	+	15	46	♀	0.42	3.6	+++
6	61	♀	0.33	0.5	++	16	50	♀	0.46	0	+++
7	61	♂	0.34	6.3	+	17	56	♀	0.57	8.0	+
8	68	♂	0.35	0	+++	18	15	♂	0.79	8.7	+
9	23	♀	0.36	7.0	—	19	53	♂	0.98	1.6	++
10	47	♂	0.36	1.2	+++	20	52	♀	1.10	0.5	++

Data obtained previous to beginning treatment; taken from Ayers and Bailey.

even more, may be noted without the appearance of any sugar in the urine. Although some cases with definite nephritic symptoms retain the power of secreting a urine of high sugar content, severe nephritis appears to reduce markedly

644		THE JOURNAL OF LABORATORY AND CLINICAL MEDICINE

the permeability of the kidney for sugar; and it is only when these latter cases are excluded from the above table that there appears to be any relation between the hyperglycemia and glycosuria. Although this table probably gives an exaggerated impression of the occurrence of nephritis in diabetes, since the cases were those needing hospital care, it is not believed that the importance of this subject has been fully appreciated, although previously discussed by the older workers. [3, 18] Fitz[19] has presented evidence to show that impaired renal function exists in many cases of advanced diabetes. Williams and Humphreys[11] have made a study of the blood sugar threshold in diabetes and have observed in general that as age advances, the threshold rises. In connection with treatment they state: "Our experience has lead us to the conclusion that it is desirable to maintain the blood sugar level as nearly normal as possible even though severe restrictions in diet may be necessary for the purpose, notwithstanding the fact that in most cases the high threshold will permit of a much more liberal diet without the appearance of sugar in the urine." In discussing the high blood sugars which are observed in some diabetics on a protein-fat diet, Mosenthal[8] has suggested that this may merely be a protective measure to adjust carbohydrate metabolism for the more advantageous utilization of glucose.

It is worthy of note in this connection that several interesting contributions dealing with the action of certain salts on the permeability of the kidney for sugar and the sugar threshold have come from Hamburger's[20] laboratory.

NEPHRITIS

It has been recognized for some time that many cases of severe nephritis show high figures for blood sugar. We have presented several papers giving such data,[14, 17] while Williams and Humphreys have made this subject the topic of a special paper.[11] They found that the range of the blood sugar levels was from 0.08 to 0.25 per cent, varying directly with the severity of the disease.

TABLE IV

BLOOD SUGAR OBSERVATIONS IN SEVERE NEPHRITIS

CASE	AGE	SEX	DATE	SUGAR	CREATININE	UREA N
				PER CENT	MG. TO 100 C.C.	MG. TO 100 C.C.
1. E. M.	39	♂	12/ 4/15	0.225	21.5	129
			12/ 7/15	0.180	21.8	129
2. J. B.	34	♂	1/26/17	0.195	8.2	53
			2/23/17	0.114	7.9	61
			2/27/17	0.120	7.5	45
			3/ 2/17	0.117	6.6	44
3. F. F.	8	♂	12/18/17	0.106	6.1	106
			12/21/17	0.150	5.9	93
4. A. N.	27	♀	3/11/18	0.181	8.6	97
			3/19/18	0.131	9.4	102
			3/22/18	0.120	12.6	110
			3/26/18	0.161	12.1	110
5. M. D.	30	♀	5/27/20	0.121	6.5	42
			6/ 1/20	0.121	5.5	43
6. F. M.	57	♀	6/ 3/20	0.153	4.8	59
			6/18/20	0.096	3.5	43
7. A. D.	66	♀	6/ 5/20	0.163	2.8	30
8. M. I.	75	♀	6/16/20	0.172	7.0	121
			6/21/20	0.190	5.7	147

Hamman and Hirschman[6] have studied the sugar tolerance in nephritis and state that in many cases there is a profound change in carbohydrate metabolism, the blood sugar curve after the ingestion of glucose resembling the "diabetic curve." When there is marked interference with renal function very small amounts of sugar or none appear in the urine, although the blood sugar may go above 0.2 per cent. Bailey[10] has presented data on a very interesting case of nephritis where the blood sugar rose to 0.3 per cent before a slight glycosuria occurred. No satisfactory explanation of the hyperglycemia has been offered, although the suggestion has been made that some disturbance in the adrenals or other endocrine glands may be responsible for both the high blood pressure and the increased blood sugar. As already noted Myers and Killian[14] have observed an increased diastatic activity of the blood in this condition. Hyperglycemia data in nephritis are given in Tables I and IV. It should perhaps be noted here that Morgulis and Jahr[21] have criticized the findings of high blood sugars in nephritis on the basis of error due to interference of creatinine in the sugar estimation. While there is no doubt that the creatinine does influence some of the blood sugar findings, the error is much less than they imply and does not invalidate the deductions that have been made. This criticism has been further discussed in connection with the method below.

ENDOCRINE CONDITIONS

That cases of hyperthyroidism frequently show high blood sugars (although not often in the fasting state), and that alimentary glycosuria may be readily provoked in this condition has been recognized for some time. Blood sugar observations obtained after glucose tolerance tests have given us much more definite information regarding the carbohydrate tolerance of individuals with endocrine disorders than the older studies made on the urine. Experimental

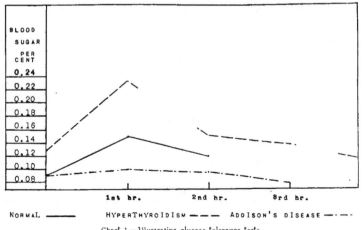

Chart 1.—Illustrative glucose tolerance tests.

proof that hypoglycemia results from hypo-endocrine function was obtained by Janney and Isaacson[9] in the case of the thyroid, where hypoglycemia regularly developed after thyroidectomy. Low blood sugar values, figures ranging from 0.06 to 0.09 per cent, have been reported in myxedema,[5] cretinism.[9] Addison's disease, pituitary disease and other less clearly defined conditions such as muscular dystrophy. The last mentioned condition has been discussed by Janney, Goodhart and Isaacson[22] and McCrudden and Sargent.[23] Altogether twelve cases were reported, the blood sugars ranging from 0.064 to 0.086.

CARBOHYDRATE TOLERANCE TESTS

The advent of a simple method for blood sugar has made possible the estimation of the blood sugar concentration at short intervals after the administration of carbohydrate, usually glucose. With this method of study it has been possible to obtain much more consistent data regarding the carbohydrate tolerance than with similar tests formerly carried out on the urine, chiefly for the reason that the threshold point of renal excretion is not here a factor in the test. This test has served to put many of our older views, especially those regarding glucose tolerance in endocrine conditions, on a more firm foundation. A number of the papers to which reference has already been made present data obtained with this method of study. The papers of Hamman and Hirschman,[6] and Williams and Humphreys[11] nicely demonstrate the great value of this method particularly in cases of diabetes and nephritis. Bailey[10] has presented quite extensive data on a few cases covering a wide variety of conditions and emphasizes the value of obtaining blood specimens at quarter hour intervals during the first hour and at half hour intervals thereafter until the sugar concentration returns to normal. With this technic the character of the curve is very clearly brought out. In practical work, however, this large number of determinations is not always possible. As a rule four sugar estimations at one hour intervals will serve to show the type of curve, despite the fact that the highest point in the curve may frequently be missed.

The method employed in this laboratory by Killian[21] is as follows: The patient is given, the first thing in the morning, a standard breakfast consisting of two slices of bread, one egg in any form and one cup of water. Two hours after this breakfast the patient empties the bladder and then receives 200 c.c. of water to drink. One hour after this a specimen of blood and a specimen of urine are taken to serve as controls. The patient then takes glucose, 1.75 grams per kilo of body weight in 50 per cent solution. Specimens of blood are now taken every hour for three to four hours, the sugar determined as described below and a curve plotted. Following the taking of glucose a 24-hour specimen of urine is collected and the glucose determined with the Benedict methods, by titration if the amount is large, otherwise by the colorimetric method.[25]

It is not possible in the compass of the present paper to describe in detail the characteristics of the different types of curves obtained, although an idea of the curves observed in hyper-and hypo-endocrine conditions may be obtained from Chart I. This chart presents unpublished observations of Killian, showing a severe case of hyperthyroidism and a case of Addison's disease contrasted with a normal.

A large number of methods have been described for the estimation of blood sugar. Although many of these methods determine the reducing power of the blood (presumably in large part glucose) with a high degree of accuracy, and have given us considerable insight into this phase of carbohydrate metabolism; nevertheless, most of them have been so technical as to require special equipment and training, and are therefore not suited to clinical purposes. S. R. Benedict, who introduced the most satisfactory tests we possess for sugar in urine, has performed, in collaboration with Lewis,[1] a similar service for the sugar of the blood. The general principle and technic of this method are far simpler than those of any other method, and for this reason it is particularly well suited to clinical purposes. The method is dependent upon the fact that very small amounts of glucose react with picric acid and sodium carbonate to produce a red color (sodium picramate). In the actual test the picric acid serves the additional purpose of precipitating the proteins of the blood. As has been pointed out by Myers and Bailey,[17] the technic of Lewis and Benedict may be considerably simplified by a lower dilution of the blood, so that the direct picric acid filtrate may at once be used for the colorimetric estimation without evaporation. This method is the one described below.

There has recently been so much discussion of blood sugar methods that some remarks should be made regarding four other methods, which have recently been introduced, and also regarding certain criticisms which have been made of the picric acid method. Höst and Hatlehol[26] have just presented some very interesting comparative data on the methods of (1) Bang and Hatlehol[27] (Bang's most recent method), of (2) Hagedorn and Jensen,[28] of the (3) Myers-Bailey modification[17] of the Lewis-Benedict method and of the method of (4) Folin and Wu.[29] (The other of the four methods referred to above is the new titration method of McLean.[30]) Höst and Hatlehol find that the first two methods which are titrimetric agree quite closely, but give somewhat lower results than the second two which are colorimetric. This is true of the diabetic bloods in particular, the picric acid method giving the highest results. It is worthy of note that the duplicate determinations with this method were particularly satisfactory. While these differences are theoretically very interesting and will probably be suitably explained, they are so small as to possess no clinical significance in themselves.

Höst and Hatlehol have given the technic of the method of Hagedorn and Jensen which is very neat and requires only 0.1 c.c. of blood. The method of Folin and Wu is adapted to their tungstic acid blood filtrate and requires the equivalent of 0.2 c.c. of blood. Although this method gives results which are slightly lower than with the Benedict method, it is probably subject to somewhat the same sources of error. It nicely fits their scheme of blood analysis but as an individual determination it requires more time and attention than the picric acid method. They have recently introduced certain improvements.[31]

A year ago Morgulis and Jahr[21] offered certain criticisms of the Lewis-Benedict method, directed especially to the influence of creatinine. They stated: "It is probable, therefore, that the Lewis-Benedict method is applicable to normal bloods when the creatinine concentration is about 1 to 3 mg. per 100 c.c., but under pathologic conditions when the creatinine level may rise to 10 to 40 mg. per 100 c.c., the sugar analysis by the Lewis-Benedict method loses its value as a quantitative procedure." Criticism was made of results obtained with either the original Lewis-Benedict method or our modification of it, although Morgulis and Jahr employed Benedict's new picric acid sodium picrate reagent,[32] this being much more sensitive to creatinine than the picric acid alone, owing to the

TABLE V

INFLUENCE OF CREATININE ON THE ACCURACY OF THE BLOOD SUGAR ESTIMATION

GLUCOSE PLUS CREATININE			PICRIC ACID REAGENT					PICRIC ACID-SODIUM PICRATE REAGENT
			READINGS MADE AT ONCE	SUGAR FOUND	READINGS MADE NEXT DAY	SUGAR FOUND	READINGS CALCULATED	SUGAR FOUND
MG. TO 100 C.C.			MM.	MG.	MM.	MG.	MM.	MG.
1.	100 +	5	14	107	14.5	104	14.3	113
2.	100 +	10	13	115	13.4	112	13.6	122
3.	100 +	20	12	125	12.7	118	12.5	150

The colorimetric readings made at once (as soon as the solution had cooled), were made roughly. Since the sodium picramate color formed from glucose does not appreciably fade, we frequently make these readings on the next day. These second readings were made with considerable care. Readings calculated on the basis of the same color development for creatinine as sugar agree very well with these figures. The readings in the case of the sodium picrate reagent were taken on two days with little change in the values.

presence of hydroxide. In their experiments they found that creatinine gave 3 to 5 times as much color as glucose. In our first paper[33] on the subject in 1915 we stated: "It is well to remember, especially in uremia, that each mg. of creatinine present in the blood introduces an error of approximately the same magnitude in per cent," i.e., gives the same amount of color as glucose. This is borne out by the data in the table above. For example, a blood showing 20 mg. creatinine would raise a blood sugar from 0.100 to 0.120 per cent. It is perfectly apparent that this would not account for blood sugars of from 0.15 to 0.25 per cent. In six years we have encountered only 10 cases with over 20 mg. creatinine, and only one of these exceeded 30 mg. out of about 125 cases having over 5 mg. creatinine. In view of the fact that creatinines as high as 20 mg., to say nothing of 40 mg., are seldom found, and also the findings given in Tables IV and V, it is apparent that creatinine does not invalidate the findings of hyperglycemia in nephritis, at least when the method below is employed. In this particular. Benedict's most recent blood sugar method would appear to be more subject to error from creatinine than his original method or our modification of it, but as Benedict[25] has recently pointed out in connection with the estimation of the sugar content of normal urine, it is perfectly possible to completely remove the creatinine and other interfering substances with charcoal or completely dissipate the color derived from the creatinine with the aid of acetone.

Method[17].—To 8 c.c. of distilled water in a 20 c.c. cylindrical centrifuge tube are added 2 c.c. of the well-mixed oxalated blood (or oxalated plasma). This is then stirred with a glass rod until the blood is thoroughly hemolyzed, after which about 0.5 grams of dry picric acid (sufficient to completely precipitate the proteins and render the solution saturated) is added. The mixture is thoroughly stirred at intervals of several minutes until it is uniformly yellow, after which it is centrifuged and the supernatant liquid filtered into a dry test tube through a small 4 cm. filter paper. (As indicated in the preceding paper on creatinine, the sugar estimation may be combined with the creatinine, both estimations being carried out on portions of the same picric acid filtrate.)

Three c.c. of filtrate are pipetted into a tall, narrow test tube 12 x 200 mm., (sugar tube) graduated to 3, 4, 10, 15 and 20 c.c., 1 c.c. of saturated (22 per cent) sodium carbonate is added, and the tube heated in a beaker of boiling water for 15 to 20 minutes. Simultaneously 3 c.c. of a 0.02 per cent solution of glucose in saturated picric acid (keeps permanently) is treated with a similar amount of sodium carbonate in a sugar tube and heated at the same time as the unknown. This serves as the standard. Under the action of the heat and alkali the yellow sodium picrate is converted to reddish-brown sodium picramate in proportion to the amount of sugar present. The solutions are now cooled to room temperature either by allowing the tubes to stand or by placing them in a beaker of water. The solution in the standard tube is made up to exactly 10 c.c. with water employing a pipette, preferably with a rubber bulb, so as not to overrun the mark. The unknown tube is now diluted to 10, 15 or 20 c.c. (or some other definite volume in a graduated cylinder) that approximates the color of the standard. It is best to allow a little time to elapse before color comparisons are made.

The standard may conveniently be set at the 15 mm. mark on the colorimeter (Bock-Benedict, Kober or Duboscq). Since the 3 c.c. of blood filtrate employed are the equivalent of 0.6 c.c. of blood and the 3 c.c. of standard solution contain 0.6 mg. of glucose, the proportions are the same as though 100 c.c. of blood and 0.1 gram of glucose were employed. For the calculation the following formula may be used:

$$\frac{S \times D \times 0.1}{R \times 10} = \text{blood sugar in per cent,}$$ in which "S" represents the depth of the standard (15 mm.), "D" the dilution of the unknown, 0.1 the strength of the standard in grams, calculated on the basis of 100 c.c of blood, "R" the reading of the unknown and 10 the dilution of the standard.

ESTIMATION OF BLOOD SUGAR WITH THE TEST TUBE COLORIMETER

The test tube colorimeter is particularly well adapted to the blood sugar determinations.

Method.—For the blood sugar estimation one may use 3 c.c. of the same filtrate as employed for the creatinine estimation (see preceding paper). If only the sugar is desired the following technic may be used: 2 c.c. of the well-mixed oxalated blood are treated with 8 c.c. of water (4 volumes) in a 20 c.c. cylindrical centrifuge tube. After the corpuscles have been laked, about 0.5 gm. of dry picric acid is added and the mixture stirred at intervals with a glass rod until it is a light yellow. When the protein precipitation is complete, the tube is centrifuged and the supernatant fluid filtered through a small filter paper.

Three c.c. of the filtrate are now pipetted into a test tube (or the right-hand tube of the colorimeter) and 1 c.c. of saturated sodium carbonate (22 per cent) added. To another test tube (or the left hand tube of the colorimeter) add 3 c.c. of 0.02 per cent glucose solution in saturated picric acid (standard) and 1 c.c. of the saturated sodium carbonate. The tubes are now placed in a beaker of boiling water for 15 to 20 minutes, then removed and allowed to cool. The standard is made up to the 10 c.c. mark in the left hand tube with water. The unknown is diluted with water with the aid of the diluting pipette, inverting after each addition, until identical in color with the standard. Since the equivalent of 0.6 c.c. of blood is employed and 0.6 mg. of glucose is used as a standard, the proportion is the same as though 100 c.c. of blood were used and 0.1 gram of glucose. This being the case, the reading in the unknown tube gives the percentage of blood sugar directly, i.e., a reading of 9 c.c. being equivalent to 0.09 per cent sugar, a reading of 25 c.c. per cent, etc.

ESTIMATION OF THE DIASTATIC ACTIVITY OF THE BLOOD

As indicated above, the diastatic activity of the blood may often furnish information not disclosed by the blood sugar alone. For this reason directions are given for the determination.

Method[14].—Two 2 c.c. samples of oxalated blood are taken, one being employed as a control. The control tube* is made up to 10 c.c. with distilled water, and the tube to be employed for the test to 9 c.c. Both tubes (20 c.c. cylindrical centrifuge tubes) are now placed in a water bath arranged to maintain a constant temperature of 40° C. As soon as the contents of the tube have been brought to this temperature, 1 c.c. of 1 per cent soluble starch† (or glycogen) is added to the second tube, the contents are mixed, and the incubation carried out for exactly 15 minutes at 40° C. After the incubation has been completed, about 0.5 gram of dry picric acid is at once added to each tube and the mixtures are stirred. When the proteins are precipitated, the tubes are centrifuged and the yellow supernatant fluid is filtered. The sugar in 3 c.c. portions of the filtrate is now estimated as described above for the blood sugar. Correction is made for the sugar originally present in the blood (with the aid of the control) and for the slight reducing action of the soluble starch, if any exists. It has seemed most convenient to record the results in terms of the percentage of the soluble starch (10 mg.) transformed to reducing sugars (calculated as glucose) by the 2 c.c. of blood employed.

The following formula may be used for the calculation of the reducing sugar content of the control (C) and test (A) specimen $\dfrac{S \times D \times 2.0}{R \times 10}$ = mg. of reducing sugar in terms of glucose for 2 c.c. of blood, in which "S" represents the depth of the standard (15 mm.), "D" the dilution of the unknown in c.c., 2.0 the strength of the standard in mg. compared to 2 c.c. of blood, "R" the reading of the unknown in mm. and 10 the dilution of the standard. The difference between the results of the control and test specimens times 10 gives the percentage transformation of the starch to reducing sugar (diastatic activity), provided the soluble starch requires no correction. For example, a diabetic blood having 0.26 per cent blood sugar would give a control of 5.2 mg. Suppose the test specimen gave 9.8 mg. reducing sugar and the soluble starch contained 6 per cent reducing substance, 9.8 – (5.2 + 0.6) times 10 would give a diastatic activity of 40.

REFERENCES

[1]Lewis and Benedict: Proc. Soc. Exper. Biol. and Med., 1913, xi, 57; Jour Biol. Chem., 1915, xx, 61.
[2]Bang: Biochem. Zeitschr., 1913, lvii, 300.
[3]Bang: Der Blutzucker, Wiesbaden, 1913.
[4]Hopkins: Am. Jour. Med. Sc., 1915, cxlix, 254.
[5]Geyelin: Arch. Int. Med., 1915, xv, 975.
[6]Hamman and Hirschman: Arch. Int. Med., 1917, xx, 761.
[7]Denis, Aub and Minot: Arch. Int. Med., 1917, xx, 964.
[8]Mosenthal, Clausen and Hiller: Arch. Int. Med., 1918, xxi, 93.
[9]Janney and Isaacson: Arch. Int. Med., 1918, xxii, 160.
[10]Bailey: Arch. Int. Med., 1919, xxiii, 455.
[11]Williams and Humphreys: Arch. Int. Med., 1919, xxiii, 537, 546, 559.
[12]Allen, Stillman and Fitz: Monographs of the Rockefeller Institute for Medical Research, No. 11, 1919, (October).
[13]Benedict, Osterberg and Neuwirth: Jour. Biol. Chem., 1918, xxxiv, 258.
[14]Myers and Killian: Jour. Biol. Chem., 1917, xxix, 179.
[15]DeNiord and Schreiner: Arch. Int. Med., 1919, xxiii, 484.
[16]Bailey: Am. Jour. Med. Sc., 1919, clvii, 221.
[17]Myers and Bailey: Jour. Biol. Chem., 1916, xxiv, 147.

*If a sugar estimation is being made simultaneously, there appears to be no good reason for running a control, since a 15 minutes' incubation results in no very appreciable change in the blood sugar. The control may, however, be made the basis of the blood sugar estimation.

†Many preparations of soluble starch on the market contain reducing sugar. Starch containing much in excess of 6 per cent reducing sugar is not suitable for this work. For some time we have employed soluble starch prepared by the method of Small[3] from potato starch. This is practically free from reducing sugar. Glycogen is free from reducing sugar and theoretically is to be preferred. Practically, good soluble starch gives the same results and is much less expensive.

[18]von Noorden: Metabolism and Practical Medicine, English Ed., 1907, iii, 529.
[19]Fitz: Arch. Int. Med., 1917, xx, 809.
[20]Hamburger: Brit. Med. Jour., 1919, i, 267.
[21]Morgulis and Jahr: Jour. Biol. Chem., 1919, xxxix, 119.
[22]Janney, Goodhart and Isaacson: Arch. Int. Med., 1918, xxi, 188.
[23]McCrudden and Sargent: Arch. Int. Med., 1918, xxi, 252.
[24]Killian: Proc. Soc. Exper. Biol. and Med., 1920, xvii, (Feb.).
[25]Benedict: Proc. Soc. Exper. Biol. and Med., 1920, xvii, (May).
[26]Höst and Hatlehol: Jour. Biol. Chem., 1920, xlii, 347.
[27]Bang and Hatlehol: Biochem. Zeitschr., 1918, lxxxvii, 264.
[28]Hagedorn and Jensen: Ugesk. Læger, 1918, lxxx, 1217.
[29]Folin and Wu: Jour. Biol. Chem., 1919, xxxviii, 81.
[30]MacLean: Biochem. Jour., 1919, xiii.
[31]Folin and Wu: Jour. Biol. Chem., 1920, xli, 367.
[32]Benedict: Jour. Biol. Chem., 1918, xxxiv, 203.
[33]Ayers: Chemical Composition of the Blood, 1915, p. 29.
[34]Small: Jour. Am. Chem. Soc., 1919, xli, 113.

BACILLUS INFLUENZÆ IN NORMAL AND PATHOLOGIC THROATS*

By Lloyd Arnold, M.D., Nashville, Tenn.

THE Bacillus influenzæ (Pfeiffer) has been studied with renewed vigor during the past two years. It was considered as an etiologic factor in the acute respiratory disease which was pandemic in 1918, by many observers. In view of the difference of opinion that now exists on this point, it was thought advisable to make a few observations in this locality on the prevalence of B. influenzæ in average normal throats, in cases of acute rhinitis, and in throats of patients suffering from "influenza"—which was epidemic in Nashville in February, 1920.

HISTORICAL

Pringle and Huxham in 1743 named a disease, which they thought was due to the influence of atmospheric conditions—sudden changes—influxus, or influenza. Pfeiffer[28] was the first to find a microorganism that could be regarded as the cause of this condition. He found just after the 1889-92 pandemic, a short, small, gram-negative bacillus, aerobic, hemophilic, reaching maximum growth in about 24 hours at 37° C., no growth occurring at temperature below 28° C. nor above 42° C.

Wassermann[41] in 1893 believed that if Pfeiffer's bacillus was found in a throat, this individual suffered from influenza, and that it was never found in healthy individuals, and was always associated with influenza.

Kretz[16] in 1897, found the B. influenzæ in throats of patients several months after an attack of influenza. This author named such individuals "Influenza carriers."

Ortner[25] in 1903, believed that influenza was always caused by Pfeiffer's bacillus, but it could under some conditions be demonstrated in patients not suffering from influenza. This worker called attention to the fact that influenza had never entirely disappeared from Europe since the pandemic of 1889-90, but had been endemic ever since, and that cases had occurred in the region of Vienna every winter and spring since that time.

Rosenthal[33] in 1900 and 1903, found B. influenzæ in the larynx and trachea in about 20 per cent of all healthy persons examined; from this he concluded that this was a saprophyte, and not a pathogenic form.

The B. influenzæ had a rather wide distribution in this country previous to the pandemic in 1918. Lord[20, 21] in 1902 found it in pure culture in 30 per cent of the cases of nontuberculous lung infections in this period. Holt[12] in 1910 found it in 63 per cent of acute bronchitis or pneumonia during the winter and spring in New York City. This author also records that 23.2 per cent of 185 cases, not suspected—patients and nurses—were carriers of B. influenzæ. Woll-

*From the City Hospital Laboratory, Nashville, Tenn.

stein[40] in 1906 found this organism in many nontuberculous lesions of the respiratory tract in children in New York.

Hastings and Niles[11] in the period from 1903 to 1911, found this bacillus in the upper respiratory tract in many pathological conditions.

Luetscher[19] in 1915, at the Johns Hopkins Hospital found, in his studies on some 600 cases of nontuberculous infections of the respiratory tract the pneumococcus and B. influenzæ as the cause of 91 per cent of the infections of the bronchi and lungs; of these B. influenzæ alone in about 30 per cent; in infections of larynx 20 per cent, and in infections of the head 13 per cent.   During the pandemic of 1918 the B. influenzæ has been demonstrated in the sputum, nasal secretions, and in nasopharynx in a high percentage of cases where proper methods have been used.   In England McIntosh,[23] Fildes and Thompson,[8] Mathews,[22] Eyre and Lowe,[7] and others found it in the majority of cases examined.   In Germany, Papamarku,[30] Levinthan,[17] Hundeshagen,[13] and others.

Some work has been done in this country on the number of carriers of this organism.   Lord, Scott and Nye[18] found in 34 healthy Harvard S. A. T. C. recruits, 76 per cent carriers of B. influenzæ.

Opie and coworkers[24] found 35.1 per cent Pfeiffer's bacillus in the mouths of healthy men examined at Camp Funston.

Park and Williams[26] found 40 per cent of nurses carriers of B. influenzæ, also that 41 per cent of patients not suffering from respiratory troubles admitted to wards were positive.   Pritchett and Stillman[29] found 43 per cent of normal individuals examined to be carriers.

Winchell and Stillman[38] found 40 to 46 per cent of 100 normal individuals examined monthly from December, 1918, to June, 1919, were carriers. They found from a comparison with studies carried on previous to the pandemic, that there were no more carriers during the epidemic period than there were previously.

Wahl, White and Lyall[37] found that B. influenzæ when experimentally implanted in the nares of healthy men disappeared in 24 to 72 hours, but multiplication took place rapidly and remained for a considerable length of time, two weeks or more, when in the nasopharynx, and was very resistant to disinfectants.

Wollstein[39] found two general morphologic forms of B. influenzæ, a short and a long type.   Cultural strains are of the short type, meningeal strains belong to the long type, but these become shorter on artificial cultural medium.   This author considers the moisture present in the cultural medium has a great influence on the morphology.   Many workers have substantiated these findings. The author has noticed these characteristics repeatedly.   There has also been found on continuous transplants a long filamentous looking form, which we took for contamination.   It resembles certain fungi morphologically.   Wade and Manalang[36] have studied this form and consider it a form of B. influenzæ.

Park[27] tested by agglutinin absorption about 100 strains of B. influenzæ and found that the strains isolated from the same case give the same immunologic reactions, but seldom occurred with strains from different individuals.   Park concludes, "that influenzæ bacillus, like the pneumococci, have gradually through the years altered on the mucous membranes of healthy carriers into many strains which, while having many characteristics in common are still different in their susceptibility to specific immune substances and perhaps other reactions." Park found that one colony from a plate culture made from several strains may show two different strains immunologically, but separated when thoroughly shaken up before plating.

Many workers have shown that B. influenzæ was capable of producing variable amounts of toxins. Huntoon and Hannum[14] showed that certain conditions of symbiotic growth intensified the liberation of the toxin. Roos[32] found that the symbiosis of streptococci and B. influenzæ increased the virulency of the latter tenfold. This was first observed by Jacobson.[15]

METHODS OF ISOLATION OF BACILLUS INFLUENZÆ

1. *Hemophilic Property Alone.*—Blood agar plates. Pfeiffer found pigeons blood more advantageous than human's blood. Davis found that in mediums containing as little as 1:180,000 of hemoglobin the organism may continue to grow. Czaplowski[5a] found the organism grew better when very small amounts of blood were added to the medium, hardly enough to tint, than when large quantities were added. Ghon and Preyss[10a] found that hemoglobin in smaller amounts than was demonstrable with the spectroscope was sufficient to promote growth.

Rivers[31] found rabbits' and cats' blood produced better growth than human blood. Fitzgerald and Cohen[9] obtained good growths by heating the blood to 80° C. for three minutes. Mathews[22] showed a very profuse growth occurs when blood has been digested with an excess of trypsin for 5 days at 37° C. Fleming[10] recommends treatment of blood with acid and neutralizing with alkali, this medium giving a simple and good differential medium.

2. *Symbiotic Relationship for Growth.*—Cantani[4] showed the favorable influence of other organisms upon the growth of B. influenzæ on artificial mediums. Organisms now used are B. subtilis, staphylococci, streptococci. Roos,[32] Brown and Orcutt[3a] both have developed differential methods in this manner.

3. *Special Differential Mediums.*—Bernstein and Lowe[7] used Churchman's observation that gentian-violet inhibited growth of gram-positive organisms. These authors have used this dye in concentration of 1:5000 in blood agar plates. Avery[1] after considerable experimentation used sodium oleate in 1:1000 concentration in blood agar plates, serum-free blood being used. Winchell and Stillman,[38] using Avery's method, found that the best results were obtained when the P_H of the medium was between 7.2 and 7.5.

TECHNIC

Avery's sodium oleate method was used, great care being taken in the adjustment of the P_H value. This latter was the most important point in the success of the method. The Barnett and Chapman[2] colorimetric method was used. Swabs were taken from the posterior nasopharynx and immediately smeared across a poured and surface dried Avery Sodium Oleate Blood Agar Plate, being distributed by means of a bent glass spreader. Plates were inverted and incubated forty-eight hours. It was found that the colonies were better developed and as contamination and spreaders were few, this was more satisfactory than a shorter incubation period. Colonies looking like B. influenzæ were picked, stained by Gram method and tested for hemophilic property.

October, 1919, to January, 1920, 80 apparently normal throats were examined by this method, 28 were positive, making 35 per cent carriers of B. influenzæ.

In November, 1919, there occurred a slight epidemic of acute pharyngitis and rhinitis in this locality. Of 45 such cases that were examined, 35 were positive, making 77.7 per cent positive.

In February, 1920, there was a recurrence of the "influenza" epidemic in this locality, lasting some two weeks. During this time 104 cases were selected at random from the patients entering the hospital, diagnosed as "influenza" in the acute stage. Many of these cases had been sick several days before admission. Of the 104 cases, 90 were positive, making 87.5 per cent positive.

EXPERIMENTS ON THE VIABILITY OF BACILLUS INFLUENZÆ

Nasal secretions, known by cultural methods to contain B. influenzæ, were taken up with cotton swabs.

No. 1 swab left at room temperature for 4 hours. Culture positive.
" 2 swab left at room temperature for 6 hours. Culture positive.
" 3 swab left at room temperature for 8 hours. Culture positive— one colony.
" 4 swab left at room temperature for 10 hours. Culture negative.
" 5 swab left at room temperature for 12 hours. Culture negative.
Room temperature was 22.5° C. day time, but no sun light.

Nasal secretions, known by cultural methods to contain B. influenzæ, were taken up on sterile gauze, placed under a bell-jar on a glass plate, at room temperature.

No. 1 Culture made after 6 hours. Positive.
" 2 Culture made after 12 hours. Positive.
" 3 Culture made after 18 hours. Positive—few colonies.
" 4 Culture made after 24 hours. Positive—one colony.
" 5 Culture made after 36 hours. Negative.
" 6 Culture made after 48 hours. Negative.

DISCUSSION

It would seem that the percentage of carriers of B. influenzæ (35 per cent) is about the same in Nashville as in New York, Boston, Camp Funston, and elsewhere. Stillman states that the carriers were not numerically increased during the recent pandemic of influenza. Lyall found when B. influenzæ were planted on the nasopharynx they were very resistant to antiseptics and remained for weeks. Stillman found some 84 individuals constant carriers of Pfeiffer's bacillus, over a period of seven months. In cases of acute rhinitis and pharyngitis, we found 77.7 per cent of 45 cases, all occurring within the hospital during a period of ten days, were positive to B. influenzæ. In February, 1920, during the recurrence of the influenza epidemic in Nashville, of the 104 cases run 87.5 per cent were positive to Pfeiffer's bacillus.

A percentage of 87.5 during the apex of an epidemic was lower than was expected to be found, especially since acute upper respiratory disorders gave

77.7 per cent. The same media and the same technic were used for both observations. In a subsequent paper on the throat flora previous and during this February, 1920, epidemic of influenza, this question will be dealt with in detail.

CONCLUSIONS

Bacillus influenzæ is present in 35 per cent of normal throats in this vicinity. Bacillus influenzæ was present in 77.7 per cent of 'bad colds"—acute rhinitis and pharyngitis.

Bacillus influenzæ was present in 86.5 per cent of the cases in the recent—February, 1920—epidemic of influenza in Nashville.

Bacillus influenzæ, in nasal secretions from acute rhinitis, directly exposed to the air, are not viable if planted on artificial culture medium after 10 hours; if exposed to light, but desiccation prevented, are viable for 24 hours.

With Avery's sodium oleate blood agar plates, we have a reliable method of isolating the B. influenzæ.

REFERENCES

[1]Avery: Jour. Am. Med. Assn., 1918, lxxi. 2050.
[2]Barnett and Chapman: Ibid., 1918, lxx, 1062.
[3]Bernstein and Lowe: Jour. Infect. Dis., 1919, xxiv, 129.
[3a]Brown and Orcutt: Jour. Exper. Med., 1918, xxviii, 659.
[4]Cantani: Zeitschr. f. Hyg., 1901, xxx, 29.
[5]Crowe and Thacker-Neville: Bull. Johns Hopkins Hosp., 1919, xxx, 322.
[5a]Czaplowski: Centralbl. f. Bakteriol., I.O., 1902, xxxii, 667.
[6]Davis: Jour. Infect. Dis., 1907, iv, 73.
[7]Eyre and Lowe: Lancet, London, Oct. 12, 1918.
[8]Fildes and Thompson: Lancet, London, 1918, ii, 699.
[9]Fitzgerald and Cohen: Centralbl. f. Bakteriol., 1911.
[10]Fleming: Lancet, London, 1919, i, 139.
[10a]Ghon and Preyss: Centralbl. f. Bakteriol., 1902, xxxii, 96.
[11]Hastings and Niles: Jour. Exper. Med., 1911, xiii, 639.
[12]Holt: Arch. Int. Med., 1910, v, 449.
[13]Hundeshagen: Deutsch. med. Wchnschr., 1918, xliv, 1181.
[14]Huntoon and Hannum: Jour. Immunol., 1919, iv, 167.
[15]Jacobson: Arch. de med. exper., 1900, xiii, 425.
[16]Kretz: Wien. klin. Wchnschr., 1897, x, 877.
[17]Levinthal: Berl. klin. Wchnschr., 1918, lv, 712; Ztschr., f. Hyg. u. Infektk., 1918, lxxxvi, No. 1.
[18]Lord, Scott, and Nye: Jour. Am. Med. Assn., 1919, lxxii, 188.
[19]Luetscher: Arch. Int. Med., 1915, xvi, 657.
[20]Lord: Boston Med. and Surg. Jour., 1902, cxlvii, 662.
[21]Lord: Ibid., 1905, clii, 574.
[22]Mathews: Lancet, London, July 27, 1918.
[23]McIntosh: Lancet, London, 1918, ii, 695.
[24]Opie, et al: Jour. Am. Med. Assn., 1919, lxxii, 108.
[25]Ortner: Deutsch. Klin., 1903, ii, 417.
[26]Park and Williams: Am. Jour. Pub. Health, 1919, ix, 45.
[27]Park: Jour. Am. Med. Assn., 1919, lxxiii, 318.
[28]Pfeiffer: Deutsch. med. Wchnschr., 1892, xviii, 28; Ztschr. f. Hyg., 1893, xii, 357.
[29]Pritchett and Stillman: Jour. Exper. Med., 1919, xxix, 259.
[30]Papamarku: Deutsch. med. Wchnschr., October 24, 1918.
[31]Rivers: Bull. Johns Hopkins Hosp., 1919, xxx, 129.
[32]Roos: Jour. Immunol., 1919, iv, 189.
[33]Rosenthal: Comp. rend. Soc. d. Biol., 1900, liii, 266.
[34]Rosenthal: Ibid., 1903, lv, 1500.
[36]Wade and Manalang: Jour. Exper. Med., 1920, xxxi, 95.
[37]Wahl, White and Lyall: Jour. Infect. Dis., 1919, xxv, 419.
[38]Winchell and Stillman: Jour. Exper. Med., 1919, xxx, 497.
[39]Wollstein: Jour. Exper. Med., 1915, xxii, 445.
[40]Wollstein: Ibid., 1906, viii, 681.
[41]Wassermann: Deutsch. med. Wchnschr., 1893, xix, 1201.

THE LOCALIZATION OF HALLUCINATIONS*

BY H. I. GOSLINE, M.D., HOWARD, RHODE ISLAND

IN THE consideration of localization of any sort, is it not a desirable condition if not an essential one, that we know the ground in which our localization is to take place? That we do not know our ground any too well when we consider the central nervous system, I take to be almost axiomatic. Necessarily, much of the evidence upon which our conception of the structure of the central nervous system is built, is in the nature of indirect evidence. It has proved utterly impossible to trace nerve fibers from start to finish. However, with the uncertain tools of indirect evidence neuropathology has succeeded in building up a fair conception of the structure of the centripetal pathways, the centrifugal pathways and to a certain extent the arrival platforms for sensations and the departure platforms for motion.

That there must, at least logically, be a connection between the sensory arrival platforms and the motor departure platforms seems rarely to have concerned the anatomists. Under the spell of old forms of psychology they have preferred to look for association tracts and centers for abstract ideas or concrete ideas. Flechsig thought he had found the association tracts in the brains of his fetus;[1] Campbell thought he had found the centers for concepts and for concrete ideas in the so-called silent areas of the brain.[2] But, strangely enough, the discovery does not seem to have led very far, or to have suggested any new lines of advance. So far, it has proved barren from a practical standpoint.

In lieu of better histopathologic methods which seem rather slow in coming, it occurred to the writer that one might more easily attack the problem from the psychologic side. This side seemed especially hopeful for several reasons. First, there were some aspects that had been neglected even from the point of view of elementary logic. I have named one aspect above in the connection which I mentioned as necessarily existing logically between the arrival and the departure platforms. Another ran as follows: How do you expect to correlate symptoms with anatomy until you are sure that your symptoms are indivisible? In other words that they are elementary? The thought also must have arisen somehow that most any one could propound psychology of some of the ancient sort.

However, a thorough search revealed that it was not necessary to propound any psychology of an ancient sort but that with the institution of laboratory methods, a psychology had already grown up which might offer some outlook.[3] That psychology seems to have reduced all mental processes to four simple or elementary processes, sensation, association, reaction and inhibition, and it is these processes that can be correlated with our anatomy. Strangely enough, a

*From the Department of Pathology, State Institutions, Howard, Rhode Island.
Read at the meeting of the New England Psychiatric Society, held at the Danvers State Hospital, March 25, 1920.

set of logical deductions from this psychology made lucid the structure of the gray matter of the cortex as well as that of the white matter of the brain.

Before proceeding to the structure deduced from this psychology let me emphasize the fact, if it requires any emphasis, that this set of plans of the central nervous system is only a logical deduction, has not been proved anatomically and is so new as not to have been put to the pragmatic test. However, I will ask your forbearance, while I inflict it upon you, assuring you that a thorough search of both the psychologic and anatomic literature has failed to reveal one iota against it and has actually revealed a great deal for it by a mere mental recasting of some of the facts as we have known them for many years.

Following is the paradigm of the central and peripheral nervous system:

The Individual

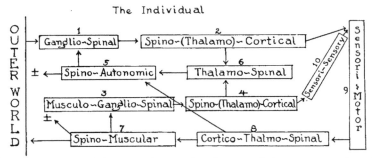

One, two, three, and four are the centripetal parts of the apparatus. five, six, seven, and eight are the centrifugal parts and nine and ten are the connecting parts deduced from the psychology we mentioned.

The detail of the visual system is then as follows:

Visual Sphere

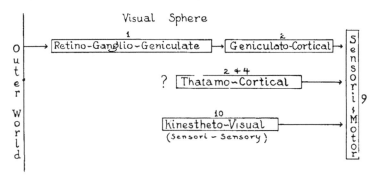

This single example can serve as a paradigm for the construction of the rest of the nervous system, for anyone who is interested enough to take the time and trouble.

Let us leave the anatomic field for the moment and recall to your memories some axioms relating to function. May it not be assumed that the following thesis is axiomatic? Sensations depend upon the structure and function of the peripheral and central apparatus and upon the condition of the consciousness. If the structure is so altered as to be that of the dead substance, it may be assumed that the function will be completely lost. That is apparently not the state of the nerve structure in the case of hallucinations, for function is retained and in fact some of the structures are functioning without apparent stimulus. One would scarcely suppose a paralysis of function in a case where function was taking place without adequate cause. One would more logically assume an overactivity. The question of whether the overfunction is due to irritation by direct involvement of the paths concerned or by removal of the effects of other paths is an extremely attractive one. It has previously been presented to you under the title of "Hyperkinesis by Defect"[4] and I feel that our newer psychology bears this assumption out. Common examples of this condition are known to you all. The exaggeration of the reflexes when the spinal reflex arc is retained and the inhibitory control of the corticospinal tracts is removed, is used by all of you daily in the phenomenon of the patella reflex. I am assuming for the purposes of this paper that the same phenomenon is universal in the nervous system; that, in other words, there is a mutual inhibition of neurones which seek a final common path[5] and that this phenomenon is born in the nerve tissue, is a function of nerve tissue, is part of the machinery of our bodies. Naturally, I am not denying at the same time that changes in the blood supply, poisons, et cetera may cause conditions of excitation in the paths concerned or that exciting conditions in the sense organs may play a part, if only to act as points of departure for excitations. But what I do wish to emphasize is the state of irritability in the sense centres as against a defect in the sense centres and that the irritability may be due not only to direct contact with irritating conditions but also to the removal of the inhibitions of neurones seeking a final common path through the sensory centre.

Referring again to our diagrams, you can see anatomically for yourselves how an injury of the spinocortical neurone or of the thalmocortical neurone may allow the one or the other to overact thus overstimulating the sensorimotor neurone. The defect, the pathologic anatomy is not to be expected or looked for then in the sensorimotor neurone but in the spinocortical or the thalamocortical neurone. We are not to expect changes in the cerebral cortex in this case but in the subcortical white matter.

Let us make the attempt to localize from the symptoms presented by our patients. We can omit for the purposes of this paper the absent function in the blind or the deaf as well as the artificial performance of function under the electric current. We might also do well to omit the hallucinations which are to a certain extent dependent upon pathologic conditions in the external apparatus. In this group we may consider the unilateral visual hallucinations which do not show hemiopic limitation, hallucinations that may be made to disappear by covering one eye, those which move with the movements of the eyes, which may be doubled by prisms or by lateral pressure on the orbit, or that may appear larger or smaller by looking through an opera glass, or that may appear in the mirror. Cases of a similar sort have not been reported in the other senses.

The following sources of hallucinations are psychologically possible, adhering to the laboratory type of psychology which has been worked out within the last twenty-five years. The sensations, the associations, the reactions and inhibitions may be disordered. These are the only possibilities. Naturally, these disorders are not revealed immediately to the senses of the observer but appear to him in the form of disordered perceptions, disordered ideas, disordered activities. disordered inner states. The personality, consisting as it does in an intricate interplay of these complex mental functions, is disintegrated in direct proportion to the disintegration in these complex functions. By an analysis which I cannot present at this time, but which can be found in print in the near future and which can be made by yourselves from the proper sources, all these complex mental functions are reduced to the simple processes sensation, association, reaction and inhibition.[6] The specific sensations involved in any given case must be determined from the productions of the patient. So also the specific localization must be derived in every case from the productions of the patient. It is the purpose of this paper to point out in general the simple functions involved in the common hallucinations of our patients.

Let us consider the visual sphere first.

Only a few of the symptoms as we find them may be directly correlated with our anatomy as presented in the charts. Even the simplest objects of visual hallucinations such as the seeing of patterns, flowers, animals reveal the elements of size and shape and we know from our psychology that these are given to our consciousness by the sensations which arise from the action of the eye muscles. May it not be then, that a disorder of the kinesthetic centre for the eye muscles will produce a visual hallucination of varying size, shape and position? The only essential is that the sensorisensory neurone be disturbed from the kinesthetic centre for eye muscle movements to the arrival platform for visual sensations. Perhaps the presence of size, shape and position is evidence of the intactness of that sensorisensory neurone and it is the sizeless, shapeless, and positionless hallucinations that mean a destruction of the sensorisensory neurone. Of the same nature are the hallucinations of birds flying behind one. of a knife seen behind one, of being able to look from behind into ones own body. Nocturnal visions of radiant figures belong here as do the seeing of coins, wire, woven threads or the active, gay crowds of the alcoholic. Of the same nature are the microscopic visual hallucinations of the cocaine addict, the countless similar, tiny individuals, animals, holes in the wall and little points that they see.

Naturally, in some of the examples mentioned you will see another complex mental function. the emotions or the feelings, appear. Patterns appear beautiful to some and hence have an esthetic value. Flowers and animals frequently have emotional equivalents. May not fear be at the bottom of the hallucination of a knife behind one? But the emotions themselves as well as the esthetic attitude are given to our consciousness through our reactions. To remove or to overstimulate the pathways from our emotional centers to our visual arrival platforms may then cause visual hallucinations by the process of excitation or that of hyperkinesis by defect.

Turning to the auditory sphere we may assume that the process of hyperkinesis by defect is working in the case of hallucinations whose content is meaningless words, repeated over and over. But in this case the defect is in the functions which give meaning to the words. Our psychology analyzes the perception of meaning into reaction. That is to say, our reaction to an object of perception, to an idea which stands for an object of perception is the thing which gives the perception or the idea its meaning; it is the reaction to a combination of sensations which unifies them into a perception and which gives the perception its meaning. In the example of hallucination just given, then, the defect is in the reactive mechanism or in its sensory arrival platforms or in connections between the sensory arrival platforms for the reaction sensations and the sensory arrival platform for the auditory sensations.

Alcoholics can at times hear the buzzing of a fly ostensibly held in the hand placed at their ear. The attention is directed toward the hearing of an imaginary sound. The attention is a function of the reaction mechanism. The discharge of the reaction mechanism and its sensory results are in this case able to stimulate the sensory mechanism for audition. The same is true for the hearing of imaginary telephone conversations by the alcoholic. The localization is to be expected and looked for in the reaction mechanism or in the sensory arrival platforms for the reaction mechanism or in the sensorisensory neurone connecting these arrival platforms with the arrival platform for the auditory sense.

The combination with the muscle sense which gives the space perception seems to exist in the case of auditory hallucinations as well as in that of the visual hallucinations. Of this sort are the voices that are placed in the abdomen, breast, head, ears, in the wall, or in the bed in which the patient lies.

On the other hand, the localization may be entirely in the sensory arrival platform for the auditory sense, that is, in the sensorimotor neurone in the case of hallucinations of different pitch, of different tone coloring, in the soft, whispering, faint, or the loud, piercing hallucinations, or in the short broken remarks, the loud shouting, the crackling, or the bell-tone hallucinations. Do we not see the peculiar features of audition itself in the pitch and tone-coloring? Is not soft, whispering faint or loud and piercing merely differences of intensity which are not peculiar to anything but audition itself? Even remarks, shouting and crackling are combinations of tones and noises, the two categories which comprise all sounds to which the human machine is sensitive.

In the case of a patient whose hallucinations are different in the two ears, it would be necessary to analyze in the same way. It might happen that the same elements were effective in each side or that they were different. In case they differed we should expect to find the lesion in different loci in the two sides of the brain.

The presence of a speech defect should lead one to consider the possibility of a single lesion producing the two disorders, that is to say, the speech defect and the auditory hallucinations. In the brain the two pathways lie very close together in the white matter.

In the case of hallucinations of smell, one might think as we did with those of sight and sound, of a lesion in the sensory arrival platform for smell, if the smell is always the same and often repeated, without other concomitant phenomena to lead us to look elsewhere.

The localization is to be determined as pointed out above in the case of a patient who describes objects ostensibly placed in the closed hand but not really placed there. The disorder is in the attention. The irritation of an overacting reaction mechanism influences the arrival platform for the tactile sense and causes it to react with an hallucination.

Disorders of the kinesthetic senses may be seen in the following examples and may be submitted to the same processes of analysis for the purpose of localization. The chief ones are feelings of stiffness, of change in the skin or soft parts, of being filled up, sewed up, drawn in, feelings of electricity, of metamorphosis, of inner petrifaction, of drying up, of loss of the head, mouth, stomach. The feeling of being possessed may have an emotional background and the feeling that words are spoken by others in the patient's own tongue seem to point directly to localization in the arrival platform for the sensations from the muscles of the tongue.

In the individual case the analysis is aided by other observations on the patients. Symptoms never occur singly and the final localization is to be made from the analysis of all the symptoms. For example in the cases of hallucination already cited, some patients cut off all other stimuli in order to follow the hallucinations, others produce lively sensations in order to get rid of the hallucinations, while still others stop up the ears, making it appear that outside noises increase the native irritability of the central arrival platforms. Some hallucinations are worse at night or in the loneliness of the prison cell. In these cases the attention and the emotions should be analyzed. In other words the localization should be thought of in the reaction mechanism.

Some cases of hallucination apparently occur by the process of association. In the analysis of the association process it comes out that no new paths are involved and least of all paths connecting all sense arrival platforms directly with one another as we have always assumed till now. All associations take place by contiguity or by similarity. The first means that they must occur together or in immediate succession and the second means that they must have sufficient elements in common to give the feeling of similarity. In other words similarity is a function of the reaction mechanisms. We also know that things are associated in the mind if they have occurred recently, frequently, are emotionally important or are impressive, that is to say, if they have some attention value. Recency and frequency are matters of time and repetition. Emotion and attention values might make us suppose that there are connections between the sensory arrival platforms and the centres for emotions on the one hand and the reactions on the other. We have already been led to make this conclusion previously from other considerations. It is by the process of association that the normal person presents himself the visual picture of the cat whose mee-owing he hears. So we can enumerate the seeing of colors with the hearing of certain sounds, the pain at seeing others suffering pain, the feeling in the larynx when hearing a hoarse singer, the tickling at the suggestion of being tickled, the warding off a blow. Dreams also make a transfer of the senses. The original sense equipment plays a part in some of these cases, depending on whether the individual concerned ordinarily and habitually used visual, auditory or kinesthetic imagery, in other words, depending on his inborn mechanism.

In the case of hallucinations by association in the visual sphere we have the hearing of tones from a tuning fork or from a hand organ which produce visual hallucinations. A glance or a movement may produce peculiar feelings of tension or of restfulness in some patients. A case is presented where a deaf, blind boy heard bells playing a melody when he moved his eyes in rhythm toward the right. Auditory hallucinations have been produced by stroking different parts of the body. From our presentation above we do not need to consider recency, frequency or contiguity. In the first instance, the hallucinations may be due to these very things or they may be produced by the fact that the emotional re- action to the sounds was similar to that produced by the vision. The disorder in his case would not be true hallucination though practically impossible to differentiate from one. It would be more in the nature of a feeling that the visual impression took place than a real visual impression such as occurs in a true hallucination. In the second case, the visual impression produces a muscle sensation. The balance may be taken to be disturbed in the emotional control, in the thalamocortical neurone. In the third case, the overstimulation of the sensory arrival platform for audition from the sensory arrival platform for muscle sensations is apparent. In the fourth case we have an instance similar to the first one but the part functioning is the tactile sphere.

The analysis is not always given directly from the hallucinations but light may be thrown upon the processes at fault from other fields. Ideas may all be grouped under memory, imaginative and general ideas. There are no ideas which may not be grouped in one of these three groups. And the ideas can be reduced to sensations, association, reaction and inhibition. In this way several disorders which are somehow related to hallucinations and which are sometimes difficult to distinguish from them in practice, are of use to the analyst. In the disorder known as "double thinking" the "thoughts come out loud." A word thought of is heard spoken outside or as a sort of inner speaking. "Inner voices" are not hallucinations, either; they are like the voice of conscience, between hearing and having a presentiment. To these inner voices belong the sugges- tions, the world speech, thoughts, telephoning and telegraphing. They may at- tach themselves to another person and a silent dialogue ensues.

In cases where it is impossible to give the content verbatim, we are more likely concerned with convincing thoughts than with true hallucinations. These thoughts are ascribed to strange influences, are often considered supernatural. God or Christ gives the patient a charge or a promise, explains to him a secret of his personality. These phenomena appear dreamy and transcendental to the patient.

While these are not true hallucinations and so will not take our time for analysis here, is it not apparent that practically the same factors are at work in them as have already been outlined in the analysis of the true hallucinations? And, since these same phenomena together with others appear in the hallucinated patient, is it not apparent that the one aids in limiting the analysis of the other to certain ultimate and definite neurone systems? It is these phenomena which have led some to say that hallucinations may be imaginative ideas of extreme sensory vividness and which have led other authors to speak of imaginative hal- lucinations, psychic hallucinations, pseudo-hallucinations and apperception hal- lucinations.

Some hallucinations can be influenced by forms of will tension. They may disappear with work and return with leisure. An inhibition of thinking and will may be at the bottom of these cases. The hallucinations may be independent of the will and of the train of thought, giving the feeling that they are strange, independent. come from the outside. Thus their subjective origin is hidden from the patient. But a psychological analysis of will, attention and thought itself shows that the fundamental disorder in these cases is in the reaction mechanism plus the ideas and the ideas are reduced to the processes of sensation, association, reaction and inhibition.

The last group of complex mental functions that may act in the causation of hallucinations is that of the inner states which comprise the feelings, the emotions and the attitudes. This group offers the chief difficulties to analysis both because it comes into the majority of all hallucinations and because the reaction mechanisms upon which it depends for its existence are so complicated. The reaction mechanisms concerned in the emotions apparently involve the vegetative nervous system and the glands of internal secretion as well as some of the glands provided with a duct. It is apparent then, that we have gone about as far as we can at the present time and in the present state of our knowledge if we are able to say that the disorder is probably in the vascular-glandular system rather than in the central nervous system, in a given case. We have gone still further if we can say that it is probably in the nature of an irritative lesion or of a destructive lesion with hyperginesis by defect as the essential process at bottom of the condition.

The attempt will be made to present all hallucinations in accordance with the latter viewpoint and in some cases to classify them more exactly under the former category.

We know that hallucinations often agree with the thoughts, fears and wishes of the patient and for this reason they seem to be so powerful. The emotional undercurrents in the form of secret hopes and dim longings stand out, causing the absence of perception of real stimuli, a sort of negative hallucination which occurs in the hysteric. In such cases, also, the hallucination or disorder is frequently in a single sense. It is not due to lack of attention, failing attention, or distracted attention. It is not due to clouding of consciousness, to disorder of the sense organ or to disorder of conduction to the brain. The simplest, commonest way of describing it without committing oneself is to call it psychogenic.

The attempt in this paper is made to further analyze "psychogenic" and necessarily commits one to certain views although they are only logical ones.

The following hallucinations are taken to have an emotional background and hence, on the basis of our diagrams, we must assume a hyperkinesis of the thalamocortical neurone by defect of the sensorisensory neurone or an overaction of the thalamocortical neurone from some other cause. This other cause may lie in the vegetative nervous system or the glands of internal secretion. In the hysteric we have already mentioned absence of function of the blindness, the deafness, the absence of the sense of touch or anesthesia. Hallucinations of a single sense, whether of sight, sound, taste, smell, touch, or of general sensibility are to be thought of as hysterical in origin. In such patients the neglect of one side of a bilateral visual hallucination will present to the observer as a unilateral visual hallucination. Hysterics also see veiled forms, dead relatives, men with long knives.

In the visual sphere the following hallucinations show a strong emotional factor: the nocturnal "visions" of God, Christ, the angels, the dead, flowers, fearful faces, the devil, shadow plays, wild animals; the alcoholic hallucinations of rats, goblins, numberless creeping vermin, butterflies, birds, black dogs, wolves, looking in at the window, on the bed covers, dark shadows, blood, the face of a corpse, men hanging from a tree; the epileptic hallucinations of seeing fire, frightful forms, heavenly visions.

In the auditory sphere the same is true of the hearing of the voices of relatives, faithless lovers, hateful neighbors, God, the devil; hearing confused crying, pleasing music and singing. The epileptic hears threats, shooting, war-crys, promises, and angel music. The circular depressions hear single short remarks of a disquieting content. Some schizophrenics hear exciting, gladdening voices at first.

Some patients taste unappetizing, harmful things, such as human flesh in the mouth, dirt, arsenic, cantharides given them by their enemies. They smell poisonous vapors which are made to kill them and the odor of sulphur which comes from the devil.

The common assumption in all these cases is that the abuse, the insults, the jeers, the cries of abused relatives, the threats, the commands only excite, torment the patient and make him suspicious, dangerous, anxious, confused, or make him run away and do senseless, unnatural acts. On the contrary may it not be that these hallucinations only echo the woes of the patient? It is the woes of the patient that color his visual, his auditory, his tactile, his olfactory, his gustatory, his thermic, his algesic, and his kinesthetic hallucinations. On the basis of the James-Lange theory[7] of emotion and of the action theory of introspective psychology is it not more likely that the reaction mechanism is disordered than that the sensations are disordered and are upsetting the reaction mechanism? It is on the basis that this is a correct assumption that I would have you look in these cases for pathology in the sensorisensory neurone of a destructive sort or for pathology in the thalamocortical neurone of an irritative sort, or for pathology in the glands of internal secretion or in the controlling nervous mechanism of the vegetative nervous system.

The fear reaction may have its basis in a disorder of the chromaffine system but farther than this we cannot go at the present time with any degree of certainty.

A few examples of hallucinations colored by removal of the emotional control and consequent overaction of the sensorisensory neurone have been cited above in the paragraphs on the origin of the hallucinations in the sense centers. To these may be added the indifferent, senseless auditory hallucinations of some cases of dementia precox or the case of a patient who slaps her abdomen because she is hard inside and takes douches because she is black inside.

Another group of productions of great assistance to the analyst is that of the illusions or those productions in which an illusion is mixed in with an hallucination so inextricably that it is impossible to tell where one begins and the other leaves off practically. For the purposes of this sort of analysis a separation into hallucinations and illusions lacks point because more information is gathered and more light is cast on the localization by leaving them together. However, the determination of an illusion is at times of value in pointing to an irritation in the external apparatus or in the first sensory neurone, the ganglio-spinal neurone. Such cases are those caused by the endogenous retinal light or the endotie noises. Others in the visual sphere are conditioned and determined to a certain extent by uneven lights as in the case of alcoholics who read off words and numbers from a clear sheet, or by specks on a smoothe surface on which the alcoholic sees animals. In these cases also, in the delirious state, hallucinations can be produced by pressing on the eyes.

In the auditory sphere the beat of the carotid pulse is at times the apparent cause of rhythmic hallucinations. Soft noises like the dripping of water or the sighing of the wind may cause the hallucinations. In the tactile sphere hallucinations can be produced in some alcoholics by pressing on the skin.

In the following example perhaps it is the attention that is disordered. The patient says that pictures shown to him hide real objects or only let the real objects shimmer through.

In the following examples the memory and the attention both seem to be affected. The patient recognizes relatives in strangers or does not recognize his own relatives as such.

The attention has already been analyzed. The memory renews previous perceptions and hence the analysis of the perceptions involved should lead to the proper localization.

The following mixtures of illusion and hallucination have an emotional background and their analysis should proceed on the same plan as that of the hallucinations themselves. And in making the final estimate of the localization in any given case, these should certainly be used for the valuable aid that they give in fixing the localization of the cause of the true hallucinations. In the visual sphere, towering tree-tops and scurrying mists are specters to the patient. When eating, he sees moulds in his food and little heads cut off with moving eyes, and he sees wiggling worms. Objects about are distortions, skulls; they move and change themselves; people change faces and forms and make faces at the patients.

In the auditory sphere, but still conditioned by the emotions, we may group the following examples: the idea of danger from water produced by roaring and ringing in the ears; the ringing of bells, the scratching of a pen, the whistling of an engine, the barking of a dog, the creaking of a wagon or of some boards may be insulting words or reproaches against the patient; noises mean the crying of the patient's children, crackling means the fires of hell; behind his back words refer to him, remarks accompany his every action and openly expose the most hidden occurrence of his past; the voices insult, threaten, bless, especially if indistinctly heard; wagons creak and rumble in an unusual way and tell stories; swine grunt names and give wonderful attestations; dogs insult and bark reproaches; hens cackle them; geese and ducks quack names, phrases and fragments of references.

Most of the examples above, if not all, give evidence of the overaction of the thalamocortical neurone and, as in the case of the true hallucinations, this should lead us to expect an irritative lesion of this neurone or a destructive lesion of the sensorisensory neurone which would produce an overaction of the thalamocortical neurone by the process of hyperkinesis by defect.

SUMMARY

On the basis of laboratory psychology all mental functions can be reduced to the simple processes, sensation, association, reaction and inhibition. On the basis of this psychology the hallucinations are reduced to simple processes and the results are correlated with the anatomy of the nervous system. Psychology is carried into psychopathology for the purpose of making anatomic localizations.

The writer attempts to conclude from the patient's symptoms as to whether the pathologic process is an irritative one or a destructive one.

CONCLUSIONS

1. That it is possible to judge from the patient's symptoms as to the localization of hallucinations in any given case.

2. That the localization is usually in one of three foci, namely, the sensorimotor neurone, the sensorisensory neurone, or the thalamocortical neurone.

3. That the symptoms are evidence of hyperkinesis which takes place either by direct irritation of the neurone in question or by defect of any other neurone which seeks a final common path with the neurone in question.

4. That the symptoms of the patient are sufficient to tell the observer which process is at work, if he keeps the tenets of the psychology upon which the analysis is based, firmly in his mind.

REFERENCES

[1]Flechsig. Paul: Gehirn und Rückenmark—Wilhelm Engelmann. Lepsig. 1876.
[2]Campbell. A. W.: Histological Studies on Cerebral Localization—Proceedings of the Royal Society, 1903.
[3]Munsterberg. Hugo: Psychology, General and Applied, Appleton and Co., New York, 1914.
[4]Southard. E. E.: Literature Referring to "Hyperkinesis by Defect" and "Cortical Simplification."
[5]Sherrington, C. I.: The Integrative Action of the Nervous System, New York, 1911.
[6]Gosline, Harold I.: The Anatomical Implications of the Introspective Psychology, to be published.
[7]James, William: Textbook of Psychology.
The main body of the paper is a readaptation of Emil Kraepelin. Psychiatrie. 8te Auflage, Bd. I, Teil 2. "The Signs of Mental Disorder," a translation of the above is in preparation.

LABORATORY METHODS

THE ALKALIMETRY OF WHOLE BLOOD—A PRELIMINARY STUDY*

By John B. Rieger, S.M., M.D., Detroit, Mich.

IT SEEMS fair to assume that the alkali content of the circulating blood is in equilibrium with that of the tissues. A depletion of blood alkali therefore spells a corresponding depletion of alkali throughout the body. The methods devised on this basis for the estimation of the degree of acidosis have generally depended on the measurement of the bicarbonate content of the blood-plasma or the carbonic acid content of the alveolar air. Since increased pulmonary ventilation is really a compensatory process and demands for its maintenance an increased hydrogen-ion concentration of the blood, these methods will not detect the slighter grades of acidosis, such as may be caused by kidney lag. Such lag may be due to impairment of renal function, increased production of acid or both. When due to increased production of acid and the kidney function is normal, the index of acid excretion, devised by Fitz and Van Slyke[1] is the most delicate indicator of acidosis that we have. The test tells us nothing, however, about the amount of acid remaining unexcreted in the blood.

THE ACID-FIXING POWER OF THE BLOOD

For convenience, the acid-fixing power of the blood may be termed 'oxy-'desis" (ὀξύ, acid; δέσις, to bind).† It is evident that the first effect of kidney lag is a back-up of acid salts (or basic salts) in the blood-stream, and the condition of acidosis or alkalosis may then be said to exist regardless of the acidity of the urine, the rate of ventilation, the carbonic acid content of the blood or of alveolar air. The hydrogen-ion concentration of the blood varies within such narrow limits in health that it may be said to be a constant. The oxydetic power of a unit volume of blood likewise represents an equilibrium between acid and base that in health approaches constancy. Indeed its relation to the hydrogen-ion concentration is much the same as the rim of the wheel to its hub. Henderson[2] believes that acidosis is even more common in pathologic states than fever. If oxydesis be a constant in health as the observations thus far made seem to indicate, any fall below the established figure will mean an impairment of renal function, an excessive production of acid or a depletion of the alkali-store of the body. Conversely if in certain pathologic conditions there occur an excessive production of alkali, and under the new conditions the kidney be able to selectively secrete basic phosphate, any increase beyond the normal oxydetic value of the blood will denote alkalosis, with perhaps kidney lag.

*From the clinic of Drs. Hugo A. Freund and Bruce C. Lockwood.
†Suggested by Dr. Max Ballin.

Jour. Lab. & Clin. Med., v, No. 10.

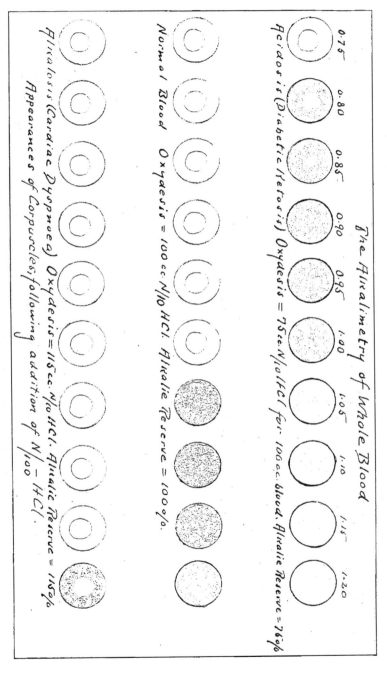

The Alkalimetry of Whole Blood

Acidosis (Diabetic Ketosis) Oxydesis = 75 cc. N/10 HCl for 100 cc. blood. Alkalic Reserve = 76%

Normal Blood   Oxydesis = 100 cc. N/10 HCl. Alkalic Reserve = 100%.

Alkalosis (Cardiac Dyspnoea) Oxydesis = 115 cc. N/10 HCl. Alkalic Reserve = 115%
Appearances of Corpuscles, following addition of N/100 HCl.

0.75   0.80   0.85   0.90   0.95   1.00   1.05   1.10   1.15   1.20

A SIMPLE METHOD OF BLOOD ALKALIMETRY

Ten test tubes are set up in a rack. To the first is added 9 c.c. of an 0.85 per cent salt solution (chemically pure salt in distilled water) and 1 c.c. whole, fresh oxalated blood (avoid citrate). A Folin blood pipette or a 1 c.c. differential bacteriologic pipette may be used for charging the successive tubes. The blood is mixed with the saline by drawing it up in the pipette a few times, and bubbles are avoided by always keeping the tip of the pipette below the surface of the fluid. One c.c. of the diluted blood is placed in the bottom of each tube, avoiding the sides, and then starting on the left N/100 hydrochloric acid is added with a 2 c.c. differential pipette, increasing the amount by 0.05 c.c. with each tube. The tip of the pipette should be poised at least two inches above the surface of the blood to insure rapid diffusion of the acid, which should be dropped directly into the blood and not touched off on the sides of the tubes. The tube once charged should be immediately shaken and the set should not again be disturbed until the cells have completely settled. They should be kept in a cool place where there are no fumes. If no acidosis be suspected the first tube may be started with 0.70 c.c. acid, the last thus receiving 1.15 c.c. About fifteen minutes are required to charge the tubes and from one to two hours for settling, depending on their diameters. The last tube which shows the erythrocytes sharply settled in the center without any evidence of hemolysis in the supernatant fluid, gives the oxydetic value of the blood. The next tube to the right will generally show the corpuscles scattered over the bottom in an irregular manner giving a speckled appearance and in the tubes following, slight hemolysis will be noted. Sometimes hemolysis occurs without evident agglutination or swelling of the corpuscles. This will vary with their fragility. The oxydetic value of whole blood is then the greatest amount of acid that can be added to a unit volume without damage to its corpuscles. The bloods of fifty random subjects who considered themselves in good health and who gave no evidence of impaired kidney function, showed with the exception of two, an oxydesis of one hundred, i.e., 0.1 c.c. of blood can absorb 1.0 c.c. of N/100 hydrochloric acid, and 100 c.c. of blood absorbs 100 c.c. of N/10 acid, under the conditions described.

SOURCES OF ERROR

Sodium oxalate, in spite of careful purification, and in a concentration of 10 mg. to five c.c. of blood, has an appreciable buffer action, because of the weakness of oxalic acid compared with sodium hydroxide as a base. The erythrocytes of fresh blood, containing no oxalate are invariably damaged by 1.0 c.c. N/100 acid, but not by 0.95 c.c., while oxalated blood first shows an excess of acid in the 1.05 c.c. tube.

For the collection of blood, one ounce salt mouth bottles are utilized, and to each is added 1.0 c.c. of a 1 per cent solution of sodium oxalate, that has been several times recrystallized from distilled water. The bottles are gently warmed in an oven, to evaporate the water, and the oxalate is thus spread over a large surface, clumping is obviated, and the corpuscles are not damaged.

The syringe and needle used should have been boiled in distilled water and dried before use, to avoid dilution of the blood. The blood should not be used if it has stood more than an hour at room temperature. Placed immediately in an ice-box it is available for twenty-four hours.

Any kind of test tubes may be used, but they must be thoroughly cleansed in chromic acid and finally in distilled water, dried and stoppered as in bacteriologic work. The pipettes must be accurately calibrated and deliver clean. Test tubes of from ⅝ to 1 inch diameter and 6 to 8 inches in length have been preferred because the cells settle more rapidly the shallower the layer of blood.

When carefully performed, this method of alkalimetry is one of precision, and any inaccuracy in measurement or contamination of glassware is made evident by the presence of "sports" in the series, showing hemolysis or agglutination out of order. It is not of course academically correct to say that a unit volume of blood will fix a certain amount of acid, as determined by damage to the erythrocytes. It requires about 0.05 c.c. of N/100 acid to agglutinate the washed corpuscles and the oxalate somehow accounts for 0.05 c.c. more. However, the method gives promise of service in the diagnosis of early stages of acidosis, the prognosis of the more severe grades and the early recognition of impairment of renal function. Dr. Freund and the present author will report elsewhere the results obtained with alkalimetry on the blood of patients representing a variety of pathologic conditions as determined by other laboratory tests.

REFERENCES

[1]Fitz and Van Slyke: Jour. Biol. Chem., 1917, xxx. 389.
[2]Henderson, L. J.: Oxford Medicine, 1, Part 4, p. 389.

VARIATIONS IN THE WASSERMANN REACTION*

By Eric R. Wilson, A.B., Los Angeles, Cal.

WE FEEL that the acceptance of a positive Wassermann of blood serum showing either a weakly-positive up to a two-plus reaction as a final diagnosis in cases giving a negative history and symptoms and deeming this sufficient indication for immediate antiluetic treatment, without first considering the possible variations which are bound to occur under any and all circumstances, is doing a gross injustice to the average patient.

In a great many cases which we have observed giving negative symptoms and history, a positive blood serum reaction has been obtained varying from a decided negative with one antigen to a pronounced two-plus reaction with another kind of antigen.

As to the different kinds of antigens employed. We have found the ordinary alcoholic extracts of normal organs to be inferior in every respect to that of the acetone-insoluble extract of beef heart, and this in turn to be inferior to an alcoholic extract of normal organs reinforced with cholesterin. The writer invariably uses both the latter antigens in all Wassermann serologic tests.

The cholesterinized extract gives a quicker, sharper, and more sensitive reaction than the acetone insoluble antigen to such an extent as that of giving a faint but decided positive reaction with some normal blood sera.

Again it has been shown that a positive Wassermann is present in other diseases such as leprosy, hepatic disease and scleroderma, which are far remote from syphilis.

*From the Department of Pathology, Bacteriology, and Laboratory Diagnosis, College of Physicians and Surgeons, University of Southern California.

We have observed that from twenty-four to seventy-two hours after either chloroform or ether anesthesia a normal blood serum will sometimes yield a positive reaction.

A point of great interest is the variation of a reaction over short periods of time, especially is this true in the variation from a weakly-positive or suspicious reaction to one decidedly negative over a period of from seven to sixteen days.

We cannot help but believe that some of the variations are accounted for to a greater or lesser degree by metabolic irregularities, especially when the physiologic balance of lipoid metabolism becomes disturbed.

We cannot too strongly emphasize that the tubes used for collecting the samples of blood to be tested be sterilized and that all sera should be tested as soon after collection as possible. We have repeatedly demonstrated that anti-complimentary substances develop in the sera if it be kept for considerable time, which not only inhibit hemolysis in the antigen and control tubes but certain substances are formed presumably by bacterial growth or bacterial action on some substance in the blood serum creating an inhibition of hemolysis in the antigen tubes alone, causing perhaps a negative serum to become positive.

In conclusion we earnestly plead that all facts be considered which may cause these variations before accepting as final a positive Wassermann test in which both history and symptoms are known to be negative.

BIBLIOGRAPHY

Kolmer: Infection. Immunity and Specific Therapy, 1917, W. B. Saunders Co., pp. 443-447.
Craig: The Wassermann Test, 1918.

SOME REMARKS ON THE QUESTION OF THE LEUCOCYTES IN ANAPHYLAXIS OF SERUM SICKNESS

By Jacob Rosenbloom, M.D., Ph.D., Pittsburgh, Pa.

IN a recent article Barach[1] has reported a study of the changes in the leucocytes in a case of serum sickness with a delayed anaphylactic reaction.

In this case he reports that *no* eosinophilia was present and on this account he states that eosinophilia is not a criterion of anaphylactic reaction.

I would like to call attention to the fact that *acute* anaphylactic shock and the ordinary serum sickness are characterized by a leucopenia with a reduction of the polynuclear cells and *no* change in the eosinophiles.[2] We expect eosinophilia in this relation only in cases of *nonacute* sensitization and as the case reported by Barach is an acute one, eosinophilia would naturally not be present.

REFERENCES

[1]Barach: Leucocytes in Anaphylaxis of Serum Sickness. Jour. Lab. and Clin. Med., 1920, v, 295.
[2]Bienenfeld: Das Verhalten der Leukozyten bei der Serumkrankheit. Jahr. f. Kinderheilk., 1907, lxv, 174.
Herrick: The Eosinophilia of Bronchial Asthma with Report of a Case Showing Extreme Blood Changes, Jour. Am. Med. Assn., 1911, lvii, 1836.

A MACHINE FOR SHAKING BLOOD COUNTING PIPETTES*

By Russell L. Haden, M.D., Detroit, Mich.

IN LABORATORIES where many routine red and white blood counts are done each day much time is consumed in shaking the pipettes by hand. A pipette shaking machine in use at the Mayo Clinic has been described by Little. This machine carries only two pipettes at a time and is rather complicated.

For the past two years we have used in our laboratory a pipette shaking machine designed and made for us by Eberbach & Son Company, of Ann Arbor, Michigan. We have found that much time is saved by its use and that more satisfactory preparations are obtained in the counting chamber, due to the more uniform suspension of cells in pipettes shaken mechanically.

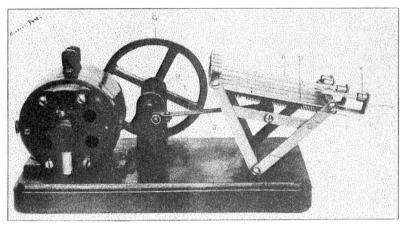

Fig. 1.

Fig. 1 shows all the essential details of the instrument. The base is a heavy cast iron block measuring 10 x 5½ x 1 in., set on rubber supports to diminish vibration. A one-sixteenth horse power motor is fastened to one end. On the other end is a pipette holder block (A). Each holder (B) is separate and can be adjusted to any length pipette by means of an arm (C) sliding in a groove and held in place by a spring (D).

The pipette holder block is attached to the base by a metal V-shaped frame (E) with shaft at (F).

Between the motor and pipette holder block there is a 4 in. wheel (G) connected by a belt to the spindle of the motor. To the counter shaft (H) of the

*From the Laboratory Department, Henry Ford Hospital, Detroit, Mich.

wheel is attached a crank (I) which is connected with the under part of the pipette holder block by a straight metal piece (J).

The pipettes are held in place by small cups (K) on the holders. Each cup is half filled with a solid soft rubber plug which prevents leakage of fluids and breakage of pipettes. It is necessary to have a rheostat to control the speed of the motor. This is placed under the laboratory table. The switch is in a similar position.

With the machine in motion the pipettes have a to and fro motion through an arc similar to that described in shaking pipettes by hand.

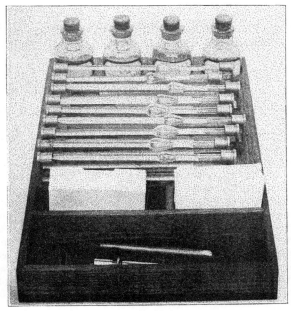

Fig. 2.

The block can be made to hold six or eight pipettes if desired. The machine can be easily adapted for other shaking purposes.

A spring clamp fitting over the cups of the outer holders enables one to use an Erlenmeyer flask. A small test tube can be used by putting a match stick through the cork and fitting it into the cup.

Similarly a frame to contain small bottles held in place by the pipette holder has been used.

The very convenient pipette holders have been made use of to hold pipettes on a tray used in collecting blood for counts in the hospital wards.

The tray Fig. 2 is shown in the accompanying photograph. It measures 6 x 10 x 1 in. The holder is similar to those on the shaking machine. The spring securing the sliding arm in the groove is placed on the upper instead of under side of the holder. Four holes are bored in one end of the tray to hold 20 c.c. bottles containing N/10 hydrochloric acid, Hayem's solution, dilute acetic acid, and alcohol. Compartments at the other end are provided for cover slips used in making blood films, and for pipette rubbers, blood lancet, and camel's hair brush.

The tray assembles in a convenient way everything needed to do blood counts. The holders prevent leakage of the fluids from the pipettes after filling, and diminish breakage.

A SATISFACTORY METHOD OF DEMONSTRATING GASTRIC MOVEMENTS ON A SMALL ANIMAL. COMPARATIVE STUDIES II*

By T. L. Patterson, M.A., M.Sc., Iowa City, Ia.

RESULTS of recent studies on the movements of the empty and filled stomach in some of the lower animals would make it seem desirable to record briefly a method of demonstrating gastric activity, inasmuch as it is quite satisfactory even in the hands of an amateur.

The methods of registering gastric movements in both hunger and digestion which have been conducted largely on man and the higher laboratory animals make it inconvenient for many of the smaller institutions to adopt due to a lack of proper facilities and equipment. Furthermore, in the case of the larger laboratory animals it requires several days of training before the animals are even in a condition for giving normal physiologic reactions, which is more time than can ordinarily be allotted to a single laboratory experiment. In addition, any disturbing influence, such as noise, tends to affect the animal, leading immediately to a more or less prolonged inhibition of the gastric movements, so that again, these animals in which quietness plays such an essential role are not best adapted for general laboratory use, and especially where the classes are of considerable size.

The method I have devised is based on three general principles: 1. On the balloon method of registration. 2. On an easily obtainable animal, the bullfrog (Rana catesbiana), the common species of frogs not being suitable on account of their smallness. 3. On the operation of stomostomy.

This very simple operation, requiring but a few moments for its completion after the anesthetization of the animal and without aseptic precautions, consists of making a circular opening on one side between the ramus of the inferior maxillary near the posterior angulosplenial region and the anterior cornua of the hyoid bone through the skin, the submaxillaris (mylohyoideus) muscle and the lining membrane of the pharyngo-oral cavity of about 8 mm. in diameter (Fig. 1). This operation may be bloodlessly performed, provided care is taken to avoid injury to the superficial mandibular vein (Vena maxillaris inferior)

*From the Physiological Laboratory, Queen's University, Kingston, Canada.

which courses along the insertion of the submaxillaris muscle and turns inwards at its hinder border to join the lingual vein.[1]

The gastric balloon is constructed from the lower portion of a condom which is of very delicate rubber, so that it will record definitely the stomach's activity. This is securely tied to one end of a long, flexible rubber tube (outside diameter 4 mm.), which contains a short piece of glass tubing (6-8 mm. in length) and of such a size as to slip easily into the lumen at the end of the tube thus preventing its occlusion. The balloon after being connected to the tube as above should be about 6 cm. in length (Fig. 2).

The stomostomy usually heals in from three to four days so that the animal is ready for physiologic study and the fast should be commenced a day or so previous to the operation. Through this opening the balloon may be introduced

Fig. 1.—Ventral view of frog's head showing location of stomostomy at S.

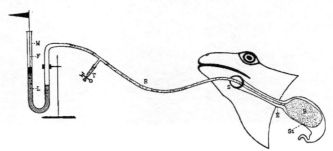

Fig. 2.—Diagram showing method of recording gastric movements of the frog's stomach. B, rubber balloon in stomach. M, manometer. F, cork float with recording flag. L, manometer liquid (water). R, rubber tube connecting balloon with manometer. . T, side tube for inflation of stomach balloon. S, stomostomy. E, esophagus. St, stomach.

by means of a glass seeker and then by opening the frog's mouth it may be carefully pushed into the stomach with the seeker through the short esophagus, which may be greatly enlarged, yet when empty is completely closed by folding of the walls. To accomplish this, set the frog against the side of a sink or box, grasp it with the left hand around the shoulders and body, then with the forefinger of the same hand raise the head slightly and proceed as above. The balloon should be inflated two or three times after its introduction into the stomach in order to straighten out the folds before being connected with the manometer. In this manner the small rubber tube lies under the free edge or at the side of the tongue, passes through the stomostomy to the side tube and thence to the manometer carrying the float. In this position the balloon may be inflated through the side tube until the manometer indicates a pressure of about 2 cm. which has proved to be the best pressure for recording stomach movements of this animal. By this method, the stomach pressure fluctuations are transmitted by air transmission to the surface of the liquid in the manometer and recorded graphically by the writing point of the float on a 50 to 60 minute drum, without any danger of it being interrupted by the animal biting on the rubber tube, as would be the case if the tube passed between the jaws. The animal during the experiments or when tracings of the gastric movements are being recorded may be placed in a small laboratory sink about 7 x 10 x 5 inches, or if this is not available any other small compartment may be used. In either case, the bottom should be covered with filter paper, kept well moistened and the top covered with the exception of a very small opening to admit air and the rubber tube or tubes of the apparatus.

With this arrangement the animal is well concealed from most disturbing influences and the sinks or other compartments being darkened by opaque covers,

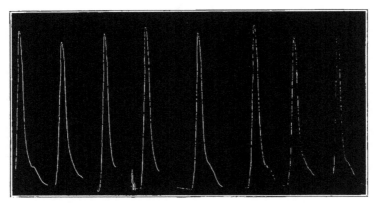

Fig. 3.—Normal contractions of the empty stomach of the frog after a fast of four days.

the animal feels itself securely hidden and will remain quiet for long periods of time unless directly disturbed which always leads to a more or less prolonged inhibition of the gastric movements.[2,3] The introduction of the balloon itself will lead to a temporary inhibition lasting usually from 20 to 50 minutes and if the animal is being used for the first time typical and regular contractions of the stomach may not be obtained for a much longer period. The best way to deal with a new animal is to introduce the balloon and then leave it entirely alone, unless it throws out the balloon in which case replace it as often as it occurs.

The gastric hunger contractions of the frog are practically continuous, with no indication of any periodicity, while the tonus changes of the stomach musculature are so slight as to be practically a negligible factor and for this reason only one type of hunger contraction is exhibited. This particular type of contraction shows an average duration of about one and three-fifths minutes, and the intervals between the contractions vary from sixteen to thirty-three seconds. These contractions are remarkably strong, sustaining a column 15 to 22 cm. high.

The contraction phase is abrupt, while the relaxation is slower. The curve is perfectly smooth, showing no smaller superimposed waves and no indication of the contractions falling into groups separated by periods of relative quiescence, as is the case in all the higher animals (Fig. 3). The amplitude of these contractions increases during prolonged fasting, but there is no obvious increase in tonus.

For the digestive movements, the cannibalistic bullfrog may be fed a couple

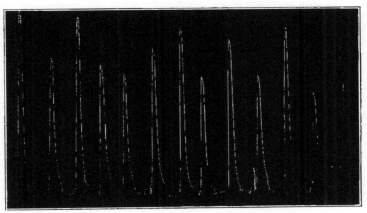

Fig. 4.—Normal digestive peristalsis of the frog's stomach four hours after feeding two live grass frogs.

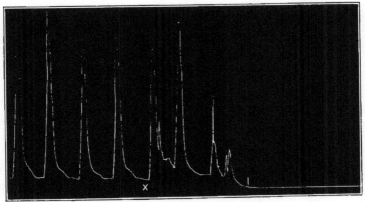

Fig. 5.—Normal contractions of the empty stomach of the frog after a fast of five days, showing inhibition from introducing directly into the stomach at X, 5 c.c. of 0.5 per cent solution of hydrochloric acid.

of live grass frogs and the balloon reintroduced into the stomach after thirty to sixty minutes to allow sufficient time for the asphyxiation of the ingested frogs. The digestive peristalsis when compared with the normal hunger records shows but very little change from the stomach of the animal in hunger, the only observable variation being a slight increase in the rate of the contractions (Fig.

4). Figs. 3 and 4 probably show the maximal variation of increased rate, for more often there is much less differentiation between these two conditions.

The inhibition of the gastric hunger contractions may be studied on the frog by introducing slowly through a second rubber tube, one end of which is attached to the balloon end of the first tube, such substances as water, sodium carbonate, 1 per cent solution, and hydrochloric acid, 0.5 per cent solution, in amounts of about 5 c.c. These substances invariably produce temporary inhibition, the duration depending on the nature of the substances introduced, it being the most marked in the case of the acid and least with the water (Fig. 5). These inhibitory effects may also be produced on the digestive movements of the frog in the same manner, but such substances do not inhibit the digestive peristalsis in the higher animals.

REFERENCES

[1]Ecker, A.: The Anatomy of the Frog (transl. by George Haslam), Oxford, 1889, pp. 34, 62, 64. 242.
[2]Patterson, T. L.: Am. Jour. Physiol., 1916, xl. 140.
[3]Patterson, T. L.: Am. Jour. Physiol., 1916, xlii, 56.

The Journal of
Laboratory and Clinical
Medicine

VOL. V.   JULY, 1920   No. 10

Editor-in-Chief: VICTOR C. VAUGHAN, M.D.
Ann Arbor. Mich.

ASSOCIATE EDITORS

DENNIS E. JACKSON, M.D.	CINCINNATI
HANS ZINSSER, M.D.	NEW YORK
PAUL G. WOOLLEY, M.D.	DETROIT
FREDERICK P. GAY, M.D.	BERKELEY, CAL.
J. J. R. MacLEOD, M.B.	TORONTO
ROY G. PEARCE, M.D.	AKRON, OHIO
W. C. MacCARTY, M.D.	ROCHESTER, MINN.
GERALD B. WEBB, M.D.	COLORADO SPRINGS
WARREN T. VAUGHAN, M.D.	BOSTON

EDITORIALS

Pneumoperitoneum and Abdominal Diagnosis

INFLATION of the peritoneal cavity for diagnostic purposes is a relatively recent innovation. The first instance on record, however, in which this method was employed on human beings occurred eighteen years ago, when Kelling introduced oxygen into the abdominal cavity in a case of ascites and in one of gastric carcinoma.

Oxygen inflation of body cavities as an adjuvant in the use of the roentgen ray has long been in use. The lungs, naturally air-containing, indicated to the early observers the advantages, and air injection into the bladder, the renal pelves, and joint capsules has become quite a common procedure. Conversely, the x-ray has frequently been employed to control lung collapse in artificial pneumothorax. Air inflation of the stomach has been used in roentgenology for study of that organ as well as surrounding organs, particularly for the diagnosis of pericardial effusion. The air-containing colon throws the spleen into good relief on the x-ray plate. Ventriculography, the raying of air-filled cerebral ventricles, has been decidedly helpful in cases of internal hydrocephalus and in the diagnosis and localization of certain brain tumors.

The pioneer workers in pneumoperitoneum introduced air or oxygen into the abdominal cavity in cases of ascites after withdrawing the fluid, employing therewith the method of endoscopy or laparoscopy.   Using the Jacobus endoscope in the same manner as the urethroscope and cystoscope are used, they were able to study the appearance of the abdominal organs, particularly the liver, over a limited area and without operation.   This method never proved extremely successful and could be used in such a small number of cases that it has never come into general practice.

Later it was found that gas could without harm to the patient be introduced into the peritoneal cavity of nonascitic individuals.   Roentgenograms of individuals so treated have shown that the parenchymatous organs of the abdomen and pelvis, particularly the liver, spleen and kidneys, may be brought into as clear detail as are the heart and lungs in thoracic plates.   The following types of diseases have been diagnosed by this method: carcinoma of the liver; hepatic cirrhosis; other tumors and irregularities of the liver and spleen; peritoneal carcinosis and cancer nodules on the diaphragm; gall stones and other lesions in the region of the gall bladder; peritoneal adhesions, particularly to the anterior abdominal wall; carcinoma of the ascending colon; cystic ovaries and uterine myomata; enlarged mesenteric glands; echinococcus cysts of the liver.

Detail of the kidneys, while not as clear as that of the liver and spleen, is decidedly better than that of the ordinary renal plate.

The technic of gas inflation has been variously described by different authors.   The patient must be prepared as for bismuth studies, the intestines being thoroughly cleansed and the bladder emptied.   The patient lies on his back. The skin of the abdomen is scrubbed and painted with iodine over the area selected for paracentesis.   This point is usually a little to the left of and below the umbilicus.   If adhesions are supposed to be present in a certain area or if there is a scar of an old operation it is important to avoid such area.   The skin is anesthetized with an ethyl chloride spray, an ordinary lumbar puncture needle is passed in obliquely, and cautiously pushed through the fascia into the peritoneum. The stylet is removed, the needle connected by a sterile rubber tubing to an oxygen tank, and sufficient oxygen is allowed to flow into the cavity until the abdomen becomes dome-shaped or the patient complains of distention or mild painful sensations between the shoulders.   The gas is then cut off and the needle withdrawn.   From two to four liters of oxygen are usually required.   The injection should take from ten to twenty minutes' time.

The volume of gas may be controlled and measured in a system of bottles similar to those used in producing artificial pneumothorax.   The air or oxygen may be bubbled through sterile warm water.   Some German writers, notably Schmidt and Rautenberg use an ordinary air bellows to produce inflation.   The tendency appears to be towards simpler methods, but these should not be adopted at the price of increased risk of infection.   With an oxygen tank the volume administered may be measured by attaching a rubber bag similar to that used in gas-oxygen outfits.   As a rule the oxygen or air is not sterilized.   During abdominal operations the peritoneum is exposed to nonsterile atmospheric air and this of itself does not result in infection.   No untoward results in infection have so far been reported following pneumoperitoneum.

There seems to be little or no danger of injuring a loop of intestines.   If a needle be passed through the abdominal wall of a rabbit the intestines are found to always recede before the sharp point. After death the intestines are easily punctured in this way. Pneumoperitoneum practiced on well over two hundred cases has resulted in no reports of injury to the intestines. Care in introducing the needle slowly and the usual surgical asepsis should of course always be rigidly observed.

Schittenhelm suggests a method of puncture which should appeal as enabling the operator to know definitely when the point of the needle has entered the peritoneal cavity. He has attached to the lumbar puncture needle an all-glass syringe containing physiologic salt solution. During the slow passing of the needle through the abdominal wall, gentle pressure is exerted on the plunger of the syringe. When the liquid flows easily the cavity has been reached.

Fluoroscopic examination is quite satisfactory. Plates are especially valuable. For best results it is important to take plates through several planes and with the patient in different positions. The principle to be borne in mind throughout is that the organ to be studied should be in the highest possible plane so that it will be surrounded by air and the intestines will fall away and not obstruct the view. For studies of the liver and spleen the patient should be upon his abdomen and the head end of the table should preferably be slightly raised. For plates of the right or left kidney he should lie on his left or his right side as the case may be, the tube should be in front of his abdomen and the plate at his back. For pelvic studies he should lie on his abdomen and the foot end of the table should be raised about 15 degrees. The intestines will then fall out of the pelvis. The tube is placed beneath the table and focussed on the promontory of the sacrum. Studies of the anterior abdominal wall for adhesions or other pathology of the peritoneum, are made with the patient supine, the rays being directed transversely through from side to side.

For examination of the stomach Schmidt recommends air inflation of that organ just preceding inflation of the peritoneal sac. Transverse plates with the patient supine after such preparation show excellent pictures of such conditions as carcinoma of the lesser curvature. Colonic inflation in the same way will often show pathology in that portion of the intestines or will improve the picture of the spleen or left kidney.

The procedure is not without some inconvenience to the patient. With a gas-filled abdomen he frequently suffers an unpleasant feeling of distention or he may complain chiefly of dyspnea. If he stands up he may have rather severe pain in the region of the shoulders, particularly the right. The gas is usually resorbed within 24 to 48 hours, but the patient, if he does not remain in bed, may be quite uncomfortable for three or four days. Two remedies for this drawback have been suggested. Schmidt uses a special needle of the same size and shape as a lumbar puncture needle and bevelled at the tip, but with a solid tip and a stopcock at the proximal end of the needle. The air enters the peritoneal cavity through a side slit just behind the solid tip. After the abdomen has been filled, he leaves the needle in place with stop cock closed. When the examination is completed he opens the cock and allows the air to slowly escape. Gentle pressure in the flanks aids in the deflation.

Alvarez uses instead of air or oxygen, carbon-dioxide gas. This is absorbed very rapidly and produces no apparent ill effects. It is usually all absorbed within a half hour—so rapidly in fact that considerable skill is required to take all necessary plates before too much of the gas has disappeared.

Pneumoperitoneum represents a diagnostic method of value equal to that of bismuth studies. The two methods are not competitors. Whereas, the latter is useful in the study of pathology of the stomach and intestines, the former enables us to gain further information of the parenchymatous organs of the abdomen. With the exception of some discussion of the temporary discomfort of the patient, all reports so far have been very favorable to the procedure. It is certainly a valuable diagnostic method, but the enthusiasm of the pioneer workers must not allow us too great a sense of security. A new method that fills so great a need as does this will probably be used very widely and at times perhaps a little carelessly. A few unnecessary accidents have been known to bring good methods into disrepute. Thorough physical examination should always precede the operation, particular attention being devoted to study of the cardiovascular apparatus. Carbon dioxide would not be used where there is any possibility of a tendency to acidosis. Until the technic has been mastered cases should be treated as hospital patients and watched during return to normal.

REFERENCES

Stein, Arthur, and Stewart, William H: Roentgen Examination of the Abdominal Organs Following Oxygen Inflation of the Peritoneal Cavity, Ann. of Surg., 1919, lxx, 95.
Stewart, W. H., and Stein, A.: (Same Title), Am. Jour. Roent., 1919, vi, 533.
Schittenhelm, A.: Reviewed in Am. Jour. Roent., 1919, vi, 584.
Rautenberg, E.: Pneumoperitoneale Röntgendiagnostik, Deutsch. med. Wchnschr., 1919, No. 8, p. 203.
Schmidt, Adolf: Ein Neues Verfahren zur Röntgenuntersuchung der Bauchorgane, Deutsch. med. Wchnschr., 1919, No. 8, p. 201.
Alvarez, Walter C.: California State Jour. of Med., February, 1920.
Whitman, Armitage.: Oxygen Inflation of the Peritoneal Cavity: a Personal Experience, Jour. Am. Med. Assn., 1920, lxxiv, 1021.

—*IV. T. V*

Recent Work On Vitamines

EVEN when the requirements of the animal body for calories and protein building stones are fully met, the diet will fail to maintain health unless it also contains substances of unknown chemical nature called "accessory food factors" or "vitamines." These are entirely of plant origin, and require to be taken only in very small quantities to display their beneficial action. They do not become rapidly destroyed in metabolism, but may remain attached to the tissues for a sufficient time so that carnivorous animals obtain them indirectly.

Serious and prolonged absence of certain vitamines from the dietary may hinder the growth of young animals or may be the cause of serious disease in adults. Great advancement in our knowledge of vitamines had been made in recent years, particularly through the work of F. Gowland Hopkins and Hariette Chick,[1] Osborne and Mendel,[2] Funk[3] and McCollum.[4]

There are at least three different vitamines which are characterized partly by the nature of the diseased condition which their absence from the diet occasions, and their influence on the growing animal, and partly by their solubilities.

The human diseases which are known definitely to be due to the absence of one or other of the vitamines are beriberi, scurvy, and rickets, and accordingly three vitamines are distinguished:

1. Antiberiberi or antineuritic vitamine (also called water-soluble "B" growth factor).

2. Antirachitic vitamine (also called fat-soluble "A" growth factor).

3. Antiscorbutic vitamine.

Investigation of the distribution of these factors among the various foodstuffs, and their degree of stability towards heating, etc., has been very materially facilitated by the fact that certain of the lower animals suffer diseases like those seen in man when vitamines are absent from the diet. This renders it possible to prosecute the investigations intensively and under scientifically controlled conditions, thus affording us the knowledge which enables us to alleviate human suffering.

The Antiberiberi or Antineuritic Vitamine.—Beriberi is a disease characterized either by wasting, anesthesia and paralysis, or by excessive edema. Pathologically, it is a form of severe neuritis. It is common in rice-eating communities, and the first clue to its precise cause was afforded by the observations that it does not occur among people who take unmilled rice, and that it disappears in those who take "polished" rice when the millings, or a watery extract of them, (pericarp and germ) are added to the diet. It was observed by Eijkman that the poultry of a prison where beriberi cases occurred exhibited symptoms very like those of the human disease, and further investigation showed extensive nerve degeneration to exist in the affected animals. Pigeons fed on polished rice develop exactly the same symptoms so that experimental investigation soon rendered it possible to determine with accuracy which foodstuffs prevent beriberi, and the further properties of the active substance.

Meanwhile McCollum and Davis[4] discovered that the absence of the same water-soluble vitamine interfered seriously with the growth of young animals. The withdrawal of the vitamine causes an immediate cessation of growth followed by a period during which the body weight remains more or less constant, but ultimately declines. During this stage muscular incoordination is a prominent symptom, and death ultimately occurs. This vitamine disappears from the organism immediately it is withdrawn from the food and the animal cannot synthesize it.

This vitamine is present in abundance in the seeds of plants and the eggs of animals. It is very plentiful in yeast and in yeast extracts, which may therefore be added to the diet when there is risk of its deficiency. It is absent from bread made with white wheat flour, but beriberi is rare in people living on this food, since other foodstuffs containing the vitamine are usually also taken. Beriberi is unknown where rye bread is a staple food.

The Antirachitic Vitamine (Fat-soluble "A" Factor).—The first inkling to the existence of this factor we owe to Stepp who found that mice could not live for long on foods from which all fatty substances had been thoroughly extracted by alcohol and ether. If the extract was restored to the extracted food, this again became adequate. Hopkins then showed in carefully controlled work that animals (rats) not only failed to grow, but declined and died when they were fed on artificial diet composed of the purified constituents of milk, although they might eat voraciously. The addition of a few drops of milk, insufficient to raise the energy or protein-value appreciably, invariably caused normal growth to return. Osborne and Mendel also found that although rats grew for about two months upon a diet containing protein, protein-free milk, starch and lard, they ultimately declined, but that this decline could be avoided by substituting butter for the lard, and that the active substance was concentrated in the butter-fat portion of the butter. Later work by various investigators showed that most animal fats, but not those of plants, contain this essential, and it was hence called fat-soluble A factor vitamine. Lard does not contain it, so that young animals fed with this as the only fat of an otherwise perfect diet fail to grow. An important difference will be observed in the curve of growth of young animals in the diet of which the factor B is alone deficient, namely that a small amount of growth continues for a time after the removal of the proper diet. This indicates that there must be some reserve of the fat-soluble vitamine in the body, and that it is only after this is exhausted that growth entirely ceases and decline then sets in.

When the reserves of the fat-soluble vitamine are exhausted, not only do the young animals fail to grow, but they become highly susceptible to bacterial disease, one symptom of which is a very characteristic eye infection (xerophthalmia) which begins with a swelling of the lids, and later develops into a purulent conjunctivitis, often leading to blindness. Administration of some fat-soluble vitamine in the diet dispels the eye symptoms usually within a few days. When the dietary of adult animals contains none of this vitamine the eye symptoms also develop, the general condition greatly deteriorates and the animals become extremely susceptible to bacterial infections, particularly those affecting the lungs, and from which they readily succumb. Adults are, however, much less susceptible to the absence of the fat-soluble vitamine than growing animals. This may be because of great storage capacity for it.

At the same time it is worthy of note that there is reason to believe that the condition known as war edema is due to a deficiency of this vitamine. It may be stated here that when both the A and B factors are absent from the diet young animals immediately cease to grow and develop the nervous symptoms due to the absence of the B factor, from which they usually succumb before the symptoms due to the absence of the A factor have had time to develop.

A most important relationship probably exists between this vitamine and the occurrence of *rickets*. Thus, when the puppies of large dogs are fed with separated milk, bread, linseed oil, yeast and orange juice, they grow at a normal rate, but in about six weeks develop undoubted symptoms of rickets (bones defectively calcified so that the long bones bend, swelling at the epiphyses, a rosary at the costochondral junctions, the ligaments loose, general lethargy and loss of muscular tone). In this diet both the water-soluble and the antiscorbutic factors are present in abundance (the yeast and the orange juice), but the fat-soluble factor is very low. Evidently linseed oil contains a sufficient trace of this factor to allow of an abnormal form of growth in puppies. When animal fats, such as cod liver oil or butter, are substituted for the linseed oil in the above, or a similar diet, rickets does not occur. It should be noted, however, that lean meat and meat extracts contain more of the antiscorbutic factor than can readily be attributed to the amount of fat in them.

There are two main sources for the fat-soluble vitamine, (1) certain animal fats, and (2) green leaves. It is particularly abundant in cream, butter, beef fat, fish oils (particularly cod liver oil and whale oil) and egg yolk. It is absent or present only in traces in most vegetable oils, such as linseed, olive, cotton seed, but in some of them such as peanut oil it is present in larger amounts.

Its presence in green leaves stands out in contrast to its absence from root vegetables. It is also present in certain cereals and pulses.

The Antiscorbutic Vitamine.—That this, at one time so prevalent, disease is definitely due to the absence in the dietary of some vitamine has been known in a general way for a long time. It used to be very common among the crews in the days of sailing ships, and nautical history records many interesting observations by captains and ship's surgeons showing that it could be prevented by adding certain fruits or the juices of fruits or vegetables to the daily ration. Indeed lime juice became a regular part of the mariner's ration. Great progress was made in the investigation of the precise distribution and behavior of the antiscorbutic vitamine by the discovery that guinea pigs develop the disease when all green stuff was removed from the diet and the animals were fed on grains and water or autoclaved milk. The symptoms appear in about 20 days, up to which time if young animals are used the growth curve continues. The symptoms of *postmortem* findings, similar to those seen in man, (tenderness and swelling in the joints, swelling of the gums, loosening of the teeth, tendency to hemorrhages and fractures of the bones). The curve of growth declines, and the animal dies usually about the 30th to 40th day. Important work is being done in the Lister Institute in London to determine the minimal amounts of various foodstuffs that are required in the scurvy diet to prevent the occurrence of the disease.

Regarding distribution it may be said that this vitamine is found in nature in all tissues which are actively undergoing metabolic change. It is abundant in growing green leaves, in fruits and in germinating seeds. But it is absent, or present only in traces, in dormant seeds, or in plant tissues that have been dried. It is also present, though less abundant, in fresh animal tissues and in milk. Although potatoes do not contain much of this vitamine, a diet composed mainly of them is seldom scorbutic because of the large quantities that are usually consumed. Canned vegetables and meats only contain traces of it because it is destroyed by the heating process. Canned fruits, however, contain more of it because it is preserved by the acid.

REFERENCES

[1]Hopkins, F. Gowland, and Chick, Hariette: Med. Research Committee National Health Insurance, Special Report No. 38, 1920, H. M. Stationary Office, Imperial House, Kingsway, London, W. C. 2.
[2]Osborne, T. B., and Mendel, J.: Jour. Biol. Chem., 1917, xxxi, 144.
[3]Funk, C.: Ergebnisse der Physiologie, 1913, xiii.
[4]McCollum, E. V.: Harvey Lectures, 1919, J. B. Lippincott Co., New York.
—*V. C. V.*

The Financial Support of Medical Education

IT IS highly gratifying to note the liberal way in which medical education in this country is being supported. These financial provisions are coming from the state and from private endowment, and both are welcome and at the same time are evidences of the high appreciation placed on the medical profession both by governmental agencies and by private individuals.

Under the influence of Thomas Jefferson the State of Virginia was, if we remember correctly, the first in the Union to make provision for the education of medical students. When the territory of the Northwest was partitioned and divided into territories, which subsequently became states, provision for state medical education was made by Indiana and Michigan. For many years the University of Michigan Medical School was the most important and prominent of all state university medical schools. This institution was opened in 1850 and has now passed through seventy years of its existence. The Legislature of 1919 made, without a dissenting vote, liberal appropriation for the medical school. This indicates that after seventy years of trial the state is satisfied, or at least well pleased, with the work which has been done by its medical school. During these seventy years state medicine has developed gradually, but constantly and healthfully, in Michigan. From time to time the Legislature of the State has passed acts which have provided for the treatment of certain people in the state, either at state or county expense. There is not in the state a cross road from which some individual has not come to University Hospital, received treatment and been benefited thereby. University Hospital is, therefore, regarded by the legislature as one of the most efficient institutions in the state. From every county patients are sent to this hospital each year. Poor people of respectability are kept from passing into the bounds of pauperism by being relieved of their physical disabilities. One act of the legislature provided for the treatment of children whose parents or guardians are unable to pay. This worked so well and the beneficial results were so in evidence that a few years later an act was passed to provide free hospital service and medical and surgical treatment for persons afflicted with a malady or deformity which can be benefited by hospital treatment who are unable to pay for such care and treatment, and for pregnant women unable to pay for such care and treatment and for the children of such pregnant women born during the period of hospital care, and providing for the expense thereof, and prescribing the jurisdiction of the probate court in said cases. This law also has been found beneficial to the people of the state at large. Recently the State of Iowa has in sum and substance copied these laws, and still more recently this has been done in the State of Wisconsin. Most of the state universities in the Northwest and in the West have their medical schools and so far as we know they are liberally supported by their respective legislatures. This indicates an appreciation of medical education on the part of the public that is highly gratifying. Very recently the Legislature of Wisconsin in special session has appropriated, as we understand, more than $1,000,000 for a state hospital, and has provided for the development of a four-year medical school at Madison. The splendid work already done in that institution in the two-year course justifies this enlargement. We hope that the appreciation of state medicine will continue to grow and that the time will soon come when every community will have its hospital where all classes of people may be examined by experts in the different lines of medicine and surgery and from which health work will radiate throughout the country. The State of Illinois has made an appropriation for its medical school and, as we understand it, the university authorities have already planned large developments, including ample hospitals, laboratories, and equipment.

In former centuries universities were founded for the most part for the purpose of teaching some religious dogma or creed. We had not only Protestant and Catholic universities, but the former were divided among Unitarians, Congregationalists, Presbyterians, and so on *ad infinitum*. Some universities have been built and endowed for the purpose of perpetuating the name of some wealthy man. All of these purposes have been laudable and have been much to the benefit of mankind at large. State universities, however, are built and supported by the people and for the purpose of making better citizens. It is not a function of the state university to admit feeble-minded or the vicious, or even to coddle its students. The state makes provision elsewhere for those of these classes. The purpose of a state university is not to make shyster lawyers or quack doctors, nor is it its purpose to enable men and women to make an easy living. The sole justification for the existence and continuance of state universities is that they provide a better citizenship. When the ordinance of 1787, providing for the territory of the Northwest, was written, its framers expressed one of their purposes in the following statement: "Religion, knowledge and morality being necessary to good government and to the happiness of mankind, schools and the means of education shall forever be encouraged." The country for which provision was then being made was at the time for the most part a wilderness of primeval forests and unbroken prairies. It has since become the very heart and core of the nation and is now appropriately called "the valley of democracy." It is pleasing to think that the spirit of the framers of the ordinance of 1787 has never perished, but has been and still is with us. The time has come for us to write into a new ordinance: there shall be no physical suffering among our people, which human skill can relieve, allowed to go unrelieved. Descartes said centuries ago, in sum and substance, that if man is ever brought to the highest possible degree of physical, mental, and moral perfection it must be through the agency of preventive and curative medicine. There is no better index to the intelligence of a people than the attention which is given to the relief of suffering among its people.

We now turn to the equally gratifying evidences of the appreciation of medical education shown by wealthy men. Mr. Rockefeller continues to give from his boundless millions for the support of medical education, and he has given wisely. During the past few months several millions have been distributed among the medical schools in this country and in Canada. The latest thing that has been done by the Rockefeller Foundation, aided by Mr. Eastman, is the very liberal provision made for a medical school in connection with the University of Rochester. This is an old institution and one which has made a highly honorable record, and we rejoice greatly that it is now to be supplied with ample provision for a medical school. Medical education is costly and there are none too many good medical schools in this country; and what is more gratifying than anything else is that practically all these schools are good ones. It is often said that we have too many physicians already in this country. Some one figures out that we have about one doctor for every seven or eight hundred inhabitants, and calls attention to the fact that no such abundance of doctors exists in any of the European countries. If medicine is going to reap its richest rewards, and it can do this only by rendering its greatest service, there must be more skilled physicians than there are at present. One doctor to eight hundred persons convinces most of us that there are already too many physicians. Probably there are, under the system of practice now in vogue, but if state medicine is to come, and we would be loath to think it possible for it to fail to come, we shall need many times the number of physicians we now have. The army regulations provide for seven medical officers for every one thousand enlisted men and the enlisted medical corps is ten per cent of the force. It is a safe estimate to say that among 100,000,000 people the number of those daily sick is not less than 3,000,000. We shall leave it for some one else to compute how many doctors and nurses would be necessary to give the best attention to these people. The army regulations provide that hospital beds shall number not less than five per cent of the strength of the command. There will probably never be so large a demand for hospital beds among civilian populations, but the number now in existence will need to be multiplied many times.

Besides attending to the physical needs of the people, medical research must be provided for more abundantly in the future than is done at present. We know but little as yet concerning the diseases that most commonly afflict us. What do we know about measles? How much have we done to restrict this disease? What is its cause? How much is the death rate in this disease affected by secondary infections? What can we say about the accuracy of any morbidity statistics that we have pertaining to this disease? What is the average death rate in uncomplicated measles? What is the death rate in measles complicated with pneumonia? Are there epidemic waves of measles, and if so, what do we know about the periodicity of these waves? What can we do to forestall or to modify an epidemic of this disease? These are simply samples of the innumerable illustrations that might be employed to show the depth of ignorance in which we still find ourselves so far as knowledge of one of the most common of the communicable diseases of infancy and childhood is concerned.

In expressing our high appreciation of the financial support now being given to medical education in this country, let us not forget that this appreciation will grow greater or smaller according to the service rendered by the profession to the well being and development of the people. While we are happy that the people at large, as represented by state and municipal governments, and great individual philanthropists, are bestowing upon the profession their favors with a liberal hand, let us see to it that the profession justifies this confidence.

The Spontaneous Disappearance of Yellow Fever from Certain Localities

CARTER[1] says that yellow fever has spontaneously disappeared from certain small ports in the West Indies, South and Central America. He says that for the spread of yellow fever in a community the following three factors are needed: (1) The presence of a person or persons in the early stages of a yellow fever attack, (2) a sufficient number of active stegomyia, (3) the presence of susceptible persons. These factors must be operative at the same time. The stegomyia acquires the infection by biting a patient in the early stages of the disease. This mosquito must then transmit the virus to a nonimmune. If there are no susceptible persons the disease dies out for want of soil in which to grow. Susceptibles must be not only present, but must be present under certain conditions of time and place with relation to mosquitoes infected from other persons with the disease. If in a given community there are no susceptible persons complying with these conditions yellow fever will disappear; in other words, yellow fever will disappear as soon as the already infected mosquitoes die. It follows, therefore, that the immigration of susceptible material to yellow fever localities is necessary for the continuance of the disease. The ports which have been spontaneously freed from this disease receive little or no immigration of susceptible persons. It has been observed that other localities have suffered less and less from yellow fever as their prosperity declined and the arrival of traders and others decreased. The decline of the sugar industry in some of the West Indian Islands has led to this result. The withdrawal of European garrisons and fleets from the endemic area of yellow fever has resulted similarly. Even the War has helped to stamp out yellow fever on account of the commercial depression felt most keenly in certain small places in the endemic area. Carter believes that in time yellow fever may be entirely exterminated. He says that many of the higher forms of life have permanently disappeared from the earth, some of them even in our own times. He thinks this might be made an international basis for the extermination of a virus which has proved itself so pathogenic to man and which in the past has taken heavy toll of human life.

—V. C. V

Fatal Anaphylaxis Following the Prophylactic Administration of Antitetanic Serum

GURD and Roberts[2] report the case of a soldier who, a few hours previously had received several small bomb wounds on both hands, the right thigh, and the left calf. All wounds were in and of themselves unimportant and the patient was apparently in good condition, being a well built man of about thirty years of age, with normal pulse and temperature. Inasmuch as the soldier had not received antitetanic serum before being wounded, he was given at 11:15 A.M. 5 c.c. of antitetanic serum subcutaneously over the right pectoralis major muscle.

[1] Ann. Trop. Med. & Parasitology, xiii, 4.
[2] The Lancet, London, April 3, 1920.

There was no disturbance until 1:30, when the soldier began to vomit and had a bloody diarrhea. Between 1:30 and 5 P.M. he vomited eight times and had six bowel movements. At the last-mentioned hour his pulse was 104 and his temperature 102.8°. The collapse continued during the night and at 6 A.M. on the next day the pulse was feeble and the beat 180. Death resulted at 10:30 A.M. on that day. The authors state:

"In so far as we are able to discover, the patient had not been previously wounded, nor had he received at any other time injections of horse serum. That he was an individual presenting a natural hypersensitiveness to horse serum is therefore a fair assumption. The fact that the same person is not infrequently sensitive to more than one foreign protein in all probability offers an explanation of the patient's history of repeated attacks of vomiting and bloody diarrhea. * * * That symptoms of respiratory spasm were not noted clinically is explained in part by the fact that, owing to pressure of work, the patient was not under constant supervision, and, more particularly, because the splanchnic reaction was predominant and so weakened the patient that expiratory dyspnea was not sufficiently evident to be noted by the sister in charge of the case. Deficient oxygenation of the tissues during life was evidenced by the extreme degree of cyanosis. It is now definitely established that man reacts to anaphylactic shock in one or other or both of two ways, in addition to the well-known cutaneous phenomena. Either he reacts in the manner which characterizes the phenomenon in the dog; i.e., splanchnic dilatation, drop in blood pressure, cardiac failure, and death—or in the way in which the typical reaction occurs in the guinea pig; i.e., bronchiole spasm, expiratory dyspnea, and death from arrest of respiration."

This case illustrates the necessity of giving first a minute dose of serum of any kind whenever administered.

—V. C. V.

The Diagnosis of Malaria

O'CONNELL[1] calls attention to the frequent want of harmony between the clinical and microscopic diagnosis of malaria. He mentions three cases diagnosed clinically as sunstroke but which were found by microscopic examination to have been malignant malaria; five cases of dysentery were found to be malarial enteritis; cases diagnosed clinically as relapsing and typhus fevers were shown to be malaria with relapses; cases believed at first to be influenza, on account of the prevalence of that disease, were subsequently shown to be malignant malaria. On the other hand, in Palestine, malaria is highly prevalent and here the microscope upsets all ideas of clinical experience. Parasites are found swarming in the blood of some, especially children, who exhibit no rise of temperature, and who are to all appearances in good health, whilst another suffering from what is clinically a typical malarial fever, not even one parasite can be found in the blood. Consequently, it is possible that the subsequent discovery of parasites in a patient's blood does not mean that the original clinical diagnosis of another disease must necessarily have been an error. Furthermore, failure to find parasites in the

[1]The Lancet, London, February 28, 1920.

blood during the first days of a primary attack of malaria does not exclude the possibility of the disease being malaria. The absence of parasites from the blood during the first few days of a primary attack of malaria was doubtless the reason that there were some who, when Laveran announced he had discovered parasites in malarial blood which were the cause of the fever, asserted that the bodies he discovered were not parasites but pseudoparasites. Their late appearance in the blood was given as a reason for regarding them as an effect and not the cause of the fever.

—V. C. V

Tuberculosis Research Fellowship, University of Minnesota

TO encourage study of the means for the prevention and cure of tuberculosis, the Hennepin County Tuberculosis Association of Minneapolis, Minn., announces that it has set aside a fund for the support of a tuberculosis research fellowship in the Graduate School of the University of Minnesota. The candidate for the fellowship must be a graduate of a Class A medical college. He will be expected to devote himself to research in some problem concerned with the causes, prevention, or cure of tuberculosis. No teaching or other service will be required. The fellowship yields $750 the first year and progressively increasing amounts to be appropriated for the second and third years as conditions warrant. Inquiries and requests for application blanks should be addressed to the Dean of the Graduate College, University of Minnesota, Minneapolis, Minn.

United States Training Corps for the Promotion of the Health of Women

THE United States Training Corps for Women is an organization incorporated under the laws of the State of Illinois not for pecuniary profit. From its inception the purpose of the organization met with the warmest commendation and support from official Washington and the leaders of constructive thought and action.

The organization had its origin in the necessity for conducted physical exercise brought about by the crowded office and housing conditions in Washington during the war, when many women were summoned to Washington to fill government positions vacated by men called to the colors. Thirty-five hundred office women were organized into thirty companies, or three regiments. They were given military drill, taught to stand erect, to breathe properly, and were given practical talks on health, hygiene, and sensible dress. The result in health and efficiency was so marked that it commanded the attention of the heads of the departments of the government, and at their suggestion and advice, the United States Training Corps was organized November 22, 1918.

A bill is at present pending to authorize the Secretary of War to grant the use of land and camp equipment to the United States Training Corps, and to detail army officers for service at recreational camps. When this bill passes, plans have been made for the establishment of five large recreational health camps for women to be located in the East, in the Southeast, in the West, in the Middle-West, and in the South. It is also planned to locate camps outside large industrial centers where women employees may live during the summer and go to and from their work. They will be under the direction of trained military leaders who will give the military drill and setting-up exercises adapted to women.

The first camp was conducted during the month of August, 1919, at Lake Geneva, Wisconsin, and proved to be a success. Camp No. 2 for 1920, will be held at Asheville, N. C., July 15, to August 25. The site selected is on a beautiful wooded knoll across the Country Club from the Grove Park Inn, commanding a wonderful view of the Asheville valley. While the spot is secluded and well adapted to the development of camp morale, it is within easy access of the train.

The purpose of the organization is to promote the health, efficiency and happiness of society, professional, home, and business women, and to send them home physically and mentally fit. Setting-up exercises for children in the public schools and in parks will also be emphasized. Any woman, twenty years of age or over, is eligible for membership, provided she brings a certificate from her physician stating that she has no communicable disease and is physically able to take exercise.

The Journal of
Laboratory and Clinical
Medicine

| Vol. V. | St. Louis, August, 1920 | No. 11 |

ORIGINAL ARTICLES

RUBBER TUBING AS A FACTOR IN REACTION TO THE BLOOD TRANSFUSION

By George J. Busman,* M.D., Rochester, Minn.

IN an article in the *Journal of the American Medical Association*, April 10, 1920, Dr. John H. Stokes and I described reactions of patients receiving intravenous injections of arsphenamine and alkaline solutions through a certain brand of rubber tubing. These reactions were characterized by chills, with a sharp rise in temperature coming on from thirty minutes to one hour after intravenous injection, and nausea, vomiting, diarrhea, pain in the head and back, and varying degrees of prostration. The reactions appeared in crops, so to speak, and then disappeared for a time, only to recur in the very midst of what seemed a period of flawless technical accuracy.

The results of a preliminary study of the possible causes of such reactions led us to the following conclusions:

1. A certain widely distributed brand of so-called pure gum rubber tubing seems to contain, when new, a toxic agent responsible for a definite type of reaction following the intravenous administration of arsphenamine, and possibly alkaline solutions and transfusion mediums.

2. The toxic substance gradually disappears from the tubing on use.

3. A pure gum rubber tubing can be made which does not produce reactions even when new.

4. The toxic substance is apparently removable in the first instance by soaking the tubing for six hours in normal sodium hydroxide solution and rinsing.

5. The toxic substance is not destroyed in the ordinary process of sterilization by boiling for from one-half to one hour; is not soluble in water or removable by irrigation; appears in toxic amounts in arsphenamine, neoarsphenamine, and dilute sodium hydroxide solution merely by passing them through a new tube 80 cm. long, enroute from container to vein, and is not apparently associated with the mechanically removable debris from the inner surface of the tube.

*Fellow in Dermatology and Syphilology, The Mayo Foundation.

6. The reaction can be induced in typical form in dogs.

That a certain number of persons have been observed to experience a somewhat similar reaction following blood transfusion by the citrate method led me to study the possible relation of this reaction to new rubber tubing. The transfusion reaction in question, although not so severe as that following the intra-

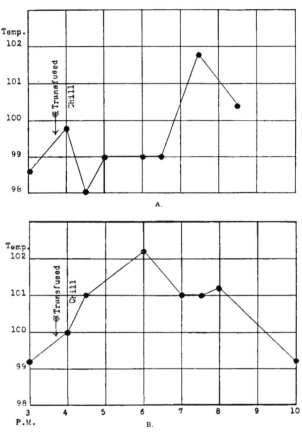

Chart 1. - Tubing reaction in man following transfusion by the citrate method in which new tubing had been used. Note that both patients developed a chill about one half hour after transfusion, followed by rise in temperature.

venous administration of arsphenamine through new tubing, consists of a chill coming on from one half to one hour after injection, a gradual rise in temperature (Chart 1), varying grades of prostration, and occasionally nausea and vomiting.

Considering the fact that the toxic substance is present in sufficient amounts to produce reactions in patients receiving the first ten to twenty-five injections of arsphenamine given through a new tube, 80 cm. in length, it is conceivable that if the toxic substance is soluble in blood or transfusion mediums a number of patients receiving blood transfusion through a new tube would show reaction. Since this number of transfusions in most clinics or hospitals would extend over a relatively long period, the reaction would have less tendency to occur in crops, and could even be a continuous feature of the work if another new tube were used before all the toxic agent had been removed from the old one.

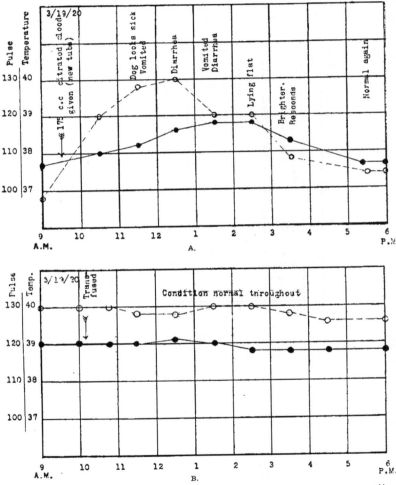

Chart 2.—A. Tubing reaction in a dog transfused through a sterilized new "pure gum rubber" tube with 175 c.c. of his own citrated blood. Note the fever, rise in pulse rate, vomiting and diarrhea. B. Control dog, which received an equal amount of his own citrated blood through "pure gum rubber" tube that had been in use for some time. Absolutely no reaction occurred. Solid line temperature; broken line pulse, in both charts.

The striking success of our efforts to duplicate in dogs the reactions following intravenous injections of arsphenamine led me to use the dog in my study of
the transfusion reaction. In order to approach as nearly as possible the technic
of transfusion in man, the experiments were performed with rigid asepsis. The
glassware used was Pyrex or Jena. About 80 cm. of the gum rubber tubing of 4
mm. internal diameter used in routine transfusion work were employed. This
tubing is identical with that employed in our arsphenamine work. It was boiled
for one-half hour and rinsed before using. Old tubing was used as a control
against the new in each experiment. Blood was drawn with continuous stirring

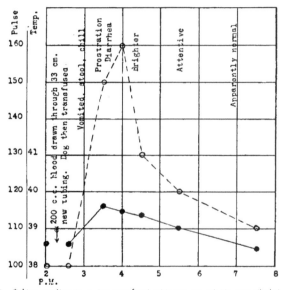

Chart. 3.—Tubing reaction in a dog transfused with 200 c.c. of his own titrated blood that had
been drawn from the vein to the container of sodium citrate solution through a sterilized new "pure
gum rubber" tube, 35 cm. in length. Note the chill, fever, diarrhea, vomiting, and prostration characteristic of the tubing reaction. A control dog that was transfused with 200 c.c. of his own citrated blood
that had been drawn from the vein to the container of sodium citrate solution through an equal length
of an old tube, showed no effect. Solid line temperature, broken line pulse.

into sterile flasks containing 2 per cent sodium citrate solution until a concentration equivalent to 30 c.c. of citrate solution to 250 c.c. of blood was reached. In
every instance, each dog was transfused with his own blood. Experiments as
follows were performed:

Experiment 1.—Two large healthy dogs were each transfused with 175 c.c.
of their own citrated blood, one through a new piece of tubing and the other
through a used piece of the same tubing. The dog that received his own blood
through the new tubing developed a severe reaction. The dog that received his
own blood through the used tube showed no change of pulse rate and temperature, and gave no clinical evidence of a reaction. About one hour after the injection the reacting dog showed a rise of pulse rate and temperature followed by

nausea, vomiting, diarrhea with tenesmus, prostration, rigor and tremors (Chart 2). The total rise in temperature was one degree centigrade and the increase of pulse rate, 30 per minute, the highest points being reached from three to four hours after the injection. The reaction subsided in about six hours.

Experiment 2.—The dog that had received his own blood through an old tube one week before, was given it through a new piece of tubing. A reaction occurred, although by the use of an old tube this dog had escaped reaction in the previous transfusion. In the same manner the dog that received his own blood through an old tube and showed no reaction had reacted severely the previous week to his own blood through a new tube.

Experiment 3.—A piece of the new tubing, 33 cm. long, was attached to a cannula inserted into the jugular vein of a dog and 200 c.c. of blood drawn through it from the vein to the flask containing the citrate solution. The same dog was then transfused with this blood through an old tube and a severe reaction resulted (Chart 3). This reaction began in about one-half hour with nausea, vomiting, rigor, diarrhea with cramps, sudden rise in temperature and pulse rate, followed by severe prostration. All evidence of the reaction disappeared in about six hours. The control dog whose blood was drawn through an old tube, citrated, and transfused through an old piece of tubing, showed no ill effects. It is apparent, therefore, that blood can take up the toxic agent from the tubing before citration, merely in passing from the vein to the container of citrate solution.

Experiment 4.—Two dogs each received 100 c.c. of a 0.23 per cent sodium citrate solution, one through a new tube and the other through an old one. The dog receiving the injection through the new tube developed a fatal reaction (Chart 4) characterized by vomiting, nausea, diarrhea with cramps, chills, rise in temperature and pulse rate, and prostration with death in three hours after injection.

Necropsy findings in this animal revealed only a severe, passive congestion of all organs, together with marked hemorrhages into the intestinal canal. The control dog that received the same amount of the sodium citrate solution through a used tube showed no effect.

Experiment 5.—The scrapings, dust, and debris mechanically removable from the inside of a sterilized tube, even when present in sufficient quantity to produce visible turbidity, induced no reactions in dogs when injected in suspension in distilled water, or 0.18 per cent sodium hydroxide solution, through a used tube.

Experiment 6.—Two hundred cubic centimeters of neutral redistilled water injected intravenously into dogs through new tubing induced no reaction.

Our previous observations have indicated that new tubing can be rendered harmless and incapable of producing reaction by soaking for six hours in normal sodium hydroxide solution.

SUMMARY

1. The brand of supposedly pure gum rubber tubing which in preliminary experiments by Stokes and Busman produced reaction in arsphenamine administration is apparently also able, when new, to produce reaction if used in blood transfusion work.

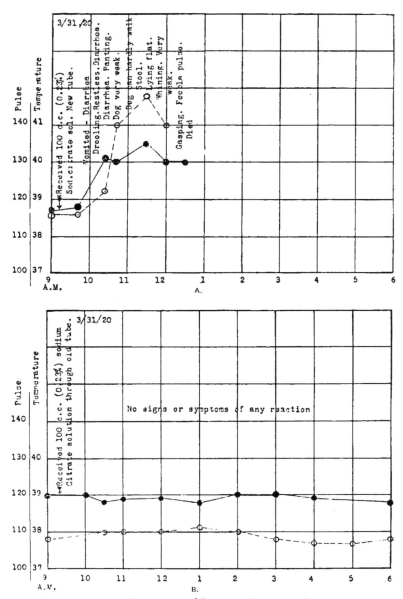

Chart 4.—A. Tubing reaction in the dog followed an intravenous injection of 100 c.c. of 0.23 per cent sodium citrate solution given through a new "pure gum rubber" tube. Note the vomiting, diarrhea, fever, high pulse rate, prostration and death. B. Control dog that received an equal dose of the same sodium citrate solution, but through a used "pure gum rubber" tube. Absolutely no reaction occurred. Solid line temperature; broken line pulse.

2. The toxic substance is taken up in sufficient amounts to produce reaction in patients receiving transfusions of citrated blood through 80 cm. of new rubber tubing of 4 mm. internal diameter.

3. Enough of the toxic agent is taken up by 250 c.c. of normal uncitrated blood drawn through as little as 35 cm. of new tubing (internal diameter 4 mm.) enroute from the vein to the container of citrate solution, to produce marked reaction when given through an old tube. It is not, therefore, necessary that whole blood be citrated to absorb the toxic principle.

4. The mechanically removable debris from the inside of new sterilized tubing does not produce reactions when given in suspension in distilled water or 0.18 per cent sodium hydroxide solution.

5. Further experiment confirms the observations previously recorded, that the toxic agent can be removed from the new tubing by soaking it in normal sodium hydroxide solution for six hours.

6. It should be specifically stated that no attempt is made to propose rubber tubing as an explanation of all transfusion reactions which present chills, fever, prostration, and so forth. Tubing is merely proposed as one factor.

7. The identity and toxicology of the poisonous principle is under investigation.

I desire to acknowledge the cooperation of my Chief, Dr. John H. Stokes, in the arrangement of this material.

CHEMICAL CHANGES IN THE BLOOD IN DISEASE*

V. Carbon Dioxide Combining Power

By Victor C. Myers, Ph.D., New York City

A LTHOUGH the phenomena of acidosis or acid intoxication would now appear to have been satisfactorily explained, it is only within the past five or six years that this has been accomplished. Progress in this subject has been particularly rapid since the advent of chemical methods of blood analysis. Of the different methods suggested to serve as an index of the degree of acidosis, the CO_2-combining power of the blood would appear to give the most reliable as well as the most useful information. The introduction by Van Slyke[1,2] of a relatively simple method of estimating the CO_2-combining power of blood plasma has given considerable impetus to the use of this determination as a practical clinical method. It is the object of the present paper to touch upon only the salient features of acidosis with particular emphasis on this method. For a more detailed discussion, reference may be made to the paper of Van Slyke and Cullen.[3]

The term acidosis, although originally coined by Naunyn to apply to the ketosis of diabetes, has come to be used in a much broader sense with the development of our knowledge of this subject. Obviously, acidosis may result either from an abnormal formation of acid substances, such as is found in diabetes, or from a decreased elimination of normally formed substances, as in nephritis. Under conditions of health, the blood is uniformly maintained at a constant slightly alkaline reaction through the influence of the bicarbonate, phosphate and proteins of the blood.

The carbonates of the blood have been called by L. J. Henderson the first line of defense. Increased pulmonary ventilation, as occurs with dyspnea or hyperpnea, serves to increase the excretion of carbon dioxide, thus keeping the reaction of the blood within normal limits. In conditions of acidosis, other acids may combine with the bicarbonate, robbing the body of its alkali reserve. Under ordinary conditions, however, the kidneys are able to secrete an acid urine from a nearly neutral blood through the medium of acid phosphate, constituting a second means of defense. From the investigations of Marriott and Howland[1] it appears that it is just this factor which breaks down in the acidosis of nephritis. They have found the inorganic phosphates of the blood serum increased to many times the normal in nephritic acidosis, although nephritic cases without acidosis did not show this change. Other means of defense against acidosis are the blood and body proteins, which are able to take up considerable amounts of acids without marked change in reaction, and the ability to form alkali, i. e., ammonia. The latter factor is of considerable importance in the

*From the Laboratory of Pathological Chemistry, New York Post-Graduate Medical School and Hospital.

acidosis of such conditions as diabetes and pernicious vomiting, but apparently of little significance in nephritis.[5]

DETERMINATION OF DEGREES OF ACIDOSIS

A number of different criteria have been suggested as a measure of the degree of acidosis: (1) lowered carbon dioxide combining power of the blood; (2) lowered alveolar carbon dioxide tension; (3) decreased affinity of hemoglobin for oxygen; (4) reduced alkalinity of the blood (Sellard's test); (5) increased hydrogen-ion concentration of the blood; (6) increased intensity of urinary acidity (hydrogen-ion concentration), and (7) the retention of alkali by the body in cases in which the kidney is capable of rapidly excreting an excess of alkali. Yandell Henderson[6] has also suggested the very simple test of holding the breath. A normal person can hold the breath 30 to 40 seconds without an especially deep inspiration, but the period diminishes in proportion to the reduction in the blood alkali.

All of these methods have furnished valuable information in the development of our knowledge of this subject, but the first, second and seventh have yielded information of special clinical value. Although the carbon-dioxide tension of the alveolar air may readily be ascertained with the Friderica[7] or the Marriott apparatus,[8] the information is not as reliable as the carbon dioxide combining power of the blood determined by the Van Slyke method. That the bicarbonate depletion may roughly be determined by administration of sodium bicarbonate has been pointed out by Sellards,[9] and by Palmer and Henderson,[10] and this method has been in practical use for several years. Normally from 5 to 10 gm. of sodium bicarbonate are sufficient to change the reaction of the urine, but in acidosis of advanced nephritis the deficiency may amount in exceptional instances to as much as 100 gm. of bicarbonate or more.

Palmer and Van Slyke[11] have recently studied this question in connection with the carbon dioxide combining power of the blood. They found that in most pathologic cases the urine did not become more alkaline than blood until a higher plasma bicarbonate had been reached than in normal individuals. This would result in the giving of unnecessary and possibly injurious amounts of bicarbonate, if the administration was continued until the urine turned alkaline, as has

TABLE I
THE CO_2-COMBINING POWER OF BLOOD PLASMA IN NORMAL SUBJECTS AND IN ACIDOSIS*

CONDITION OF SUBJECT	CO_2 CAPACITY OF PLASMA	FURTHER DROP OF CO_2 PERMITTED BEFORE INTERRUPTING FAST IN ALLEN TREATMENT OF DIABETES
	c.c. to 100	
Normal resting adult,** extreme limits	77-53	To 45 volume per cent
Mild acidosis, no visible symptoms	53-40	Drop of 10 to 5 volume per cent
Moderate acidosis, symptoms may be apparent	40-31	Drop of 3 to 2 volume per cent
Severe acidosis, symptoms of acid intoxication	Below 31	Fast interrupted in 6 to 12 hours unless CO_2 rises with fasting and alkali
Lowest CO_2 observed with recovery	16	

*Compiled from Stillman, Van Slyke, Cullen and Fitz,[13] and Allen, Stillman and Fitz.[14]
**The figures for normal infants are about 10 volume per cent lower.

been the usual clinical procedure. The bicarbonate retention may therefore indicate a much more severe acidosis than actually exists. Palmer and Van Slyke advise carefully controlling the therapeutic use of sodium bicarbonate. They have calculated that taking 42 pounds as the unit of weight, 0.5 gm. of sodium bicarbonate will raise the plasma carbon dioxide 1 per cent by volume. In view of this, it is possible to calculate the amount of alkali required to restore the plasma bicarbonate to normal.

The normal range for the carbon dioxide combining power of the blood in the adult, as shown by Van Slyke, Stillman, and Cullen,[12] is from 53 to 77 c.c. of carbon dioxide per hundred c.c. of plasma. For normal infants the figures are about 10 c.c. lower than in adults. An idea of the findings for the CO_2 in acidosis of varying degrees of severity may be obtained from Table I.

ACIDOSIS IN DIABETES

That acetone bodies appear in the urine in large amounts in cases of diabetes with acidosis has long been recognized and their amount taken as an index of the acidosis. Later it was noted that these cases showed a high output of ammonia and this was likewise employed to determine the severity of the acidosis. As indicated above, these findings led to some confusion because they could not be applied to the acidosis of nephritis. The defective oxidation of the fats in diabetes results in the formation of the acetone bodies, acetone, diacetic acid and β-hydroxybutyric acid. The reaction of these organic acids with the sodium bicarbonate of the blood, results in the taking up of sodium by the acids and the setting free of the CO_2, thus robbing the body of its alkaline reserve. What may happen in this respect in diabetes is shown in Table II.

TABLE II

ILLUSTRATIVE FINDINGS FOR THE CO_2-COMBINING POWER OF BLOOD PLASMA IN DIABETES

CASE	AGE	SEX	DATE	CO_2 COMBINING POWER	BLOOD SUGAR	REMARKS
				c.c. to 100	per cent	
1. B. S.	46	♀	8/25/15	12	0.42	Death in coma
2. U. W.	49	♂	2/27/19	25	0.79	Death in coma
			3/ 1/19	12	1.33	
3. A. F.	20	♂	11/12/18	32	0.86	Marked lipemia. Cholesterol
			11/19/18	39	0.41	0.64 per cent, left hospital improved
4. J. G.	51	♀	6/20/19	59	0.24	Improved
			6/28/19	46	0.24	
			7/ 7/19	55	0.25	
5. R. G.	45	♀	9/11/17	36	0.22	Improved
			9/18/17	52	0.20	
			10/ 9/17	53	0.19	
6. M. B.	27	♀	2/ 9/17	33	0.22	Marked improvement
			2/16/17	45	0.23	
			2/20/17	55	0.19	
			2/27/17	54	0.16	
			3/ 9/17	50	0.18	
			3/27/17	60	0.14	

The first two cases died in diabetic coma with CO_2-combining power figures of 12. Case 3 illustrates the findings in a case of severe diabetes, who was still up and about. This patient was referred to the writer (as a member of the Medical

Advisory Board) as to his availability for the Army, although the fact that he had diabetes was known. Except for shortness of breath and slightly impaired vision, this patient appeared to feel very well. At his own request he was admitted for a short stay in the hospital. The data on Case 4 and 5 illustrate the findings in the average case of diabetes, the latter showing a moderate acidosis. In Case 6 there was a gradual restoration of both the CO_2 and sugar to praetically normal.

The body is ordinarily able to handle quite large amounts of acids without a marked drop in the alkaline reserve. The tests for acetone and diacetic acid in the urine in diabetes and other conditions are valuable diagnostically, but they tell little concerning the severity of the acidosis. To secure this information it is necessary to resort to such tests as the carbon dioxide combining power of the blood.

In the treatment of diabetes, in particular by the Allen method so commonly employed, acidosis is more to be feared than hyperglycemia, and should be more carefully followed. With the fasting treatment the hyperglycemia is obviously effectively combated, but sometimes, as pointed out by Allen, Stillman and Fitz,[14] patients react to fasting with an increase of acidosis, occasionally to a dangerous degree. Rules which they have laid down to follow as to the drop in CO_2 permissible in this connection are given in Table I.

Both Allen and Joslin are opposed to the extensive use of sodium bicarbonate in the treatment of diabetic acidosis, believing that when not severe the condition may be more satisfactorily treated in other ways. Allen states[14] that fasting checks the acetone body formation and that accordingly the great majority of cases of acidosis can be treated by this means alone, and alkali holds no more than a minor adjuvant position. He has shown, however, that occasionally its use is of definite value either in combating a long and stubborn acidosis, or in combating coma in certain severe cases. Here it may save life.

ACIDOSIS IN NEPHRITIS

Many cases of renal disease show a more or less pronounced acidosis. In a recent report Chace and Myers[15] have concluded that all fatal cases of chronic nephritis with marked nitrogen retention show a severe acidosis, sufficient in many instances to be the actual cause of death. Their experience would lead them to believe that not even moderately severe acidosis was encountered in cases of nephritis without considerable nitrogen retention. Cases of acute nephritis may occasionally show a severe acidosis. To illustrate the importance of acidosis in nephritis, three groups of two cases each are tabulated in Table III. The first two patients suffered from severe chronic nephritis, showing marked nitrogen retention and acidosis. It is worthy of note that Case I was up and about at the time of the first analyses, while Case 2 after a short stay in the hospital, was at home for a period of seven weeks feeling improved. In both of these cases there was a very severe acidosis, and at the end the CO_2 dropped to such a low level as to be incompatible with life. The observations of Whitney[16] make it evident that such low figures may be the direct cause of death. As these patients did not receive alkali (until after the last recorded test), the CO_2 obviously fell to a

TABLE III

ACIDOSIS IN CHRONIC AND ACUTE NEPHRITIS*

CASE	AGE	SEX	DATE	CO₂ COMBINING POWER C.C. PER 100	CREAT- ININE, MG. PER 100 C.C. BLOOD	UREA NITROGEN, MG. PER 100 C.C. BLOOD	REMARKS
1. E. M.	39	♂	11/30/15	24	17.5	97	
			12/ 4/15	21	21.5	129	
			12/10/15	26	22.3	132	
			12/17/15	15	24.2	150	
			12/24/15	12	26.7	200	Death in chronic nephritis apparently due to acidosis; no alkali given
2. A. N.	27	♀	3/12/18	31	8.6	97	
			3/26/18	28	12.1	110	
			4/16/18	23	11.2	78	
			5/ 7/18	25	15.2	76	
			5/24/18	12	17.0	148	
3. W. W.	30	♂	2/11/16	23	8.5	55	
			2/23/16	21	12.5	76	
			3/ 7/16	52	10 4	60	Acute exacerbation of chronic nephritis; clinical improvement coincident with rise in alkali reserve; alkali given for a time
			4/ 7/16	54	9.5	39	
			5/10/16	22	9.6	56	
4. J. McC.	56	♂	12/28/15	20	5.1	64	
			1/ 8/16	55	4.5	39	
			1/11/16	58	5.4	39	
			2/ 4/16	40	4.8	36	
5. M. McA.	44	♂	1/25/16	22	4.6	71	
			4/11/16	45	2.7	17	
			5/ 8/17	..	2.4	17	
6. W. C.	49	♂	1/15/16	22	3.5	44	Severe acidosis in acute nephritis with complete recovery
			1/17/16	58	4.1	62	
			1/19/16	56	3.2	53	
			1/28/16	..	1 9	19	
			6/11/18	..	1.8	16	

*Taken from Chace and Myers.¹⁵

lower level than would otherwise have been the case. The findings in these two cases are the lowest we have encountered, the figures more often falling between 20 and 30 during the last days of life.

Cases 3 and 4 on admission to the hospital showed pronounced symptoms of acidosis. Although both patients died about one month after leaving the hospital, they showed considerable clinical improvement, this being coincident with the rise in the CO_2-combining power of the blood plasma.

The last two patients were cases of acute nephritis, showing severe acidosis (very marked dyspnea), but ending in complete recovery. Although this type of case is apparently not frequently encountered, it furnishes an interesting contrast to the preceding two groups. Case 6 was admitted supposedly in "uremic" coma. On estimating the blood creatinine and urea, however, we were surprised at the comparatively slight nitrogen retention, but an estimation of the CO_2 of the blood plasma disclosed the apparent difficulty. Two infusions of sodium bicarbonate, 12 grams each, on the fifteenth and sixteenth produced quite remarkable clinical results, and in less than two weeks the blood findings were normal.

That cases of Asiatic cholera develop a severe acute nephritis and a fairly large percentage, uremia is well known. Sellards[17] has obtained most favorable results by the administration of alkali to these cases, markedly lowering the mortality rate.

It may also be noted here that cases of severe pneumonia frequently show considerable nitrogen retention, and often severe acidosis, as shown by the CO_2-combining power of the blood. We have many observations in substantiation of this.

ACIDOSIS FINDINGS IN CHILDREN

The subject of acidosis occurring with infantile diarrhea is one that has recently received considerable attention, especially at the hands of Howland and Marriott,[18] Chapin and Pease,[19] and Schloss and Stetson.[20] Howland and Marriott have shown that the acidosis found in many cases of severe diarrhea not of the ileocolitis type is not due to the presence of acetone bodies, but apparently is due to deficient excretion of acid phosphate by the kidneys, as is the case in nephritis. The administration of sodium bicarbonate will often bring about a cessation of the almost characteristic hyperpnea and cause the laboratory tests to give results that are found with normal infants. Nevertheless, the child may die. Schloss and Stetson have applied the Van Slyke method to a quite extensive series of cases. In 27 normal cases the figures ranged from 46 to 63 c.c. CO_2 per 100 c.c. of plasma, while in 17 out of 19 cases of diarrhea with toxic symptoms his figures ranged from 13 to 38. The acetone bodies of the blood have been studied by Moore.[21] In cases of diarrhea without ileocolitis there is only a moderate increase in acetone bodies, while with ileocolitis the amount of acetone bodies is very large.

TABLE IV

CASES ILLUSTRATING ACIDOSIS IN CHILDREN*

CASE	AGE	SEX	DATE	CO_2 COMBINING POWER	BLOOD SUGAR per cent	DIAGNOSIS, REMARKS
	mo.			c.c. to 100		
1. A. N.	2	♀	9/26/15	22	0.09	Gastroenteritis; acidosis; death
2. W. R.	3 1/2	♂	1/20/15	24	0.10	Gastroenteritis; acidosis; death
3. Y. W.	1 1/2	♀	II/ 9/17	24	....	Gastroenteritis; acidosis; death
4. M. K.	10	♂	10/19/17	25	....	Gastroenteritis; acidosis; death
5. J. T.	4	♂	10/13/15	26	0.10	Malnutrition; recovery
6. H. C.	8 1/2	♂	11/15/15	28	0.09	Malnutrition; acidosis; recovery
7. J. M.	12	♀	11/ 3/17	28	....	Gastroenteritis and rickets; vomiting; improvement
8. P. K.	10	♀	11/24/15	33	0.11	Lobar pneumonia; acidosis; death

*Taken from Chapin and Myers.[22]

Table IV presents observations on a few of our cases. It will be noted that the plasma CO_2 ranged from 22 to 25 in the first four cases and that these cases all proved fatal.

ACIDOSIS AS THE RESULT OF ANESTHESIA

It is a matter of common observation that urine voided following ether anesthesia gives positive tests for acetone bodies in the urine. More recently it has been shown by Morriss,[23] and others that the anesthesia results in a lowering of the CO_2-combining power of the blood. From this coincidence it was natural to attribute the decreased alkaline reserve to the acetone body formation. Experiments carried out by Short[24] in this laboratory indicate, however, that acetone bodies are not formed promptly enough during the anesthesia to account for the decreased plasma bicarbonate. Data are given in Table V on illustrative cases showing the CO_2-combining power of blood plasma before and after ether anesthesia. As will be noted the drop in CO_2 ranged from 4 to 17 volume per cent. From these observations it is apparent what would happen if cases

TABLE V

INFLUENCE OF ETHER ANESTHESIA ON THE CO_2-COMBINING POWER OF BLOOD PLASMA*

CASE	AGE	SEX	CO_2 COMBINING POWER c.c. to 100 c.c.		TIME OF ANESTHETIC	OPERATION
			PREOPERATIVE	POSTOPERATIVE	min.	
1. E. C.	36	♂	53	49	26	Hemorrhoidectomy
2. W. D.	37	♂	69	60	40	Inoperable carcinoma of stomach
3. E. C.	51	♀	51	45	45	Femoral hernia
4. A. B.	36	♀	54	40	70	Carcinoma of the breast
5. W. C.	50	♂	62	52	43	Inoperable carcinoma of bladder
6. S. A.	40	♀	58	41	43	Right nephrectomy

*Taken largely from Short.[24]

of severe diabetes or nephritis with low figures for the CO_2 were operated on under general anesthesia. According to Morriss the drop in the CO_2 is more pronounced after chloroform than ether. A few unpublished observations which have been collected by Killian in this laboratory indicate that the drop in CO_2 is much less after spinal or gas-oxygen anesthesia. Morriss has pointed out that the preliminary administration of sodium bicarbonate increases the alkali reserve, although the most noteworthy effect of this treatment is to lead to higher values for this factor of safety at the conclusion of the anesthetic. Another method of combating the postoperative acidosis has been suggested by Henderson, Haggard and Coburn,[25] viz., the administration by inhalation of carbon dioxide properly diluted with air. This serves for one thing to increase the breathing and more rapidly remove the anesthetic from the blood, also to restore the preoperative CO_2-combining power.

ESTIMATION OF THE CO_2-COMBINING POWER OF THE BLOOD

As already pointed out, the estimation of the carbon dioxide combining power of the blood is probably the most reliable means of ascertaining the severity of acidosis. We have long had methods of estimating the CO_2 of the blood, although the subject did not receive much attention previous to the work of Barcroft and Haldane.[26] Many important contributions have emanated from

Haldane's laboratory, but it remained for Van Slyke[2] to develop a method so simple that it could readily be employed for clinical purposes. For the extraction of the gas, Van Slyke has made use of a Torricellian vacuum, with which the gas is easily and completely extracted in a closed chamber without any loss. The objection has been raised to the Van Slyke method that determinations made on plasma are not as reliable an index of acidosis[27] as those obtained with whole blood. (The Van Slyke method may be employed for whole blood, but the apparatus is easily gummed up and not readily cleaned.) Henderson and Morriss[27] have described a method of gas analysis, which may be applied to whole blood as well as plasma. Their method is, however, theoretically less exact than that of Van Slyke. That the CO_2 tension of the alveolar air yields results that are evidently less reliable than the CO_2-combining power of blood plasma is brought out in data presented by Peters.[28]

In the Van Slyke method the plasma from oxalated blood is shaken in a separatory funnel filled with an air mixture, the CO_2 tension of which approximates that of normal arterial blood. In this way it is combined with as much CO_2 as it is able to hold under normal tension. A known quantity of the saturated plasma is then acidified within the gas pipette, and its CO_2 liberated by the production of a partial vacuum. The liberated CO_2 is then placed under atmospheric pressure, its volume carefully measured and the volume corresponding to 100 c.c. of plasma calculated.

Method[2, 3]—The blood plasma may be obtained from the blood specimen collected for routine blood analysis as already described* provided a portion of this specimen is centrifuged as soon as secured.** The plasma is then pipetted off. Better, the blood may be drawn into a special centrifuge tube containing a little powdered potassium oxalate under some paraffin oil (see Fig. 1). By a gentle rotating motion the blood is mixed with the oxalate and then centrifuged as soon as possible, and the plasma pipetted off. In case the CO_2 capacity cannot be determined at once, the plasma is transferred to a paraffin lined tube, covered with oil, stoppered and placed on ice where it will keep unchanged for a week. To determine the CO_2-combining power, the plasma is saturated with carbon dioxide at alveolar tension. This can conveniently be done by placing about 3 c.c. of plasma (at room temperature) in a separatory funnel of about 300 c.c. capacity, and the funnel filled with alveolar air from the lungs of the operator. In order to bring the moisture content down to saturation at room temperature, the air is passed through a bottle full of glass beads before it enters the funnel (see Fig. 1). The operator, without inspiring more deeply than normal, expires as quickly and as completely as possible through the glass beads and separatory funnel. The funnel is closed just before the expiration is finished, and is shaken for one minute in such a way that the plasma is evenly distributed about the walls, forming a thin layer which quickly approaches equilibrium with the CO_2 in the air. After the shaking has lasted a minute, a fresh portion of alveolar air is run into the funnel and the shaking completed. The funnel is now placed in an upright position so that the plasma may drain into the narrow space at the bottom of the funnel and from which it may be readily pipetted.

The Van Slyke apparatus is illustrated at the left in Fig. 1. It consists essentially of a 50 c.c. pipette with three-way stopcocks at top and bottom, and a 1 c.c. scale on the upper stem, divided into 0.02 c.c. divisions. The bottom of the apparatus is connected with a leveling bulb filled with mercury by means of a heavy walled rubber tube. The chamber, d, serves to draw off the solutions after the CO_2 has been extracted from them, while c serves for the subsequent release of the vacuum by the entrance of mercury. The apparatus is made of strong glass, in order to stand the weight of mercury without danger of breaking, and is held in a strong screw clamp, the jaws of which are lined with thick pads of rubber. To prevent accidental slipping of the apparatus from the clamp, an iron rod covered with a piece of rubber tubing should be so arranged as to project under cock f and between c and d. Capillary a is used for convenient removal of solutions from the apparatus. It is of advantage to have a small large-necked bottle clamped to the stand in such a position as to be under the mouth of this tube. Three hooks or rings at the level 1, 2, and 3 serve to hold the leveling bulb at different stages of the analysis. Practically the only source of difficulty with the apparatus is in the entrance of air through the stopcocks. It is essential, therefore that both cocks should be properly greased (a mixture of paraffin and vaseline works very well) and air tight. It is also necessary that the cocks (especially f) should be held in place so that they cannot be forced out by pressure of the mercury. For this purpose strong rubber bands work very well.

Before beginning a determination it is necessary to test the apparatus for tightness and freedom from gases. The entire apparatus (Fig. 1), including the capillaries above the upper stopcock, is filled with mercury, and the mercury bulb then lowered to position 3, so that a Torricellian vacuum is obtained, the mercury falling to about the middle of d. The leveling bulb is then raised again. If the apparatus is tight and gas-free the mercury will refill it completely and strike the upper stopcock with a sharp click, but in case there is any gas in the apparatus this will serve as a cushion. Should this be the case, the apparatus must be repeatedly evacuated until the gas has all been removed.

For the determination, the apparatus, including both capillaries above the upper stopcock, is entirely filled with mercury by placing the leveling bulb of mercury in position 1, and turning stopcock c. The cup at the top is next washed free of acid with carbonate-free ammonia water,* by employing a few drops of the ammonia water, a drop of phenolphthalein and about 1 c.c. of distilled water. This is then all removed but a drop or two, with the aid of a pipette. With an Ostwald-Folin pipette 1 c.c. of the plasma from the separatory funnel is allowed to run into the cup b of the apparatus, the tip of the pipette remaining below the surface of the solution in the cup during the transfer, and under the thin film of slightly pink solution. The final drop of plasma is expressed by closing the top of the pipette with the forefinger of one hand, and warming the bulb with the palm of the other.

With the mercury bulb at position 2 and the stopcok f in the position shown in the figure, the plasma is admitted from the cup into the 50 c.c. chamber, leaving just enough above the stopcock e to fill the capillary so that no air is introduced when the next solution is added. The cup is now washed with two portions of about 0.5 c.c. each of water, care being taken that no air enters the apparatus. A small drop (about 0.02 c.c.) of caprylic alcohol is next added to the cup and permitted to flow entirely into the capillary above c, and finally 0.5 c.c. of 5 per cent sulphuric acid is run in. It is not necessary that exactly 1 c.c. of wash water and 0.5 c.c. of acid shall be used, but the total volume of the water solution introduced must extend exactly to the 2.5 c.c. mark on the apparatus if the special formulas of Van Slyke and Cullen in Table VI are to be used. After the acid has been admitted a drop of mercury is placed in b and allowed to run down the capillary as far as the stopcock in order to seal the latter. Whatever excess of the sulphuric acid remains in the cup is washed out with a little water.

The mercury bulb is now lowered and hung at position 3, and the mercury in the pipette is allowed to run down to the 50 c.c. mark, producing a Torricellian vacuum in the apparatus. When the mercury (not the water) meniscus has fallen to the 50 c.c. mark, the lower cock is closed, and the pipette is removed from the clamp. Equilibrium of the CO_2 between the 2.5 c.c. of water solution and the 47.5 c.c. of free space in the apparatus is obtained by turning the pipette upside down fifteen or more times, thus thoroughly agitating its contents. The pipette is then replaced in the clamp. By turning the lower

*It is convenient to have a set of five dropping bottles with ground in pipettes and rubber bulbs. The set consists of 1 per cent carbonate-free ammonia water, 1 per cent alcoholic phenolphthalein, distilled water, caprylic alcohol and 5 per cent sulphuric acid.

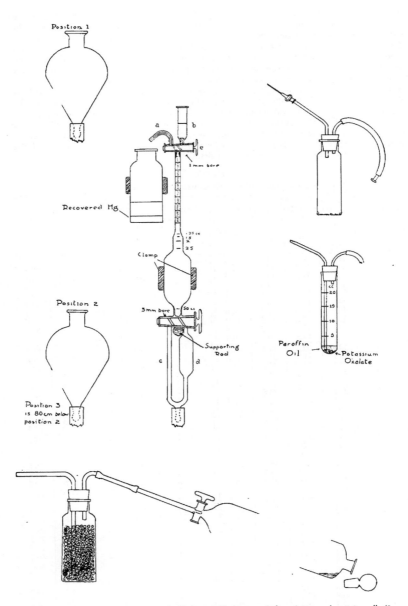

Fig. 1.—Showing Van Slyke apparatus at left, blood bottle and centrifuge tube employed in collecting blood at right, and apparatus used in saturating blood plasma with carbon dioxide.

stopcock, *f*. the water solution is now allowed to flow from the pipette completely into *d* without, however, allowing any gas to follow it. The leveling bulb is then raised in the left hand, while with the right the stopcock is turned so as to connect the pipette with *c*. The mercury flowing in from *c* fills the body of the pipette, and as much of the calibrated stem at the top as is not occupied by the gas extracted from the solution. A few hundredths of a c.c. of water which could not be completely drained into *d* float on top of the mercury in the pipette, but the error caused by reabsorption of carbon dioxide into the small volume of water is negligible if the reading is made at once. The mercury bulb is placed at such a level that the gas in the pipette is under atmospheric pressure, and the volume of the gas is read off on the scale. In order to have the column in the pipette exactly balanced by that outside, the surface of the mercury in the leveling bulb should be raised until it is level with the mercury meniscus in the pipette, and then, for entire accuracy, raised above the latter meniscus by a distance equal to 1/14 the height of the column of water above the mercury in the pipette.

TABLE VI

TABLE FOR CALCULATION OF CO₂-COMBINING POWER OF PLASMA*

OBSERVED VOL. GAS X $\frac{B}{760}$	C.C. OF CO_2, REDUCED TO 0°, 760 mm., BOUND AS BICARBONATE BY 100 C.C. OF PLASMA.				OBSERVED VOL. GAS × $\frac{B}{760}$	C.C. OF CO_2, REDUCED TO 0°, 760 mm., BOUND AS BICARBONATE BY 100 C.C. OF PLASMA.			
	15°	20°	25°	30°		15°	20°	25°	30°
0.20	9.1	9.9	10.7	11.8	0.60	47.7	48.1	48.5	48.6
1	10.1	10.9	11.7	12.6	1	48.7	49.0	49.4	49.5
2	11.0	11.8	12.6	13.5	2	49.7	50.0	50.4	50.4
3	12.0	12.8	13.6	14.3	3	50.7	51.0	51.3	51.4
4	13.0	13.7	14.5	15.2	4	51.6	51.9	52.2	52.3
5	13.9	14.7	15.5	16.1	5	52.6	52.8	53.2	53.2
6	14.9	15.7	16.4	17.0	6	53.6	53.8	54.1	54.1
7	15.9	16.6	17.4	18.0	7	54.5	54.8	55.1	55.1
8	16.8	17.6	18.3	18.9	8	55.5	55.7	56.0	56.0
9	17.8	18.5	19.2	19.8	9	56.5	56.7	57.0	56.9
0.30	18.8	19 5	20.2	20.8	0.70	57.4	57.6	57.9	57.9
1	19.7	20.4	21.1	21.7	1	58.4	58.6	58.9	58.8
2	20.7	21.4	22.1	22.6	2	59.4	59.5	59.8	59.7
3	21.7	22.3	23.0	23.5	3	60.3	60.5	60.7	60.6
4	22.6	23.3	24.0	24.5	4	61.3	61.4	61.7	61.6
5	23.6	24.2	24.9	25.4	5	62.3	62.4	62.6	62.5
6	24.6	25.2	25.8	26.3	6	63.2	63.3	63.6	63.4
7	25.5	26.2	26.8	27.3	7	64.2	64.3	64.5	64.3
8	26.5	27.1	27.7	28.2	8	65.2	65.3	65.5	65.3
9	27.5	28.1	28.7	29.1	9	66.1	66.2	66.4	66.2
0.40	28.4	29.0	29.6	30.0	0.80	67.1	67.2	67.3	67.1
1	29.4	30.0	30.5	31.0	1	68.1	68.1	68.3	68.0
2	30.3	30.9	31.5	31.9	2	69.0	69.1	69.2	69.0
3	31.3	31.9	32.4	32.8	3	70.0	70.0	70.2	69.9
4	32.3	32.8	33.4	33.8	4	71.0	71.0	71.1	70.8
5	33.2	33.8	34.3	34.7	5	71.9	72.0	72.1	71.8
6	34.2	34.7	35.3	35.6	6	72.9	72.9	73.0	72.7
7	35.2	35.7	36.2	36.5	7	73.9	73.9	74.0	73.6
8	36.1	36.6	37.2	37.4	8	74.8	74.8	74.9	74.5
9	37.1	37.6	38.1	38.4	9	75.8	75.8	75.8	75.4
0.50	38.1	38.5	39.0	39.3	0.90	76.8	76.7	76.8	76.4
1	39.1	39.5	40.0	40.3	1	77.8	77.7	77.7	77.3
2	40.0	40.4	40.9	41.2	2	78.7	78.6	78.7	78.2
3	41.0	41.4	41.9	42.1	3	79.7	79.6	79.6	79.2
4	42.0	42.4	42.8	43.0	4	80.7	80.5	80.6	80.1
5	42.9	43.3	43.8	43.9	5	81.6	81.5	81.5	81.0
6	43.9	44.3	44.7	44.9	6	82.6	82.5	82.4	82.0
7	44.9	45.3	45.7	45.8	7	83.6	83.4	83.4	82.9
8	45.8	46.2	46.6	46.7	8	84.5	84.4	84.3	83.8
9	46.8	47.1	47.5	47.6	9	85.5	85.3	85.2	84.8
0.60	47.7	48.1	48.5	48.6	1.00	86.5	86.2	86.2	85.7

*Taken from Van Slyke and Cullen.³

By means of Table VI the readings on the apparatus can be directly transposed into c.c. of CO_2 chemically bound by 100 c.c. of blood plasma. This table takes into account the air which enters the apparatus dissolved in the water, etc. The barometer reading and room temperature are taken at the time of the determination. For convenience in the calculation, values are given in Table VII for the ratio $\frac{barometer}{760}$ over the range usually encountered.

TABLE VII

BAROMETER	$\frac{BAROMETER}{760}$	BAROMETER	$\frac{BAROMETER}{760}$
732	0.961	756	0.995
734	0.966	758	0.997
736	0.968	760	1.000
738	0.971	762	1.003
740	0.974	764	1.006
742	0.976	766	1.008
744	0.979	768	1.011
746	0.981	770	1.013
748	0.984	772	1.016
750	0.987	774	1.018
752	0.989	776	1.021
754	0.992	778	1.024

From an inspection of Table VI it will be observed that the difference between the readings and actual values of CO_2 gas bound is roughly 12. When we first began the use of their apparatus, Drs. Van Slyke and Cullen suggested to us that a correction of 12 would give sufficiently accurate results for clinical purposes, thus eliminating the use of the table or a calculation. We have frequently done this. Somewhat greater accuracy might be obtained by deducting 10 from readings 20-35, 11 from readings 36-40, 12 for readings 51-70 and 13 for readings 71-85.

After the determination has been finished, the leveling bulb is again lowered without opening the upper stopcock, and most of the mercury is withdrawn through c. The water solution from d is readmitted and, the leveling bulb being raised to position 1, the water solution, with a little mercury, is forced out of the apparatus through a. The apparatus is now ready for another determination. It is not necessary to wash it out, since the few drops which remain in it attached to walls hold no measurable amount of carbon dioxide. When not in use the entire apparatus should be filled with water.

REFERENCES

[1]Van Slyke, Stillman and Cullen: Proc. Soc. Exper. Biol. and Med., 1915, xii, 165.
[2]Van Slyke: Jour. Biol. Chem., 1917, xxx, 347.
[3]Van Slyke and Cullen: Jour. Biol. Chem., 1917, xxx, 289.
[4]Marriott and Howland: Arch. Int. Med., 1916, xviii, 708; also Denis: Ibid., July, 1920.
[5]Marriott and Howland: Arch. Int. Med., 1918. xxii, 477.
[6]Henderson, Y.: Jour. Am. Med. Assn., 1914, lxiii, 318.
[7]Friderica: Berl. klin. Wchnschr., 1914, li, 1268.
[8]Marriott: Jour. Am. Med. Assn., 1916, lxvi, 1594.
[9]Sellards: Bull. Johns Hopkins Hosp., 1914, xxv, 141.
[10]Palmer and Henderson, L. J.: Arch. Int. Med., 1913, xii, 153; 1915, xvi, 109.
[11]Palmer and Van Slyke: Jour. Biol. Chem., 1917, xxxii, 499.
[12]Van Slyke, Stillman and Cullen: Jour. Biol. Chem., 1917, xxx, 401.
[13]Stillman, Van Slyke, Cullen and Fitz: Jour. Biol. Chem., 1917, xxx, 405.
[14]Allen, Stillman and Fitz: Monographs of the Rockefeller Institute for Medical Research, No. 11, October, 1919.
[15]Chace and Ayers: Jour. Am. Med. Assn., 1920, lxxiv, 641.
[16]Whitney: Arch. Int. Med., 1917, xx, 931.
[17]Sellards: The Principles of Acidosis and Clinical Methods for Its Study, Cambridge, Mass., 1917, p. 55.
[18]Howland and Marriott: Am. Jour. Dis. Child., 1916, xi, 309; Bull. Johns Hopkins Hosp., 1916, xxvii, 63.

[19]Chapin and Pease: Jour. Am. Med. Assn., 1916, lxvii, 1351.
[20]Schloss and Stetson: Am. Jour. Dis. Child., 1917, xiii, 218.
[21]Moore: Am. Jour. Dis. Child., 1916, xiii, 244.
[22]Chapin and Ayers: Am. Jour. Dis. Child., 1919, xviii, 555.
[23]Morriss: Jour. Am. Med. Assn., 1917, lxviii, 1391.
[24]Short: Jour. Biol. Chem., 1920, xli, 503.
[25]Henderson, Y., Haggard and Coburn.: Jour. Am. Med. Assn., 1920, lxxiv, 783.
[26]Barcroft and Haldane: Jour. Physiol., 1902, xxviii, 232.
Barcroft and Higgins: Ibid., 1911, xlii, 512.
Barcroft: The Respiratory Function of the Blood, Cambridge, Eng., 1914.
[27]Henderson and Morriss: Jour. Biol. Chem., 1917, xxxi, 217.
Haggard: Ibid., 1920, xlii, 237.
[28]Peters: Am. Jour. Physiol., 1917, xliv, 84.

ON CHLORIDE METABOLISM*

By H. F. Host, M.D., Christiania, Norway.

ALTHOUGH Justus von Liebig, the founder of the modern system of nutrition, pointed out in the middle of the last century the value of salts in the diet, and later on Voit and Forster in the "seventies" on the basis of experiments carried out by Forster, emphasized the importance of the mineral salts in the organism, the chemical investigations of metabolism have for a long time dealt chiefly with the organic food stuffs, while little interest has been evinced for the inorganic substances in the diet until the last few decades.

Among the soluble substances the chlorides are in majority in nature, and are also the most predominant in the fluids of the human organism. According to the investigations of Stuber the chlorides constitute about three-fourths of all the electrolytes in the human body.

Chlorine exists in the body chiefly combined with Na and K, partly also with Ca, Mg, and ammonium. The K salt is chiefly found in the cells, while the Na salt is for the most part in the fluids.

The importance of the chlorides is partly due to their general physicochemical influence, partly to some special qualities.

The life and activity of the protoplasm depend upon certain physicochemical qualities of the fluids in the body: fixed osmotic pressure and fixed hydrogen-ion concentration. Minimal changes in the pressure and in the hydrogen-ion concentration exist, but the changes need not be great to destroy life. Both the absorbed foodstuffs and the intermediate metabolism tend to change the pressure and the reaction of the blood and the tissue fluid, but in consequence of the rapid diffusion and the great dissociation of the salts, especially the chlorides, the osmotic pressure and the hydrogen-ion concentration are very stable.

Together with many other salts the chlorides are always to be found in the living cells, and the investigations of Loeb suggest that the chlorides are necessary for the development of the animal cell.

Like many other salts the chlorides act as catalysts, but the opinion of Voit that the chlorides influence the general metabolism has not been confirmed.

The chlorides are of special importance for the production of the hydrochloric acid of the stomach. Opinions still differ as to how this acid is produced, but its origin from the chlorides of the diet, with the chlorides of the blood serving as an intermediate link, cannot be disputed. This is proved by the fact that the production of hydrochloric acid ceases in animals on salt-free diet.

Owing to the ability of the organism to keep the osmotic pressure constant, there is an intimate correlation between chloride and water metabolism. Widal and Javal have pointed out that by great changes in the chlorides of the diet, the amount of the chlorides in the body may vary about 12 gm., while at the

---

*Lecture given at the University of Christiania. Christiania. Norway.

same time the water content varies 1½-2 liters. But on ordinary diet and under physiologic conditions the chloride and water content of the body are fairly constant.

Determination of the total amount of the chlorides in an adult person is not yet made. But we have several analyses of newborn children, in whom has been found an average of 0.30 per cent. If from this we calculate the amount in adults and remember that adults have a little less water and therefore also less chlorides than newborn children, we shall find that the amount of chlorides in a person weighing 70 kilos is between 100 and 200 gms.

The chlorides are found chiefly, but not exclusively, in the fluids of the body. Uncertainty still exists as to whether the chlorides exist as adsorbed to the protoplasm of the cells. Some authors are of the opinion that at least in pathologic conditions the chlorides are partly adsorbed to the cells. But all agree that the chlorides mainly circulate in dissociated compounds in the organism.

The concentration of the chlorides in the blood has been the subject of considerable research:

Blood, per cent: 0.44 Rumpf.
0.6-0.7 Georgpulos.
0.45-0.47 Schmidt, Wanach.
0.49 McLean, Van Slyke.
0.45-0.50 Gettler, Baker.
Serum, per cent: 0.46-0.58 Hefter, Siebeck.
0.597-0.614 McLean, Van Slyke.
0.56-0.64 Gettler, Baker.
0.46-0.65 Ayers, Fine.

By means of Bang's micro method I have examined the conceneration of the blood chlorides in several healthy men and women, as a result of which I have found the concentration to vary between 0.44 and 0.48 per cent. Bang's method is correct within 5 per cent.

The concentration of the chlorides in the serum I have found to vary between 0.55 and 0.60 per cent. This great difference between the concentration in blood and serum shows that the chlorides exist chiefly in serum, to a much less degree in the corpuscles.

It has been impossible to determine the chloride concentration of the tissue fluid. But since the chlorides easily permeate the membranes of the organism, the chloride concentration of the tissue fluid is probably the same throughout the body and not much different from the concentration in serum. In patients suffering from pleuritis I have determined the chloride concentration 16 times, and always found the same values as in serum.

In consequence of the chlorides being found chiefly in the fluids of the organism, the chloride content of the organs depends much on their water content. The cells of the stomach form perhaps an exception. According to Rosemann, the cells of the stomach have a special affinity for chlorides, for which reason they can store chlorides between the periods of secretion, so that the chloride content of the fasting stomach is higher than that of the blood. Apart from this the chloride concentration in the organs is approximately proportional to their water content. In recent years the chloride content of the organs has been examined by several investigators, as a result of which it has been found that the chloride concentration varies between 0.1 and 0.4 per cent. The greatest concentration has been found in the lungs and in the skin, which according to Wahlgren contain ⅓ of all the chlorides of the body. On the other hand, on a salt poor diet the chloride output is chiefly due to the skin, while other organs do not lose any salts.

The amount of chlorides with which the body is supplied varies a great deal in proportion as salt is added to the food. It has long been known that some nations use much salt in their food, while others do not use salt at all. Sallust tells us that the Numides despised salt, and Plutarch was astonished to find that the priests in Egypt did not salt their food. Widal and Javal point out that the tribes still leading a nomadic life do not use salt, and that they begin to do so only when they settle and follow agricultural pursuits. Also many other authors point out that vegetarians, on the average, use more salt than meat eaters. According to the theory of Bunge the reason is that vegetables contain mainly K salts, especially potassium carbonate, which reacts in the organism with sodium chloride, forming sodium carbonate and potassium chloride. The carbonate is excreted, while the potassium chloride is retained and substitutes the sodium chloride. To compensate for this loss, vegetarians are disposed to salt their food. This theory of Bunge is denied by several authors. According to Forel, a sect of vegetarians, living at Locarno, do not use salt at all. Some herbivorous animals, for instance the hare and the rabbit, do not eat salt. Widal therefore agrees with Lapique, that vegetarians use salt simply to impart a greater flavor to their diet.

Although the chloride content in the diet varies, not only with the individual, but also with the nation, some authors have nevertheless tried to calculate the average intake of chlorides in the diet. Dastre estimates that Europeans, on the average, have about 17 gm. sodium chloride in their diet per day. Laache estimates 10-15 gms. for Norwegians.

It has long been a well-known fact that the salt in the food is mainly due to the use of salt as a condiment and as a food preserver. The amount of chlorides we get in our food does not therefore correspond to the amount necessary for the organism.

Sodium chloride is common in nature, and all our foodstuffs contain some chloride. The need of the organism is therefore always satisfied by the chlorides which the foodstuffs contain. Dastre pointed out that neither animals nor human beings can be put on their chloride minimum without the salt of the food being extracted.

The chloride minimum for human beings has not yet been determined with certainty. During inanition the chloride output decreases rapidly in the first few days, later on it diminishes slowly. Luciani found in Succi from the fourth to the thirtieth day of inanition an average daily output of 0.66 gm.

The output during inanition does not, however, represent the need of the organism. Bunge is of the opinion that the organism needs one or two grams of chlorides per day on ordinary diet, and Mayer has shown by experiments made on himself, that it is possible to live and feel well on 1.25 gm. per day, at least for some weeks.

The chlorides are excreted mainly through the kidneys. A small portion is excreted through the skin and the intestines. In healthy persons the excretion from the skin and the intestines is so small that it need not be taken into consideration in examination of the metabolism. In case of diarrhea, however, the excretion from the intestines may increase a great deal. Javal found in a patient suffering from nephritis and diarrhea an excretion of 9.51 gm. chlorides in the feces in 24 hours.

Under physiologic conditions the chlorides are excreted rapidly, provided that the intake does not surpass a certain upper limit; 10 to 15 gm. chlorides are as a rule excreted in two or three days. Even a much greater amount of chlorides can be excreted in a short time. Lemierre and Digne found in a patient with hysteric polyuria an excretion of 80 gm. in twenty-four hours.

To determine the power of chloride excretion of the kidneys the organism must be in chloride balance. An exact equilibrium cannot be obtained and it cannot therefore exactly be determined when the surplus of chlorides is excreted.

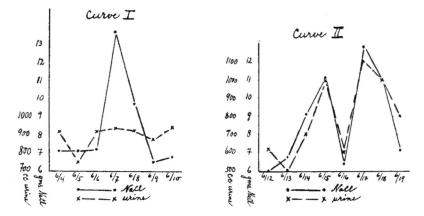

The water content of the organism is of importance for the excretion of the chlorides, because the power of concentration of the kidneys may vary even under physiologic conditions. Some people may excrete the surplus of chlorides without an increase of the diuresis, while others get an increased output of water, so the concentration of the urine does not change. The chloride output is then, as a rule, small on the first day; but if a great portion of water is taken together with the chlorides, the salt is excreted much faster.

Curve I demonstrates the former type of chloride excretion. The person experimented on was a convalescent, whose urine was normal. He lived on a constant diet, containing about 7 gm. chlorides. As will be seen from the curve, the majority of the 10 gm. added are excreted on the first day, the rest being excreted the following day. The diuresis is practically unchanged.

Curve II demonstrates the latter type of excretion. The person experimented on suffered from slight rheumatic pains without any objective findings. The urine was negative. The diet was the same as in the case of the first person. As will be seen, the curves for the excretion of water and chlorides are almost parallel, and the excretion of chlorides reaches its maximum on the second day. When the experiment is repeated in such a way the 1000 c.c. water is given with the salt, the greater part of the salt is excreted on the first day. On account of his small power of concentration this individual cannot excrete the chlorides as fast as the former person, unless a fair amount of water is given with the salt. It is often seen that the concentration power of the kidneys increases when greater amounts of salt are added to the diet for some

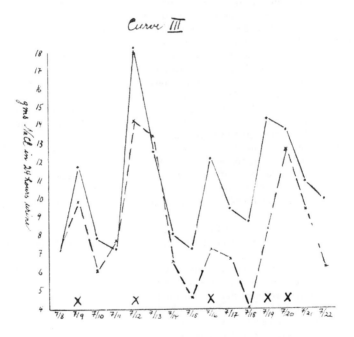

Curve III

time. The concentration of the chlorides will, however, never surpass a certain upper limit, which Ambard has found to be 2.2 per cent.

As will be seen, the organism rapidly excretes the surplus of salt, provided that this surplus does not surpass a certain upper limit, and, consequently the chloride excretion will be proportional to the intake of chlorides. I have examined the chloride excretion in two persons, living on ordinary hospital diet. As will be seen from the curves, the excretion varies considerably from day to day, viz., from about 4 to about 18 gm. The days on which salt flesh or salt fish are given are marked "X" on the curve, and it will be observed that the excretion of chlorides is much greater on the "salt days" than on the other days.

THE PATHOLOGY OF CHLORIDE METABOLISM

It has long been recognized that concentrated solutions of chlorides, or chlorides in substances taken per os, act toxically, owing to the irritation on the stomach and the intestines. Of late years some authors, for instance Finkelstein and Schaps, have emphasized that even dilute solutions, especially when used intravenously or subcutaneously, act toxically, producing the so-called "salt-fever," which was supposed to be due to influence on the temperature centre. Several other authors, among them Jorgensen, have however never got increased temperature when fresh distilled water was used for the injections, while increased temperature often happened when the distilled water had been kept for some time. These authors therefore are of the opinion that the "salt fever" is due to bacteria. · These experiments coupled with our experience of the "salvarsan fever," which is now generally looked upon as bacterial in origin, makes it probable that salt fever also is due to bacterial products.

As far as we know, the chlorides do not alter their constitution during their passage in the organism. The changes we know in the chloride metabolism are therefore only of a quantitative nature, consisting of a diminished or an increased amount of chlorides in the organism.

Diminution of the chlorides of the organism is little known and is obviously not of great importance. French authors, for instance Mestrezat, emphasize that the chlorides in the cerebrospinal fluid are diminished in tuberculous meningitis. I have confirmed this in two cases. In 7 patients suffering from nontuberculous diseases I found the concentration of the chlorides bettween 0.68 and 0.72 per cent, while in two cases of tuberculous meningitis the concentration was 0.59 and 0.61 per cent, respectively.

Far better known and investigated is the increased concentration of chlorides in the organism.

Increased concentration due to increased intake, which Widal and Javal have produced, is of no pathologic interest. All other kinds of increased concentration are due to *retention*.

The retention may be a direct one, due to retention of molecular chloride, of −Cl, or of the cations with which −Cl forms salts, especially +Na, or the retention may be an indirect one, due to retention of water. Owing to the osmotic pressure a retention of water is followed by a retention of chlorides.

A retention of molecular chlorides is possible only when the molecules are adsorbed to the tissue or circulating protein, the dissolved chlorides being nearly all dissociated. The theory on the "adsorbed chlorine" which is due to French authors (Marie, Ambard, Beaujard), is not yet proved. The theory is to explain the so-called "dry retention." It has been known for a long time that patients suffering from nephritis often retain much chlorine without corresponding amounts of water. René Marie has published a case in which 158 gm. of chlorides were retained and only 7.8 liters water, that is, a retention of about 2 per cent salt solution. Such a retention seems inconsistent with a constant osmotic pressure, unless some part of the chlorides was adsorbed. It must be remembered that the determination of the water retention is difficult, the patient in question often being in a state of inanition. Of importance is also the fact that small variations of the osmotic pressure may happen, and further that the pressure does not increase proportionally to the retained chlorides, because the dissociation decreases, and finally, that the organism may diminish its content of other electrolytes.

A chloride retention may be due to a retention of −Cl or +Na, or of both ions. Most authors have not determined to which ion the retention is due. Salkowski has, however, found a pronounced Na-retention in pneumonia, and v. Wyss has published a case of nephritis with edema, in which the edema was due to a retention of Na. The patient was cured when he received hydrochloric acid. A secondary retention of −Cl may be due to sodium bicarbonate, which Widal and Lemierre have found in diabetes, and which v.Wyss has demonstated in healthy persons. −Cl is then, according to v. Wyss, retained to neutralize +Na, while Widal supposes that the bicarbonate diminishes the permeability of the kidneys to chlorine. This is made probable by the fact that magnesium sulphate (Widal) and sodium phosphate (L. A. Meyer) may produce retention of −Cl.

The primary retention of water is little known. In many pathologic conditions water is retained, but chlorides are retained at the same time, so that it is difficult to decide which is retained first.

An increase of the chloride content of the organism may be found in several pathologic conditions, the principal of which are:

1. Fever.
2. Decompensation of the heart.
3. Anemia and cachexia.
4. Nephritis.

In fever Redlenbacher found as early as the middle of the last century a pronounced diminution of the chloride output, which on cessation of the fever was followed by an increase. This was confirmed by many authors, among them Röman who found a diminished output in spite of abundant supply. The diminished output is accordingly not due to diminished intake, but to a retention, which is parallel to the water retention. In pneumonia the chloride retention is well known, but where the chlorides are accumulated is not yet known, the chloride content of the exudate being too small to account for the retained chlorides.

The cause of the chloride retention in fever is not yet known. A retention due to the kidneys is often difficult to exclude. Many years ago v. Leyden stated that a chloride retention might exist without any focal infection. The "general influence" of the fever is therefore looked upon as the cause of the chloride retention.

In decompensation of the heart the cause of the retention is due to stasis and edema.

In cachexia, for instance in cancer, several authors, among them v. Müller and Bohne believe they have found a diminution of the chloride output. The investigations of Gärtig and especially of Laudenheimer have, however, shown that there is no special relation between cancer and chloride metabolism. In most cases the diminished output is due to diminished intake of food. In other cases the cause is edema and transudates.

In addition to cancer some authors such as v. Limbeck and Biernacki have found an increased concentration of the chlorides in the blood in chlorosis and anemia.

TABLE 1

NAME	AGE	DIAGNOSIS	CHLORIDE CONCENTRATION IN BLOOD (AND SERUM). DUPLICATE ESTIMATIONS. PER CENT.					
O.A.	25	Anemia	5/17	0.54	0.53	5/19	0.54	0.54
M.S.		Sec. anemia	6/26	0.54	0.54	6/27	0.56	0.55
		(post. hemorrh.)				(serum :	0.60	0.61)
G.O.		Anemia pernic.	7/11	0.58	0.58	7/15	0.59	0.59
I.G.	30	Anemia.	7/22	0.61	0.61	7/23	0.57	0.58
S.	50	Anemia pern.	9/11 ·	0.56	0.57	(serum	0.62	0.63)
L.S.	15	Sec. anemia.	9/12	0.54	0.55	(serum	0.60	0.60)
R.		Sec. anemia. (post. hemorrh.)	9/12	0.54	0.55	(serum	0.62	0.63)
L.	56	Sec. anemia. (cencer vent.)	7/17	0.53	0.55			
S.		Sec. anemia. (cancer vent.)	7/22	0.55	(serum: 0.66	0.60)		

In several patients suffering from cancer and from primary and secondary anemia I have examined the chloride concentration in blood and in serum (see Table 1).

As mentioned above I have found the normal chloride concentration in the blood between 0.44 and 0.48 per cent and in the serum between 0.55 and 0.60 per cent, that is, the concentration in the serum is about 0.1 per cent greater than in the whole blood. As is evident from Table 1 I have found the chloride concentration of the blood in cancer and in anemia greater, in some cases much greater than the normal, while the concentration in the serum is about normal or only slightly increased. It appears from this that the increased concentration in the blood is not due to retention, but chiefly to the anemia, which has reduced the formed, relatively chlorine-poor elements in relation to the blood fluid.

Since Böhme, toward the close of the "nineties," demonstrated chloride retention in several pathologic conditions, among them uremia, the relation between the *chloride retention and nephritis* has been the subject of many investigations.

Since the experimental studies on animals by Heineke and Meyerstein, as well as by Schlayer and Takayasu, and the clinical and pathologicoanatomic investigations, especially by v. Monakow, it is taken for granted that the nitrogenous products are excreted through the glomeruli, while chlorides and water are excreted through the tubuli. In some of v. Monakow's cases, where the glomeruli were much degenerated, the chloride output was normal, while the N-excretion was much diminished. On the other hand, in cases where the tubuli were affected, the N-excretion was normal, while the chloride excretion was decreased.

It is in cases where the pathologic process is in the tubuli, the pure and the combined nephrosis (Volhard and Fahr) that we find anomalies in the chloride metabolism, while in pure nephritis the chloride output is normal. Most cases of acute glomerulonephritis are, however, in the beginning combined with nephrosis; in other words, the process is at first diffuse, later on confined to the glomeruli.

The chloride retention in nephritis may be due to the *kidneys*, the *peripheral vessels* or the *tissue*.

The experiments by Schlayer and Schmid have demonstrated that the kidneys, at least in experimental nephritis, may bar the chloride excretion: in nephritis, due to intoxication with chromium, blood containing increased amounts of chlorides circulates in the kidneys without the chlorides being excreted. In human beings conditions are not so clear. Widal and Javal emphasize that the chloride retention in nephritis is mainly due to the kidneys. On the other hand other authors, as Achard and Ribot, point out that the chloride retention may be independent of the kidneys.

I have examined the chloride content of blood and urine in 9 patients suffering from acute nephritis. All the 9 patients had been taken ill suddenly. They had cephalalgia, edema, increased blood pressure, retention of urea in serum and had protein, blood and casts in the urine. All these 9 cases were typical of glomerulonephritis. In the present paper I shall report in detail only the experiments with 3 patients.

CASE 1.—J. H. Seaman, nineteen years old. The patient was taken suddenly ill a few days before admission to the hospital, with weakness, dyspnea, and edema.

Status on admission to the hospital: Puffiness of the face, edema in the sacrolumbar region and in the lower extremities. Systolic blood pressure 145. Urine: albumin, casts and red and white corpuscles. Urea in serum: 0.065 per cent.

Diet: 1000 c.c. milk, 200 gm. bread and 100 gm. butter. This diet contained about 7 gm. salt.

TABLE 2

DATE	WEIGHT	DIURESIS	NaCl in: 24 HOURS URINE	BLOOD %	
6/6	74.9	730	6.50	0.54	Blood pressure 140
6/7	74.3	905	6.66	0.53	
6/8	74.0	730	4.30		
6/9	73.6	850	3.91	0.53	Blood pressure 125
6/10	73.7	1000	4.70		
6/11	73.3	1400	3.67	0.51	
6/12	73.3	1350	6.21	0.52	
6/13	72.0	1000	6.36		
6/14	70.3	1400	10.64	0.58	+5 gm. salt in 500 c.c. water.
6/15	69.7	1300	10.70		
6/16	68.3	1400	12.00	0.52	
6/17	68.0	1500	12.53		
6/18	66.5	2000	13.40	0.50	
6/19	65.0	2200	14.04		
6/20	64.9	2100	16.88	0.45	
6/21	64.2	2200	14.30	0.45	

This patient, who lived on a constant diet, containing about 7 gm. salt, retained some chlorides during the first week, but on the day the patient was given 5 gm. salt in addition to the diet, the chloride output increased and continued to be high until the edema disappeared about three weeks later. The chloride concentration in the blood, as will be observed, was greater than normal, between 0.51 and 0.54 per cent, during the first week. On the day 5 gm. salt were given, the concentration in the blood increased and 6 days later the chloride content of the blood was normal.

CASE 2.—A. S., working man, sixty-one years old. Six days before admission to the hospital he suddenly experienced weakness and dizziness. In the evening of the same day he developed edema in the lower extremities, the day after also in the face.

When he came to the hospital he had edema in the extremities, in the sacrolumbar region and in the face. Some râles in the lungs; temperature normal; urine: albumin and casts; systolic blood pressure 175; urea in serum 0.13 per cent.

Diet: 1000 c.c. milk, 200 gm. bread and 100 gm. butter, containing about 7 gm. chlorides.

The chloride metabolism of this patient was similar to that of the first patient. In the first six days he retained some chlorides, but suddenly, in this case

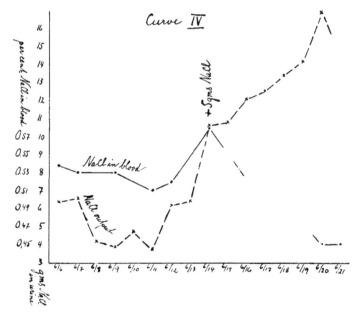

the day after he got 10 gm. salt, the chloride output rose and was much increased until the edema was gone. The concentration of the blood chlorides was much the same as in the first patient. The first days the concentration was 0.55-0.56 per cent, reached its maximum coincident with the rise in the chloride output, after which it decreased and reached its normal value in the course of five to six days.

CASE 3.—A. B., female, thirty-nine years old. Twelve days before entering the hospital she was suddenly taken ill of cephalalgia, nausea and edema in the lower extremities. On the day of admission she was pale, had some râles in the lungs and edema in the legs. In the urine was found albumin, blood and casts. She was put on a diet consisting of 1500 c.c. milk, 100 gm. bread and 50 gm. butter, containing about 5 gm. chlorides.

In this patient we find the same conditions as in the two previous ones. The chloride output was, however, already going on when the examination began. The curve and the table therefore only show how the chloride output decreased until the edema was gone, when the output corresponds to the intake. At the same time the chloride concentration in the blood fell to the normal value.

Of the remaining 6 patients suffering from nephritis whose chloride metabolism I have examined, I will report on one case later. None of the five was cured during the stay in the hospital. Four of the patients had protein and

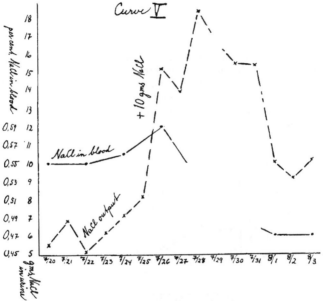

TABLE 3

DATE	WEIGHT	DIURESIS	NaCl in: 24 HOURS URINE	NaCl in: BLOOD %	
7/20	71.6	950	5.61	0.55	
7/21		1250	6.75		
7/22		775	5.20	0.55	
7/23	71.5	870	6.25		Blood pressure 180.
7/24		900	7.20	0.56	
7/25		975	8.20		+10 gm. salt in 500 c.c. water.
7/26		1200	15.22	0.59	NaCl in serum 0.67%.
7/27	71.3	1475	13.87		
7/28	70.9	1600	18.62	0.53	NaCl in serum 0.63%.
7/29	69.9	2600	16.64		
7/30	67.2	1900	15.50	0.49	NaCl in serum 0.60%. Blood pressure 170.
7/31	66.6	2000	15.40		
8/1	65.0	1400	10.08	0.47	
8/2	64.0	1300	9.18		Blood pressure 150.
8/3	63.6	1200	10.20	0.47	

TABLE 4

DATE	WEIGHT	DIURESIS	NaCl in: 24 HOURS URINE	BLOOD %	
6/23				0.51	
6/24				0.51	
6/25	61.5	1350	11.61		Blood pressure 155.
6/26	60.1	1500	11.40	0.48	
6/27	58.5	1500	10.20		Blood pressure 155.
6/28	57.3	1100	7.35	0.46	
6/29	56.8	1100	7.62		Blood pressure 140.
6/30	55.9	1175	6.23	0.46	
7/1	55.6	900	5.50		Blood pressure 120.
7/2	55.2	1100	5.20	0.46	

blood in the urine more than four to five months. In these patients the edema disappeared, but in all the chloride concentration of the blood kept higher than the normal, between 0.51 and 0.56 per cent, and the chloride output was delayed.

In contrast to the increased chloride concentration in anemia and cachexia, the chlorides in nephritis are increased both in blood and in serum. The concentration in serum in nephritis I have found between 0.60 and 0.68 per cent.

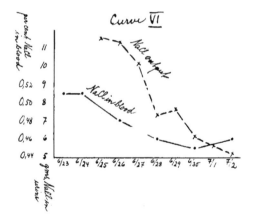

Summing up the results of these examinations it is evident that the chloride concentration in the blood in 9 patients suffering from nephritis with and without edema is high, while at the same time the chloride output is incomplete. In 3 of the patients the output suddenly rises and continues to be great until the retained chlorides and water are excreted and at the same time the chloride concentration in the blood falls to the normal value. There can accordingly be no doubt that the cause of the chloride retention in these cases of nephritis is mainly to be found in the kidneys, which to a certain extent bar the way for the chlorides. When this barrier gives way more or less suddenly, the retained chlorides and water rush out.

In two of the patients the chloride excretion began when the patients began 5 and 10 gm. salt, respectively. It is difficult to decide whether there is any relation of cause or not. Mohr has several times seen that retained chlorides have been excreted when the patients have received a single fairly large dose of salt.

When the chloride retention is caused by lesions of the peripheral vessels, we may at least theoretically differentiate between a primary chloride retention, and a retention due to retention of water. Practically speaking it is, however, impossible to distinguish between the primary retention of water and the primary retention of chlorides. The result is in both instances the same: augmentation of the fluid in the tissue, which we call edema, when it is demonstrable clinically.

A special form of retention is that which the French call "preedema" or "postedema," the Germans "latent edema."

CASE 4.—H. B., office clerk, thirty-four years old. The last month before admission he felt weak and had shortness of breath. On entering the hospital he had slight swelling of the feet, which had completely disappeared on the following day. From that day no edema was to be found. In the urine were found protein, casts and blood corpuscles.

Diet: 1½ liters milk, 100 gm. bread and 50 gm. butter, containing about 5 gm. salt.

TABLE 5

			NaCl in:		
DATE	WEIGHT	DIURESIS	24 HOURS URINE	BLOOD %	
6/11	62.3	2000	19.12	0.52	Blood pressure 185.
6/12		1600	17.60	0.51	Blood pressure 180.
6/13	57.2	1525	14.21		
6/14		925	9.81	0.50	Blood pressure 165.
6/15	57.0	1100	9.50		
6/16		550	6.38		
6/17	53.3	500	4.14	0.45	
6/18	53.2	750	4.75	0.46	
6/19	53.2	700	5.20		
6/20	53.2	675	5.50	0.45	

The patient had the usual symptoms of acute hemorrhagic nephritis. The day he came into the hospital he had slight edema of the ankles which disappeared the following day. The day before the examination began he had no edema and no hydrops of the serous cavities. Nevertheless the patient, living on a diet containing about 5 gm. salt, excretes in a week about 55 gm. salt and 9 kilos of water. At the same time the chloride concentration of the blood sinks to the physiologic level, quite in the same way as with the other patients. This relatively large amount of water has accordingly been stored in the deeper parts of the organism and has been demonstrable only by controlling the weight of the patient.

The pathogenesis of edema has been the subject of many investigations. It is not probable that a retention due to the kidneys is sufficient to produce edema. Cohnheim and Lichtheim, transfusing large amounts of water into the vessels, got no edema.

To get edema it is therefore supposed necessary, in addition to the retention from the kidneys or without it, to have a lesion of the peripheral vessels or a pathologic change of the tissue or a combination of both.

In edema, where the retention is supposed to be due to the tissue, the fluid is by some authors thought to be stored intracellularly, by others to be stored extracellularly.

In intracellular retention the colloids of the cells are supposed to have an increased affinity to water due to some intoxication. Iscovesco, who is the inventor of this theory, emphasizes, that it is of great importance for the patho-

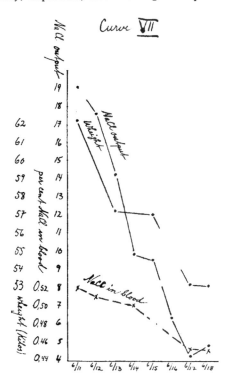

genesis of the edema. Fischer, having the same theory, is of the opinion that the increased affinity to water is due to acid intoxication of the tissue. The theory of the edema caused by the colloids of the cells has not gained much credit. The general opinion is that the edema is caused by extracellular retention of water.

Most authors agree that besides the retention due to the kidneys there must be a lesion of the peripheral vessels to produce edema, but opinions differ much as to the importance of these two causes. While some authors look upon the chloride retention as the main cause of the edema (Widal, Strauss and others),

others attach less value to this retention, or look upon it as a consequence of the edema, while the affection of the peripheral vessels is considered of the greatest importance to the pathogenesis of the edema (Albu, Richter a.o.).

Cohnheim, who first pointed out the importance of the extrarenal factors, supposed that the cause was inflammation in the vessels in the skin and in the muscles, which produced an increase of the exudation from the capillaries to the tissue. Heineke and v. Monakow found that the chloride concentration in edema was greater than in serum. This, they find, favors the belief that the edema is due to an active secretion from the vessels.

A greater concentration of chlorides in the edema than in serum does not prove a secretion from the vessels. When the vessels get more permeable, the smallest molecules, especially the chlorides, will of course, first pass through the wall of the vessel, so that also passive transudation may explain an increased concentration in edema. That protein with its big molecules has a concentration of 5-7 per cent, while the concentration in edema only is about ½ per cent goes to prove the same theory.

Senator, and later Schlayer and Hedinger, have extended the theory of Cohnheim to the effect that first the lesion is localized in the vessels of the kidneys, later on in the peripheral vessels, especially in those of the skin. The cause of this lesion is not known.

The importance of the extrarenal factors has been emphasized especially by the investigations of Achard and Ribot. These authors found that the chloride concentration in the blood in several patients suffering from nephritis was not increased, nay, that it was now and then decreased, in spite of the presence of extensive edema. This goes to prove that the chloride retention may be independent of the kidneys.

To sum up, it will be seen that the chloride retention in nephritis appears to belong to two categories:

In the first in which the chloride concentration of the blood is increased, the retention is mainly due to the kidneys, while the extrarenal factors are of minor importance.

In the second in which the chlorides of the blood according to Achard and Ribot are not increased, the cause is entirely or essentially extrarenal, in the capillaries or even in the tissue.

I shall not discuss in detail the clinical applications of chloride metabolism. The edema we find mainly in two types, which evidently correspond to the above-mentioned two types of chloride retention. The edema, which is chiefly due to the kidneys, is, as a rule, extensive, and often disappears rapidly, while the edema which is stable for a long time, is evidently mainly due to other causes than the kidneys.

Opinions differ as to the symptoms of the increased chloride concentration in the blood. Already in 1840 Rilliet and Andral had pointed out that convulsions may arise when the edema is resorbed. Later on, especially Widal and his coworkers reported several symptoms, for instance increased blood pressure, cephalalgia, convulsions, and unconsciousness, which they attributed to the increased chloride concentration of the blood. It is probable, however, that all these symptoms are not due to the hyperchloremia, but to some other pathologic conditions, which exist along with the increased chloride concentration.

I have determined the chloride concentration of the blood in two patients suffering from uremia, which represented a combination of the "real uremia" and the "eclamptic uremia" (Volhard and Fahr). Both patients had increased urea in the blood, 0.247 and 0.340 per cent respectively. They were somnolent, had a systolic blood pressure above 200 and had convulsions. In one case the chloride concentration in the blood was 0.44 per cent, consequently quite normal, while in the other it was 0.59 per cent, which is the greatest concentration I have found in the blood.

Uremia with increased blood pressure, unconsciousness and convulsions may exist in patients with normal chloride concentration as well as in patients with much increased chloride concentration, which does not go to prove any relation between the chloride concentration and the above mentioned symptoms.

As to the *therapy* of chloride metabolism, Toulouse and Ritchet emphasized in the latter part of the 19th century the importance of limiting the quantity of salt in diet in cases of epilepsy, but salt-poor diet cure did not become general in the clinic until Strauss, some years later, pointed out the significance of the chlorides for the renal and cardiac edema, and Widal and Javal demonstrated in the same period the importance of the chlorides for the edema and the albuminuria in nephritis. Besides in kidney and in cardiac diseases the restriction of chlorides is of importance in some other diseases, for instance, in cirrhosis of the liver (Finsen) and in diabetes insipidus (Tallquist and Erich Meyer). But the salt-poor diet is not of equal significance in all cases of nephritis. In some cases the addition of chlorides seems to remove the edema, while, on the other hand, the salt-poor diet often does not influence it at all. As a rule, the addition of salt will, however, increase the edema, while the edema often disappears when the chlorides of the diet are restricted, which Widal, in particular, has demonstrated.

REFERENCES

Achard, Ch.: Pathogenie de l'oedeme, Paris, 1914.
Achard, Ch., and Ribot, A.: Action compareé du bicarbonate de soude et du chlorure de sodium sur l'hydratation etc, Bull. et Mém. de la Soc. méd. des Hop. de Paris, March 31, 1912.
— Action compareé du chlorure de sodium et du bicarbonate de soude sur une assite cirrhotique, ibid., Feb. 28, 1913.
— Retention chlorurée hypochloremique dans les nephrites hydropigènes, La Semaine Med., 1913, p. 409.
Albu, Albert, and Neuberg: Physiologie und Pathologie des Mineralstoffwechsels, 1916.
Hefter, Julie, and Siebech, R.: Untersuchungen an Nierenkranken u. s. w., Deutsch. Arch. f. klin. Med. cxiv, 497.
Hoesslin, Kashiwado: Experimentelle Untersuchungen über Kochsalzwechsel und Nierenfunktion, ibid., cii, 520.
Mohr, L.: Zeitschrift für klinische Medizin, i.
v. Monakow: Beitrag zur Funktionsprüfung der Niere, Deutsch. Arch. f. klin. Med., cii, 248.
— Beitrag zur Kenntnis der Nephropatien I, II und III, Deutsch. Arch. f. klin. Med., cxv and cxvi.
v. Muller, Fr.: Bezeichnung und Begriffsbestimmung auf dem Gebiete der Nierenkrankheiten, Veröffentlichungen aus dem Gebiete des Militärsanitätswesens Heft 65.
V. Noorden: Handbuch der Pathologie des Stoffwechsels, 1916.

Richter: Die Nierenwassersucht, Deutsch. med. Wchnschr., 1910, No. 38.
Rosemann: Beiträge zur Pathologie der Verdauung, Pflügers Arch., cvi, p. 609.
Schlayer, Takayasu: Untersuchungen über die Funktion kranker Nieren beim Menschen, Deutsch. Arch. f. klin. Med., ci, 333.
Schlayer: Untersuchungen über die Funktion kranker Nieren, ibid., cii, 311.
Scholz, Henkel: Zur Frage der Chlorretention, ibid., cxii, 334.
Stuber: Ueber Diabetes insipidus, ibid., civ, 344.
Widal, Javal: La Cure de Dechloruration, 1913.
v. Wyss: Ueber Oedeme durch. Natrium bicarbonicum, Deutsch. Arch. f. klin. Med., iii 93.
Gettler, Baker: Micro-Analysis of the Human Blood, Jour. Biol. Chem., 1916, xxv.
Ayers, Fine: The Post-Graduate. 1914-1915. Jour. Biol. Chem., 1915, xx, 391.
McLean, Van Slyke: Jour. Biol. Chem., 1915, xxi.

BLOOD SUGAR TOLERANCE AS AN INDEX IN THE EARLY DIAG-NOSIS 'AND ROENTGEN TREATMENT OF HYPERTHYROIDISM*

BY ERIC R. WILSON, A.B., LOS ANGELES, CAL.

THE blood sugar tolerance as an aid in the early diagnosis of hyperthyroidism cannot be minimized, and is most valuable as an index to the degree of toxicity brought about bv increased thyroid secretion. This latter fact is forcibly demonstrated by the return to normal of the blood sugar tolerance in individuals showing an abnomal curve after series of roentgen ray teatments.

TECHNIC OF BLOOD SUGAR TOLERANCE TEST

Patient having fasted the night before was weighed and a sample of blood taken for the determination of the initial blood sugar at 9 A.M. The patient was then given 1.75 grams per kilo body weight of glucose in from 250 to 350 c.c. of distilled water.

The blood sugar was determined by the Lewis-Benedict method. Fehling's solution was used in determining the sugar in the urine.

The physical findings of the five patients coming under our observation and upon which this report is based, were similar in all cases, some being slightly more pronounced in one case than in the others.

All were unmarried women between the ages of 23 and 33.

	BEFORE ROENTGEN THERAPY		AFTER 2 SERIES ROENTGEN TREATMENTS		AFTER COMPLETION 3 SERIES ROENTGEN TREATMENT		
	BLOOD SUGAR TOLERANCE CURVE	SUGAR IN URINE AFTER ADMINIS-TRATION GLU-COSE	BLOOD SUGAR TOLERANCE CURVE	SUGAR IN URINE AFTER GLUCOSE ADMINISTRATION	BLOOD SUGAR TOLERANCE CURVE	SUGAR IN URINE AFTER GLUCOSE ADMINISTRATION	GENERAL IM-PROVEMENT
Case 1	Abnormal	Sugar in 1-1½-2 hr. spec.	Approaching Normal	Neg.	Normal	Neg.	Gen. Improve-ment marked
Case 2	Abnormal	Sugar in 1-1½-hr. spec.	Approaching Normal	Neg.'	Practically Normal	Neg.	Gen. Improve-ment Fair
Case 3	Abnormal	Sugar in 1½-2 hr. spec.	Approaching Normal	Sugar in 1 hr. spec.	Practically Normal	Neg.	Gen. Improve-ment marked
Case 4	Abnormal	Sugar in 1½-2 hr. spec.	Approaching Normal	Neg.	Normal	Neg.	Gen. Improve-ment marked
Case 5	Abnormal	Sugar in 1-1½-2 hr. spec.	Abnormal very slight improvement	Sugar in 1½ 2 hr. spec.	Nearer Normal than previous curve	Neg	Improvement marked at times Slight gen. improvement

*From the Department of Pathology, Bacteriology, and Laboratory Diagnosis, College of Physicians and Surgeons, University of Southern California, Los Angeles, Cal.

Distinct lagging of the upper eyelids was noticed at one time or another in all five cases; this sign being slightly more pronounced in cases Nos. 1 and 3.

Case No. 5 was the only one showing a decided exophthalmos.

The thyroid gland was found to be slightly enlarged in all the five cases, this being decidedly pronounced during menstruation; only in one case did we notice a marked hypertrophy of the gland existing continually.

Tremor of the hands was occasionally found to be absent. We found this sign largely dependent upon the degree of irritability and general feeling of well-being of the patient as to whether it became pronounced, absent or only slight in character.

Warm and moist hands was a sign constant in all cases.

The pulse rate was repeatedly taken and in all cases prior to the time of roentgen treatment was found to be above 110 beats per minute. There was usually a marked increase over this found, under the slightest excitement.

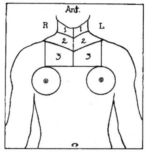

Fig. 1.

The apex beat was found to be forceful in all cases, but only in one was it found to be slightly displaced. The carotids were noted to beat violently under the least excitement, and only occasionally could a blowing murmur be heard over the base of the heart in one or two cases.

The subjective symptoms were in all cases very similar in that there was a general feeling of muscular weakness, lack of "pep," easily tired on exertion, shortness of breath, and occasional palpitation.

All cases gave histories of disturbed menstrual function.

TECHNIC OF ROENTGEN THERAPY (ADMINISTERED UNDER THE DIRECTION OF F. W. HOWARD TAYLOR, M.D.)

The neck below the hyoid bone is anteriorly divided into six sections as shown in Fig. 1; three to the right and three to the left of the median line. Posteriorly these subdivisions do not extend downward as far as they do anteriorly, and are better divided into two areas on each side of the median line. One of these areas is treated every second day, alternating first on one side and then the other, the same with the areas posteriorly which are not treated until the anterior portion has been gone over once. A ten inch spark gap, 3 mm. aluminum filter, ten inch skin distance and thirty milliampere-minutes was used on each area. A rest of three weeks was given the patient when these areas anteriorly and posteriorly had been treated as above outlined. This then constituted the first series. A second and third series was given, and in all early cases seemed sufficient to bring the blood sugar tolerance curve back to normal.

COMPARISON OF THE BLOOD SUGAR TOLERANCE CURVE BEFORE AND AFTER X-RAY
TREATMENT

As will be noticed in a normal control case the blood sugar after administration of glucose rises rapidly reaching its height in one-half to three-quarters of an hour; descends rather rapidly, approaching the normal fasting level, (or it may remain slightly above this level) between one and a half and two hours (Curve No. 2).

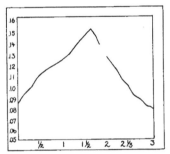

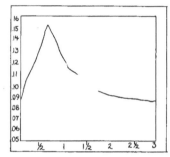

Fig. 2.—Curve No. 1 illustrating typical blood sugar tolerance after ingestion of glucose in case of hyperthyroidism.

Fig. 3.—Curve No. 2 of blood sugar tolerance after ingestion of glucose. Normal control case.

In cases of hyperthyroidism, the blood sugar rises gradually, reaching its height in one to one and a half hours after the administration of glucose; it falls rapidly and does not reach the fasting level (or slightly above this level) until between two and one-half to three hours after the glucose solution has been administered (Curve No. 1).

The urine gave positive tests for glucose in all cases; this was usually most marked in the one and one-half to two hour specimens after the administration of the glucose solution.

THE COMPARISON OF THE CURVES

Curve No. 1 (Fig. 2), illustrating a typical hyperthyroid curve of the blood sugar tolerance after the ingestion of glucose as outlined in the first part of this article. differs so radically from curve No. 2 (Fig. 3), a typical normal control curve, that no further comment than the above is deemed necessary. Curve No. 3 (Fig. 4) demonstrates a typical blood sugar tolerance curve in a case of hyperthyroidism responding favorably to roentgen therapy after two series of treatments. As will be noted in this latter curve. its tendency is to approach the normal. In all but one case, after three series of roentgen treatments had been completed, the blood sugar tolerance curve had practically returned to normal. We found that a slight deviation of the curve might exist and it still be considered normal.

The subjective symptoms in all cases showed marked improvement from after the second to the fourth x-ray treatment. The pulse became slower. A decided improvement in muscular weakness was noticed: the return of "pep" was spontaneous, while shortness of breath was greatly relieved. Menstrual function, which had previously been abnormal gradually returned to what had been normal for the individual.

DISCUSSION

In cases of hyperthyroidism the rate of body metabolism is increased, this increase is roughly proportional to the severity of the clinical manifestations. This fact accounts for the clinical symptoms commonly present, such as, loss of weight, warm moist skin and slight elevation of body temperature. The toxic

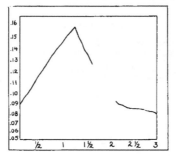

Fig. 4.—Curve No. 3 of blood sugar tolerance after ingestion of glucose in case of hyperthyroidism after 2 series of x-ray treatments.

effect of oversecretion of the thyroid on the cardiovascular system is possibly due to stimulation of the cardiac accelerator nerves. The nervous symptoms are produced by excessive toxic secretion, and the increased irritability and nervousness in turn may tend to greater thyroid secretion, thus establishing a vicious circle. The tolerance for glucose administered by mouth is diminished, which depends on variable factors, namely, the rapidity of absorption from the alimentary tract, or the inability of the body to remove an excess of glucose from the circulation, this is due in larger part to failure of the liver to perform its normal glycogenic function when excessive quantities of sugar are taken by mouth. There may be some influence affecting the threshold limit at which the kidneys begin to excrete the excess of sugar in the urine. It is most probable that all these factors enter into this diminished tolerance for glucose, and particularly the latter in producing the temporary glycosuria. It has been repeatedly demonstrated that there exists an interrelation between the glands of internal secretion, and just as excessive thyroid secretion materially affects ovarian secretion which manifests itself clinically by disturbed menstrual function, so might excessive thyroid secretion cause marked disturbance of the pancreas in its control over carbohydrate metabolism.

Nevertheless, whatever may be the mechanism directly or indirectly causing this impaired glucose tolerance (the causative factor being the hypersecretion of the thyroid gland), an abnormal glucose tolerance exists early in the disease, making it a diagnostic sign of importance, as well as an index in roentgen therapy.

CONCLUSIONS

The blood sugar tolerance test is of distinct importance in the early diagnosis of hyperthyroidism. That seemingly advanced cases of hyperthyroidism will respond but moderately to roentgen therapy, as shown by the blood sugar tolerance test. An abnormal blood sugar tolerance curve when due to hyperthyroidism will tend to approach the normal under roentgen therapy, indicating that excessive toxic secretion is lessened.

Clinical manifestations of hyperthyroidism may be lessened, but an abnormal blood sugar tolerance curve may exist after series of roentgen treatments.

The blood sugar tolerance curve is an index to thyroid hypersecretion in those cases in which toxic secretion has manifested itself by a decreased glucose tolerance.

BIBLIOGRAPHY

Smith, F. M.: Jour. Am. Med. Assn., Dec. 13, 1920.
Janney, N. W., and Isaacson, V. I.: Blood Sugar Tolerance Test, Jour. Am. Med. Assn., 1918, lxx.
Lewis, R. C., and Benedict, S. R.: Jour. Biol. Chem., 1920, lxi, 15.
Monographic Medicine, New York, D. Appleton & Co., 1918, i, 641-643.

LABORATORY METHODS

NUTRITION EXPERIMENTS WITH RATS. A DESCRIPTION OF METHODS AND TECHNIC*

By Edna L. Ferry**

INTRODUCTION

Several years ago we published descriptions of the devices and technic employed in our nutrition experiments with white rats.[1] Since then experience and revised plans of study have brought about various improvements in the outfit and methods used. Inasmuch as inquiries received from time to time have indicated that other workers are interested in our experimental methods it has seemed worth while to describe in detail some of their features.

For the successful outcome of feeding experiments the maintenance of hygienic conditions and a supply of healthy stock are essential factors. Where a large number of animals are to be fed it is important to reduce to a minimum the labor involved, and we believe that the apparatus and methods which we have used contribute to this end. In general all parts of cages and food and water containers should be strictly interchangeable so that no time is lost because some one piece does not fit into its proper place.

CAGES

The cylindrical cages (Figs. 1 and 2) used for the experimental animals are 9 inches in diameter and 8 inches high, made of ¼ inch mesh galvanized wire netting, the raw edges being bound with sheet zinc. The cage has no bottom but is set in an ordinary enamel-ware pan with sides 2¾ inches high and about 9½ inches in diameter at the bottom. The sides of the commercially obtainable pans should flare sufficiently to make it possible to stack them compactly for storage. As food containers we use cups of porcelain 2⅞ inches in diameter and 1¾ inches high, such as are attached to bird cages; the water holders are 2 oz. bar glasses (see Fig. 1). In assembling the various parts five or six sheets of paper napkin are introduced into the bottom of the pan to absorb the urine or any water that is spilled. This paper is covered with two discs of ⅛ inch mesh

*From the Laboratory of the Connecticut Agricultural Experiment Station, New Haven, Connecticut.

This paper represents the experience gained in connection with the nutrition investigations conducted by Dr. Thomas B. Osborne and Dr. Lafayette B. Mendel under the auspices of the Carnegie Institution of Washington, D. C., and the Connecticut Agricultural Experiment Station.

**This paper was prepared by Miss Ferry and was nearly ready for the printer when she became seriously ill and died. By her death biological science has lost one of the most promising and enthusiastic of the younger women who are engaged in this field of work. All who were associated with Miss Ferry in the many activities in which she was interested and in which she excelled have experienced a personal loss which they will feel deeply. We ourselves wish to here acknowledge the debt we owe to Miss Ferry for the ability and devotion with which she cooperated with us in the numerous investigations with which during the past decade we have been engaged.—T. B. O. and L. B. M.

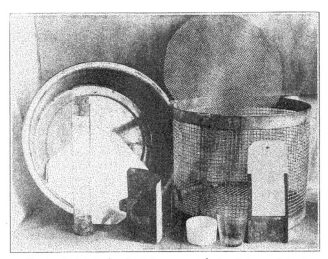

Fig. 1.—Showing the individual parts of the cages and feeding devices used for the experimental animals. The cage and cup holder are made by the Herpich Company, New Haven, Conn. The food cups are obtained from the A. B. Hendryx Co., New Haven, Conn., who also are now prepared to furnish the cages, as well as the accessories illustrated in Figs. 1-6. The netting discs and zinc card holders are cut out in the laboratory.

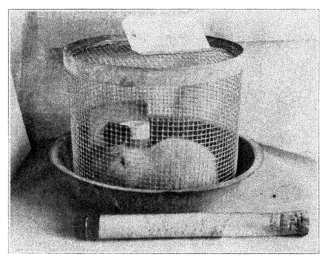

Fig. 2.—Showing the experimental cage in use. The strip on the back of the cup holder hooks over the edge of the pan, thus holding it firmly in position. If a rat acquires the habit of pulling out the glass and spilling the water, a wire hook can be inserted through the back of the holder just above the top of the glass to hold the latter securely.

wire netting to prevent the animals from obtaining access to the sheets. Over the edge of the pan is hooked the specially shaped cupholder (shown in Fig. 1) with food and water containers in place and its bottom resting on the wire disc. The animal can now be placed in the pan and covered with the wire cage.

This arrangement of the cage and its parts presents the following advantages: it simplifies the process of cleaning and it eliminates covers and doors, thus facilitating handling the animals. As the entire cage can be lifted up when the food is placed in the holders, or the rat removed, there is much less danger of being bitten than when the hand must be inserted through a small opening either in the top or the side.

To clean the parts before they are sterilized the cage and cupholder need merely to be rinsed; the wire discs are boiled in water, after which the debris attached to them can easily be removed by rinsing under the faucet. The pans and cups are readily cleaned with a brush. It is our custom to wash and sterilize the cages of the experimental animals with live steam in a large tank twice a week.

Experience has demonstrated that, except for rats with young, "bedding" is unnecessary if the temperature of the environment is suitable. Our rat rooms are usually maintained at a temperature of 65-70° F.

In order to obtain rats of known age and vigor we have found it advantageous to raise our own, and for this purpose a breeding colony of about 200 animals is maintained. These are kept in rectangular cages, 18 inches long, 12 inches wide, and 8 inches high (Figs. 3 and 4). The front and sides of the cage are made of ½ inch mesh galvanized wire netting, reinforced along the top, bottom and corners with strips of zinc. The back and top are made of sheet zinc, the top being attached to the back by hinges which make it possible to open the entire top of the cage. The top is held closed by a small brass catch in front. The bottom of the cage is made of heavy netting with a 1 inch mesh. The cage rests in a galvanized pan 18½ inches long, 12½ inches wide and 1 inch deep. To absorb moisture the bottom of the pan is covered with one or two sheets of thin blotting paper held in place by ⅛ inch mesh wire netting.

These cages are washed under a faucet, using a brush whenever necessary, and are sterilized with steam once a week. Fresh papers are put in the pan twice a week and the sheets of wire netting are boiled to remove the adherent dirt. The coarse netting on the bottom of the cage permits the feces and debris of the food to fall through into the pan when the cage is lifted. This makes it possible to renew the papers and boil the sheet of fine netting as often as may be desirable without handling the rats. In these larger cages the water cups are like those used in parrot cages and are slipped in through an opening in the front of the cage. Usually four rats are kept in one cage. No bedding is used.

Either just before or just after a litter of young is born the mother is removed to a special cage, 9 inches square and 9 inches high (Figs. 5 and 6). This is like the larger ones except that it has no bottom because the very young rats were sometimes crushed on the heavy netting of the large cages. The fine wire netting is left as a separate sheet so that it may be boiled to facilitate cleaning. In these cages water is furnished in a glass drinking tube, inserted through a hole in the top of the cage as shown in Figs. 5 and 6. This prevents the rat from spilling the water and thus wetting the bedding. Crepe paper strips obtained from the Denison Co. are used for bedding. They have proved much more satisfactory than cotton, because threads of wet cotton may become wound tightly around the legs or tail of a newborn rat and cause the loss of a member. When the young rats are about three weeks old they are transferred with the mother to one of the larger cages to afford them better opportunity for exercise. The mother is left with her young until they are at least four weeks old.

STERILIZATION OF CAGES

The cages are sterilized in a galvanized tank 3′ 6″ long, 2′ 5″ wide, and 2′ 5″ high with hinged top. It holds 12 large breeding cages or 36 round experi-

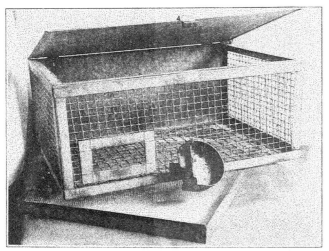

Fig. 3.—Showing the individual parts of the cages used for the animals in the stock colony. The cages and pans are made by the Herpich Company and the water cups are obtained from A. B. Hendryx Company, both of New Haven, Conn.

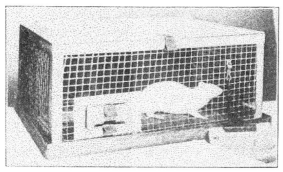

Fig. 4.—Showing the cage of the stock colony in use.

mental cages at once. The steam enters through a pipe at the back of the tank. At one end, near the top is inserted a piece of stove pipe, the free end of which passes to the outside of the building through a window. At the opposite end of the tank, at the bottom, is attached an electric blower or fan. After the steam has been passed into the tank for 10 minutes the current of air is turned on, and the steam blown out of doors before the tank is opened. The escape of large quantities of steam into the room is entirely avoided. A pipe drains the condensed steam away from the tank.

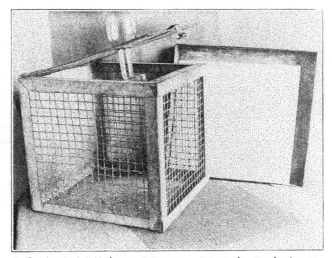

Fig. 5.—Showing the individual parts of the cages used for the breeding females. The cages and pans are made by the Herpich Company, New Haven, Conn., and the water tubes by E. Machlett & Sons, New York.

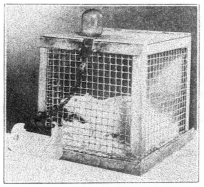

Fig. 6.—Showing the breeding cage in use.

FOOD

The food of the experimental animals is made into a coherent paste which the rats will not scatter. When fat is used, the finely ground protein, carbohydrate and salts are mixed thoroughly, stirred into the melted fat and the entire mixture passed repeatedly through an electric food chopper. Such a water-free food is practically sterile and can be kept for several weeks without any apparent deterioration.

When the foods are to be prepared with water, the dry ingredients are thoroughly mixed, usually by passing them through the food chopper, and enough water is added to each day's ration to make it the proper consistency. Each morning the food which is left over is removed from the food cup and dried in an oven. At the end of the week the daily residues are collected, weighed, and their weight deducted from the total amount of the dry ingredients given to the animals. In the process of drying, the residues lose about 8 to 10 per cent of moisture, but allowance can be made for this in computing the food intakes.

The food of the animals in the stock colony consists of "dogbiscuit" made by the Potter and Wrightington Co., Charles River Ave., Boston, from a formula furnished them by Professor Castle. Once or twice a week these animals are given fresh vegetables of some kind, usually carrots when they can be obtained. Nursing mothers and young rats under four to five weeks of age receive in addition a milk food paste made as follows:

	per cent
Milk powder	60
Starch	12
Lard	28

WEIGHING

The rats are weighed on a spring balance shown in Fig. 7. The dial reads from 0-1000 grams in 5 gram divisions. Although the readings between the 5 gram divisions must be estimated, the errors made during a long experiment are negligible. Where many animals are to be weighed the use of a spring balance saves time.

Food enough for a week or more for each rat is put into a heavy glass tube 10 inches long and $1\frac{1}{8}$ inches in diameter with a cork at each end (see Fig. 2). From this tube the food is forced out into the cup as desired, by using one cork as a plunger. At the beginning and end of each weekly period the tube, cup and food in them are weighed on a spring balance (see Fig. 7). The scale on this balance reads from 0-400 grams in 2 gram divisions. The little pan for holding the tube and cup is made of sheet aluminum.

The most satisfactory methods for marking the food tubes and cups of the individual rats are as follows: The number of the animal is written on the tube with indelible ink and then covered with a thin coat of shellac; in the case of the cups, the glazing is removed from a small spot with an emery wheel, the number of the rat is then written on the rough spot with pencil and covered with shellac. The shellac prevents the numbers from being accidentally washed off, but they can be removed easily by soaking in dilute alkali.

GENERAL CONDUCT OF EXPERIMENTS

Each morning the food and water cups are taken out of the cup holders and placed on top of the individual cages. The water glasses are collected, for washing and filling, in large trays with wire netting bottoms. A wheeled table such as is used in hospitals, greatly facilitates distribution of the containers. The food

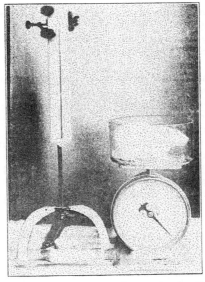

Fig. 7.—Showing the devices used in weighing the food and the rats. The food balances are made by the Chatillon Company, New York. The rat balance was obtained from Chas. Forschner & Sons, New York.

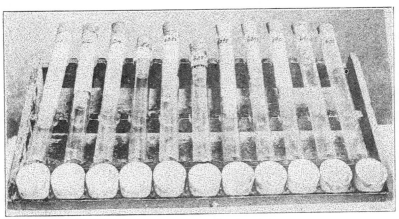

Fig. 8.—Showing tray for food tubes in use.

cups and tubes of those animals whose food is to be weighed are collected in trays (see Fig. 8) and weighed. The remaining food cups are filled without removing them from the tops of the cages, the tubes of food being kept at the left of each cage.

Vitamine or other preparations which are to be fed apart from the basal ration are offered in additional cups introduced into the cages. Recently the use of carefully prepared compressed tablets of these accessory materials has been found most convenient.[2] Formerly small sized scoops were used to measure portions of these products.

At night a strip of board about 4 inches wide is placed along the tops of series of cages to prevent any of the animals from tipping up the latter and escaping.

On Saturday enough food is put into the cups to last until Monday, so that on Sunday it is necessary merely to supply any desired accessory food and water.

By having enough clean cages it is possible for three persons to weigh the animals, chart the weights of the rats, to clean and sterilize the cages at the rate of almost three per minute.

The rats are weighed first when about three weeks old; thereafter the stock rats are weighed once a week and the experimental animals twice a week. The young rats are usually started on experimental diets when they are between 30 and 40 days old and weigh from 50 to 80 grams. Animals weighing decidedly less than the average for their age are never used in diet experiments.

IDENTIFICATION

In the stock room where several animals are kept in each cage the individuals are distinguished by staining patches of their fur with different nonpoisonous colors. By using two colors and marking different parts of the body it is easily possible to identify a dozen or more animals in a single cage.

The cages containing the experimental animals are arranged in numerical order. The color of the correspondingly numbered location sign serves to indicate the days on which each animal and its food are weighed. The number of the rat is printed on a tag which is inserted in a zinc holder placed on the top of the cage. The holder keeps the rat from destroying the tag, and also is heavy enough to prevent the tag from being knocked off accidentally.

BREEDING

In breeding the animals, three females are usually mated with one male, care being taken to select only vigorous individuals and to avoid inbreeding if possible. A female which has successfully raised a litter of young is not remated until three or four weeks after the young are weaned, and she has regained the weight lost during the lactating period. Females more than a year old are discarded for breeding purposes, but males are frequently used until they are nearly two years old.

RECORDS

The records of the experiments are kept in a loose leaf notebook, the pages of which are numbered serially to correspond with the rats. At the top of the page is recorded the sex, date of birth, and parentage of the animal and the purpose of the experiment. Below are columns for the date, weight of the rat, weight of the food + tube + cup, and amount of food eaten. There is also space for the formula of the ration used and comments on the condition of the animal, or reasons for making any changes in the diet (Fig. 9). To facilitate a rapid survey of the changes in body weight and food intake a corresponding record is kept in the form of graphic charts (see Fig. 10).

RAT 4082.

Parents 3503 ♀ and 3437 ♂
Born Feb. 10, 1917   Female
    Diet: Soy cake + starch + lard
    Purpose: To study growth on soy cake as the sole source of protein, inorganic salts, water-soluble vitamine and fat-soluble vitamine.

Date 1917	Weight gm.	Tube + cup +food gm.	Food eaten gm.	
Mar. 1	33			
8	48			
14	60	269		Soy cake 37.5%
15	57	266		Starch 42.5
				Lard 20.0
15	57	266		
19	58			
22	58	239	27	
22	58	239		
26	61			
29	59	208	31	
29	59	294		
Apr. 2	61			
5	63	262	32	
5	63	262		
9	69			
12	74	209	53	
12	74	303		
16	74			
19	78	250	53	
19	78	233		Food changed to study effect of improving the inorganic salts in the diet.
23	100			
26	110	171	62	Soy cake 37.5%
				Salt mixture 4.5
26	110	253		Starch 38.0
30	121			
May 3	124	185	68	

Fig. 9.—Showing a specimen page from the laboratory notebook.

In addition to these records a card catalogue which gives the ancestry for three or four generations is kept. This is useful as a guide in selecting animals for mating so as to avoid close inbreeding. These cards show not only the ancestry of the individuals but also the progeny resulting from each mating, and in the case of experimental animals a list of the different diets used and the dates between which each was fed, thus giving in tabular form a brief resume of the history of each rat (Fig. 11).

INDEXES

The following indexes have proved very useful:

1. An alphabetical list of the proteins or other food factors which have formed the topics of investigation, together with a numerical list of the rats fed on the corresponding diets.

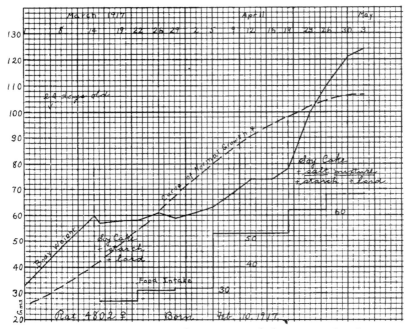

Fig. 10.—Showing a specimen page from the laboratory book of body weight charts.

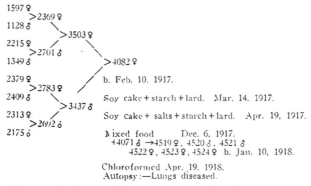

Fig. 11.—Showing a specimen card from the heredity catalogue.

2. A list of the experimental animals classified according to the types of experiments which they represented, such as "growth," "maintenance," "protein minimum," "amino-acids," etc.

3. A chronological, classified record of the new experiments begun, and changes made during each month. This last is chiefly useful when it is desirable to review the work from an historical standpoint. The importance of records of this sort becomes apparent in investigations, such as ours, where several thousand animals have been employed.

REFERENCES

[1]Osborne, T. B.. and Mendel, L. B.: Feeding Experiments with Isolated Food-Substances. Carnegie Institution of Washington, 1911. Pub. 156, pp. 53; Ein Stoffwechselkäfig und Fütterungsvorrichtungen für Ratten. Ztschr. f. biol. Technik und Methodik, 1912, lxxx, 307.

[2]An illustration is afforded in the paper of Osborne, T. B., and Mendel. L. B.: The Occurrence of Water-Soluble Vitamine in Some Common Fruits, Jour. Biol. Chem., 1920, in press.

A NEW FORM OF ETHERIZING DEVICE FOR USE IN ANIMAL EXPERIMENTATION*

By G. Raap, A.B., A.M., and D. E. Jackson, Ph.D., M.D., Cincinnati, Ohio

IN recent years a number of forms of ether valves, etherizing devices, and artificial respiration machines have been described, among which may be mentioned those by Guthrie,[1] Jackson,[2] Gates,[3] Hoyt,[4] Sollmann[5] and others. In the present article we wish to describe briefly a new form of etherizing apparatus

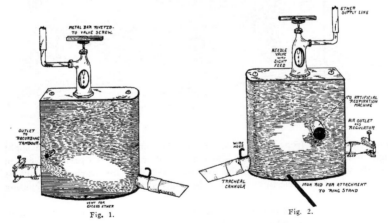

Fig. 1.   Fig. 2.

which we have recently devised. This apparatus is well adapted for use with all the ordinary types of artificial respiration machines, such as those of Gates,[3] Jackson,[6] Hoyt,[4] Stewart and Rogoff,[7] Meltzer,[8] Hanzlik,[9] Fells[10] and Higgins,[11] or even with an ordinary hand bellows.

*From the Department of Pharmacology, University of Cincinnati Medical School, Cincinnati, Ohio.

As shown in Figs. 1 and 2 the device consists of a brass box held in position as shown in Fig. 3 by a stand and clamp, permitting of adjustment in height from the table according to the size and position of the animal operated on. The box is curved on the bottom to fit the surface of the animals neck and jaws. Fig. 4 shows the box with the top and end removed to illustrate the arrangement of the interior which contains a U-shaped strip of woven wire gauze with four or five layers of ordinary cotton gauze sewed over the outside of it. This serves to give ample evaporation surface and to deflect any currents of air which might otherwise become insufficiently laden with ether vapor. Into one side of the box is soldered a short tube one half inch in diameter, to which the rubber hose from the artificial respiration machine may be attached. The tracheal cannula

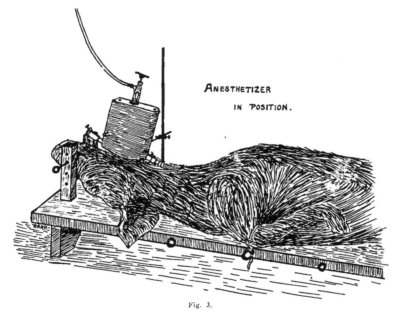

ANESTHETIZER

IN POSITION.

Fig. 3.

is attached to the front of the box, near the bottom and is inclined at a slight angle to facilitate rapid insertion into the incised trachea. To permit of use in animals smaller or larger than the average sized dog, the tracheal cannula is supplied with removable tips which can be attached to suit the animal (including cats).

Into the side of the box nearest the operator is soldered a short piece of one-fourth inch tubing to which the rubber tube leading to the respiratory tambour is attached. A very small hole is made in the bottom of the box near the tracheal cannula opening. This hole permits escape of any pure ether which might accidentally fall to the bottom of the box, thus preventing the ether from getting into the trachea or lungs.

The air outlet and regulator, which, as shown, consists of a short rubber tube supplied with an adjustable screw clamp, is placed opposite the tracheal cannula, and is so situated as to allow the animal a very free air-way through which to breathe. By slightly opening or closing the screw clamp the amplitude of the respiratory tracing (tambour) can instantly be adjusted to any desired height.

Ether is supplied from a reservoir (mercury bulb or aspirator bottle) hung about 12 or 15 inches above the animal and arranged to prevent unnecessary evaporation by means of a small air ingress tube as shown in Fig. 5. A rubber

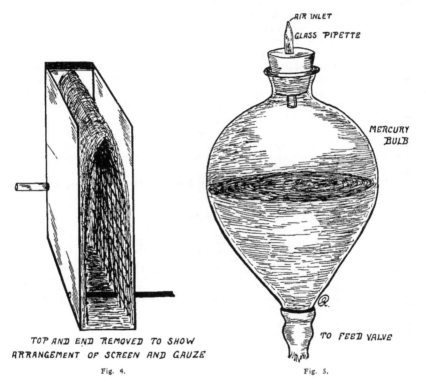

Fig. 4.

TOP AND END REMOVED TO SHOW
ARRANGEMENT OF SCREEN AND GAUZE

AIR INLET

GLASS PIPETTE

MERCURY BULB

TO FEED VALVE

Fig. 5.

tube conducts the ether to a small sight feed needle valve which is soldered into the top of the box. Thus the supply of ether breathed by the animal can be very quickly and accurately regulated by a simple adjustment of the needle valve. This works equally well for either natural or artificial respiration, or if changes are quickly made from one to the other. But if artificial respiration is given, a pinchcock must be placed on the tambour tube to prevent an excess of air being forced from the box into the tambour, thus injuring the rubber membrane over the tambour.

The artificial respiration machine may be attached before the operation is begun and started and stopped at any time by means of an electric switch.

One special advantage secured by attaching the tambour directly to the apparatus is the avoidance of changes in the character and amplitude of the respiratory tracing due to changes from the abdominal to the thoracic type of breathing, or vice versa. These spontaneous changes always affect the character of respiratory tracings obtained by means of a stethograph tied around the chest or abdomen of an animal.

The device has been of great value in open chest work in which cardiac, lung or pulmonary pressure tracings were to be made. This is due to the fact that the rate and extent of lung inflation always remains constant, because there is no change in the dead space of the tubes, etc., through which the air is supplied to the animal, and ether can be given or stopped at any desired moment.

It is advisable to coarsely adjust the needle valve before the experiment is begun. The ether supply tube can then be closed off completely with a pinch cock until the tracheal cannula is inserted. A small wire hook is placed on the tube just above the attachment of the replaceable cannula tip. Around this hook the string used to tie in the cannula tip is fastened, thus preventing the cannula from being pulled out of the trachea.

The device uses less ether to carry on anesthesia than is usually required with an ordinary ether bottle. It is especially useful for students, since the confusion of changing from ether to air or vice versa in case of accidents, etc., is almost entirely eliminated.

The device may be obtained from the Max Wocher & Son Co., 19 West Sixth St., Cincinnati, Ohio.

REFERENCES

[1]Guthrie, C. C.: Jour. Am. Med. Assn., Sept. 9, 1911, p. 887.
[2]Jackson, D. E.: Jour. Am. Med. Assn., Feb. 17, 1912, lviii, 475 and 476.
[3]Gates, F. L.: Proceedings. Jour. Pharmacol. and Exper. Therap., 1915, p. 611.
[4]Hoyt, J. T.: Jour. Physiology, Sept., 1901, xxvii.
[5]Sollmann, T.: Laboratory Guide in Pharmacology, 1917, p. 257, Figs. 58 and 59.
[6]Jackson, D. E.: Experimental Pharmacology, 1917, St. Louis. C. V. Mosby Co., pp. 473, 475, Figs. 360-364.
[7]Stewart, G. N., and Rogoff, J. M.: Jour. Lab. and Clin. Med., 1918, iv, No. 2, p. 73.
[8]Meltzer, S. J.: Med. Rec. New York, July 7, 1917.
[9]Hanzlik, P.: Jour. Lab. and Clin. Med., 1916, i, 688.
[10]Fells, G. E.: New York State Med. Jour., 1916.
[11]Higgins, J. A.: Jour. Lab. and Clin. Med., 1919, iv, No. 12, p. 737.

The Journal of Laboratory and Clinical Medicine

VOL. V.	AUGUST, 1920	No. 11

Editor-in-Chief: VICTOR C. VAUGHAN, M.D.
Ann Arbor, Mich.

ASSOCIATE EDITORS

DENNIS E. JACKSON, M.D.	CINCINNATI
HANS ZINSSER, M.D.	NEW YORK
PAUL G. WOOLLEY, M.D.	DETROIT
FREDERICK P. GAY, M.D.	BERKELEY, CAL.
J. J. R. MacLEOD, M.B.	TORONTO
ROY G. PEARCE, M.D.	AKRON, OHIO
W. C. MacCARTY, M.D.	ROCHESTER, MINN.
GERALD B. WEBB, M.D.	COLORADO SPRINGS
WARREN T. VAUGHAN, M.D.	BOSTON

EDITORIALS

Major General Gorgas

WILLIAM CRAWFORD GORGAS was born at Mobile, Ala., October 3, 1854. His father, Josiah Gorgas, was born in Pennsylvania in 1818, graduated at the United States Military Academy at West Point in 1841 and was assigned to the Ordnance Corps. He served with credit in the Mexican War with the rank of captain. When the Civil War began he cast his lot with the Confederates and was made head of the Ordnance Department with the rank of Brigadier General. One of the buildings in which General Josiah Gorgas manufactured gun powder, now unoccupied and falling into decay, stands near Macon, Ga. After the Civil War General Josiah Gorgas was elected Vice-Chancellor of the University of the South and later became President of the University of Alabama.

William's mother was Amelia Gayle, the daughter of John Gayle, governor of Alabama from 1831 to 1835. He was a presidential elector in 1836 and in 1840 and afterwards served in Congress.

William took his collegiate degree at the University of the South in 1875 and his medical degree at Bellevue Hospital Medical College, New York City, in 1879. As a student at Bellevue he listened to the first course of lectures given by Dr.

William H. Welch, who had recently returned from his European studies and who was destined to become the father of scientific medicine in this country. General Gorgas frequently referred to Dr. Welch as his revered and beloved teacher, and it is more than probable that the lectures of Dr. Welch stimulated the spirit of research in young Gorgas, as later courses of lectures by the same distinguished man have stimulated hundreds of others at Johns Hopkins. After serving one term as an intern in Bellevue Hospital, Gorgas entered the Medical Corps of the Army. In 1881 Gorgas and Crowder were young officers at the post at Brownsville, Texas. In that year an epidemic of yellow fever prevailed at this post. An order was issued that no officer should come in unnecessary contact with a case of yellow fever. Crowder was officer of the day and on making the rounds he found Gorgas making an autopsy on a man who had died from this disease. Crowder told Gorgas to wait while he secured his sword. Gorgas continued his dissection and Crowder, properly equipped, came back to the hospital, placed Gorgas under arrest, and carried him to the calaboose. The spirit shown by Gorgas in making this autopsy continued with him throughout life and made him the greatest expert on yellow fever the world has ever known and will secure for him the honor of having eradicated this disease from many parts of the world. From their Brownsville days Crowder and Gorgas remained fast friends and during the World War there was the closest affiliation between the office of the Surgeon General and that of the Provost Marshal General. Both Gorgas and Crowder delighted in telling the story of the former's arrest by the latter at Brownsville in 1881.

In 1898 Captain Gorgas went with the Fifth Army Corps to Santiago and while there was promoted to the rank of major. In the Santiago campaign Gorgas had charge of the Yellow Fever Hospital and it was largely through his skill in the management of this disease that the death rate in our Army in Cuba from the disease was so low. In charge of the yellow fever patients at Siboney he was untiring in his efforts to limit the spread of the disease and to properly treat the sick. The sight of his kindly face was a stimulant which did much to tone up the muscles exhausted by the exercise imposed upon the body by *el vomito negro*. His kindly words to his patients served as better tonics than any named in the pharmacopeia. As one of his patients at that time the writer testifies to the kindness and skill of Gorgas from personal experience. At Siboney Gorgas contracted typhoid fever and was seriously ill for several weeks. After his recovery in the fall of 1898 he became chief sanitary officer of Havana. In this position he was in closest touch with Major Reed and his associates in their investigations concerning the transmission of yellow fever. After Reed had demonstrated the truth of the theory of Finlay and had incriminated the stegomyia, it was believed that the fight against this disease was to be waged by immunizing susceptibles by the bites of infected mosquitoes, but this did not prove practical. To Gorgas belongs the credit of having originated and executed methods for the extermination of the stegomyia. He carried this out so successfully in Havana that the city for the first time in several hundred years was free from the disease.

When the building of the Panama Canal was undertaken Colonel Gorgas was made chief sanitary officer of the Zone. It is no exaggeration to say that his work on the Zone rendered the building of the canal possible. It is estimated that for every tie on the Panama railroad the French left a skeleton on the Zone. Gorgas so improved the sanitary condition of this death laden region that it became healthier and showed a lower death rate than any community in the United States; indeed, on the Canal Zone Gorgas demonstrated that malaria and yellow fever might be banished from the tropics and the fairest and most fruitful regions of the world might become fit and even delightful habitations for man.

After the completion of the Isthmian canal Gorgas was made Surgeon General and in his honor the rank attached to this office was raised from a brigadier to a major generalship.

It is exceedingly fortunate that during the World War General Gorgas occupied the position of Surgeon General of the Army. Everybody knew of him, was acquainted with the work he had done and had implicit confidence in him both as a skilled sanitarian and as a man of honor. During the war his chief concern was the welfare of the soldier. He personally inspected all the camps and a notification that any camp had an undue amount of sickness was sufficient to bring General Gorgas to it with the greatest speed. In making his inspections he insisted that he and those who accompanied him should take at least one midday meal in the hospital unannounced and with the purpose of ascertaining by personal experience how the patients were fed. He not only adhered to this rule himself, but insisted that all inspectors should do the same. The skill and devotion of General Gorgas to the welfare of the enlisted men resulted in the mobilization of a great army with a smaller death rate than had hitherto been known in the annals of military medicine.

General Gorgas was deeply interested in the Medical Reserve Corps and it was largely through their knowledge of his work and their faith in the man that more than thirty thousand civilian physicians immediately offered their services to him. At the beginning of the war the highest rank that a Reserve officer could secure was that of major. General Gorgas prepared with his own hands a bill providing for increased rank in the Reserve Corps and personally appeared before Congressional committees to secure the passage of this bill. In this he was successful. He was not content to visit the camps in this country, but made a tour of those in France.

General Gorgas' splendid work has received universal recognition. Before the War he was called by the British Government to South Africa to advise as to the methods necessary for the eradication of infectious pneumonia on the Rand. He was given degrees by many universities in this country and by the University of Oxford. He received many decorations, both in this country and abroad. His great ambition was to completely eradicate yellow fever and after his term as Surgeon General had expired he went to South America as a health commissioner for the International Health Board of the Rockefeller Foundation. At that time and for many years previously Guayaquil had been a hot bed and breeding-place for this disease. He succeeded in completely stamping out this disease at that place. A few months ago yellow fever was reported on the west coast of Africa and General Gorgas was asked by the British Government to visit that region and determine whether or not the reported disease was yellow fever, and if so how it could be eradicated. On his way to South Africa he was stricken with a cerebral hemorrhage in London and there died.

Certainly if service to his fellow man be a measure of greatness, General Gorgas' name will take a place with those of Pasteur, Koch, Ross, Reed, and others of this class. We mourn his death, but we recognize the fact that he built for himself, for the medical profession, and for the world at large, a monument more lasting than one of stone or bronze.

To know General Gorgas was a high privilege and an education in and of itself. He was as gentle as a woman, but at all times inflexible in his adherence to what he believed to be right. He would listen with the greatest patience and deference to any suggestion, but he always acted in accordance with the dictates of his intelligence and his heart. Companionship with him was heightened by the vein of true wit and humor which ran through much of his conversation and his writings. His book on Sanitation in Panama is interspersed with stories which would have done credit to Mark Twain.

It was his custom to begin or to end his interviews with some humorous remark. The sparkle in his eye always foretold some humorous suggestion. After a conference with the writer he once said: "This is your judgment and it is mine, but remember that your judgment and mine have at times been at fault. Do you recollect that you and I recommended the burning of the village of Siboney in 1898 in order to stamp out yellow fever? I have often wondered how many infected mosquitoes were destroyed in that conflagration."

His story of the stampede among a group of distinguished sanitarians, who while visiting the hospital in Havana and standing around a jar filled with mosquitos some one accidentally displaced the top of the jar and set free the host of winged insects, is only equaled by that of the turkey gobbler at the hospital at Ancon that became blind from swallowing the quinine capsules surreptitiously dropped in the bushes by the laborers to whom they were issued as a daily ration. We hope that Mrs. Gorgas will publish his letters. In doing so she would confer a favor and, indeed, we may say, a boon upon the medical profession. They would display the inner man of one who has done great things for the good of mankind and one we all delight to honor.

In 1885 General Gorgas married Marie Cook Doughty, of Cincinnati, who has accompanied him on many of his journeys in search of infection and has intelligently helped him in his work. They have one daughter, the wife of Colonel W. D. Wrightson, who was one of General Gorgas' chief aids on the Canal Zone, chief of the Sanitary Corps during the War, and since that time an assistant to General Gorgas in his work in Central and South America.

The Medical Corps of the Army, the medical profession of this country and of the world, all who are interested in the eradication of disease and the alleviation of human suffering, recognize the greatness of the man and his work and deeply mourn his death. May his life be an incentive to the young men in our profession.   —*V. C. V.*

Prevention of Goiter

WHILE it is possibly true that the majority of goiters one sees so frequently in children in grade schools, and high schools; in adolescents in colleges and offices, and in adults in the market places and department stores, wherever there are crowds, are benign, i.e., they produce no symptoms, nevertheless, they are abnormalities which have in them vicious potentialities. If it were possible to suppress them, to keep the thyroids within bounds morphologically as well as physiologically, the community would be better off. At least the cosmetic effect would be good, and also possibly the morbidity rate would be reduced in certain directions. Just how far the latter would be true cannot be estimated as yet, but in the course of years a valuable statistical material will have gathered in the city where Marine has commenced his experiment. There are many apparently harmless conditions (and an abnormally enlarged thyroid may be one of them), which are expressions of variations in structure and metabolism which tend in the direction of diseased conditions, the connections of which are not at present understood. These directions and connections may be learned in the future by following and studying the vital statistics of districts in which the attempt is made to reduce the incidence of abnormality. In goiter districts such studies should have much value with reference to the prevalence of thyroid states, and may also point out other states and relationships of which we do not know.

It is not frequent that a physiologic experiment on a large scale is made in the community, at least it is not frequent that such an experiment is planned and carried out for a specific purpose. Such a one Marine and his co-workers have made. After years of study and experiment on thyroid states, Marine devised a scientific experiment upon a community, and in successive years has checked up the results and published them for the benefit of other communities in which the incidence of thyroid enlargement is high. The result is a valuable contribution to preventive medicine.

In his most recent report Marine gives the records of 2305 pupils in the public schools who have not taken the prophylactic treatment, and 2190 pupils who have. Of the 1182 pupils with thyroid enlargement at the first examination and who took the prophylactic, 773 thyroids have decreased in size, while of 1048 pupils with thyroid enlargement at the first examination and who did not take the prophylactic, 145 thyroids have decreased in size. The only presumptive error in these figures is due to the fact that many pupils listed as not taking the prophylactic have taken iodine in one or another form outside the school jurisdiction. The figures are striking.

The treatment used by Marine consists in administering 2 grams of sodium iodide, given in 0.2-gram doses daily for ten consecutive school days, repeated each spring and autumn. An ounce of syrup of the iodide of iron or hydriodic acid given over a period of two or three weeks and repeated twice yearly might be as efficacious. The sodium iodide treatment Marine believes has prevented enlargement of the thyroid in more than 99 per cent of the children in his district.

In the practical application of the preventive treatment, Marine and Kimball say, one must keep in mind the three periods when simple thyroid enlargements most commonly occur, i. e., (1) fetal, (2) adolescent, and (3) pregnancy. Prevention of goiter in mother and fetus is as simple as that occurring during adolescence and probably smaller amounts of iodine could be used. for instance, 1 gram of sodium iodide distributed over a month. At this period the problem is one for physicians alone. The problem during the second period is, however, a public health problem for state, county, and municipal boards of health. The existing system of organization of schools, public and private, is sufficient to handle the details without aid or expense. Physicians in industrial medicine can render important service by practical and educational methods. It seems that the maximum of prevention with a minimum of effort would be obtained by giving the treatment between the ages of eleven and seventeen years.

So far no untoward effects have been observed as a result of the treatment. No obvious case of exophthalmic goiter has developed, although such cases have been carefully watched for. Less than 0.5 per cent of the cases have shown symptoms of iodism, practically all of them mild.

REFERENCES

Marine and Kimball: Prevention of Simple Goitre in Man. Arch. Int. Med., 1920, xxv, 661. See also Jour. Lab. and Clin. Med., 1917, iii, 40; Arch. Int. Med., 1918, xxii, 41.
Kimball, Rogoff, and Marine: Jour. Am. Med. Assn., 1919, lxxiii, 1873.

—*P. G. W.*

Significant Phenomena of Influenza Pandemics

WITH the development of greater refinements of investigation many novel features of pandemic influenza have been recognized. Many of them apparently corroborate existing theories of epidemiology while others call for further explanation or different interpretation.

Before the days of bacteriology the contagiousness of the disease was little discussed. Its infectiousness was, in fact, not universally established until the epidemic of 1889-90. Watson recorded "instances * * * too numerous to be attributed to mere chance in which the complaint has first broken out in those particular houses of a town at which travellers have arrived from infected places."[1] Parkes[2] commented on the frequency with which first cases had been introduced or imported and also how often the townspeople nearest the invalids had been infected. Leichtenstern recorded many such isolated examples.[3] Some of the earlier observers, especially Haygarth in 1775 and 1782, Falconer in 1802 and Baker in 1814, collected so many instances in support of this that they became convinced that its propagation was due entirely to human intercourse.[4]

In the literature of the period there were many examples reported from personal experience to show that influenza is transmittted from man to man. Two objections had to be met, however, before this view was generally accepted. It had been claimed by some that the disease spread more rapidly than individuals could travel and again that instances were on record of cases occurring spontaneously in isolated communities. Abbott records an example of the latter.[5]

"An impression having gained some credence that influenza had appeared on board the squadron of naval vessels which sailed from Boston in December, 1889, while on their course across the Atlantic and before their arrival in Europe, a letter was addressed by the writer to the Bureau of Medicine and Surgery of the United States Navy for information upon this point to which a reply was received, as follows:

" 'The "Chicago," "Boston," "Atlanta" and "Yorktown" left Boston December 7, 1889, for Lisbon, Portugal. The first three arrived at Lisbon on December 21 without having touched at any port *en route*. The "Yorktown" arrived at that port December 23, having stopped about twenty-four hours at Fayal, Azores. * * * Influenza first appeared on the "Chicago" December 23, on the "Boston" December 28, on the "Atlanta" December 30, and on the "Yorktown" December 28.'

"Influenza was prevailing in Lisbon at the date of arrival of the squadron."

Many similar reports of epidemics on ships at sea and in other isolated communities have, in the same way, been shown to be distortions of the actual facts.

Other facts which have aided in establishing the contagiousness of influenza have been the frequent "immunity" of remotely isolated groups or of segregated individuals, such as lighthouse-keepers and inmates of quarantined institutions, as well as the tendency of outbreaks to follow the gathering of crowded public assemblages.[5]

Another argument formerly raised against the contagious character was the claim that it broke out in mass attacks—that large numbers became ill on the same day, without the occurrence of isolated antecedent cases. The first cases of such epidemic diseases as the plague became a matter of record because of the accompanying high mortality, while in influenza with its relatively low mortality, the record usually begins only after a comparatively large mass of individuals has been attacked. Detailed studies of the Munich epidemic of 1889,[6] and numerous similar studies of the recent epidemics have shown a period of two or three weeks of steadily increasing numbers of cases before the height of the epidemic was reached.

The Epidemic of 1889-90 was first recognized as such in October, 1889, when it appeared in Northern Russia. It first occurred in St. Petersburg in the last week of October. In the following month cases appeared in Paris, Vienna, and Berlin, and it did not reach London until December. South America was reached in January, 1890. This does not indicate more rapid progress than the rate of human travel of that period. The period of greatest mortality at Stockholm followed that at St. Petersburg by three weeks, that of Berlin, by yet another week. This period for Paris was a week later than for Berlin, that for London another week later, and that for Dublin three weeks later than that for London. The week of highest mortality in Dublin was later than that for New York or Boston.

The earlier epidemics progressed even more slowly. That of 1762 prevailed in Germany in February, in London in April, in France in July and in America in October. Epidemics have varied not only in rapidity of spread but also in extent of spread. Of the 72 epidemics on record since the thirteenth century, thirteen have spread to nearly all inhabited parts of the earth. Between 1847 and 1889 there was no pandemic, but the disease had prevailed in more or less limited areas, as at Paris and Strassburg in 1857-58 and in 1867. This appears to have been true for all periods.

It has been more difficult to trace the site of origin of the last epidemic and its direction of spread. Several factors have contributed to this, the principal of which are the speed of modern travel, the character of modern commerce, and the existence of war. The channels of the commerce of today radiate nearly from all points to all other points of the civilized world. An epidemic breaking out in Turkestan or Sweden could be carried as directly and nearly as rapidly to New York or Singapore as to Naples, Lisbon or Liverpool. No longer are there a few preeminent lanes of travel such as there were in 1580, when the epidemic spread clearly from Constantinople to Venice and on to Hungary and Germany, finally finding its way to Norway, Sweden, Denmark and Russia. The war has made it difficult to know accurately the date and direction of spread in enemy countries. The broad dissemination of trade with belligerent countries adds to the difficulties of following routes of travel and of spread.

The autumn epidemic has been reported as being at its height in October, 1918, in such widely separated localities as the United States, England, France, Brazil, Greece, India, Japan and Korea. There was no such rapid wide dissemination as this in previous epidemics. It may be a question whether the spring of 1918 with its much milder epidemic was not the actual period of spread from an endemic focus to all parts, and whether the autumn epidemics consisted in recrudescences of the disease already planted in these localities. This point will be discussed later.

Influenza was recognized in the United States Army in this country in March and April of 1918.[7-8] There is also good evidence that the civilian population was attacked at the same time in certain localities. The first outbreak in the American Expeditionary Forces is recorded as in April and May, 1918, the first cases being near a port of debarkation. The second epidemic occurred in September and October and the third recrudescence in February, 1919.[9] In Greece the disease first appeared toward the end of May, 1918. The severe form appeared in September.[10] A mild epidemic passed through Spain in the early spring of 1918, then visited France and probably extended into Germany. It was mild in the two former countries. By July it had become relatively severe in Germany.[11] In England an epidemic was prevalent in June and July[12] and in Scotland in July and August.[13] A mild epidemic occurred in certain parts of Britain in May. Recurrence occurred in October and November, 1918, and in February and March, 1919.[4-10] Japan was afflicted with the mild form of the disease in the spring of 1918 and it had invaded India by August.

Thus we see that a mild and rather less highly contagious form of the disease had planted its seed in nearly all countries during the spring and early summer. Since then we have had a severe recurrence in 1918, a less severe one in 1919, and yet another in 1920.

The tendency to recurrence is characteristic of epidemic influenza. Can we go farther and state that the curves of incidence tend to vary in any set fashion with the successive recurrences? Greenwood[12] describes the salient features of the primary epidemic as, first, a rapid and quasi-symmetrical evolution, and, second, a frequency very closely concentrated around the maximum. In other words the duration is short, the rise to a peak rapid and the subsequent fall equally rapid. He shows that in the July-August, 1918, epidemic in Great Britain nearly 80 per cent of the total incidence in the localities studied was grouped within three weeks time. This was also true for the primary attack of 1889. In contradistinction a secondary epidemic affects, according to Greenwood, a relatively small proportion of the population, is slower in reaching its maximum, and thereafter declines slowly and irregularly, more slowly than it increases. The distribution of the curve is less symmetrical and there is less concentration around the maximum. A secondary epidemic is characterized by a much higher fatality than a primary one.

In England from 1889-94 there were four epidemics. The first was primary in character, the second secondary, and the third, while reverting to primary type in respect to symmetry remained of the secondary type as regards mortality. The epidemic of 1676 appears to have caused more deaths than the primary one of 1675. That of 1679 reverted to the primary type. One hundred years later, in 1782, a summer epidemic occurred in London, followed the next year by another which appears to have been of about equal severity. The pandemic of 1847-48 appears on the contrary to have been a single primary epidemic without recurrence.

If we accept Greenwood's classification we must conclude that the autumn of 1918 epidemic in this country partook of the nature of a primary epidemic in most localities as regards symmetry and explosiveness, but affected a much larger number of people and was much more highly fatal than the spring epidemic. That of 1920 was equally explosive, but less severe. The epidemic in Detroit illustrates the manner of the last recurrence.[14] On the 27th day of the 1920 epidemic the death rate had returned nearly to normal and the epidemic had run its course. There had been 11,202 cases with 1,642 deaths. On the 27th day of the 1918 epidemic there had been 16,423 cases, 1286 deaths, and the epidemic had not run its course. The second outbreak was of shorter duration and affected a smaller number of the population, but had been more highly fatal.

Greenwood alludes to the fact that the epidemic constitution of a secondary influenza period is pneumonic, as contrasted with a primary period which is usually without serious complications. This was true in England, in America, in Europe, as exemplified by the experience in the American Expeditionary Forces. There the spring epidemic was so mild as to be designated by the descriptive title "three day fever." If the secondary epidemic should occur in the winter it might well be most severe, while in the summer it could be very mild.

Is there any tendency to regularity in the interepidemic intervals? Brownlee[15] after studying the records of 1889-94 and the intervening years concluded that for some reason influenza periods tend to recur at thirty-three week intervals after the primary epidemic, and that the favorable season for its occurrence is from January to the end of May. Should the thirty-third week fall in other than these winter months the epidemic may be mild or even missed, reappearing after another eight months' interval. Epidemic influenza does not assume a form which causes any large number of deaths until a bronchitic or pneumonic constitution has been established. The fatal form is usually a disease of the winter or spring.

Reasoning thus, Brownlee was able to predict correctly the date of the recent 1920 epidemic. He did not attempt, however, to explain the short interval between the two epidemics of 1918. He speaks of the second as "aberrant." In other words it does not fall within his classification. October is not a high respiratory disease month. The epidemic should have been mild.

Stallybrass[16]; has confirmed Brownlee's thirty-three week periodicity and suggests an explanation for the aberrant October epidemic. Using periodograms with a thirty-three week basis, and plotting deaths from influenza and respiratory diseases from January, 1890, through January, 1920, he finds that the most definite thirty-three week periodicity is shown during the years 1890-99. During this period there is one maximum, when all thirty-three week periods are superimposed, which occurs at the seventh week of the cycle. Beginning about 1899 a new maximum appears in the nineteenth week of the cycle, which continues to recur until the culminating point is reached in the week ending October 26, 1918. An additional sixty-six weeks carries the date forward to the first week in February, 1920. The maximum at the seventh week of the periodogram during the years 1899-1913 is greatly diminished from that in 1890-98. The periodogram for 1914-1919 shows clearly both maxima, that in the seventh and that in the nineteenth weeks. The interval 1914-1919 was chosen for separate tabulation because from 1914 onward there was a progressive increase in the annual number of influenza deaths, with the single exception of 1917.

There is still a third small but definite maximum in both the early and late periodograms, at the twenty-seventh to the twenty-ninth week. The twenty-ninth week of the cycle falls on May 18, 1918, and on January 10, 1919. Crests of influenza deaths actually occurred in Liverpool on May 18, 1918, and January 3, 1919. There were also outbreaks in the Grand Fleet, in Spain, Glasgow, and other places in May, 1918.

Stallybrass bases his figures chiefly on death rates in Liverpool, Brownlee, on those of London.

It becomes apparent that there are probably three sets of phenomena, each with thirty-three-week cycles, the first reaching its crests in May, 1918, and January, 1919, the second in October 1918, and, after sixty-six weeks, February, 1920, and the third in July, 1918, and March, 1919. Crests of influenza waves occurred in all of these months, at one place or another and sometimes all in the same locality. These observations go one step farther toward explaining the "aberrant" October epidemic. This particular outbreak falls about the nineteenth week and, therefore, is in the cycle which has become increasingly prominent since 1900.

Stallybrass remarks, "if it should prove correct that there are three strains of the influenza virus, each with a periodicity of about thirty-three weeks, and that simultaneously all three strains became enhanced in both virulence and infectivity, then we are faced with a phenomenon without exact parallel, although the behavior of the meningococcal viruses during the war present some points of similarity."

In addition to the thirty-three-week cycle, there is evidence of a larger, basic cycle of about ten years' range. Epidemic crests have been reached in England in 1789-90, 1802-03, 1830-32, 1840-41, 1848-51, 1854, 1869-70, 1879, 1890, 1898, and 1918-20.

Are the sporadic interepidemic cases encountered by the practitioner of medicine and diagnosed as influenza, the same disease as that which we have been discussing? Are they due to the same cause? This is a vital question in the epidemiology of the disease. Some have taught that there is somewhere far away, perhaps in Turkestan, an epidemic focus where the disease smoulders for years occasionally flaring up and covering the earth with its conflagration. It has even been suggested that we search out this "foyer" and by appropriate procedures in that locality, eradicate the disease forever.

But if the disease is constantly with us in milder form, its eradication would not be so easy a matter. No disease is more characteristic, or conforms more nearly to type than does epidemic influenza. The symptoms are clear cut, the manner of spread is constant, and the epidemic as a whole has the definite features previously described. The sporadic case has the same quite clear-cut clinical symptomatology, but fails to manifest the one feature most characteristic of epidemic influenza—a high degree of contagiousness. Further, although the symptoms in themselves are characteristic, there is no one pathognomonic sign by which one may say "this is a case of influenza," and, finally, other disease conditions frequently resemble it so much as to cause error in diagnosis.

Thus, while probably not all sporadic cases diagnosed influenza are in reality that disease, yet there have been plenty of instances thoroughly studied by the best clinicians, where no other diagnosis could be accepted. Such observations as those of Brownlee and Stallybrass also indicate that the disease is always with us in mild form. Then there is the added significance of local outbreaks, limited to an institution or a town or a small section of country, but not becoming pandemic. These do not trace their origin to Turkestan. Examples are numerous. Outbreaks in Paris and Strassburg in 1857 and 1867 have already been referred to.

An excellent example of an epidemic limited to an institution was described in 1869 by Webster.[17] The number of inmates was about five hundred, of whom one-fourth were attacked, and a large part of these applied for treatment. These cases usually presented the following symptoms: *Prostration*, often so great as to require patients to take to their beds. *Chills* with great sensibility to cold. *Headaches* and frequently *vertigo*. *Fever* apparently higher than that which is common in the early stages of typhoid. *Insomnia, anorexia* and *thirst*. Cough and expectoration in all cases. No physical signs were detected in the lungs where they had been previously healthy. The acute stage ran its course in from three to five days, and subsided gradually, leaving the patient weak and with an obstinate cough, which did not yield for weeks or months. Not every case presented all these symptoms. There was every degree from very severe to light cases. They agreed in one characteristic, that the constitutional disturbance was primary and was out of proportion to the local catarrhal lesion. The epidemic ran its course in about a month, the epidemic influence growing weaker, the severer cases occuring in the first weeks of the epidemic. There were no fatal cases. There were a few cases of pneumonia and pleurisy, and in every case of phthisis the rational symptoms and the physical signs were greatly aggravated for a time. There had been no cases, either of pneumonia or of pleurisy prior to this epidemic. There was at the same time a prevalence of "colds" in the neighboring city of Augusta, Maine, but they lacked the severe constitutional symptoms which prevailed at the asylum.

There was no pandemic of influenza at the time of this outbreak, but there are records of local epidemics in England in 1869.

Assuming that a disease similar to influenza is present in greater or less degree during interepidemic periods, can the virus infecting these mild cases become the cause of the fearful pandemics, or must we still have recourse to Turkestan?

The answer to this question lies in the future. We have quoted Brownlee and Stallybrass as giving evidence of its constant presence. It will be objected that their figures are for all respiratory infections, that in interepidemic periods pneumonia and bronchitis may alone make the total numbers. While this is true, the fact remains that there is a close correlation between the waves of the periodogram and the actual dates of the recent recurrences. Perhaps it would be more correct to say that the respiratory infections, including influenza tend to recrudesce in thirty-three-week cycles.

The periodogram as used by Brownlee and Stallybrass is not without possible error. The including of the large 1918 wave so overshadows all previous waves as to distort the entire picture.

We are presented with a variety of facts concerning the origin and manner of spread of pandemic influenza,—facts many of which seem directly contradictory. What information we possess of former pandemics indicates geographic progression from an initial focus. Description of the site and size of this focus is usually vague. Evidence presented within the last year or two, on the contrary, emphasizes the constant presence in many localities of an infectious phenomenon whose salient characteristics are a tendency to periodicity and occasional outbreaks of respiratory pandemics with no break in the periodic cycle. Finally, and to further complicate the picture, we know that during the severe 1918 epidemic there was geographic progression. Pandemic influenza entered the United States in August and September, 1918, at Boston and Camp Devens and spread thence, south and west, to cover the entire country.[18] It entered Connecticut at New London and appears to have spread from there, northwest and west, spreading more rapidly along the more highly-travelled routes.[19] The spread from Spain across France and Germany has been described.

In 1918, the epidemic very evidently spread across the United States from city to city, from east to west. In 1920 this spread was not so evident. The disease was first reflected in the total mortality in Kansas City during the week ending January 17, 1920. The following week increase was recorded in Chicago, New York and Milwaukee, and still a week later in Detroit, Boston, San Francisco and Philadelphia. The mortality increase in New Orleans did not commence until the week ending February 14th.[20] The earlier cases appear to have been in the central area of the continent, and quite unrelated to still earlier epidemies reported in Europe, particularly in Spain.

Certainly pandemic influenza is a contagious disease spread by personal contact, capable of traversing entire continents in remarkably short time, but spreading no faster than the present means of human travel. Surely also the spread is from some focus. But the question, that recent epidemiologic work has raised is whether we must still assume one far off endemic focus, or whether the primary focus may occur wherever and whenever all conditions, biologic, telluric, meteorologic, become propitious to an increase in virulence of the disease virus?

If the latter be true, there might conceivably be two or more simultaneous primary foci, or, if there be more than one virus, each with its own periodicity, more than one epidemic might manifest itself in the same focus or locality.

Such a conception is not entirely new. Leichtenstern[21] in 1896 suggested the possibility of two endemic foci, one in Eastern Europe or Asia and the other in North America. He also considered the secondary epidemics as arising from many foci, left after the spread of the primary waves.

The mechanism which produces an increased virulence may be more easily understood from a consideration of the following remarks by Theobald Smith.[22]

"During the elimination of the more virulent races of microorganisms, there goes on as well a gradual weeding out of the most susceptible hosts. In a state of nature in which medical science plays no part, there must occur a slight rise in the resistance of individuals, due to selection and perhaps acquired immunity, which meets the decline of virulence on the part of microbes until a certain norm or equilibrium between the two has been established. This equilibrium is different for every different species of microorganism, and is disturbed by any changes affecting the condition of the host or the means of transmission of the parasite. One result of the operation of this law is the low mortality of endemic as compared with epidemic diseases. Certain animal diseases while confined to the enzootic territory, cause only occasional, sporadic disease, but as soon as they are carried beyond this territory, epizootics of high mortality may result. Climate in some cases enters as an important factor, but the most important, perhaps, is the *slight elevation in virulence brought about by a more highly resistant host.* The most susceptible animals are weeded out, and the rest strengthened by non-fatal attacks. *The virulence of the microbe rises slightly to maintain the equilibrium.* In passing to a hitherto unmolested territory, the disease rises to the level of an epizootic until an equilibrium has been established.

"In the more or less rapid changes in our environment due to industrial and social movements the natural equilibrium between host and parasite established for a given climate, locality, and race or nationality is often seriously disturbed and epidemics of hitherto sporadic diseases result."

An example of increasing virulence from such changing conditions, is the experience in the army camps with the streptococcus. This microorganism became so exhalted that, whereas, it was at first but a secondary invader, it soon became the cause of primary disease.

With our present knowledge the assumption of widespread endemic influenza with multiple primary foci and any attempted explanation thereof must be but mere conjecture.

REFERENCES

[1]Watson, Thomas: Principles and Practice of Physics. 1872, ii, 71.
[2]Parkes, E. A.: Reynold's System of Medicine, 1876, i, 35.
[3]Leichtenstern, O.: Nothnagel's Specielle Pathologie, 1896, iv, Thiel I., 1-195.
[4]Abbott, Samuel W.: The Influenza Epidemic of 1889-90, 21st Annual Report of State Board of Health of Massachusetts, (Pub. Doc. No. 34), 1890, pp. 307-384.
[5]For an example during the recent epidemic, see. Stanley, L. L. Influenza at San Quentin Prison, California, U. S., Public Health Reports, May 9, 1919, xxxiv, 19.
[6]Leichtenstern, O.: (Loc. cit.).
[7]Vaughan, V. C.: An Explosive Epidemic of Influenzal Disease at Fort Oglethorpe. Jour. Lab. & Clin. Med., 1917, Vol. iii, 560.

[8]Vaughan. W. T. and Schnabel. T. G.: Pneumonia and Empyema at Camp Sevier, Arch. Int. Med., 1919, xxii, 441.
Also: Opie, E. W., et al.: Pneumonia at Camp Funston, Jour. Am. Med. Assn., 1919, lxxii, p. 109.
[9]Longcope, W. T.: Survey of the Epidemic of Influenza in the American Expeditionary Forces, Jour. Am. Med. Assn., 1919, lxxiii, 189.
[10]Filtzos, T. C.: Epidemic Influenza in Greece, Public Health Reports, Mar. 14, 1919.
[11]Vaughan, V. C.: The Influenza in Germany, Jour. Lab. & Clin. Med., 1918, iv, 83.
[12]Greenwood, M.: The Epidemiology of Influenza. Brit. Med. Jour., 1918, ii, 563.
[13]Dunlop, J. C.: Notes on the Influenza Mortality in Scotland During the Period July, 1918, to March, 1919. Edinburgh Med. Jour., 1919, xxii. 403, xxiii, 46.
[14]Vaughan, Henry F.: Influenza in Detroit, Weekly Health Reports, Commissioner of Health, Detroit, 1920.
[15]Brownlee, Jno.: The Next Epidemic of Influenza. Lancet, London, Nov. 15, 1919, p. 856.
[16]Stallybrass, C. O.: The Periodicity of Influenza, Lancet, London, (Feb. 14) cxcviii. 372.
[17]Webster, J. O.: Report of an Epidemic of Influenza. Boston Med. and Surg. Jour., 1871, New Series, vii, 377.
[18]Soper, George A.: The Influenza Pneumonia Pandemic in the American Army Camps During September and October, 1918, Science, N. S. xlvii, 451.
[19]Winslow, C. E. A., and Rogers, J. F.: Statistics of the 1918 Epidemic of Influenza in Connecticut, Jour. Infect. Diseases, 1920, xxvi, 185.
[20]Vaughan, H. F.: (Loc. cit.).
[21]Leichtenstern, O.: (Loc. cit.).
[22]Smith, Theobald: American Medicine, 1904, p. 711.

—W. T. V

The Rationale of Narcotic and Antipyretic Therapy

THE therapeutist of today may look back with tolerant amusement on those ancient pioneers who, believing in the doctrine of signature, were wont to prescribe liverwort for disease of the liver and milk weed as a galactagogue. These early followers of the art believed that from the shape or color of a leaf, a root, a blossom, from a superficial resemblance to some organ of the human anatomy, they might divine what malady the Creator had intended be cured thereby. In those days there were nearly as many remedies from which to choose as there were varieties of plants. Many of them used quite empirically were found to be highly beneficial. Today the drugs of proven value scarcely number half a hundred.

The physiologic action of most of the members of the latter group is now well known. A few of proven worth are still accepted as valuable empirical remedies. Pharmacologic knowledge has been gained chiefly through laboratory experiments on animals; to a lesser extent through observations of the effect on disease in man. Quite unconsciously we are still using some drugs whose physiologic action is well known, entirely empirically so far as concerns their manner of action on the particular symptom to be relieved.

Thus one may dissertate at great length on the action of morphine as a myotic and concerning its action in slowing the respiration or lessening peristalsis. But we do not give morphine to contract the pupils or to slow the respiration. We administer it empirically to relieve pain, and that it accomplishes better than any other drug. Here we are not dealing with its ability to alter the function of a particular organ so much as with its action on psychic processes.

D. I. Macht and his co-workers have in recent years studied this problem, which they designate "psychopharmacology," and Macht has recently published (Bull. Johns Hopkins Hosp., May, 1920) a summary of their results.

They first studied quantitatively the extent of analgesia produced by the various opium alkaloids. They determined the sensory threshold value for pain by electrical stimulation on various parts of the skin and mucous membranes before and after the administration of the drugs. Martin and others had previously determined that the threshold of electrocutaneous sensation is quite constant in normal individuals and is subject to physiological, diurnal, nocturnal and fatigue variations. The present investigators found a normal pain threshold which remained constant for many hours in succession and with but slight diurnal and nocturnal variations.

They then administered the drug to be examined either subcutaneously or intramuscularly, the subject being ignorant of the nature of the drug. These experiments were conducted under constant conditions and were suitably controlled. They concluded that the narcotic drugs administered in moderate therapeutic doses fell in the following order with respect to their analgesic power, beginning with the strongest: morphine (10 mgs.), papaverin (40 mgs.), codeine (20 mgs.), narcotin (30 mgs.), narcein (10 rugs.), and thebain (10 mgs.). In one subject with morphine idiosyncrasy they discovered that small doses rendered him hypersensitive to pain. This confirms the common experience of persons who are not relieved by morphine but are thereby rendered more sensitive.

They further found that certain combinations produced greater analgesia than either drug given separately. Thus, narcopthin, (morphine and narcotin meconates), produced distinct analgesia in 5 mg. doses, while 5 mg. of morphine or 10 mg. of narcotin alone failed to produce this effect.

Attention was next directed to the local or peripheral action of the opium alkaloids, a subject concerning which there has been considerable difference of opinion. Dionin or ethyl morphine is well known to be a powerful local anesthetic and is used as such in ophthalmic surgery. Monkhtar demonstrated a local action on sensory nerve terminals. Pal discovered accidentally that papaverin placed on the tongue produces numbness. Macht and his associates found that the opinum alkaloids, when applied to the skin or the mucous membranes, affected the sensory nerve endings with a resultant raising of the threshold for pain. The most efficient was papaverin. Narcotin, morphin, narcein, codein and thebain followed in the order of efficiency. They also found that analogous to the results after subcutaneous injection pantopon, (a mixture of the total opium alkaloids), exerted an affect greater than that produced by the same amount of either morphine or papaverin.

Thus we see that opium acts both as a poison on the central nervous system and to some extent on the peripheral nerves. The old empirical local application of opiates to relieve pain appears to have a rational basis.

The common antipyretics when studied in the same manner as the opium derivates were also found to produce a certain degree of analgesia of central origin, but of lesser degree than the latter. Acetanilid, acetphenetidin and pyramidon were found to be especially effective in this group. They were administered by mouth.

In an investigation of the effects of opium derivates on psychologic reaction time, the simple reaction to touch, light and sound stimulation was tested first under normal conditions and second after injection of a drug. All experiments were carefully controlled. Complex reaction time or associated reaction time was also determined by having the subject add given numbers, etc. In this manner the action of the opium alkaloids on the higher brain centers was studied.

Small doses of morphine (4-6 mg.) produced a primary stimulation with shortening of the simple reaction time and a lesser number of errors made in the computation of mathematical problems. This primary effect was followed in a half hour or more by a stage of depression with prolongation of the reaction time. With doses of 8-15 mg. of morphine the stage of stimulation was very short and the depression became the dominant feature, with delayed reaction time and a greater number of mistakes in the association tests.

In four out of seven experiments with pantopon, a mixture of the hydrochlorides of all the opium alkaloids, and containing 50 per cent of morphine, the narcosis and prolongation of the reaction time was greater than that produced by an equal amount of morphine.

With very small doses of morphine, only the primary stage was observed.

In all experiments the simple reactions were less affected than the association tests, indicating an action especially on the higher functions of the brain.

The effect of the antipyretics on the reaction times was quite different. There was no primary stimulation effect, except possibly after small doses of quinine, and in ordinary doses these drugs produced little effect on the reaction time, tending if anything to delay it slightly. Such depression was noticed particularly in the case of pyramidon. This corresponds to the common experience that it is a more powerful analgesic than the other antipyretics. It is interesting that when there was a depressant effect it was more marked in the simple reactions to light, sound and especially touch than on the higher association processes, although there was some impairment of the latter. Thus, the absolute readings in case of the mathematical calculations were sometimes actually improved, the depressant effect being seen only in the greater number of errors committed. These reactions were the reverse of those found for the opiates and suggest some lower synapse as the seat of action of the coal tar derivates.

In the neuromuscular test of continuous tapping with a brass stylus it was found that less than 5 grains of phenacetin, antipyrin, acetanilid and quinine showed a tendency to improve the tapping rate, while doses of 8 or more grains tended to impair the efficiency in the test. Pyramidon, salol and aspirin had no appreciable effect.

Morphine and pantopon injected subcutaneously produce a definite narrowing of the field of vision, whereas the antipyretics tend if anything to increase it slightly. It is difficult to establish the mechanism of these phenomena. Macht suggests that constriction of the pupil in the case of opium, vasomotor changes produced by the antipyretics, specific effects upon the retinal ganglia and nerves, and the central cerebral effects must all be considered.

The acuity of hearing was increased by antipyrin, pyramidon and quinin and decreased by acetanilid, salol and aspirin. A remarkable synergistic action was seen in some drugs as in acetanilid and sodium bicarbonate. Taken alone, the former decreases the acuity of hearing while the latter has no effect whatever. The two taken together produce a definite improvement in auditory perception.

Morphine administered to albino rats who had previously learned to negotiate an experimental labyrinth produced a marked impairment of the memory habit and activity. But even after a prolonged narcotization the animals ultimately recovered all of their "intellectual" activities. Macht suggests that this is hopeful evidence for ultimate recovery in the cure of drug addicts. While we welcome all such evidence we must bear in mind that the psychologic reaction is much more complex in humans than in rats, or at least than the recognizable reactions in these animals.

—*W. T. V.*

The End Results in Cases of Focal Infections

CONSIDERING the enthusiasm which attaches to focal infection, it is perhaps no wonder that many almost crimes are committed in its name. Has a patient an ache or a pain? He must have a diseased tonsil or a carious tooth, or a root abscess, or an infected sinus. So, it will be easier to take out the tonsils and make the diagnosis later, or take out the teeth or drain a sinus, and, if the symptoms cease, all well and good; if they do not, well, let's look farther. Focal infection has become an excuse for snap-shot diagnosis. It occupies, in some quarters, the same position as does the exploratory laparotomy. It deserves to be said very emphatically that the state of affairs pictured above is not a general one, albeit too general. Rather it is itself a sort of focal infection that truly causes aches and pains in the body medical. The treatment is obvious.

The contrary state of affairs also exists. There are physicians who decry the emphasis,—any emphasis, indeed— upon focal infections. Such an attitude is probably a more serious one than that of the positive enthusiast, for after all a man is not damaged save only temporarily by the loss of his teeth or tonsils.

Between these two extremes of absolute faith and clinical agnosticism lies a mean. How much truth and how much poetry is there in the whole situation?

Fontaine* has taken 100 cases, and discusses them from the standpoint of the end results. In each case the relation of the focus of infection to the symptoms in question has depended upon: (1) the absence of any other demonstrable cause for the symptom; (2) the failure to cure the symptom by all other methods than the one used, and (3) prompt and continued relief, with no return of the symptom, on the cure or eradication of the focus of infection. Be it said in passing that Fontaine evidently studied his cases and that the conclusions were arrived at largely through the cooperation of a group of specialists. Great reliance was placed on roentgenograms.

In this series the teeth were the most common source of infection, and all sorts of dental conditions were included. Most common, however, were either apical abscesses or granulomas at the roots of devitalized teeth. Next in order of importance were tonsils, and in this group the small fibrous, or submerged, tonsils were quite as frequently involved as the visible sort. The sinuses were of least importance.

The most frequent symptom was pain, for which relief was sought in 42 per cent of the cases, and it occurred, usually, in the muscles of the neck, back,

*Fontaine: Jour. Am. Med. Assn., 1920, lxxiv, 1629.

chest or limbs. The painful areas were not affected by changes of temperature nor were they often associated with tenderness. These symptoms were most frequently associated with dental lesions.

Fever was the symptom second in importance to pain, and was present in 18 per cent of the cases. It seldom exceeded 101° F., was not often accompanied by chills, and in a few cases was accompanied by night sweats. Such cases suggested incipient tuberculosis. In them the foci were equally distributed between the teeth and the tonsils.

Chronic headaches was the dominating symptom in 4 per cent of the cases, and in each case the focus was tonsillar.

General debility with loss of weight and strength occurred in about 10 per cent of the cases. This syndrome was, as a rule, observed in middle aged adults, and in most cases it was accompanied by obvious disease of the teeth.

Severe secondary anemia occurred in 4 per cent, and these cases were due in equal numbers to disease of tonsils or teeth.

There were 6 cases of albuminuria, four due to tonsillar foci, two to dental.

Six cases had an achylia gastrica. In all the only focal infection was in the mouth.

In 6 per cent of the cases moderate vascular hypertension (Systolic = 150 – 170) occurred. All of the patients were middle aged; most of them women. In all the focal infection was dental.

No acute joint conditions were reported. There were eight cases of chronic arthritis of the deforming type. None was benefited by attacks upon foci of infection in teeth, tonsils or sinuses.

In other words in the groups in which general debility, achylia gastrica, and hypertension were dominant, representing some 22 per cent of the cases, the teeth alone were at fault. In the headache group the tonsils alone were diseased. When pain was present, the foci were usually in the teeth. Fever and anemia were due equally to dental and tonsillar conditions, and in albuminuria the tonsils dominated the situation.

The whole report serves, it seems, to emphasize the importance of hidden foci, i. e., foci of infection that are drained only by the blood stream. Lesions that have free access to the exterior are much less apt to be associated with metastatic infection. Hence it is that root abscesses are so much more frequently productive of harm than the usual tonsillar infections.

—*P. G. W.*

The Journal of Laboratory and Clinical Medicine

Vol. V.	St. Louis, September, 1920	No. 12

ORIGINAL ARTICLES

THE INCIDENCE OF STREPTOCOCCUS HEMOLYTICUS IN A RECENT EPIDEMIC OF INFLUENZA*

By HOMER L. CONNER. MAJOR, M.C., U. S. A.

HISTORY

A T the U. S. A. General Hospital No. 19 there was made during the month of January, 1920, a nasopharyngeal survey of all the enlisted men on duty with the detachment. This survey was undertaken to find carriers of meningococci, pneumococci, streptococcus hemolyticus, B. diphtheriæ and B. influenzæ.

The survey was completed on the 29th, a total of 331 men having been examined. Just at this time when the survey was being completed, influenza began to be epidemic in Asheville. Quarantine was established at the hospital the 29th. Under its regulations nasopharyngeal cultures were taken from all classified as (a) all persons returning to the post after an absence of more than twenty-four hours; (b) all persons with respiratory disease that is acute in character; (c) all contacts to those with respiratory disease; (d) all cases suspected as possible influenza; (e) all convalescents from acute respiratory disease; (f) all attendants to patients in this hospital who might act as "carriers"; (g) all patients newly admitted to the hospital and all personnel newly joining the post.

In this period there were 822 individuals cultured a total of 2961 times.

All persons in the above classes were, in accordance with our regulations, cultured three times at intervals of forty-eight hours. Those showing streptococcus hemolyticus, pneumococcus, or B. influenzæ were quarantined until three consecutive negatives were obtained.

The number of cases detected, isolated, and diagnosed as influenza by the Medical Staff is small, being only forty-four. To this number the laboratory added twenty-seven who were carriers of the B. influenzæ.

---

*From the Laboratories, U. S. A. General Hospital, No. 19, Oteen. N. C.
Authority to publish granted by the Surgeon General, whose office assumes no responsibility as to contents.

Our first cases were among the T. B. patients, on two of whom a diagnosis of influenza was made the 29th of January. Between that time and February 12th, there were three more reported. It was among the detachment men that we had most of our cases, a total of thirty being reported. The first of these was admitted the tenth of February. Our last case was released from quarantine March 22.

We shall deal with the culturings of three periods. The preepidemic; the epidemic; the postepidemic.

The results are shown in detail in the tables which follow:

METHODS

All cultures have been taken from the posterior nasopharynx by means of sterile swabs on copper wire which could be easily bent to the required angle at the time of taking the culture. These were introduced through the mouth, care being taken not to touch other than the nasopharynx. With this swab blood plates were immediately streaked. We have used a beef infusion agar, $P_H.7.6$ as the foundation of all solid media used in this work.

This agar was kept in flasks, 200 c.c. to the flask, which was melted, and to which after the temperature of the agar had reached 90 C. was added one per cent of sterile defibrinated sheep blood. From this amount of agar twenty plates were poured, which were placed in the incubator overnight, after hardening, to test for sterility. Blood slants were made of this same mixture as needed. One plate of this "chocolate" agar was used for each person cultured, it being removed from the incubator at the time the culture was made, and after streaking with the swab it was returned immediately. After remaining in the incubator overnight at a temperature of 37° C. the plates were examined for the character of growth, smears made for Gram stain and morphology, and transfers made to Avery broth, blood and plain agar slants, or if necessary replated.

All steps and findings were carefully charted on forms prepared for that purpose.

Fished and replated colonies were incubated overnight at 37°C., then smeared and stained by Gram for morphology and purity, tested for bile solubility, and when indicated, agglutinated for type of pneumococcus according to standard methods.

Such Gram-negative bacilli as grew on blood agar and not on plain agar are classified as B. influenzæ.

TABLE I
CULTURES ON DETACHMENT MEN

Number of men cultured.	SMEAR					LOEFFLER					BLOOD PLATE								
	Spirilla	B. Fusiformis	Diphtheroids	Streptococci	Other	B. Diphtheriae	Diphtheroids	Streptococci	Staphylococci	Other	Meningococci	Strepto. Hemolyticus	Strepto. Viridans	Strepto. Indefinite	Staphylococci	Pneumococcus	B. Influenza	N. Catarrhalis	Other
331	85	18	4	298	48	1	12	178	314	97	0	20	5	185	225	95	5	2	99

PREEPIDEMIC PERIOD

Jan. 12 to Jan. 29, 1920.

During this period 331 men on duty with the detachment had cultures taken of the naso-pharynx. The results are summarized in Table I.

It should be stated that during this time there were no cases of acute respiratory disease among these men.

We therefore term the results of this survey the normal nasopharyngeal flora of these men.

EPIDEMIC PERIOD

Jan. 29 to Mar. 22, 1920

During this period there were nearly 3000 cultures taken which are classified in Tables II and III.

TABLE II

NASOPHARYNGEAL CULTURES—INFLUENZA EPIDEMIC

Date 1920	CASES AND SUSPECTS				CONTACTS				RETURN TO POST				RELEASE FROM QUARANTINE				ATTENDANTS			
	Total	Hemolytic Streptococcus	Pneumococcus	B. Influenzæ	Total	Hemolytic Streptococcus	Pneumococcus	B. Influenzæ	Total	Hemolytic Streptococcus	Pneumococcus	B. Influenzæ	Total	Hemolytic Streptococcus	Pneumococcus	B. Influenzæ	Total	Hemolytic Streptococcus	Pneumococcus	B. Influenzæ
Jan. 29 to Feb. 2	14	2	4	1	3	0	1	0	5	2	0	0	0	0	0	0	0	0	0	0
Feb. 2 to Feb. 6	29	3	1	0	6	0	0	0	30	0	1	1	54	1	3	0	70	15	4	0
Feb. 6 to Feb. 10	16	5	2	0	2	0	0	0	22	1	1	0	125	5	4	0	86	31	8	0
Feb. 10 to Feb. 14	25	8	3	1	4	2	0	0	25	3	1	0	94	11	3	0	0	0	0	0
Feb. 14 to Feb. 18	33	13	0	9	149	92	1	6	35	6	1	1	120	30	1	3	19	7	0	2
Feb. 18 to Feb. 22	18	11	0	2	109	24	0	0	42	10	0	0	148	51	0	8	46	9	0	0
Feb. 22 to Feb. 26	19	13	0	0	78	61	0	4	34	18	0	0	149	93	0	14	76	59	0	5
Feb. 26 to Mar. 1	24	12	0	0	73	47	0	3	42	25	0	1	173	25	0	1	72	47	0	3
Mar. 1 to Mar. 5	9	7	0	1	68	53	0	1	29	16	0	0	223	148	0	11	66	50	0	1
Mar. 5 to Mar. 9	4	3	0	1	48	22	0	1	2	0	0	0	112	69	0	1	48	26	0	1
Mar. 9 to Mar. 13	1	1	0	0	24	15	0	0	16	12	0	0	50	34	0	8	24	15	0	0
Mar. 13 to Mar. 17	0	0	0	0	10	2	0	0	0	0	0	0	36	14	0	4	10	2	0	0
Mar 17 to Mar. 22	5	2	0	0	12	2	0	0	0	0	0	0	37	5	0	1	12	2	0	0

It is to Table III that we especially call attention, showing as it does the progressive increase in percentage of Streptococcus hemolyticus carriers, which corresponds to the increase in number of cases of influenza detected and isolated. It shows also the decline in Streptococcus hemolyticus findings when the epidemic was on the wane, until in the postepidemic period, the number of such carriers again approaches what may be termed the normal percentage.

During this period, also, we made surveys of two complete wards, the whole nursing personnel, all detachment men on duty in the wards, the mess personnel, and the Emergency Hospital established in Asheville for the care of influenza.

The results of these surveys are given in Table IV.

Table IV also shows a seeming relationship of the streptococcus hemolyticus to influenza.

At the Emergency Hospital in Asheville, 90 per cent of the cases were carriers of this organism. The two wards were cultured, because it was from them that we were having cases reported that simulated a mild influenza like infection. The findings of so many carriers, both of the Streptococcus hemolyticus and B. influenzæ, is thought unusual. Subsequent culturings of these two wards, which

TABLE III

NASOPHARYNGEAL CULTURES

FLU PERIOD

DATE, 1920	NUMBER TAKEN	POSITIVE STREPTOCOCCUS HEMOLYTICUS	POSITIVE B. INFLUENZÆ	PER CENT STREPTOCOCCUS HEMOLYTICUS
Jan. 29 to Feb. 6	211	23	2	10
Feb. 6 to Feb. 10	251	44	0	17
Feb. 10 to Feb. 14	148	24	1	16
Feb. 14 to Feb. 18	356	160	21	44
Feb. 18 to Feb. 22	363	109	10	29
Feb. 22 to Feb. 26	356	244	23	68
Feb. 26 to Mar. 1	384	252	17	55
Mar. 1 to Mar. 5	395	274	14	69
Mar. 5 to Mar. 9	214	120	4	56
Mar. 9 to Mar. 13	115	77	8	66
Mar. 13 to Mar. 20	122	29	5	23

POST FLU PERIOD

Mar. 22 to Mar. 26	48	13	0	27
Mar. 26 to Mar. 30	31	6	0	19
Mar. 30 to Apr. 6	43	10	0	23

TABLE IV

	NUMBER CULTURED	DATE	STREPTOCOCCUS HEMOLYTICUS	B. INFLUENZÆ	PER CENT STREPTOCOCCUS HEMOLYTICUS
Nurses	87	Feb. 6	49	0	56
Orderlies	67	Feb. 6	25	0	37
Mess Men	70	Feb. 7	10	0	14
Wards	79	Feb. 14	46	6	58
Emergency Hospitals	33	Feb. 17	30	12	90

were quarantined, and from which the B. influenzæ carriers were removed, gave a progressive decrease in positive Streptococcus hemolyticus findings, and there developed no other cases of the disease or carriers of the B. influenzæ.

The survey of the nurses, orderlies, and mess men, is valuable, as it shows the incidence of Streptococcus hemolyticus to vary according to the degree of contact with patients.

TABLE V

INCIDENCE OF STREPTOCOCCUS HEMOLYTICUS IN CLINICAL CASES OF "FLU" AND IN "CARRIERS." FOUR-DAY PERIODS

DATE	1/29 to 2/2				2/2 to 2/6				2/6 to 2/10				2/10 to 2/14				2/14 to 2/18				2/18 to 2/22			
	T. B. PATIENTS	NURSES	DETACHMENT	CIVILIANS	T. B. PATIENTS	NURSES	DETACHMENT	CIVILIANS	T. B. PATIENTS	NURSES	DETACHMENT	CIVILIANS	T. B. PATIENTS	NURSES	DETACHMENT	CIVILIANS	T. B. PATIENTS	NURSES	DETACHMENT	CIVILIANS	T. B. PATIENTS	NURSES	DETACHMENT	CIVILIANS
CLINICAL CASES	0	0	0	0	0	0	0	0	2	0	0	0	0	2	8	0	2	0	10	0	3	0	8	0
POSITIVE STREPTOCOCCUS HEMOLYTICUS	2	0	0	0	0	0	0	0	2	0	0	0	0	2	8	0	2	0	10	0	3	0	8	0
POSITIVE B. INFLUENZÆ	1	0	0	0	0	0	0	0	0	0	0	0	0	2	3	0	0	0	5	0	3	0	3	0

DATE	2/22 to 2/26				2/26 to 3/1				3/1 to 3/5				3/5 to 3/9			
CLINICAL CASES	1	0	2	0	1	0	1	0	0	0	0	0	0	0	1	0
POSITIVE STREPTOCOCCUS HEMOLYTICUS	1	0	2	0	1	0	1	0	0	0	0	0	0	0	1	0
POSITIVE B. INFLUENZÆ	1	0	1	0	1	0	0	0	0	0	0	0	0	0	1	0

		Str. Hem.	B. Influenzæ
Total Cases 44	T. B. Patients	12	11	4
	Nurses	2	2	2
	Detachment	30	30	13
	Civilians	0	0	0

B. INFLUENZÆ "CARRIERS"

DATE	1/29 to 2/2				2/2 to 2/6				2/6 to 2/10				2/10 to 2/14				2/14 to 2/18				2/18 to 2/22			
	T. B. PATIENTS	NURSES	DETACHMENT	CIVILIANS	T. B. PATIENTS	NURSES	DETACHMENT	CIVILIANS	T. B. PATIENTS	NURSES	DETACHMENT	CIVILIANS	T. B. PATIENTS	NURSES	DETACHMENT	CIVILIANS	T. B. PATIENTS	NURSES	DETACHMENT	CIVILIANS	T. B. PATIENTS	NURSES	DETACHMENT	CIVILIANS
POSITIVE STREPTOCOCCUS HEMOLYTICUS	0	0	0	0	1	0	0	0	0	0	0	0	0	1	0	0	3	4	0	1	1	0	1	0
POSITIVE B. INFLUENZÆ	0	0	0	0	1	0	0	0	0	0	0	0	0	1	0	0	3	4	0	1	1	0	1	0

DATE	2/22 to 2/26				2/26 to 3/1				3/1 to 3/5				3/5 to 3/9			
POSITIVE STREPTOCOCCUS HEMOLYTICUS	1	1	3	0	0	0	4	0	0	0	4	0	0	0	2	0
POSITIVE B. INFLUENZÆ	1	1	3	0	0	0	4	0	0	0	4	0	0	0	2	0

		Str. Hem.	B. Inf.
Total "Carriers" 27	T. B. Patients	6	6	6
	Nurses	6	6	6
	Detachment	14	14	14
	Civilians	1	1	1

Nurses who are in most intimate contact show the highest percentage; orderlies whose contact is not so great rank next, and mess men whose contact is the least show the lowest percentage.

That contact has its influence is also shown in Table II, attention being called especially to "Attendants." Here again we see the progressive increase in Streptococcus hemolyticus carriers which corresponds to the increase in the number of cases of influenza. It was possible by keeping a chart of daily cultures of the individual attendants to see them give on the first day or two of contact negative findings for the Streptococcus hemolyticus. After this first day or so this organism was in most a constant finding. After a period of exposure, varying from three to twenty days, we isolated in twelve of these attendants the B. influenzæ. They were isolated, but kept on duty in the "Flu" wards. None of them became ill.

The incidence of Streptococcus hemolyticus and B. influenzæ among the individual cases diagnosed as influenza and among carriers of B. influenza is shown in Table V.

It is to be noted that with one exception Streptococcus hemolyticus was always found in the nasopharyngeal cultures of those ill with the disease, and that carriers of B. influenzæ were also always carriers of this organism.

To state the case in another way, Table VI has been prepared to show the number of individuals cultured in the different periods, and of these, the number who never at any time had the Streptococcus hemolyticus isolated from the nasopharynx.

Here again is exactly the same picture as regards the low percentage of carriers of this organism in the preepidemic period; the steady progressive rise in the epidemic period; the approach to normal again in the postepidemic period.

TABLE VI

INDIVIDUALS CULTURED

PERIOD	DATE, 1920	NUMBER CULTURED	STREPTOCOCCUS HEMOLYTICUS	PER CENT
Preepidemic	Jan. 12 to Jan. 29	331	20	6
	Jan. 29 to Feb. 8	334	100	30
Epidemic	Feb. 8 to Feb. 20	313	201	65
	Feb. 20 to Mar. 20	175	155	89
Postepidemic	Mar. 22 to Apr. 13	122	29	24

POSTEPIDEMIC PERIOD

Mar. 22 to Apr. 13, 1920

During this period we took a series of nasopharyngeal cultures from various individuals as they came into the laboratory, for comparison.

The findings are charted in the tables above.

Also during this period a small series of experiments have been begun with about 100 cultures of Streptococcus hemolyticus isolated in the epidemic and postepidemic periods from different individuals.

TYPE OF STREPTOCOCCUS HEMOLYTICUS

Under this heading, and without going into detail about experiments, which are as yet not complete, we desire to record the most noteworthy characteristics of this organism, as it was observed during the epidemic.

Our observation of this organism shows, as has been noted by others, the variation in width and color of the hemolytic zone, to be governed largely by the circumstance under which it is isolated, and the medium on which it is grown.

We noted that in the preepidemic period hemolysis was in the vast majority of instances of the narrow zone type and of a marked greenish tint. Colonies of this type could not of surety be told from pneumococci, except by transplanting to broth and blood slant, which after incubating overnight were gram stained for morphology, tested for bile solubility, and agglutinated with pneumococcus sera. During this period we found and tested in this manner 120 cultures, 95 of them being classified as pneumococci because they were bile soluble.

After the first ten days of the epidemic period it became more and more unusual to find hemolysis of this type. The hemolytic zone was broader and had lost its greenish tint.

In the postepidemic period there was a return to the narrow type, and at the end of this period it is again usual.

During the epidemic and postepidemic periods over one hundred cultures of both broad and narrow zone hemolysis, which were isolated from as many different individuals, were tested on various sugars.

We found that, with two exceptions, all reduced lactose, dextrose, mannite, dextrin, and salicin. One culture did not reduce salicin; another did not reduce dextrose or dextrin.

These same cultures were transplanted to plain broth which was incubated overnight, and to which was then added 2 c.c. of a 5 per cent suspension of sheep blood corpuscles (in normal salt solution) to observe the length of time required to produce hemolysis. This varied from two to twenty-four hours.

TABLE VII

TABLE CLASSIFIED ACCORDING TO HOSPITAL PERSONNEL, SHOWING THE NUMBER OF INDIVIDUALS CULTURED AND PERCENTAGE OF POSITIVE STREPTOCOCCUS HEMOLYTICUS—EPIDEMIC PERIOD

1920	DETACHMENT MEN			T. B. PATIENTS			NURSES			CIVILIANS		
	NUMBER CULTURED	STREPTOCOCCUS HEMOLYTICUS	% STREP.	NUMBER CULTURED	STREPTOCOCCUS HEMOLYTICUS	% STREP.	NUMBER CULTURED	STREPTOCOCCUS HEMOLYTICUS	% STREP.	NUMBER CULTURED	STREPTOCOCCUS HEMOLYTICUS	% STREP.
Jan. 29, to Feb. 10	165	63	36	95	38	40	95	51	53	0	0	0
Feb. 10. to Mar. 22,	151	99	65	144	107	74	44	41	93	78	57	73
Total	316	162	51	289	145	49	139	92	66	78	57	73

The character of the hemolytic zone, as shown on the original blood plates, be it wide or narrow, has no influence as to the length of time which it takes to produce hemolysis under these conditions.

Our experiments point to the following conclusions:

1. That repeated transplants of colonies with narrow green tinted hemolysis on artificial media never produce wide zone hemolysis.

2. That wide zone hemolysis may, in some instances, persist for three, four, or more generations on blood plates; but when it once assumes the narrow green type it so remains on this medium.

3. That width of hemolytic zone is not dependent in the length of time which it takes to produce this, but rather on passage through man or animal.

4. That streptococci with zones of broad hemolysis are virulent; that narrow green tinted hemolysis is the quiescent stage.

DISCUSSION

The sequence of events which have made this paper possible are detailed in the above tables.

We see in the preepidemic period, which just antedated the discovery of cases of influenza in the hospital, the picture of the results of a nasopharyngeal survey which does not differ from that found by many other observers under similar conditions. It was among the men on whom this survey has been made that we eventually had the greatest number of influenza cases. We can therefore follow in their cultures the change in bacterial flora, especially as regards the Streptoccus hemolyticus, which was so constant and characteristic.

We are able also to make a like statement as regards our tuberculosis patients, on a large number of whom during the spring and summer of 1919 throat and sputum cultures had been made to determine the organisms which acted as secondary invaders. The results of this survey showed that the Streptococcus hemolyticus was to be found in this disease in a percentage which varied from thirty to sixty-six, the variation depending on the severity of the disease and the amount of lung involvement. Cases that were classified as the most severe being most often carriers of this organism, and then most often in its virulent form.

We have therefore two classes of individuals on whom we had, previous to the epidemic, made throat surveys and in whom the normal percentage of Streptococcus hemolyticus carriers was known.

In preparation for a possible epidemic of influenza the quarantine regulations which we recommended, provided that carriers of pneumococcus, Streptococcus hemolyticus, and B. influenzæ should be isolated. These provisions were carried out. Within ten days after the establishment of quarantine, however, it was found that so far as our cultural findings were concerned, we had not to deal with the pneumococcus as a factor in the epidemic.

The constantly increasing percentage of positive Streptococcus hemolyticus findings, which corresponded to the increase in number of cases of influenza diagnosed suspected, was evident early in the epidemic period.

What possible influence this section of the country, or to narrow the limits, this hospital, where so many cases of pulmonary tuberculosis, known carriers of the Streptococcus hemolyticus, had on the incidence of this organism in our local epidemic of influenza we cannot state. We know that persons in direct contact with active pulmonary tuberculosis are much more often than the normal individual not so exposed, carriers of this organism. This is well shown by our surveys on nurses, orderlies, and mess men completed in the early days of the epidemic period.

In the order mentioned they are in most direct contact with known carriers of Streptococcus hemolyticus. Their cultural findings bear out the fact that contact has its influence.

That contact plays an important part in the spread of influenza we were able to show in the attendants on these cases whom we cultured every day. The first culture on assignment to a "Flu" ward would be negative for organisms which we associated with influenza, but within a day or two all commenced to show the Streptococcus hemolyticus, and in twelve, after periods varying from three to twenty days, we isolated the B. influenzæ.

The findings of Streptococcus hemolyticus were always antecedent to those of B. influenzæ. This fact brings forth a desire to speculate as to which organism is the primary infecting agent in influenza, but as this subject is outside the scope of this paper, we leave it for others to discuss, theorize on, or prove.

The results of cultures taken from individuals other than those already mentioned, classified according to status, i. e., civilian employees, duty personnel returning from leave or newly joining the Post, newly admitted patients, and visitors—show a similar increase in incidence of Streptococcus hemolyticus during the epidemic period.

We therefore assert that all individuals connected with this hospital, no matter what their status, or how great the likelihood of being chronic carriers of Streptococcus hemolyticus through contact with, or in fact being a tuberculosis patient, show in the epidemic period an increase in this carrier state. The normal for even those with the most advanced forms of pulmonary tuberculosis we have found never to be more than 66 per cent. In this epidemic we had not to deal with this class of individual. The tubercular patients who developed influenza and those exposed to the disease through contact were among those that we term ambulatory. In them our previous studies gave only twenty to thirty per cent as carriers of Streptococcus hemolyticus.

Our tables show that with one exception all cases of influenza, and all carriers of the influenza bacillus were also carriers of Streptococcus hemolyticus.

The tables which deal with, and classify the separate individuals cultured, show a percentage of positive Streptococcus hemolyticus findings, which at the height of the curve corresponds almost exactly to the findings which we obtained from cultures taken for comparison from the entire personnel of the Emergency Hospital in Asheville.

We have completed this study by showing in the postepidemic period the return to what approached, in this institution, the normal percentage of Streptococcus hemolyticus carriers.

CONCLUSIONS

1. That there was, in this locality, a direct relationship between the streptococcus hemolyticus and the influenza epidemic.

CHEMICAL CHANGES IN THE BLOOD IN DISEASE*

VI. CHOLESTEROL

By Victor C. Myers, Ph.D., New York City

DURING the past ten years cholesterol has been the subject of many varied and extended investigations, the larger number of which have been carried out on the blood. Although many of these studies have furnished information of great value regarding the physiologic and pathologic role of this interesting lipoid, they have not disclosed many deviations which can be utilized to advantage in diagnosis.

The importance of cholesterol is indicated by its widespread occurrence in the animal body. Cholesterol is obviously, therefore, a constituent of our various animal foods, from which probably much of the cholesterol of the body is derived. According to Fraser and Gardner,[1] the phytosterols of the plant foods are transformed to cholesterol in the body, evidently furnishing a portion of our supply of this substance. Whether or not cholesterol is synthesized in the body remains a disputed question. Luden[2] has clearly demonstrated the augmenting influence of animal foods, particularly eggs, butter and meat on the blood cholesterol, while Rothschild and Rosenthal[3] have advocated the use of diets low in cholesterol in the treatment of certain types of cholelithiasis with hypercholesterolemia.

Although cholesterol is a monatomic, simple, unsaturated, secondary alcohol, and further possesses the character of a complicated terpene, its close association with fat and lecithin, and the fact that it may combine with a fatty acid to form a fat makes it of special interest in this connection. Bloor,[4] in particular, has given us much useful information regarding the variations in these three lipoids in the blood. Normally the "total fat" content of the blood plasma amounts to 0.6 to 0.7 per cent, but in the severe lipemia of diabetes figures as high as 26 per cent have been observed. The cholesterol content of the blood runs fairly parallel with the total fatty acids in all cases, including lipemia, and on this account is an excellent index of the degree of lipemia in diabetes. Cholesterol occurs in the blood in both the free and combined state. Free cholesterol is present in the corpuscles and to some extent in the plasma, and the cholesterol esters in the plasma alone. Bloor and Knudson[5] have found that in whole blood the average percentage of cholesterol in combination as esters is about 33.5 per cent, and in the plasma 58 per cent of the total cholesterol. Most of the data recorded in the literature, however, are for the total cholesterol of the blood, some of the results being on the plasma or serum, others on the whole blood. Normally, the concentration of cholesterol is nearly the same in the plasma and the whole blood, although, if anything, the plasma content is slightly higher, and patho-

*From the Laboratory of Pathological Chemistry, New York Post-Graduate Medical School and Hospital, New York City.

logically it seems to be subject to somewhat greater variations. That such is the case is well illustrated in the following Table I abbreviated from Grigaut.[6]

TABLE I

DISTRIBUTION OF CHOLESTEROL IN THE BLOOD*

CONDITION	CHOLESTEROL IN PER CENT			
	SERUM	PLASMA	WHOLE BLOOD	CORPUSCLES
1. Normal man	0.168	0.168	0.159	0.141
2. Normal man	0.170	0.170	0.150	0.130
3. Normal woman	0.174	0.170	0.168	0.171
4. Normal woman	0.175	0.175	0.165	0.140
5. Carcinoma of the pancreas with jaundice	0.071	0.068	0.105	0.110
6. Pneumonia	0.098	0.098	0.110	0.150
7. Carcinoma of the liver with jaundice	0.222	0.228	0.198	0.170
8. Diabetes	0.246	0.246	0.201	0.137
9. Cholelithiasis	0.276	0.270	0.225	0.180
10. Nephritis	0.450	0.450	0.285	0.150
11. Nephritis	0.514	0.514	0.264	0.135
12. Carcinoma of the pancreas with jaundice	0.840	0.840	0.540	0.195

*Taken from Grigaut.[6]

TABLE II

THE CHOLESTEROL CONTENT OF THE BLOOD IN VARIOUS PATHOLOGICAL CONDITIONS

CASE	AGE	SEX	CHOLESTEROL	CO₂ COMBINING POWER	SUGAR	UREA N	CONDITION
			per cent	c.c. to 100	per cent	mg. to 100 c.c.	
1. H.B.	20	♂	0.82	21	0.39		
2. A.F.	20	♂	0.63	31	0.86		
			0.57	38	0.41		Diabetes, Case 1 showing
3. U.W.	49	♂	0.20		0.79		a total fat content of 7.1
			0.25	12	1.16		per cent.
4. H.R.		♂	0.34	35	0.30		
5. W.A.	45	♂	0.11	50	0.25		
6. W.F.	25	♂	0.34			100	Bichloride poisoning
7. E.E.	30	♀	0.28			33	
8. E.B.	24	♂	0.28				⎫ Nephritis
9. I.D.	17	♀	0.22			170	
10. J.W.	34	♂	0.16			63	
11. M.H.	71	♀	0.23				Arteriosclerosis
12. L.W.	62	♀	0.21				
13. D.G.	23	♀	0.24				Moderately severe pellagra
14. H.C.	44	♀	0.13				⎫
			0.16				Cholelithiasis, confirmed
15. W.L.	15	♀	0.18		.		by operation, no jaundice
			0.21				
16. F.T.	21	♂	0.21				Catarrhal jaundice
17. R.K.	51	♂	0.29				Obstructive jaundice
18. H.H.	47	♂	0.20				Carcinoma of stomach, early
19. M.L.	45	♂	0.12				Carcinoma of stomach, late
20. L.M.	34	♀	0.23				Pregnancy, 8 mos., eclampsia
21. O.G.	48	♂	0.07				⎫ Pernicious anemia,
22. F.S.	50	♂	0.07				plasma 0.065%, washed cells, 0.12% plasma, 0.065%, washed cells, 0.13%

Chauffard, Laroche and Grigaut[7] have given 0.15 to 0.18 per cent as the normal value for the cholesterol content of blood serum, figures which closely agree with the findings of subsequent workers. This would make the figures for whole blood about 0.14 to 0.17 per cent. Pathologically, many conditions have been recorded in which a hypercholesterolemia was found, while in a few conditions hypocholesterolemia has been noted. In general it may be stated that hypercholesterolemia is found in arteriosclerosis, nephritis, diabetes (especially with acidosis), obstructive jaundice, in many cases of cholelithiasis, in certain skin diseases, in the early stages of malignant tumors, and in pregnancy. The chief condition in which low values for cholesterol are found is anemia.

Figures for the cholesterol content of whole blood, which are intended to be representative of the findings in the various pathologic conditions mentioned above, are given in Table II. The figures are taken partly from Gorham and Myers[8] and partly from some of our more recent observations. Grigaut[6] has presented a most excellent discussion of the cholesterol content of blood, while the papers of Bloor[4] (includes data on other lipoids), Denis,[9] and Gorham and Myers[8] all review this general subject, including the literature.

Rothschild and Wilensky[10] give an excellent outline of the factors influencing the blood cholesterol:

1. The cholesterol content of the blood is lowered:
   (a) By a diet which is poor in lipoids.
   (b) By the occurrence of high temperatures.
2. The cholesterol content of the blood is increased:
   (a) By a diet excessively rich in lipoids.
   (b) By the presence of other diseased conditions, especially diabetes, arteriosclerosis, and nephritis.
   During pregnancy. This lasts for a variable period after evacuation of the uterus.
   (d) By the presence of obstruction in the common bile duct. If the obstruction, however, it not absolute, as indicated by the degree of accompanying jaundice, the cholesterol content of the blood may not be increased.

Although the observations recorded in Table II are given only on whole blood, with the exception of the cases of anemia, it is apparent from the data of Table I that greater variations take place in the cholesterol of the serum or plasma. Nevertheless a significant change in the cholesterol is readily evident from observations made on whole blood.

A more marked hypercholesterolemia may be found in the lipemia of diabetes than in any other condition. The lipemia of the first two cases of Table II, showing cholesterol figures of 0.6 to 0.8 per cent, was very marked. Although the ordinary case of diabetes at the present time does not show lipemia in the sense that the blood is milky, still the lipoids of the blood are increased in all types of the disease. Joslin, Bloor and Gray[11] found that the average quantity of lipoids in the whole blood with the Bloor method amounted to 0.59 per cent in 19 normal individuals, but was increased to 0.83 per cent in 30 mild diabetics, to 0.91 per cent in 37 moderately severe diabetics, and to 1.41 per cent in 55 severe cases of diabetes. This holds for all three groups of lipoids. They state, "The increase in cholesterol is significant and suggestive, and seems indeed pathognomonic of the prolonged diabetic hyperlipemia, since Bloor has found it lacking in the acute lipemia of overfeeding which is characterized by an increase in the total fatty acid alone." On this account the determination of the cholesterol alone should give valuable information regarding the lipoid content of the blood in diabetes.

Although many observers have noted and studied the hypercholesterolemia of nephritis, it is not possible as yet to give a satisfactory interpretation of these findings. In the case of arteriosclerosis, however, it is worthy of note that histologic changes have been observed in the aorta after the experimental administration of cholesterol.

Since gallstones are largely composed of cholesterol, it is reasonable to suppose that their appearance might be associated with an increase in the cholesterol content of the blood. Henes[12] has maintained that this is the fundamental and primary factor in the formation of gallstones. Although it seems quite probable that a hypercholesterolemia is presented during the early period of the formation of the calculi, analytical data show wide variations in the blood cholesterol,[3, 8, 10] the findings ranging from low normals to figures that are definitely increased. Rothschild and Rosenthal[3] emphasize the fact that in a certain group of cases the hypercholesterolemia is very persistent and operation affords only temporary relief. They believe that properly selected low cholesterol diets have been very helpful in these cases.

It is logical to expect that in obstructive jaundice the cholesterol content of the blood should be elevated and bear a fairly definite relation to the intensity of the icterus. Rothschild and Felsen[12] have shown, however, that in conditions associated with hepatic disorders the cholesterol of the blood is not increased, but usually reduced, while in so-called hemolytic icterus, there is no increase of blood cholesterol.

It would appear that in the early stages of malignancy, the blood cholesterol was somewhat elevated or normal, while in the late stages the figures are below normal. Luden[2, 14] has called attention to the fact that a diet which increases the blood cholesterol coincidently weakens the lymphoid defense. She suggests that in persons predisposed to carcinoma an increase of the cholesterol and a weakening of the lymphoid defense, such as may occur with the prolonged use of a high cholesterol diet, may perhaps result in the development of carcinoma.

The hypercholesterolemia of pregnancy is well known. Chauffard, Laroche and Grigaut[15] found that the increase begins about the fourth month of pregnancy and becomes progressively greater as full term is approached. Slemons and Curtis[16] have made the interesting observation that cholesterol esters are frequently absent from fetal blood. In this case the cholesterol is exclusively in the free form, and furthermore, the free cholesterol of both maternal and fetal blood are identical. Apparently the normal placental partition is permeable for free cholesterol but impermeable for cholesterol esters.

That the cholesterol of the blood (plasma) is lowered in anemia has been recognized for some time. When the antihemolytic action of cholesterol is recalled, it will be seen that this observation may possess some practical significance. The therapeutic administration of cholesterol in this condition has received attention from Italian investigators and has apparently been followed by beneficial results. Pacini[17] (in this country) has recently presented some interesting observations on the blood cholesterol in pernicious anemia, giving data on the whole blood, serum and cells. He found the cholesterol markedly decreased in the serum but relatively increased in the cells. He administered cholesterol in the form of lanolin as an inunction, and believed that he obtained definite benefit.

ESTIMATION OF CHOLESTEROL

Cholesterol was one of the first constituents of the blood to be determined colorimetrically. Several years before the development of the colorimetric methods of blood analysis described in the earlier papers of this series, Grigaut[6, 18] had already described (1910) a colorimetric procedure of estimating the cholesterol content of blood. In the development of the color Grigaut made use of the Liebermann-Burchard reaction, and the technic of this part of the test is still carried out essentially as he originally described it. Two years after the publication of Grigaut's method, Weston[19] described a procedure in which the Salkowski color reaction was employed. The Liebermann-Burchard reaction is better suited, however, for use in this connection. In 1913 Autenrieth and Funk[20] described a slight modification of the Grigaut technic and adapted it to use with the Autenrieth-Königsberger (Hellige) colorimeter. This modification has been extensively employed and many references may be found to work carried out with the Autenrieth-Funk method. It would seem only fair to Grigaut, however, that this method should bear his name. A number of different workers have described procedures of cholesterol extraction upon which the colorimetric method of Grigaut is applied.

In the case of the excellent but laborious gravimetric digitonin method of Windaus[21] for the estimation of total cholesterol, saponification of the cholesterol esters is necessary, since only the free cholesterol is precipitated by the digitonin. Cholesterol esters give the color reaction as well as does the free cholesterol. This fact does not appear to have been recognized until recently, since the directions for the colorimetric estimation have almost invariably called for a preliminary saponification. As pointed out by Bloor,[22] this saponification is unnecessary and the colorimetric estimation of the cholesterol thus becomes further simplified.

Bloor has suggested a method of extraction[23] for the cholesterol (and other lipoids) which is very simple and would appear to be complete, but the results obtained with the method as finally carried out (second method) are higher than those by the older methods, and rather irregular, owing apparently, to the presence in the extracts used of substances interfering with the Liebermann-Burchard color reaction for cholesterol. These high results have been criticized by Mueller[24] and Weston,[25] who are of the opinion that they are due to the admixture of brownish tints frequently obtained in the final development of the color. Luden[26] obtained similar high findings with Bloor's second method, but believed that these resulted from a combination of bile pigments and bile acids. With Bloor's first method the alcoholic ether extract was saponified with sodium ethylate, this procedure being omitted with the second method. Luden's data bearing on this point are very interesting. Our observations on this subject are in harmony with her conclusions.

Myers and Wardell[27] have described a comparatively simple method of direct cholesterol extraction which appears to yield reliable results. At any rate added cholesterol may be quantitatively recovered, and good checks obtained with the totally different Windaus method. With this method 1 c.c. of blood is mixed with plaster of Paris and dried. In addition to putting the blood into a

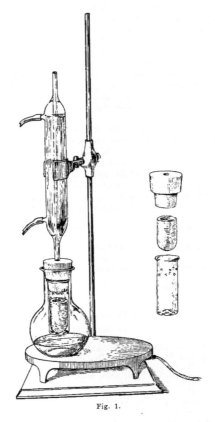

Fig. 1.

finely divided and readily extractable condition, this calcium salt apparently holds back substances which add to the color development with the Bloor technic. After reaching its greatest intensity the cholesterol color fades rather rapidly and for this reason Myers and Gorham[28] suggested the use of naphthol green B as a standard. This dye excellently matches the cholesterol color and appears to be permanent.

In carrying out the color reaction it is essential that the reagents should be anhydrous. Poor acetic anhydride will give a weak color development. For this reason it is desirable before developing a series of unknown solutions to first check the quality of reagents by developing a solution of pure cholesterol.

Method.[27]—For the determination, 1 c.c. of blood, plasma or serum is pipetted into a porcelain crucible or small beaker containing 4 to 5 gm. of plaster of Paris, stirred, and dried, preferably in a drying oven for an hour. It is now emptied into a small paper extraction shell (4 cm. long) and then inserted in a short glass tube* (2.5x7 cm.) in the bottom and sides of which are a number of small holes (Fig. 1). This is now attached to a large cork on a small reflux condenser and the tube and cork inserted in the neck of a 150 c.c. extraction flask containing about 20 to 25 c.c. of chloroform. (We have frequently run 3 to 6 extractions simultaneously on the same hot plate.) Extraction is continued for 30 min., on an electric hot plate, the chloroform made up to some suitable volume, such as 20 c.c., filtered if necessary, and colorimetric estimation carried out as follows: 5 c.c. of the chloroform extract are pipetted into a dry test tube, and 2 c.c. of acetic anhydride and 0.1. c.c. of concentrated sulphuric acid (best with 0.1 c.c. pipette) are added. After thorough mixing, the solution is placed in the dark for exactly 10 min.** to allow the color to develop, and then compared with a standardized 0.005 per cent aqueous solution of naphthol green B in a Bock-Benedict or Kober colorimeter. If the Duboscq colorimeter is used, it is necessary that the cups should be remounted in plaster of Paris, instead of balsam.

With a good grade of acetic anhydride, it has been found that when an 0.005 per cent solution of naphthol green B is used as a standard and set at 15.5 mm. on the Duboscq or Kober instrument, 0.4 mg. of cholesterol in 5 c.c. of chloroform treated with 2 c.c. of acetic anhydride and 0.1 c.c. of concentrated sulphuric acid will read 15 mm. The color curve for both the cholesterol and naphthol green B appear to fall in a straight line so that readings somewhat above or below the standard are accurate.

If a cholesterol standard containing 0.4 mg. to 5 c.c., or a naphthol green B standard of equivalent strength, are employed, the following formula may be used for the calculation $\dfrac{S}{R} \times 0.0004 \times \dfrac{D}{5} \times 100 =$ cholesterol content of blood in per cent, in which S stands for the depth of standard in mm., R for the reading of the unknown, 0.0004 the equivalent amount of cholesterol in 5 c.c. of chloroform, D the dilution of the chloroform extract from the 1 c.c. of blood, 5 the dilution of the standard and 100 the factor for 100 c.c. For example $\dfrac{15}{15} \times 0.0004 \times \dfrac{20}{5} \times 100 = 0.160$ per cent.

REFERENCES

[1]Frazer and Gardner: Proc. Roy. Soc., London (B), 1910, lxxxii, 59; Ellis and Gardner· Ibid., 1912, lxxxv, 385.
[2]Luden: Jour. Lab. and Clin. Med., 1917-18, iii, 141.
[3]Rothschild and Rosenthal: Am. Jour. Med. Sc., 1916, clii, 394.
[4]Bloor: Jour. Biol. Chem., 1916, xxv, 577; and other papers in the same journal.
[5]Bloor and Knudson: Jour. Biol. Chem., 1916, xxix, 7.
[6]Grigaut: Biologie medicale, March, 1913.
[7]Chauffard, Laroche and Grigaut: Compt. rend. Soc. biol., 1911, lxx, 336.
[8]Gorham and Ayers: Arch. Int. Med., 1917, xx, 599.
[9]Denis: Jour. Biol. Chem., 1917, xxix, 93.
[10]Rothschild and Wilensky: Am. Jour. Med. Sc., 1918, clvi, 239, 404, 564.
[11]Joslin, Bloor and Gray: Jour. Am. Med. Assn., 1917, lxix, 375.
[12]Henes: Jour. Am. Med. Assn., 1914, lxiii, 146; Surg. Gynec. and Obst., 1916, xxiii, 91.

*Originally we made these tubes from large test tubes by drawing out the tubes, blowing new bottoms (round) and then punching a number of holes with a white hot, malleable iron wire. Later we tried alundum thimbles, in which two small holes had been drilled near the top to easily permit the entrance of the chloroform vapor. Although this obviated the necessity of paper extraction shells, cups could not be found that were sufficiently porous to make a rapid extraction possible. The flat bottom tubes illustrated are an advantage in that they will stand, and the thimble cannot be sucked tight against the bottom of the tube.

**In order to get the proper temperature for color development in warm weather it is advisable either to keep the reagents in a cool place or to insert the tubes in water during the development of the color.

[13]Rothschild and Felsen: Arch. Int. Med., 1919, xxiv, 520.
[14]Luden: Jour. Lab. and Clin. Mcd., 1918-19, iv, 849, 719.
[15]Chauffard, Laroche and Grigaut: Obstetrique, 1911, iv, 481.
[16]Slemons and Curtis: Am. Jour. Obst., 1917, lxxv, 569.
[17]Pacini: Am. Med., 1918, xxiv, 92.
[18]Grigaut: Compt. rend. Soc. biol., 1910, lxviii, 791, 827; 1911, lxxi, 513.
[19]Weston: Jour. Med. Research, 1912, xxvi, 47; Weston and Kent: Ibid., 531.
[20]Autenrieth and Funk: München. med. Wchnschr., 1913, lx, 1243.
[21]Windaus: Zeitschr. physiol. Chem., 1910, lxv, 110.
[22]Bloor: Jour. Biol. Chem., 1916, xxiv, 227.
[23]Bloor: Jour. Biol. Chem., 1915, xxiii, 317.
[24]Mueller: Jour. Biol. Chem., 1916, xxv,549.
[25]Weston: Jour. Biol. Chem., 1916-17, xxviii, 383.
[26]Luden: Jour. Biol. Chem., 1917, xxix, 463; Jour. Lab. and Clin. Med., 1917-18, iii, 93.
[27]Myers and Wardell: Jour. Biol. Chem., 1918, xxxvi, 147.
[28]Myers and Gorham: Post-Graduate, 1914, xxix, 938.

THE VALUE OF THE COMPLEMENT-FIXATION TEST IN TUBERCULOSIS*

PRELIMINARY PAPER

(With Observations, Using the Hecht-Weinberg Modification)

BY ROY UPHAM, M.D., F.A.C.S., AND A. J. BLAIVAS, BROOKLYN, N. Y.

IT is a well-known fact that the antigen is the most important factor in complement-fixation work. The antigen of choice is the one that fixes complement most often in a given disease. It is the object of the writers to determine, first, which is the most delicate antigen, and second, to interpret the laboratory findings.

All cases here reported were patients that consulted one of us (Upham) for gastrointestinal disturbances and tuberculosis was not suspected. Inasmuch as a Wassermann test was made on each patient as a routine, it was thought advisable to include the complement-fixation test for tuberculosis, using the antigens of Petroff, Miller, and Fleisher-Ives. This will, of course, account for the large percentage of negatives.

METHODS EMPLOYED

The Wassermann reaction was made on each patient using both cholesterin and ether-soluble, acetone-insoluble antigens. As stated above, in the complement-fixation test for tuberculosis, the antigens of Petroff, Miller and Fleisher-Ives were used. In the complement fixation tests the results were estimated in terms of +, ++, +++ and ++++ but any result below +++ was considered negative. In the Hecht-Weinberg modification, any result below ++++ was considered negative.

The work was done separately, charted, and the laboratory had no information whatsoever regarding the patient. The temperature, weight, physical findings and x-ray examinations were made on each patient. Each patient also received from 0.5 to 2.5 milligrams of old tuberculin and the von Pirquet test.

The tables show that we have classified our cases as follows:
1. As they presented themselves.
2. Clinical tuberculosis.
3. Tuberculosis suspects.
4. Nontuberculous.
5. Other diagnoses.

Ives and Singer[1] claim that the complement-fixation test recognizes only active tuberculosis. In Table I it will be observed that cases 20 and 45 were arrested cases and still gave strong positive fixation tests. We found some cases

---

*From the Laboratories of the Prospect Heights Hospital, Brooklyn, N. Y.

TABLE I

Case No.	Name	COMPLEMENT-FIXATION TEST FOR TUBERCULOSIS			MODIFICATION OF HECHT FOR TUBERCULOSIS			H. I.*	Wassermann	H. W. G.**	
		Petroff Antigen	Miller Antigen	Fleisher-Ives Antigen	Petroff Antigen	Miller Antigen	Fleisher-Ives Antigen				
1.	J.A.B.	-	-	-				4	-		Intestinal intoxication
2.	H.M.	-	-	-	-	-	-	2	-	++	Ulcer, Asthma syphilis (?)
3.	C.B.M.	+	+	+	++	++	++	2	-	-	Intestinal intoxication
4.	I.F.W.	±	±	±	NOT MADE	NOT MADE	±	4	-	-	Gastrocoloptosis
5.	A.R.	-			NOT MADE	NOT MADE	NOT MADE		NOT MADE	NOT MADE	Cancer of stomach
6.	G.W.H	--	-	-	NOT MADE	NOT MADE	NOT MADE		NOT MADE	NOT MADE	Intestinal intoxication. Neph
7.	J.L.M.	-	-	-	-	-	-	8	-		Gastrocoloptosis, Tuberculosi
8.	E.R.G.	++	++	++	+++	++++	-	6	-	±	Tuberculosis. mucous colitis
9.	W.C.	-	-	-	+	-	-	2	-	++	Gastrocoloptosis, Syphilis (?
10.	G.A.M.	-	-	-	-	-	-	5	-	-	Cholelithiasis
11.	C.B.G.	-	-	-	+	+	+	4	-	-	Tuberculosis (?)
12.	P.R.L.	±	±	±	+	+	+	7	-	-	Subacid Gastric Catarrh
13.	C.G.	-	-	-	++	-	+	6	-	-	Intestinal Toxemia
14.	G.F.	-	-	-	++	-	+	7	-	+	Intestinal Toxemia, Nephriti
15.	S.P.G.	++	++	++	++	++	++	4	-	-	Gastric catarrh, Tuberculosi
16.	G.V.W	++++	-	-	+++	+++	+++	9	-	-	Cholelithiasis
17.	A.P.	-	-	-	-	-	-	9	-	-	Gastrocoloptosis, Tuberculos
18.	M.H.	++	-	-	+++	++	-	10	-	++++	Cancer
19.	H.R.W	+++		++	+++	+++	+++	9	-		Arrested Tuberculosis,
20.	R.T.S.	+++	+++	++	+++	+++	+++	9	-	-	Gastric catarrh
21.	J.O.	+++	+++	+++	++++	++++	++++	9	-	-	Gastrocoloptosis, Tuberculosi
22.	R.R.	+	+	+	++	++	++	3	-	-	Gastric Catarrh, Tuberculosi
23.	W.J.F.	-	-	-	++	++	++	2	-	-	Cholecystitis
24.	C.C.B.	-	-	-	++	++	++	3	-	-	Intestinal Toxemia, Nephriti
25.	J.K.	-	-	-	-	-	-	2	-	-	Gastrocoloptosis
26.	A.S.B.	++	+	+	+++	+++	+++	3	-	-	Intestinal Toxemia
27.	H.S.	-	-	-	-	-	-	8	-	-	Anemia, Tuberculosis (?)
28.	C.H.B.	-	-	-	-	-	-	4	-	-	Anemia. Tuberculosis (?) / Gastric Catarrh
29.	A.G.B.	-	-	-	-	-	-	9	-	++	Gastrocoloptosis
30.	E.H.	-	-	-	-	-	-	4	-	-	Gastrocoloptosis
31.	M.J.N.	-	-	-	+	++	-	4	-	-	Intestinal Toxemia. Anemia
32.	A.T.	-	-	-	-	-	-	5	-	-	Intestinal Toxemia
33.	J.V.L.	-	-	-	-	-	-	5	-	-	Hemorrhoids, Gastric Catar
34.	G.G.	-	-	-	-	-	-	3	-	-	Intestinal Toxemia
35.	G.R.	-	-	-	-	-	-	8	-	-	Gastrocoloptosis, Tuberculosi
36.	R.G.	-	-	-	-	-	-	4	-	-	Gastrocoloptosis
37.	G.P.R.	++	++	++	+++	+++	+++	6	-	-	Intestinal Toxemia
38.	A.M.L.	++++	++++	++++	++++	++++	++++	7	-	-	Gastric catarrh, Tuberculosi:
39.	T.M.C.	-	-	-	-	-	-	6	-	-	Gastrocoloptosis
40.	M.M.G.	-	-	-	++++	++++	++++	10	-	-	Intestinal Toxemia, Nephrit
41.	R.S.D.	-	-	-	-	-	-	3	-	-	Gastrocoloptosis, Tuberculos
42.	J.F.C.	-	-	-	+++	+++	+++		-	NOT MADE	Cholecystitis, Syphilis
43.	J.C.M.	-	-	-	NOT MADE	NOT MADE	NOT MADE	7	-	NOT MADE	Terminal Gastric Catarrh
44.	B.	++++	-	-	+++	+++		7			Terminal Gastric Catarrh
45.	R.M.W	++++	-	-	++++		+++	8	-	NOT MADE	Ulcer, Arrested Tuberculosi
46.	G.E.H.	-	-	-	NOT MADE	NOT MADE	NOT MADE		-	NOT MADE	Intestinal Toxemia, Anemia
47.	M.B.H.	-	-	-	-	-	-	7	-	-	Gastrocoloptosis, Tuberculos
48.	C.E.B.	-	·	-	-	-	-	9	-	-	Gastrocoloptosis
49.	E.W.C.	-	-	-	-	-	-	9	-	-	Intestinal Toxemia
50.	N.M.	-	-	-	-	-	-	8	-	-	Intestinal Toxemia, Tubercul
51.	M.W.	-	-	-	-	-	-	6	-	-	Intestinal Toxemia, Nephrit
52.	F.E.I.	-	-	-	-	-	-	10	·	-	Intestinal Toxemia
53.	M.K.	-	-	-	-	-	-	9	-	-	Amebic Dysentery
54.	C.S.	++++	+++	++++	NOT MADE	NOT MADE	NOT MADE		-	NOT MADE	Gastrocoloptosis, Chronic ap
55.	L.A.	++	+	++	++++	++	++++	3	-	++++	Gastrocoloptosis
56.	C.R.	-	-	-	-	-	-	2	-	-	Tuberculosis
57.	M.G.	-	-	-	·+	++	+	4	-	-	Syphilis and Tuberculosis
58.	T.J.O.	-	-	-	-	-	-	5	-	-	Tuberculosis
59.	D.	-	-	-	-	-	-	10	++++	++++	Syphilis
60.	Dr.M.	-	-	-	-	-	-	1'			Intestinal Toxemia

*Hemolytic Index.
**Hecht-Weinberg Test.

that were clinically tuberculous gave negative reactions and it was these results that led us to try the principle of Hecht.

While heating serum to 56° C. (inactivating) destroys any natural complement that may be present, it does not, however, destroy the natural amboceptor that may be present. Inactivating serum in the Wassermann test may destroy some of the syphilitic antibodies present and thus also render the test more liable to error. Heating serum in the complement-fixation test for tuberculosis may therefore also destroy some of the tuberculous antibodies present in the serum. This is only a theory of the writers and has not as yet been confirmed. The fact that in the original technic the amboceptor is not destroyed, and a titrated amount of amboceptor is added to the serum regardless of the amount of natural amboceptor present, proves that an excess of amboceptor is added to the serum. This may, of course, render a negative reaction when in reality it should be positive. Bearing this fact in mind we performed the Hecht-Weinberg modification in the complement-fixation test for tuberculosis.

LABORATORY TECHNIC

The blood was collected in the usual manner and allowed to clot. It was then centrifugalized and the serum was drawn off using a sterile pipette. The bloods were examined on the day that they were collected.

Antigens.—The antigens used in this series were:

1. Petroff's glycerine antigen which was furnished us by Petroff.

2. Miller's antigen which was generously given us by Dr. M. Kahn of Beth Israel Hospital, New York.

3. Fleisher-Ives antigen which was furnished us by Dr. G. Ives.

Complement.—Pritchard and Roderich[2] observed that guinea pigs gave a strong positive reaction and upon investigation found that the sera of the guinea pigs were at fault. The writers made complement-fixation tests on all guinea pigs and can therefore confirm the observation of Pritchard and Roderich. We then discarded those pigs that gave a positive complement-fixation for tuberculosis and used only those that gave clear-cut negative reactions.

The guinea pigs were bled from the heart and the sera of four or five guinea pigs were pooled. The complement was then diluted 1-10 using normal saline as a diluent.

Amboceptor.—The rabbit antisheep amboceptor was prepared and titrated in the usual way. Two units were used throughout the tests.

Sheep Cells.—The blood was obtained from the jugular vein into a wide-mouth bottle containing some sterile glass beads. It was then thoroughly shaken until completely defibrinated. The blood was then centrifugalized at about 3000 revolutions per minute about six or seven times. After the last time the supernatant fluid was tested for albumin using the nitric acid contact test. If there were any traces of albumin, it was centrifugalized again three times and the albumin test was repeated. A five per cent suspension of sheep cells in normal saline was used throughout the serological work.

Salt Solution.—In this work, 0.85 per cent salt solution was used. Care was taken that it was always sterile.

Glassware.—All glassware was chemically cleaned and sterilized. Although it is not absolutely necessary to have the glassware sterile, it was thought advisable to have it so throughout the serologic work.

Complement-Fixation Technic.—One unit of Complement, two units of amboceptor and one unit of the antigens were used. One c.c. of a 5 per cent suspension of sheep cells was used. After adding 0.2 c.c. of serum, then the saline, complement and the antigens, the tubes were placed in the water-bath for one hour at 37.5° C. After this time, the amboceptor and sheep corpuscles were added, the tubes were again incubated for one hour and then removed and read.

Technic for the Modification.[3]—Place 0.1 c.c. of the unheated serum into each of the twenty small test tubes which are placed in a special rack. Put 1 c.c. of the normal saline in Tube 1; 0.9 c.c. in Tube 2; 0.8 c.c. in Tube 3; 0.7 c.c. in Tube 4; 0.6 c.c. in Tube 5; 0.5 c.c. in Tube 6; 0.4 c.c. in Tube 7; 0.3 c.c. in Tube 8; 0.2 c.c. in Tube 9; 0.1 c.c. in Tube 10; 0.2 c.c. in Tube 11; 0.15 c.c. in Tube 12; 0.1 c.c. in Tube 13; 0.2 c.c. in Tube 14; 0.15 c.c. in Tube 15; 0.1 c.c. in Tube 16; 0.2 c.c. in Tube 17; 0.15 c.c. in Tube 18; 0.1 c.c. in Tube 19; and 0.3 c.c. in Tube 20.

The first ten tubes are used to determine the hemolytic index of the blood under examination. In other words. the object is to find the amount of natural complement and amboceptor in the suspected serum. With Tubes 11 to 19 the actual test is carried out. Tube 20 is the serum control tube. Now add 0.1 c.c. of a 5 per cent suspension of sheep cells to Tube 1; 0.2 c.c. to Tube 2; 0.3 c.c. to Tube 3; 0.4 c.c. to Tube 4; 0.5 c.c. to Tube 5; 0.6 c.c. to Tube 6; 0.7 c.c. to Tube 7; 0.8 c.c. to Tube 8; 0.9 c.c. to Tube 9; and 1.0 c.c. to Tube 10.

Antigen.—Dilute the titrated antigens used in the original technic with equal quantities of normal salt solution.

Place 0.1 c.c. of the diluted Petroff's antigen into Tube 11; 0.15 c.c. of the antigen into Tube 12; and 0.2 c.c. of the antigen into Tube 13.

Place 0.1 c.c. of the diluted Miller's antigen into Tube 14; 0.15 c.c. of the antigen into Tube 15; and 0.2 c.c. of the antigen into Tube 16.

Place 0.1 c.c. of the diluted Fleisher-Ives antigen into Tube 17, 0.15 c.c. of the antigen into Tube 18; and 0.2 c.c. of the antigen into Tube 19.

These nine tubes (11, 12, 13, 14, 15, 16, 17, 18 and 19) are the tubes in which the final readings are made and for that reason the antigen is added to them alone. Tube 20 being the serum control tube, received of course, no antigen. The tubes are now well shaken and placed into the water-bath for one hour at 37.5° C. At the end if this time the rack is removed from the water-bath and the last tube which shows complete hemolysis is the hemolytic index. For example, if Tube 7 is the last where complete hemolysis occurs, the hemolytic index is 7. This means that 0.1 c.c. of serum will hemolyze 0.7 c.c. of a 5 per cent suspension of sheep cells.

In order to determine the quantity of sheep corpuscles to put into Tubes 11 to 20 inclusive, we have used the same table as used in performing the Hecht-Weinberg test for syphilis. If the hemolytic index is from,

1 to 4 add 0.1 c.c. of sheep cells to Tubes 11 to 20 inclusive.
5 to 7 add 0.15 c.c. of sheep cells to Tubes 11 to 20 inclusive.
8 to 10 add 0.2 c.c. of sheep cells to Tubes 11 to 20 inclusive.

After the addition of sheep cells to Tubes 11, 12, 13, 14, 15, 16, 17, 18, 19 and 20 the contents of the tubes are well shaken and again placed in the water-bath for one hour at 37.5° C. The rack is then removed and the results read just as in the Wassermann test.

TABLE II

CLINICAL TUBERCULOSIS CASES

	COMPLEMENT-FIXATION TEST FOR TUBERCULOSIS			MODIFICATION FOR TUBERCULOSIS		
CASE NO.	PETROFF ANTIGEN	MILLER ANTIGEN	FLEISHER-IVES ANTIGEN	PETROFF ANTIGEN	MILLER ANTIGEN	FLEISHER-IVES ANTIGEN
8	+ +	+ +	+ +	+ + + +	+ + + +	–
16	+ + + +	–	–	+ + + +	+ + + +	+ + + +
18	+ +	–	–	+ + + +	+ +	–
20	+ + + +	+ + + +	+ +	+ + + +	+ + + +	+ + + +
21	+ + + +	+ + + +	+ + +	+ + + +	+ + + +	+ + + +
22	+	+	+	+ +	+ +	+ +
45	+ + + +	–	– .	+ + + +	–	+ + + +
47	–	–	–	–	–	–
56	–	–	–	–	–	–
57	–	–	–	+ +	+ +	+
58	–	–	–	–	–	–

TABLE III

TUBERCULOSIS SUSPECTS

	COMPLEMENT-FIXATION TEST FOR TUBERCULOSIS			MODIFICATION FOR TUBERCULOSIS		
CASE NO.	PETROFF ANTIGEN	MILLER ANTIGEN	FLEISHER-IVES ANTIGEN	PETROFF ANTIGEN	MILLER ANTIGEN	FLEISHER-IVES ANTIGEN
7	–	–	–	–	–	–
11	–	–	–	+ +	+	+
13	–	–	–	–	–	–
14	–	–	–	+ +	–	+
26	+ +	+	+	+ + + +	+ + + +	+ + + +
28	–	–	–	–	–	–
35	–	–	–	–	–	–
38	+ + + +	+ + + +	+ + + +	+ + + +	+ + + +	+ + + +
41	–	–	–	–	–	–
50	–	–	–	–	–	–

TABLE IV

OTHER DIAGNOSES WITH POSITIVE FIXATION TESTS

	COMPLEMENT-FIXATION TEST FOR TUBERCULOSIS			MODIFICATION FOR TUBERCULOSIS		
CASE NO.	PETROFF ANTIGEN	MILLER ANTIGEN	FLEISHER-IVES ANTIGEN	PETROFF ANTIGEN	MILLER ANTIGEN	FLEISHER-IVES ANTIGEN
19	+ + + +	–	+ +	+ + + +	+ + + +	+ + + +
37	+ +	+ +	+ +	+ + + +	+ + + +	+ + + +
40	–	–	–	+ + + +	+ + + +	+ + + +
42	–	–	–	+ + + +	+ + + +	+ + + +
44	+ + + +	–	–	+ + + +	+ + + +	–
54	+ + + +	+ + + +	+ + + +	NOT		MADE
55	+ +	–	+ +	+ + + +	+ +	+ + + +

Various workers have made different claims as to the value of the complement-fixation test in tuberculosis. Ives and Singer[1] state, "Since the manifestations of tuberculosis are of such protean character that any disease which does not permit a definite diagnosis may be suspected to be of tuberculous origin,[4] and since many tuberculous affections remain unrecognized after the application of all well-tried diagnostic methods, the desirability of a serologic test for tuberculosis, which will be equally as useful in tuberculosis, as is the Wassermann test in syphilis, is evident. It would appear that in the work of Miller and Zinsser[5] such a test has been nearly perfected. Their optimistic views regarding the test as performed by them are shared by Craig,[6] and our work further supports these views."

Pritchard and Roderich[2] conclude, "This reaction does not give as valuable or consistent information in relation to tuberculosis as does the Wassermann reaction in regard to syphilis. In some open advanced cases of pulmonary tuberculosis, no reaction occurred. An explanation of this might be that the cells have lost their power of reaction owing to their prolonged saturation with specific toxins. This test is of greatest help to us in differential diagnosis. It also acts as a stimulus to more careful observation."

Moursund[7] claims that the complement-fixation test as described by him is of no value as a diagnostic or prognostic aid. He also states that not all complement-fixation tests with bacterial antigens are specific and mentions that a large percentage of serums give cross fixation tests in the Wassermann reaction for syphilis and the complement-fixation test for gonorrhea.

CONCLUSIONS

From Table IV it will be observed that in the original complement-fixation test, there were 4.98 per cent positive reactions in diagnoses other than tuberculosis. In the modification there were 9.96 per cent positive reactions, and in the combined tests there were 11.62 per cent. In these cases further studies are being made to eliminate tuberculosis inasmuch as Case 19 had syphilis; Case 37, intestinal toxemia; Case 40, intestinal toxemia with nephritis; Case 42, cholecystitis with syphilis; Case 44, terminal gastric catarrh, Case 54, gastric-coloptosis with chronic appendix; and Case 55, gastrocoloptosis.

Of the ten tuberculosis suspects, there was one positive fixation test in the original technic. In the modification, however, there were two strong positive fixation tests. (See Table III.)

There were 11 cases of clinical tuberculosis, and of these, 4, or 39.6 per cent, were positive in the original technic. In the modification there were 6, or 59.4 per cent, positives. (See Table II.)

From Tables II, III and IV we observe that the modification gives a larger percentage of positive results than the original technic. The writers are fully aware of the fact that the cases here reported are too few in number to draw any definite conclusions, and are therefore continuing this work which will be published later.

ANTIGENS

In the original technic there were eight positive results with Petroff's antigen, 4 with Miller's and 3 with Fleisher-Ives'.

In the modification there were 14 positive reactions with Petroff's antigen, 11 with Miller's and 11 with Fleisher-Ives'.

There was not a single case in which Miller's or Fleisher-Ives' antigens were positive that Petroff's antigen was negative; on the contrary there were cases where the Petroff's antigen was positive and Miller's and Fleisher-Ives' were negative. These conclusions regarding the antigens are not final, as future experiments may prove otherwise.

We agree with Singer and Ives that a serologic test for tuberculosis that will be as useful as the Wassermann test in syphilis is desired, but in our limited experience we observed that the original technic for tuberculosis was not as valuable as the Wassermann test in syphilis. We found that in the 11 cases of clinical tuberculosis 39.6 per cent reacted positive, whereas in the modification there were 59.4 per cent positives. In other words the modification gave 20 per cent more positives than the original test. We will therefore use this modification in conjunction with the original technic with the object of perfecting the complement-fixation test for tuberculosis with the expectation that it may give as valuable and consistent information in tuberculosis as does the Wassermann test in syphilis.

REFERENCES

[1]Ives and Singer: The Complement-Fixation Test for Tuberculosis and the Wassermann Test in Pulmonary Tuberculosis, Jour. Missouri State Med. Assn., July, 1917, xiv, 284.
[2]Pritchard, J. S., and Roderich, C. E.: Complement-Fixation Test for Tuberculosis, Jour. Am. Med. Assn., Dec., 1919, lxxiii, No. 25.
[3]Blaivas, A. J.: Jour. Lab. and Clin. Med., Jan. 1920, v, No. 4.
[4]Von Ruck, S.: Southern Med. Jour., 1916, ix, 595.
[5]Miller, H. R., and Zinsser, H.: Proc. Soc. Exper. Biol. and Med., 1916, xiii, 134. Miller, H. R.: Jour. Am. Med. Assn., 1916, lxvii, 1519.
[6]Craig, C. F.: Jour. Am. Med. Assn., 1917, lxviii, 773.
[7]Noursund: Jour. Infect. Dis., 1920, xxvi, 85.

LABORATORY METHODS

BODY TEMPERATURE TAKEN IN FRESHLY VOIDED URINE

By Prof. Dr. Theodore Kasparek, Czech University of Prague, Prague, Czechoslovak Republic

I N THE course of investigations on bactericidal agents in freshly voided urine I took also its temperature and found several interesting facts, which led me to further researches in this matter.

For the purpose of determining the exact temperature of urine I have constructed a simple apparatus, consisting of an ordinary glass funnel, with a tube of 7 to 8 inches in length and 3.5 lines in diameter, so arranged as to hold an ordinary, clinical thermometer. The urine is voided directly through the apparatus, which can be placed into an ordinary urinal. In order to prevent loss of body heat, it is previously washed with about 250 c.c. of water, kept several hours in an incubator, or warmed with a properly arranged device of my own construction, at 96° F. This apparatus is manufactured and sold by the Wappler Electric Company, 162-184 Harris Ave., Long Island City, N. Y., under the name of Urothermometer with full directions for its operation.

I have obtained the following average temperatures of normal urine passed through the apparatus:

TIME	TEMPERATURE OF URINES	RECTAL TEMPERATURE	AXILLARY TEMPERATURE
Morning	97.2°-98.0°	98.2°- 98.8°	97.6°-97.6°
Noon	98.6°-99.0°	99.2°- 99.8°	97.8°-98.0°
Evening	98.2°-99.4°	98.4°-100.0°	98.4°-98.8°

In fever cases the difference of temperature between the freshly passed urine (through this apparatus) and the rectal temperature is constant and notable. In a febrile case of Morbus Basedow in which the cause of high temperature could not be recognized at the time—the difference was 0.8° and in a patient with pneumonia the same results were obtained. In several other cases the results, which are presented in Table I, show similar tendencies:

TABLE I

DISEASED CONDITION	TIME	URINE* TEMPERATURE	RECTAL TEMPERATURE
Meningitis	4:30 P.M.	99.4°	100.0°
Bronchitis	6:00 P.M.	100.6°	101.4°
Tuberculosis	7:00 P.M.	101.2°	102.0°
Pneumonia	4:00 P.M.	101.8°	102.4°
Morbus Basedow	11:00 A.M.	100.2°	101.0°
Pneumonia and Rheumatism	4:30 P.M.	102.2°	103.0°

*Obtained by catheterization.

In the following three cases (Table II) the urinary temperature was higher than the temperature by rectum. This indicates that either the urine temperature depends on some chemical or pathologic processes in the bladder, or at other portions of the urinary tract.

TABLE II

TIME	DISEASE	URINE TEMPERATURE	RECTAL TEMPERATURE
Noon	?	104.0°	98.6°
Noon	?	101.0°	99.0°
Evening	Cystitis	101.2°	99.6°

CONCLUSIONS

The results of this investigation indicate that the simple method of determining the body temperature by observation of the temperature of freshly passed urine is of practical value. This will apply principally to cases in which measurement by rectum is impossible or obnoxious, as, for instance in timid patients (children and hysterics) or in hypochondriacs, who should not be acquainted with the existence of high temperature. It may also be of value as a new diagnostic method in diseases of the urinary tract. This will depend upon a larger number of observations and will be reported in due time.

A LABORATORY CHART FOR RECORDING OBSERVATIONS ON MICROORGANISMS*

By Fred W. Tanner, Urbana, Ill.

ONE of the problems with which the instructor in bacteriology must struggle, is the manner in which the student shall record the observations made in the laboratory. The conclusion which one is quite liable to reach, is that no entirely satisfactory method exists. Each instructor must therefore work out for himself that method which is most closely adapted to the type of and amount of instruction which he may give. The object, of course, is to give the student as much practical and accurate information as possible during the time that he spends in the laboratory to acquire the basic principles of the science.

The laboratory chart described herein is a modification of the Descriptive Chart of the Society of American Bacteriologists and one received several years ago from the Laboratories of Bacteriology of the Michigan Agricultural College. Since it has been of so much assistance to us in presenting the facts of laboratory microbiology and assisting the student to know what data should be recorded, it seemed advisable to describe this chart in the literature. It is hoped that others will do the same thing. There seems to be a lack of this to one who has attempted to find in the literature much material on the teaching of microbiology.

Numerous other charts have been prepared for this purpose. Probably the first attempt at this was the effort of a Committee of the American Public Health

*From the University of Illinois, Urbana, Ill.

Association to systematize the study of bacteria. Charts upon which the various characteristics of bacteria were recorded were filed with their report as published.[1]

BACTERIA

Name of student	Desk No.
Name of organism	Isolated from
Method of Isolation	
Occurrence	
Importance	
Arrangement, *single, pairs, chains, fours, cubical packets.*	Size
Involution Forms	
Motility	FLAGELLA No. .... Attachment, *polar, bipolar, lophotrichiate, peritrichiate.* How Stained.... ....

VEGETATIVE CELLS, Medium used..	ENDOSPORES, *present, absent.*	Capsule	STAINING REACTIONS.
temp.............. ...	Location of Endospores, *central, polar.*		1-10 watery fuchsin, gentian violet, carbol fuchsin, Loeffler's alkaline methylene blue.
age............. .days.	Form, *spherical, elliptical elongated.*		Special Stains
Form, *spheres, short rods, long rods, filaments, commas, short spirals, long spirals, spindled, cuneate, clavate, curved.*	Limits of Size..........		Gram................
	Size of Majority........		Glycogen.............
	Wall, *thick, thin.*		Fat ....
	Sporangium wall, *adherent, not adherent.*		Acid fast.............
	Germination, *equatorial, oblique, polar, bipolar, by stretching, by absorption of spore wall.*		Neisser............. Metachromatic granules, sporogenous granules.

PLAIN AGAR STREAK	....days ....days ....days	*Growth,* invisible, scanty, moderate, abundant. *Form of Growth,* filiform, echinulate, beaded, spreading, plumose, arborescent, rhizoid. *Elevation of Growth,* flat, effuse, raised, convex. *Lustre,* glistening, dull, cretaceous. *Topography,* smooth, contoured, rugose, verrucose. *Optical Characters,* opaque, translucent, opalescent, iridescent.
Reaction...		*Chromogenesis*............................ ....
Incubated at		*Odor,* absent, decided, resembling........ •...........
.........°C		*Consistency,* slimy, butyrous, viscid, membranous, coriaceous, brittle. *Medium* grayed, browned, reddened, blued, greened. NOTE.—Underline terms applying to description of cultures.

PLAIN GELATIN STAB	....days ....days ....days	*Growth* uniform, best at top, best at bottom. *Line of Puncture,* filiform, beaded, papillate, villous, plumose, arborescent. *Liquefaction,* crateriform, napiform, infundibuliform, saccate, stratiform; *begins in*............. d, *complete in*................d. *Medium* fluorescent, browned........................
Reaction....		
Incubated at		
.........°C		

Page 1 of chart.

---

[1]Procedures Recommended for the Study of Bacteria with Special Reference to Greater Uniformity in the Description and Differentiation of Species. Being the Report of a Committee of Bacteriologists to the Pollution of Water Supplies of the American Public Health Association, Am. Pub. Health Assn. Proc., 1898, pp. 60-100.

The outgrowth of this early work which has been so well reviewed by Harding[2] is the Descriptive Chart of the Society of American Bacteriologists. This has passed through several revisions and with the Group Number, a numerical method for recording the salient characteristics of microorganisms, represents, probably, the most recent effort on the part of an organized society at

	.days	....days	....days	
PLAIN BROTH CULTURE				*Surface growth*, ring, pellicle, flocculent, membranous, none. *Clouding;* slight, moderate, strong; transient, persistent; none; fluid, turbid. *Odor*, absent, decided, resembling.......... ....
Reaction... Incubated at .... °C				*Sediment*, compact, flocculent, granular, flaky, viscid on agitation, abundant, scant *Medium*, fluorescent........ ....

Age of colony	................days		................days		................days	
Size of colony (Millimeters)						
Surface elevation						
	Macroscopic	Microscopic	Macroscopic	Microscopic	Macroscopic	Microscopic
AGAR COLONY		Edge of Colony Low Power Objective		Edge of Colony Low Power Objective		Edge of Colony Low Power Objective
Reaction.... .... °C	*Growth*, slow, rapid, temperature............ *Form*, punctiform, round, irregular, ameboid, mycelioid, filamentous, rhizoid. *Surface*, smooth, rough, concentrically ringed, radiate, striate		*Elevation*, flat, effuse, raised, convex, pulvinate, umbonate. *Edge*, entire, undulate, lobate, erose, lacerate. *Internal structure*, amorphous, finely, coarsely-granular, grumose, filamentous, floccose, curled.			

Age of colony	.... days		.... days		.... days	
Size of colony (Millimeters)						
Surface elevation						
	Macroscopic	Microscopic	Macroscopic	Microscopic	Macroscopic	Microscopic
GELATIN COLONY		Edge of Colony Low Power Objective		Edge of Colony Low Power Objective		Edge of Colony Low Power Objective
Reaction... Incubated at .. .°C	*Growth*, slow, rapid. *Form*, punctiform, round, irregular, ameboid, mycelioid, filamentous, rhizoid. *Elevation*, flat, effuse, raised, convex, pulvinate, crateriform (liquefying).		*Edge*, entire, undulate, lobate, erose, lacerate, fimbriate, filamentous, floccose, curled. *Liquefaction*, cup, saucer, spreading.			

Page 2 of chart.

[2]Harding, H. A.: The Constancy of Certain Physiological Characters in the Classification of Bacteria, Tech. Bull. New York, Ag. Exp. Station, Geneva, 1910.

standardizing the study of bacteria. This chart has been used by various investigators in research work. However, from the teaching standpoint, it has certain disadvantages. The matter which is given on this chart is crowded and there is no room for the various general records which a student must make. No space is left for sketching certain types of growth. Realizing this there was an effort in the society for a number of years to formulate a chart for student use. This idea culminated in the report of the committee on the Chart for Identi-

			.... days		.... days		.... days	
Litmus milk	No change							
	Acid							
	Gas							
	Acid curd							
	Rennin curd							
	Reduction							
	Alkali							
	Peptonization							

Fermentation Reactions

% OF GAS IN	CONTROL	DEXTROSE	LACTOSE	SUCROSE	GLYCEROL			
24 hours								
48 hours								
4 days								
7 days								
Total gas production								
Odor								
Acid								
Growth in closed arm								

Production of	NH_3 from peptone	
	H_2S from peptone	
	Nitrites from peptone	
	Indol from peptone	
Reduction of nitrate to	NH_3	
	Nitrites	
Diastasic action on starch	Present	
	Absent	
Chromogenesis on	Nutrient broth	
	Nutrient gelatin	
	Nutrient agar	

Page 3 of chart.

fication of Bacterial Species at the 1917 meeting of the Society of American Bacteriologists wherein was presented a "Descriptive Chart for Use in Bacteriological Instruction." It seems doubtful whether such a committee, very few of whom are actively concerned with teaching laboratory bacteriology, could most clearly realize the needs of the teacher. Those who are giving such instruction regularly and are talking with students through the academic year are probably better qualified to work out such a chart. Various other charts are being

Group Number

Special Observation:

Endospores produced 100
Endospores not produced 200.

Aerobic (Strict) 10. Facultative anaerobic 20
Anaerobic (strict) 30.

Gelatin liquefied 1.
Gelatin not liquefied 2.

Acid and gas 1 Acid without gas 2
No acid .3 No growth .4 with dextrose.

Acid and gas .01 Acid without gas .02
No acid .03 No growth .04 with lactose.

Acid and gas .001 Acid without gas .002
No acid .003 No growth .004 with saccharose

Nitrates reduced with gas .0001
Nitrates reduced without gas .0002
Nitrates not reduced .0003

Fluorescent .00001 Violet .00002 Blue .00003
Green .00004 Yellow .00005 Orange .00006 Red
.00007 Brown .00008 Pink .00009 Non-chrom-
escent .00000.

Diastasic action on potato starch, strong .000001
Feeble .000002 absent .000003

Acid and gas .0000001 Acid without gas .0000002
No acid .0000003 No growth .0000004 with
glycerin.

(Dec. 31 1914 Chart)

REMARKS

LABORATORIES OF BACTERIOLOGY
University of Illinois
URBANA   May, 1920

Page 4 of chart.

used in other institutions. The Frost Chart is probably well known to most bacteriologists. At Ohio State University and the College of Medicine of the University of Illinois such charts are being used for laboratory instruction. Copies of both of the Descriptive Charts of the Society of American Bacteriologists may be secured from Doctor J. A. Conn, Agricultural Experiment Station, Geneva, New York. The society through its committee has made a commendable effort at providing standard methods for carrying out the observations made on bacteria. Several reports have already been published.

The chart described herein, as stated above, is modified from the Descriptive Chart of the Society of American Bacteriologists. No agreement will exist with regard to what determinations should be made by the student on the various microorganisms which he studies in pure culture. The one described in this paper, we believe, contains these determinations which should be made on organisms in an introductory course in general microbiology. It must be borne in mind that our effort is to give the student the most solid foundation in technic that is possible in the time that he is with us.

It consists of a four-page printed folder 8½ by 11 inches. The student is supposed to use one of these charts for each organism which he studies and to file the charts in his notebook. Spaces are provided for recording both cultural and morphological data. Since the Group Number has been used by the Society of American Bacteriologists and since the laboratory determinations demanded in determining it are those made on microorganisms in almost every introductory course in the science, it has been included. The terms which are underlined in describing the organisms are taken from the Society Chart and a glossary is provided the student at the beginning of the semester. Other features of the chart are the spaces for making sketches. It is well known that difference of opinion exists with regard to the value of sketches. Some regard them as a waste of the student's time and probably, at times, they are very misleading especially if the student attempts to use them after he has progressed further in his course. However, anything which will help to make the student more observing of the differences in types of bacterial development is legitimate.

This chart has some disadvantages like all methods which must be used in presenting the facts of a somewhat inexact science. Copies of it may be secured, if desired, from the writer.

AN IMPROVED METHOD FOR FEEDING RABBITS BY STOMACH SOUND*

By MARTHA R. JONES, NEW HAVEN, CONN.

ALTHOUGH feeding rabbits by stomach sound is a routine procedure in many physiologic laboratories, the device described below was found to be so simple and satisfactory for introducing solutions quantitatively into the stomach that it seemed worth publication.

The rabbit is fastened on an ordinary cat board, the head holder consisting of two upright, perforated pillars through which a horizontal bar can be passed

*From the Sheffield Laboratory of Physiological Chemistry, Yale University, New Haven, Conn.

at any height desired. When handled gently the rabbits, as a rule, do not become excited. and one person can put them on the board with ease. The animal's jaws are then opened with the fingers and a pointed wooden rod about ¾ inch in diameter and 4 inches long with a ⅜ inch hole in the center passing through its short axis is inserted behind the teeth. Burette clamps attached to an iron ring stand are then slipped over the ends of the rod and fastened so that it is fixed in position. The rabbit is now able to open his mouth freely, but is prevented from ejecting the rod from behind his teeth and from biting the sound when it is introduced into the stomach. A funnel to which the sound (small

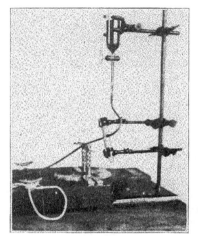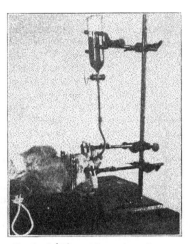

Fig. 1.—Animal board and feeding device.   Fig. 2.—Rabbit receiving a dose of sugar.

male catheter) has been attached is supported by another burette clamp. The free end of the tube is now moistened and gently forced into the stomach through the hole in the wooden rod. Usually the sound finds its way into the esophagus without difficulty. Its location, however, can be readily ascertained by gently feeling behind the trachea. The liquid is now poured into the funnel, and if desired. its rate of discharge can be regulated by means of a pinch cock. One great advantage of the device is that with a little practice one person can feed two or more animals at the same time, which is a matter of considerable importance when a large number of rabbits are being fed thick, viscid solutions that pass through the tube very slowly.

The Journal of Laboratory and Clinical Medicine

VOL. V.   SEPTEMBER, 1920   No. 12

Editor-in-Chief: VICTOR C. VAUGHAN, M.D.
Ann Arbor, Mich.

ASSOCIATE EDITORS

DENNIS E. JACKSON, M.D.	- - CINCINNATI
HANS ZINSSER, M.D. -	- - NEW YORK
PAUL G. WOOLLEY, M.D.	- DETROIT
FREDERICK P. GAY, M.D. -	- BERKELEY, CAL.
J. J. R. MACLEOD, M.B. -	- - TORONTO
ROY G. PEARCE, M.D.	- - AKRON, OHIO
W. C. MACCARTY, M.D. -	ROCHESTER, MINN.
GERALD B. WEBB, M.D. -	COLORADO SPRINGS
WARREN T. VAUGHAN, M.D.	- . BOSTON

EDITORIALS

Nonspecific Immunity

FROM the struggle between parasitic microorganisms and the forces of the animal body there evolve certain groups of phenomena which we designate by the term "disease." Infectious disease is the result of and the expression of this two-sided combat. In the study of pathological physiology we have been accustomed to observe chiefly the physical and chemical changes produced during manifest disease. But we should not limit our study of the immunologic processes to those produced during acute illness. Manifest disease is only one phase of the constant struggle between invader and host. In nature, the latter overcomes the former many times without the production of clinical disease to each time that it does with such result.

The greater portion of past research work in immunology has been devoted to studies of specific immunity produced against specific antigens. Theories based upon specificity have aided greatly in elucidating our concepts, but time and again, diverse phenomena in disease have occurred which have baffled explanation in the light of those theories.

The relative insusceptibility of city bred over rural recruits in the army even to diseases which they have not previously had is a fact concerning which

799

there can now be little doubt. There are some who believe in a relative immunity of tuberculous individuals to epidemic influenza. The clinical improvement in certain subacute and chronic diseases, such as lupus vulgaris, after the occurrence of a superimposed acute infection, as erysipelas, is a matter of common knowledge. We observe that one of the acute exanthemata rarely if ever occurs coincidently with another. Such forms of insusceptibility appear to be nonspecific in character, and it is because of these and similar phenomena that the existence of a more or less general nonspecific protective mechanism has been suggested.

That there does exist, in addition to natural and acquired specific immunity, an acquired nonspecific immune mechanism seems most probable. It is perhaps never of as great degree as the other two forms, but often confers enough protection to be the deciding factor between life and death of the individual. Thus, W. T. Vaughan and Schnabel found that among ninety soldiers with bronchopneumonia who had had no previous history of specific infections, the mortality was 47 per cent, while among 243 who had averaged nearly two previous infections apiece, the death rate was under 35 per cent. The general mortality among 234 cases of lobar pneumonia was 14.9 per cent, while of ten cases with entirely negative past histories for infectious disease, 20 per cent died. The individual who had had other infections previously, stood a better chance of winning than the one who had never been called on to fight a battle.

V. C. Vaughan and Palmer called attention to the fact that the seasoned soldier is more resistant even to newly imported infections than the recent recruit. They showed that in the army camps in 1917-1919 the men from crowded cities resisted the respiratory infections more successfully than their comrades from sparsely settled areas.

Later, Love and Davenport also showed that the communicable diseases produced the least admission and death rate in those camps which drew from areas that were prevailingly urban; that the highest morbidity and mortality rates were from camps that drew from the sparsely populated areas of the Southern Atlantic and Gulf States, and to a less extent from the sparsely settled states of the west. They demonstrated these facts mathematically by the method of multiple correlation. The results with both groups of investigators were the same not only for measles and mumps, diseases which the urban recruits had probably had in childhood, but also for pneumonia, cerebrospinal meningitis, influenza and scarlet fever, from which the majority had probably never suffered. This last fact negatives the theory that urban recruits were less susceptible to the specific infections because they had previously had them. Such an hypothesis holds good for measles and mumps, but not in general. Another explanation, the theory of the elimination of susceptibles in childhood, has much to commend it, but it only carries the solution one step farther. Why are those that remain not susceptible? Again we find ourselves face to face with nonspecific immunity.

In the study of epidemics it is often observed that the year following an epidemic of measles in a large city is one of low mortality, not only for measles, but also for whooping cough and scarlet fever.

The mechanism of nonspecific immunity is undoubtedly complex. Presumably it works on the same general principles as in specific immunity. It may be conceived of as a grade between the latter and natural immunity, having features common to both types but more closely allied to the acquired variety. Many of the processes in natural immunity are nonspecific. The intact skin and mucous membranes form the first nonspecific barrier. The physical or chemical qualities of the salivary, gastric and intestinal secretions play a part. After microorganisms have penetrated the skin the local leucocytosis combats the infection. Phagocytosis, special tissue insusceptibility, ferments or antibodies, antitoxins, bacteriolysins and precipitins all play a part in natural as well as acquired immunity and these must all be investigated in a study of nonspecific immunity.

It may be found that there are even new factors in this form of protection. According to Wooley, 3, 757 of 9,559 men who had been in camp less than five months developed influenza in the autumn, 1918, epidemic at Camp Devens, while only 1,033 of 5,943 who had seen more than five months service took sick. At Camp Lee, Lt. Wallis reports that those who had been in the service less than one month constituted only 9 per cent of the total strength, but furnished 30 per cent of the total influenza deaths; that those who had been in service over three months constituted 45 per cent of the camp population, but furnished only 23 per cent of the deaths. At Camp Custer 64 per cent of the men who had influenza had been in the service only two months.

Length of service evidently had some bearing on influenza immunity. One may explain that the older soldiers had become acclimated to their surroundings, but the fact remains beyond this, that the older soldier, no more *naturally* immune than his more recent associate, was less susceptible to the ravages of the disease, and that this relative insusceptibility was in no way specific in character. So, physical condition or metabolic equilibrium may be an additional factor to be studied in nonspecific immunity. Indeed this is a factor of other forms of immunity. Pasteur demonstrated years ago that the natural immunity of birds to anthrax could be overcome by exposure and fatigue.

Vaughan and Palmer suggest an explanation of the mechanism of nonspecific immunity which is in harmony with existing theories. The bacterial protein, when it is digested in the body is broken down into two portions; one specific, different for each different protein; and not poisonous; and the other, nonspecific, alike in all forms of protein molecules, and poisonous. By injection of the specific fraction of the bacterial molecule a true immunity can be produced against the living germ, which will protect against from two to twelve times the minimum lethal dose of that germ. It will not protect against any other. Thus is specific immunity developed by the liberation in the body of this specific antigenic fraction during destruction of the germ. The poisonous portion when injected produces no such immunity but does result in increased tolerance towards itself on the part of the body, so that sometimes as much as twice the minimum fatal dose may be injected without fatal result. It is this poisonous portion of the molecule which during destruction of the germ within the body produces the general symptoms of disease. It is the same whatever be the organism causing the disease.

So, one who has *recovered* from measles has acquired through the action of the nonpoisonous fraction of the measles virus protein, a specific immunity of high potency, and, at the same time, an increased tolerance to the poisonous fraction, nonspecific, and of low potency. Subsequent infection, say with small pox virus produces a mild attack because of the lessened susceptibility to the poison.

Here is a theory of nonspecific immunity which has the advantage of being a good working hypothesis and of being in harmony with existing theories. That theory to which new developments in immunology can be most successfully and most consistently applied will eventually be found to be the truest explanation of the mechanism of immunity.

One apparent drawback to the hypothesis is that the increased tolerance induced by the protein poison is, experimentally, of short duration, while nonspecific immunity appears to last for months or years. Further investigation will help to solve this problem.

Another explanation derived from the theories of Jobling on nonspecific protein therapy deserves mention. In it the nonspecific element is a proteolytic ferment mobilized in the blood following experimental inoculation of bacteria. This ferment has no action on bacteria, but he suggests that "if we consider the source of the intoxication as primarily due to protein split products, then a mobilization of protease may be of considerable importance in the process of detoxication, in that the toxic fragments are hydrolyzed to lower and nontoxic forms." Thus it is suggested that the nonspecific element is the ferment that helps to destroy the bacterial cell.

It is doubtful whether this form of immunity can prevent infection with a newly imported virus. But that it can mitigate the effects of the new infection seems quite probable.

The subject of local tissue immunity is difficult to study experimentally and has in the past usually been neglected for the investigation of general immunologic processes. There is some evidence pointing to local nonspecific protection. Armstrong believes that the chronic pulmonary infection with the tubercle bacillus and its accompanying secondary invaders rendered the tuberculous less susceptible to the acute respiratory infection of influenza. The Typhoid Commission in the Spanish American War concluded that temporary gastrointestinal disturbances instead of predisposing to typhoid fever, gave a certain degree of immunity against subsequent infection with this disease.

Nonspecific immunity, if such does exist, represents a radical departure from present day concepts in which specificity is the keynote. Clinical data such as those already quoted are abundant, but are so general in character that they may be misleading. Experimental evidence must be clear cut and convincing.

If the theory is corroborated many phenomena hitherto unexplained will be understandable. Much, who has written at some length in the *Deutsche Medizinische Wochenschrift*, attempts to explain thereby, results of vaccination against migraine, the use of microorganisms in the treatment of cancer, shot gun vaccines in various maladies, autoserotherapy in skin affections, high mortality among the robust in pandemics, and many other conditions. While these things may be in some manner related, one must be cautious not to endeavor to explain too great a variety of phenomena before he has proved satisfactorily that nonspecific immunity exists and how it operates.

REFERENCES

Armstrong, D. M.: Influenza Observations in Framingham, Mass. Am. Jour. Public
    Health, 1919, ix, 960.
Jobling, J. W.: The Influence of Non-specific Substances on Infections, Arch. Int. Med.,
    1917, xix, 1043.
Jobling, J. W., and Peterson, Wm.: Nonspecific Factors in the Treatment of Disease,
    Jour. Am. Med. Assn., 1916, lxvi, 1753.
Love, A. G., and Davenport, C. B.: Immunity of City Bred Recruits, Arch. Int. Med.,
    1919, xxiv, 129.
Vaughan, V. C., and Palmer, Capt. G. T., M. C., U. S. A.: Nonspecific Immunity, The Mil-
    itary Surgeon for January, 1920.
Vaughan, V. C., and Palmer, Geo. T.: Communicable Disease in the United States Army
    During the Summer and Autumn of 1918, Jour. Lab. and Clin. Med., 1919, iv, 586.
Vaughan, W. T., and Schnabel, T. G.: Pneumonia and Empyema at Camp Sevier, Arch.
    Int. Med., 1918, xxii, 440.

—*W. T. V*

Recent Researches on the Capillary Circulation

IT HAS been the custom to assume that the walls of the capillaries are incapable of constricting or dilating independently of changes of pressure in the
blood circulating in them. According to this view the magnitude of the capillary circulation depends on the amount and pressure of the blood which enters
the capillaries from the arterioles and it cannot become altered by local changes
in the capillaries themselves. A. Krogh has, however, brought forward unas-
sailable evidence to show that this view is in general incorrect. He has shown
that the capillaries possess independent powers of constricting and dilating, and
also that they are very much less in caliber when the tissue which they supply is
at rest than when it is active.

The observations from which the conclusions are drawn have been published
in two papers,[2, 3] those of the first being made on the vessels of muscles, in frogs
and guinea pigs, and those of the second on the vessels of the tongue in frogs.
The method most frequently employed to render the vessels visible was examination with the binocular microscope by reflected light, although much information
was secured by injecting intravenously a solution of India-ink, then killing the
animals and examining either fresh or fixed tissues by ordinary methods of mi-
croscopy to determine the capillaries into which the black particles have penetrated.

In resting muscle relatively few capillaries were visible, these being, however, evenly distributed to form an elongated mesh work along the muscle fibers.
In active muscle, on the other hand, many previously invisible capillaries came
into view, to disappear again when the contraction was over. These differences
could even be made out macroscopically, after injecting India-ink by the almost
black color of muscles that had been active when the animal was killed in contrast with their pale gray appearance when at rest. An observation of great interest is that the corpuscles often crowd themselves through capillaries having
diameters which are much less than those of the corpuscles. In order that they
may pass, the corpuscles become folded or sausage shaped and the capillaries
become deformed, showing marked bulgings over the corpuscles. The great
variability in the number of patulous capillaries, according to the state of activ-

ity of the tissues, indicates that alterations in oxygen supply, to meet the varying demands is probably accomplished by greater blood flow. This possibility is considered in another paper[1] in which, by mathematical calculation based on (1) the depth of tissue which each capillary supplies; (2) the rate of oxygen consumption by the tissue, and (3) the diffusion rate of oxygen, it is shown that the oxygen pressure necessary to supply the muscle fibres is so small, even during their greatest activity, that the call for oxygen can readily be met by diffusion alone. This conclusion is in conformity with the facts that the partial pressure of oxygen in the urine is the same as that in venous blood and that when a neutral gas, such as nitrogen, is placed in the pleural or peritoneal cavities it ultimately becomes mixed with oxygen up to a percentage of three or four. That no oxygen should be detectable in tissues such as muscle is explained by its immediate utilization for purposes of metabolism.

Further light has been thrown on the nature of the capillariomotor mechanism by examination through the microscope of the blood vessels, particularly of the frog's tongue, during either mechanical irritation, or the action of certain drugs. In reporting the far-reaching results which he has succeeded in obtaining on this aspect of the problem, Krogh points out that the capillaries of various tissues, just like the arterioles, differ considerably in their reactions. The exact nature of the capillariomotor mechanism must therefore be investigated for each tissue separately and general conclusions applicable to all vascular areas cannot be drawn.

When the surface of the ventral aspect of the tongue (of the frog) is scratched with a fine glass pencil, or with a hair, it can be seen, after a latent period of 10 to 15 seconds, that both the capillaries and the arterioles dilate over an area which is greater than that stimulated. The venules, however, do not show any change apart from that which can be accounted for as secondary to changes in the amount of blood flowing into them. Taken alone, the results might indicate that dilatation, or constriction, of the arterioles merely causes more, or less, blood to flow into the capillaries. That another factor is also involved, namely, independent changes in the caliber of the capillaries, was shown by the following experiment: (1) After greatly slowing down the blood flow and reducing its pressure on one side of the tongue, by partially clamping the corresponding lingual artery, mechanical irritation had its usual effect in dilating the capillaries, the blood flowed slowly into them and in place of the corpuscles having to pass as sausage-shaped bodies one by one, several could now pass side by side. When the clamp was removed no further dilatation of the capillaries occurred, although the blood current became much more rapid and several capillaries which previously had not been visible sprang into view. Of course, when the artery was completely occluded, irritation did not cause any visible change in the capillaries, but when the block was subsequently removed the arterioles and capillaries immediately became filled with blood in a dilated state, showing that the irritation produces a relaxation of the walls, but that some blood pressure is necessary to bring about an actual dilatation. (2) Sometimes it was possible to localize the stimulation so that capillaries became dilated without any change in the arterioles. In such cases the blood flow in the capillaries might actually stagnate and the corpuscles either stand still or move backwards from the venous end toward the arterial. In one case a local dilatation was noticed to occur at the arterial end of a capillary, and the venous end remaining constricted, the blood flowed into the dilated portion, but stasis occurred. The venous end of the capillary was then irritated when it opened up and the blood current through the whole capillary was reestablished. In another case a very long capillary was caused to dilate at two separate places, by mechanical stimulation, and at these places the corpuscles moved with extreme slowness, although moving quickly in the original capillary. In yet other cases the venous end of a capillary, perhaps previously invisible, could be caused, by irritation, to open up so that blood flowed back into it from the venule and, by repeated repetition of weak stimuli in front of the visible column of blood, the filling could be extended backwards until another vessel with higher pressure was reached when a current became set up in the whole length of capillary. This observation is particularly important in that it shows the state of the capillary wall to be much more important in determining the blood flow through them than the blood pressure in the arterioles. (3) Important reactions were observed to occur towards certain chemical substances. Methane (25 per cent solution) caused the capillaries to become enormously dilated and to assume a varicose appearance, while the arterioles remained unaffected. When the supplying arteriole was of narrow caliber, the blood when it enters the dilated capillary, might stagnate completely so that even after several days it was filled with a stationary mass of corpuscles. Iodine, in 1 per cent solution, caused a similar capillary dilatation, but the arteries were likewise involved, although to a less degree. The muscles of the tongue also contracted strongly when iodine was applied.

Besides the direct evidence which is furnished by the above observations much of a less direct nature was collected to show that the capillariomotor and arteriomotor mechanisms are distinct and separate. For example, pricking the wall of a small artery with a fine hair might cause this vessel to constrict while the capillaries showed the usual dilatation. Electrical stimulation did not yield satisfactory results, but local warming caused dilatation both of arteries and capillaries, and marked hyperemia. Weak acids (1 per cent acetic of pure CO_2) had an effect like that of warming. Adrenin (1 per cent adrenaline), cocaine (2 to 5 per cent), nicotine (0.5 per cent) and amylnitrite all caused the capillaries, and usually the arteries, to dilate. In certain cases, however, it was observed that adrenin caused constriction upon a few small arteries.

One of the most important questions which the above observations raise is with regard to the mechanism involved in causing the changes in the vessels. Is the effect a direct one or is it reflex, and mediated through the central nervous system? Krogh employed two methods to study this question. In one of these the tissue was bathed in a solution of cocaine that was not of sufficient strength to cause marked dilatation of the vessels. In from 30 to 60 minutes the cocaine paralyzed the local nerve endings, with the result that neither mechanical stimulation nor 1 per cent iodine could any longer bring about dilatation, and methane had much less effect than the usual. The other method consisted in observing the effects of local stimulation after cutting the nerves to the tongue (hypoglossal and glossopharyngeal) and allowing them to degenerate. Immediately after section there was often a distinct hyperemia of the corresponding side of the tongue, but local irritation was still followed by the usual response on the vessels, although this was less evident because of the hyperemia. It is considered likely that the hyperemia following cutting is due to mechanical irritation of the nerve and not to the removal of tonic constrictor impulses. Local freezing of the nerve was, for example, not found to lead to hyperemia, and freezing, of course, blocks the passage of nerve impulses. After time had been allowed for degeneration to occur (eight days) the vessels in the area supplied by the nerve reacted to stimulation much more locally than usual, that is, the effect did not spread much beyond the actual point that had been stimulated. The characteristic effect of the nerve degeneration was, therefore, sometimes a weakening and, always, a marked localization in the response of the blood vessels to mechanical and chemical stimulation.

The conclusions that are drawn from these researches are that there are nerve endings on the arterioles and capillaries and that these have a double function: the one sensory—particularly toward mechanical stimuli—and the other dilatory—that is, inhibiting the vascular tone. Some of the (sensory) endings also exist in the intervascular spaces. When the endings are stimulated the impulse travels up the branch of the nerve fiber with which the ending is connected, and when it arrives at the place of branching the impulse travels down the nerve fiber and is carried by certain of the remaining branches to the arterioles and capillaries, which it causes to dilate. The mechanism is therefore of the type known as an axon reflex. This conclusion, it will be noted, is in harmony with that adopted by Ninian Bruce[4] to explain the results of his observations on the effects which cocainization or nerve degeneration have on the vascular reactions following irritation of the cornea. They also conform with the view of Bayliss[5] that vasodilator impulses are transmitted to the blood vessels of the extremities along sensory nerves.

As a result of nerve degeneration or cocainization the endings are paralyzed, but the vessels (arterioles and capillaries) still maintain their tone and this can still be inhibited by certain forms of stimulation, particularly by methane and weak acids. This indicates that the tone does not depend on nerve impulses, the function of these being solely to inhibit, (or augment) the tone, and to mediate the spread of any change in caliber over a greater stretch of vessel. The tone, therefore, depends on a chemical action of the blood itself and when the supply of blood is cut off for some time the vessel becomes dilated, as is evidenced by the great blood flow which occurs through it when the obstruction is removed. These observations call to mind the conclusions drawn by H. H. Dale and A. N. Richards,[6] and Dale and Laidlaw,[7] concerning the locus of action of histamine and also those concerning the pathogenesis of surgical shock. They are of fundamental importance in the interpretation of many other of the problems that confront the research worker, and with the conclusions which have been drawn from them must be harmonized our views of the pathogenesis of inflammation, lymph formation and the effect of toxic substances.

BIBLIOGRAPHY

[1]Krogh, A.: Jour. of Physiol, 1919, lii, 409.
[2]Krogh, A.: Ibid., p. 457.
[3]Krogh, A.: Ibid., p. 399.

[4]Bruce, Ainian: Arch. f. Exper. Path., 1910, lxiii, 424.
[5]Bayliss, W. M.: Jour. f. Physiol, 1900, xxvi, 173.
[6]Dale, H. H., and Richards, A. N.: Ibid., 1919, lii, 110.
[7]Dale, H. H., and Laidlaw: Ibid., p. 355.

—*J. J. R. M.*

Universal Immunity to Tuberculosis

IN a recent issue of this JOURNAL a brief account was given of an experiment in preventive medicine in which a large population is serving to show that thyroid abnormalities may be greatly diminished by a simple procedure. At the same time less circumscribed work on other preventable diseases is being carried on in all parts of the world by the International Health Board and by the League of Red Cross Societies. Uncinariasis, typhus, yellow fever, malaria and plague are subjects for particular attacks. Typhoid fever is for the most part under control, and the method of control is known and is generally available. The great plagues are being fought to the death. The nations of the earth are joining hands to wipe out pestilences.

During the years of organization against disease, tuberculosis has received some large attention to be sure, but the emphasis has been placed largely upon cure, less upon prevention. Experiments in immunity have been carried on, but always under a handicap. Everywhere in the so-called civilized world the disease is endemic and therefore the possibility exists that the experiments are subject to chances of contamination from an infected environment. Notwithstanding the difficulties certain very definite data have been accumulated, and these Calmette states briefly as follows:

Infection with tubercle bacilli, so wide-spread among all civilized nations, is rare, or does not exist among savage races or among the wandering tribes in those parts of the globe which are still isolated from the great commercial routes. It is a disease of crowded social communities, its prevalence and gravity increasing with the density of the population.

It is the same with susceptible animals such as cattle. In the wild states they are free from this disease, whereas the domesticated species, obliged to live in contact with man, are affected in proportion to the closeness of the contact. In towns and in overcrowded stables, in the presence of animals or men who are ill or who, even if apparently healthy, are sowers, as it were, of bacilli, this contagion is almost inevitable. The infection is shown to have already been acquired at an early age by a great number of individuals, and the judicious use of tuberculin reactions has taught us that in New York, just as in Paris, Vienna, Berlin, or London, 55 per cent of the children who have reached their fifth year, and more than 95 per cent of adults, harbor the tubercle bacilli. This does not, however, mean that all these persons are tuberculous.

The disease tuberculosis is one thing; mere bacillary infection is another. The bacillary infection may remain occult, that is to say, it may for many years, or even during the lifetime of the subject, produce no tuberculous lesion; or it may cause a benign tuberculous lesion, liable to remain indefinitely latent. The disease tuberculosis is the result either of a single massive bacillary infection, or of frequent and copious reinfections.

Massive bacillary infection in a subject hitherto free, a young child for instance, or in adults belonging to countries free from tuberculosis, natives of Central Africa, produces severe manifestations which, developing rapidly, are almost always fatal and of various types, according to the number of the infecting bacilli, their origin, and the organs attacked. Massive infection or frequent and copious reinfection supervening on a pre-existing occult bacillary infection or a latent lesion, gives rise to resistant types of disease. The gravity of these types is in close relation to the age of the original infection and to the number and source, and hence the virulence, of the reinfecting bacilli, and also to the seat of the lesions and the anatomical relations of the organs affected.

Experiments on susceptible animals and clinical observations on human beings have justified the assertion that a mild infection occurring in childhood and remaining occult or latent for several years, endows the organism with a pronounced resistance to subsequent inoculations or reinfections. Any individual with an occult bacillary infection or with a benign and latent glandular tuberculous lesion, who is protected, either by his mode of life or by suitable prophylactic measures, from massive or frequent contaminations will retain for years, as long as he reacts positively to tuberculin, this special immunity, which is manifested by a cellular intolerance towards reinfecting bacilli.

It must, therefore, be admitted that acquired immunity to tuberculosis exists. Moreover it is known that it may be conferred artificially on susceptible animals at an early age by careful introduction into their lymphatic organs of small quantities of bacilli whose virulence has been diminished or modified so that they are no longer capable of producing tubercles. It persists as long as the symbiosis of the attenuated or modified bacilli with the lymphatic cellular elements is maintained. It ceases when they are completely eliminated or destroyed and when sensitiveness to tuberculin has disappeared.

These scientific facts show that active immunization against tuberculosis is possible. The question is to find a procedure which will be effective and harmless.

It is, as Calmette says, impossible to carry out the necessary experiments in a civilized community, because of the general environmental infection, a state of affairs which is too apt to modify or make valueless the studies. He says that the necessary conditions can be found only in aboriginal districts in which tuberculosis is nonexistent, and in which native animals can be used for experiment. He suggests an island in French Guinea where chimpanzees can be obtained and cared for by carefully selected healthy natives. These animals could be used not only for experiments in tuberculosis but also for other problems in biology and experimental psychology. Surely the opportunities offered by such an experiment station would be great. The possibilities from the standpoint of general biology are of almost inconceivable magnitude.

It is to be hoped that the plan can be adopted, and financed, and controlled under the supervision of international learned societies.

REFERENCE

International Journal of Public Health, 1920, i, 3.

—P. G. W.

Cancer Among Dye Workers

W E ARE as yet quite ignorant of the actual cause or causes of tumor growth. It may be that it depends upon a parasite, or, because of the multiplicity of tumors, upon a number of parasites. It may be that the tumor cells because of some fundamental biologic change become parasitic—are themselves parasites—and, acquiring independence of their normal environment, go forth into the wider fields of the body, become free lances, marauders, thieves and assassins. Behind such a change may be some extrinsic chemical, or physico-chemical process encouraging the anarchism. It may be true that tumors are as a rule due to a chronic irritation of a chemical nature just as, it seems, they sometimes arise because of chronic physical ones. But even so is the difference between the two processes so fundamental? One may only guess, but in so doing one might conceive that a mechanical influence acting over a certain period of time could have the same effect as a dilute chemical substance—a toxin for example. One might ask whether the "paraffin cancers" of the skin are due to the paraffin acting as a local stimulant, or whether they are an expression of long-continued mechanical stimulation permitted by the lubricant, and therefore soothing, action of the substance. Perhaps without the paraffin the irritation would lead to protective and curative measures, and therefore to prevention.

Certainly there are circumstances which point very directly to a mechanical cause for some tumors. Just as certainly there are more circumstances which point to a chemical cause. In many other cases the two cannot be separated—and this is particularly true in cancers of the gastrointestinal tract in which the growths predominate at the points where trauma is most possible, and where chemical substances formed by bacteria and by the tissues have most chances to act.

In America, where the dye industry is being established widely, we are confronted by the possibility that hitherto uncommon forms of cancer will appear, and many at least of these seem to be attributed to chemical stimulation. In this group are the urinary bladder growths which form the basis of important recent reports.

The dye workers' cancers are interesting because of the fact that they are apparently of pure chemical origin, and because they are of very long incubation. They seem to be due, in the case of the bladder tumors, to the long-continued action of a dilute material, excreted by way of the urinary tract, which affects only the mucous membrane of the urinary bladder. This irritating substance, or the ones from which it originates, may be taken into the body through the skin, the respiratory tract and the gastrointestinal tract, and is generally supposed to be aniline or fenzidine. Nassauer believes that the former alone is the specific one.

Despite the long incubation period Nassauer thinks that workmen should not be exposed for more than three months.. He also believes that by enforcement of proper rules of sanitation including personal cleanliness most of the danger can be avoided. In a factory which he has studied, in which many cases formerly occurred, no case has appeared in a period of fourteen years since the inauguration of strict hygienic requirements. It will be interesting to watch the development of studies made in dye works in America. It will be still more interesting if by taking proper care the appearance of tumors can be eliminated in our dye workers.

REFERENCES

Nassauer: Frankfurter Ztschr. of Path., 1920, xxii, 353.
Oppenheimer: München. med. Wchnschr., 1920, lxvii, 12.

—*P. G. W.*

Pellagra Among Turkish and German Prisoners of War in Egypt

BIGLAND[1] and Enright[2] report small epidemics of pellagra among Turkish and German prisoners of war in Egypt during 1916-1918. The former made a careful study of this disease in sixty-four cases. These were distributed among nationalities as follows: Turks, forty-six; Arabs, eight; Kurds, five; unknown, five. An attempt was made to determine the percentage of pellagrins among the Turkish prisoners. Bigland examined 3,823 in one camp, where he found twenty-four certainly pellagrins, and twenty-one doubtful. At another camp he examined 100 cases without finding any signs of pellagra. In still another place, he studied 470 Turkish women and children without finding any evidence of this disease. Among 4,400 cases he found sixty-four pellagrins, making a percentage of about 1.4. Inasmuch as pellagra is endemic in Egypt, Asia Minor, and Turkey in Asia and Europe, Bigland attempted to ascertain how many of these cases were chronic pellagrins. He concluded that the majority of them were suffering from the first attack.

Arsenic and adrenalin were tried as curative measures but in no instance was any apparent change secured thereby. The only thing which seemed to benefit the patients was a more liberal and varied diet. The most important point discussed by Bigland is as to food deficiency causing the disease among the Turks. He concludes that both before and for a time after capture these men had an insufficiency of food. He believes that this was the cause of the disease in most but not in all of the cases. In order to account for the appearance of pellagra among those sufficiently well fed Bigland resorts to the toxin hypothesis. He says:

"This brings me to the second supposition regarding the etiology of pellagra —viz., the presence of some toxic substance. I would suggest that such a toxin is present in these cases, and that it acts upon the intestines or the contents thereof in such a way that protein is not assimilated as it ought to be. * * * It only remains to discuss what is the nature of this hypothetical toxic substance. It must enter the body from without. It cannot be the result of a metabolic error, because the disease occurs in epidemics. It is difficult to imagine, for example, an epidemic of diabetes. It cannot be carried by the bite of an insect for reasons already stated. It has nothing to do with malaria or dysentery because pellagra

[1]The Lancet, London. May 11, 1920.
[2]The Lancet, London, May 8, 1920.

was unknown in our troops who suffered from both diseases. It may be contained in ingested material, but, if it is, it must be something common to the whole world since cases occur in such different localities. Its probable habitat is the digestive tract, as evidenced by the gastrointestinal symptoms which usually appear first, and the indicanuria, and by the fact that protein is found in the stools in abnormal amounts. It may be, however, that this toxic substance makes its effect by attacking the endocrine organs, especially the suprarenals. The similarities of pellagra to Addison's disease are too obvious to detail. The toxin is apparently of the nature of a virus, since the nervous changes show unmistakable evidence of degeneration rather than of inflammation. That this substance is not transmissible is shown by two facts: (1) That no attendant on pellagrins has ever contracted the disease; (2) the heroic experiments of Goldberger, in which feces, urine, scales from the skin, and all manner of horrible matters arising from pellagrins were eaten by volunteers with no evil results, even after injections and inoculations on mucous surfaces."

Blood cultures and bacteriologic studies of the feces, supplemented by inoculations of animals, were without results. It will be seen that on the whole Bigland confirms Goldberger's theories. He holds, with Wilson, that, although vegetable and meat proteins may be similar, they differ markedly in their nutritive value largely because the former is not assimilated so readily and so completely as the latter.

Enright studied sixty-five cases among German prisoners and comes to the conclusion that his observations are that the "food-deficiency theory" is inadequate. He says:

"I do not mean to suggest that a food deficiency can be quite excluded, but from the facts before us it can hardly be considered as of paramount importance. Obviously something more than a dietetic factor is involved. A critical analysis of the diets which these German pellagrins ate before capture and during their period of captivity prior to the onset of the eruption is sufficient to explode the food-deficiency theory as a predisposing factor. These diets were ample, both in quantity and quality, for any possible requirements, and were of such varied composition that it is perplexing to understand how they could have been improved. * * * Let us consider how the beneficial effects of a diet sufficient for a normal healthy individual, doing a normal amount of work, are liable to be counteracted. An originally good diet may be vitiated by loss through (1) abnormal expenditures of energy, (2) defective assimilation consequent on impaired digestive function, (3) absence of some internal secretion which is necessary for protein metabolism. * * * That the pellagrins suffered from defective digestive assimilation is undoubted. The incidence of malaria and dysentery was very high, and was responsible for intestinal derangement, which was a marked feature of the majority of my cases. Judging from the indicanuria commonly present and the copious foul-smelling evacuations which frequently contained undigested food material, it is evident that there was abnormal protein decomposition and that the ultimate good effects of the diet were largely vitiated or entirely lost in this matter."

Enright found among the German pellagrins a number with parotitis and he raises the question of whether the parotid gland has any effect upon protein metabolism. This is a question which he admits no one can at present answer.

—V. C. V

An Attenuated Tubercle Vaccine

RAW,[1] the distinguished tuberculosis specialist at Liverpool, thinks that human and bovine tuberculosis are separate and distinct diseases, but that the human body is susceptible to both, especially to bovine tuberculosis in the early periods of life. The two diseases are so rarely seen in the same subject that there are strong grounds for presuming that they are antagonistic to each other and that bovine tuberculosis may confer an immunity against human tuberculosis and vice versa.

Possessed of this idea Raw has secured nonvirulent cultures of both human and bovine bacilli. From these he prepares separate tuberculins. Cases of glandular tuberculosis, and all tuberculosis in children, which is evidently of bovine origin, he treats with the tuberculin made from the human type, while, on the other hand, cases of pulmonary tuberculosis, due to the human type, he treats with tuberculin made from the bovine type. He says that tuberculin should always be prepared from attenuated and nonvirulent cultures; that it should be freshly prepared and used within a week; that it should be given in graduated and increasing doses at intervals of seven days; that acute reactions are not necessary; that not less than twelve injections should be given at intervals of one week, and that the most favorable cases for treament are local lesions, but early cases of pulmonary tuberculosis may be limited and a further spread to other parts of the lungs prevented.

—V. C. V.

---

[1]British Medical Journal, April 17, 1920.

INDEX TO VOLUME V

AUTHORS INDEX

In this index following the author's name the full title of the subject is given as it appears in the Journal. Editorials are also included in the list and are indicated by (E).

Lightning Source UK Ltd.
Milton Keynes UK
UKHW040312060119
335017UK00009B/358/P

9 780332 085340